Outcomes in Radiation Therapy: Multidisciplinary Management

OUTCOMES IN RADIATION THERAPY: MULTIDISCIPLINARY MANAGEMENT

Deborah Watkins-Bruner, RN, PhD

Fox Chase Cancer Center
Cheltenham, Pennsylvania

Giselle Moore-Higgs, RN, ANP, OCN

Shands Cancer Center
University of Florida

Marilyn Haas, PhD, NP, APN-C

Mountain Radiation Oncology
Asheville, North Carolina

JONES AND BARTLETT PUBLISHERS
Sudbury, Massachusetts
BOSTON   TORONTO   LONDON   SINGAPORE

World Headquarters
Jones and Bartlett Publishers
40 Tall Pine Drive
Sudbury, MA 01776
978-443-5000
www.jbpub.com
info@jbpub.com

Jones and Bartlett Publishers Canada
2406 Nikanna Road
Mississauga, ON L5C 2W6
CANADA

Jones and Bartlett Publishers International
Barb House, Barb Mews
London W6 7PA
UK

Library of Congress Cataloging-in-Publication Data

Bruner, Deborah Watkins.
    Outcomes in radiation therapy : multidisciplinary management / by Deborah Watkins Bruner.
      p.; cm.
    Includes bibliographical references and index.
    ISBN 0-7637-1479-8
      1. Cancer—Radiotherapy. 2. Outcome assessment (Medical care)
    I. National League for Nursing. II. Title.
      [DNLM: 1. Neoplasms—radiotherapy. 2. Benchmarking. 3. Outcome Assessment (Health Care). 4. Radiation Oncology—standards.
    QZ 269 B894o 2001]
    RC271.R3 B78 2001
    616.99'40642—dc21   00-062583

Production Credits
Acquisitions Editor: Penny Glynn
Editor: John Danielowich
Production Editor: AnnMarie Lemoine
Editorial/Production Assistant: Christine Tridente
Director of Manufacturing and Inventory Control: Therese Bräuer
Cover Design: Stephanie Torta
Design and Composition: Carlisle Communications, Ltd.
Printing and Binding: Malloy Lithographing
Cover Printing: Malloy Lithographing

Printed in the United States of America
03 02 01 00   10 9 8 7 6 5 4 3 2 1

CONTRIBUTORS

Robert J. Amdur, MD
Associate Professor
Department of Radiation Oncology
University of Florida
Gainesville, FL

Terri Armstrong, RN, MS, ANP, CS
Neuro-Oncology Nurse Practitioner
MD Anderson Cancer Center
Houston, TX

Susan M. Chafe, MD, LLB, FRCPC
Radiation Oncologist
Department of Radiation Oncology
Cross Cancer Institute
Edmonton, Alberta Canada

Michael Diefenbach, PhD
Associate Member, Division of Population Science
Fox Chase Cancer Center
Philadelphia, PA

Constance Engelking, RN, MS, OCN
Executive Director/Assistant Vice President
Zalmen A. Arlin Cancer Institute
Westchester Medical Center
Hawthorne, New York

Audrey G. Gift, PhD, RN
Associate Dean of Research & Doctoral Programs
College of Nursing
Michigan State University
East Lansing, MI

Mark R. Gilbert, MD
Deputy Chair & Associate Professor
Department of Neuro-Oncology
MD Anderson Cancer Center
Houston, TX

Marilyn Haas, PhD, ANP-C
Nurse Practitioner/Outcomes Analyst
Mountain Radiation Oncology
Asheville, NC

Gerald E. Hanks, MD
Professor & Chairman, Radiation Oncology
Fox Chase Cancer Center and Temple University School of Medicine
Philadelphia, PA

J. Battle Haslam, MD
Past Medical Director
Mountain Radiation Oncology
Associates
Asheville, NC

Cherylle Hayes, MD
Assistant Professor
Department of Radiation Oncology
University of Florida College of Medicine
Gainesville, FL

Mark David Hurwitz, MD
Vice-Chief, Genitourinary Radiation Oncology
Brigham and Women's Hospital
Dana-Farber Cancer Institute
Boston, MA

Eric F. Kuehn, MD
Medical Director
Mountain Radiation Oncology
Asheville, NC

Robert B. Marcus, Jr., MD
Professor
Department of Radiation Oncology
University of Florida College of Medicine
Gainesville, FL

Cynthia Martin, ANP, MSN, RN, CS, AOCN
Nurse Practitioner-Oncology Clinical Nurse Specialist
Cobb Center for Radiation Therapy
Austell, GA

Nancy P. Mendenhall, MD
Professor & Chairman
Department of Radiation Oncology
University of Florida College of Medicine
Gainesville, FL

William M. Mendenhall, MD
Professor
Department of Radiation Oncology
University of Florida College of Medicine
Gainesville, FL

Benjamin Movsas, MD
Director of Clinical Research and
Thoracic Radiotherapy
Department of Radiation Oncology
Fox Chase Cancer Center
Philadelphia, PA

Giselle J. Moore-Higgs, ARNP, MSN
Clinical Coordinator & Nurse
Practitioner,
Department of Radiation Oncology
University of Florida
Gainesville, FL

Roberta A. Strohl, RN, MN, AOCN
Clinical Nurse Specialist
Director, Nursing Division
Department of Radiation Oncology
University of Maryland
Baltimore, MD

Carmel Sauerland, RN, MSN, AOCN
Oncology Clinical Nurse Specialist
Zalmen A. Arlin Cancer Institute
Westchester Medical Center
Hawthorne, New York

Mohan Suntharalingam, MD
Vice-Chairman, Radiation Oncology
University of Maryland at Baltimore
Baltimore, MD

Deborah Watkins Bruner, RN, PhD
Assistant Member, Population Science
and Radiation Oncology
Director, Prostate Cancer Risk
Assessment Program
Fox Chase Cancer Center
Philadelphia, PA

Thomas Whitehead, MD
Radiation Oncologist
Cobb Center for Radiation Therapy
Austell, GA

Kellie Wolk, RN, BSN, OCN
Senior Registered Nurse
Department of Radiation Oncology
University of Florida College of
Medicine
Gainesville, FL

Robert A. Zlotecki, MD, PhD
Associate Professor
Department of Radiation Oncology
University of Florida College of
Medicine
Gainesville, FL

CONTENTS

PREFACE

This book focuses on the outcomes of radiation therapy for cancer as they are experienced by adult patients. In radiation therapy, a great deal of attention is given to the measure of disease and normal tissue outcomes. These measures have been markedly improved as technology in dosimetry, treatment planning, and treatment machines has advanced. Radiation therapy has done an exemplary job in measuring the technical aspects of care through the Patterns of Care Study and other research. However, the patient's perception of his or her outcomes has been largely ignored. This book attempts to fill that void with an emphasis on outcomes as experienced and perceived by the patient. Traditional outcomes such as disease-free survival are an obvious cornerstone of the patient experience following radiation therapy; however, so too is quality of life and satisfaction with care. Herein lies the contribution of this book to the literature. We have attempted to present a comprehensive and multidisciplinary approach to the assessment and management of patient-experienced outcomes in radiation therapy including clinical, humanistic, and economic. There are measures and instruments that accurately reflect these outcomes and multiple examples are presented throughout the book. Where possible we attempted to include level one evidence (results of clinical trials) of the outcomes of interest; however, as most of us are well aware, there are many gaps in the published literature that required us (at least for now) to look to the best of lower levels of evidence. We must also acknowledge that the assessment of economic outcomes in radiation therapy, as with health care in general, is in its infancy. We hope this book will be a resource in both the clinical management of patients and the measurement of outcomes after radiation therapy. The extent to which we can improve the outcomes of therapy experienced by the patient will be proportionate to the value we place on listening carefully to the patient's perceptions. It will also be proportionate to our willingness to acknowledge that no one discipline alone can manage all of the aspects of a patient's needs following radiation therapy, and that improvement in outcomes lies in a multidisciplinary approach to care.

Deborah Watkins-Bruner
Giselle Moore-Higgs
Marilyn Haas

The authors, editor, and publisher have made every effort to provide accurate information. However, they are not responsible for errors, omissions, or for any outcomes related to the use of the contents of this book and take no responsibility for the use of the products described. Drugs and medical devices are discussed that may have limited availability controlled by the Food and Drug Administration (FDA) for use only in a research study or clinical trial. The drug information presented has been derived from reference sources, recently published data and pharmaceutical tests. Research, clinical practice, and government regulations often change the accepted standard in this field. When consideration is being given to use of any drug in the clinical setting, the health care provider or reader is responsible for determining FDA status of the drug, reading the package insert, and prescribing information for the most up-to-date recommendations on dose, precautions, and contraindications and determining the appropriate usage for the product. This is especially important in the case of drugs that are new or seldom used.

CHAPTER 1

AN OUTCOMES-BASED MANAGEMENT MODEL OF PATIENT CARE

Deborah Watkins Bruner and Gerald E. Hanks

Innovations in medical technology have spurred increased demands for utilization, yet resources to meet these demands are limited. Between 1965 and 1995 the percentage of the Gross Domestic Product (GDP) devoted to health care more than doubled from 5.7% to 13.6%. By the year 2005 the projection is for health care expenditures to comprise almost 18% of the GDP, exceeding well over $1 trillion (Braden, Cowan, Lazerby, Martin, McDonnell, Sensenig, Stiller, Whittle, Donhar, Long & Stewart, 1998; Burner & Waldo, 1995). These and other national health care trends that impact the delivery of oncology care in general affect radiation oncology specifically. Other trends include increasing risk-based compensation under the managed care mode, decreasing reimbursement with the Ambulatory Payment Classification System, and increasing patient load with the aging of the population. As hospitals and freestanding radiation facilities try to negotiate with insurers for fee-for-service, capitation, or case rates while trying to maintain quality patient care, they need to have a full understanding of the inputs (resources) and outputs (outcomes) involved in providing radiation oncology services.

An understanding of how resource consumption affects outcomes is important because even an endless stream of resources (if such a thing exists) does not guarantee the best outcomes. Health

1

care resources are subject to precepts similar to those of business resources including the classic cost-benefit curves (Figure 1–1). These curves tell us that more is not necessarily better, since at some given level of inputs the costs will outweigh the benefits of the outputs. Costs refer to human suffering as well as monetary units and benefits refer to improved clinical outcomes.

Defining Outcomes-Based Management

To understand which resources are required for a given outcome by disease, and to ensure the delivery of quality patient care, many institutions are looking to outcomes-based management models of patient care. Outcomes management has been used to define a variety of activities discussed elsewhere (Weeks, 1998). Outcomes-based management, as described here, is a method of measuring, evaluating, and improving patient care. It is closely linked to but broader based than Continuous Quality Improvement (CQI) or Total Quality Management (TQM), and it leads to evidence-based medicine. Outcomes have the additional benefit of being comprehensive since they reflect all their antecedents. Outcomes are affected not only by the intervention that was delivered to the patient, but also by a host of factors related to personal and interpersonal characteristics of both the patient and health care providers and the environment in which the care is provided (Sidani & Broden, 1998).

Figure 1–1   Marginal Benefit Derived from Use of Resources

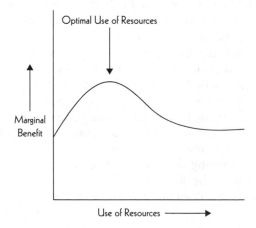

Optimal Use of Resources

Marginal Benefit

Use of Resources ———▶

A common question is, "How is outcomes-based management different from 'traditional' patient care?" Traditional patient care has been based on the best judgment of well-educated health care providers. This judgment has been highly individualized and has been based on only the broadest criteria for management. In addition, measures of effect have been ignored in all but the broadest of terms, historically focusing on morbidity and mortality. Outcomes-based management, on the other hand, is a comprehensive process that focuses on outcomes-related factors that influence the validity of conclusions in intervention effectiveness (Sidani & Broden, 1998).

It has been well documented that cancer care varies widely by geography (Nattinger, Gottlieb, Veum, Yahnke, & Goodwin, 1992), type of institution (teaching vs. nonteaching hospital) (Lee Feldstein, Anton-Culver, & Feldstein, 1994), age of patient (Newschaffer, Penberthy, Desch, Retchin, & Whittemore, 1996), race (Harlan, Brawley, Pommerenke, Wali, & Kramer, 1995), education (Smith et al., 1995), and by insurance coverage (Guidry, Aday, Zhang, & Winn, 1998; Winn, Botnick, & Dozier, 1996). For example, in a study of older women with breast cancer living in Virginia, only 66% of women between ages 65 and 69 and 7% aged 85 and older received appropriate radiation therapy after breast-conserving surgery. In addition, only 44% of those with positive lymph nodes received adjuvant therapy, although adjuvant therapy is recommended for all node-positive disease (Hillner, 1996). This study highlights the lack of uniform adherence to national guidelines, which exist for the management of breast cancer as well as many other cancer sites (Bruner, Bucholtz, Iwamoto, & Strohl, 1998; PCS Consensus Committees, 1997; Winn et al., 1996).

Adherence to guidelines for the treatment of any disease is the cornerstone of outcomes-based management. Interestingly, radiation oncologists have pioneered the development and monitoring of practice guidelines with the long-term Patterns of Care Studies (PCS). The PCS were conceived by Dr. Simon Kramer in 1969 and initially funded by the National Cancer Institute in 1971 to collect data on the processes of radiation therapy and to better understand their relationship to outcomes (Hanks, Coia, & Curry, 1997). Under the continued leadership of Dr. Gerald Hanks, the current Principal Investigator, the PCS monitor the practice of radiation oncology on a national basis and provide a continuous feedback loop of information on outcomes and information used to develop and update guidelines, as well as guide educational efforts for radiation oncologists.

Outcomes-based methodology used in the PCS and expanded by the emerging science of Health Services Research allows for patient outcomes to be tracked and analyzed in any combination of ways (i.e., by diagnosis, stage of disease, age, gender, type of insurance, treatment modality, institution, health care provider). Decisions and improvements for future patient care can be made based on the evidence derived from the outcomes measured. This creates a continuous feedback loop of information on which to further improve care.

Consumers and Applications of Outcomes

The consumers of this information are many and as health care continues to evolve, consumer sophistication in critically scrutinizing health care institutions, therapies, physicians, and health plans by their reported outcomes will only increase. In fact, it has been suggested that in order to promote a realistic societal approach to the need for priority setting and resource rationing in health care, consumers should be schooled in evidence-based medicine, one of the products of outcomes assessments. Through education consumers would learn a "healthy skepticism" for health care through full disclosure of the outcomes data on the true effectiveness of health care interventions and on the existing variation in their utilization (Domenighetti, Grilli, & Liberati, 1998). The current list of consumers of this information includes, but is not limited to:

- Patients and families
- Health care providers
- Disease management provider groups
- Health care institutions
- Health maintenance and managed care organizations
- Employers
- Accreditation agencies
- Governmental agencies
- Legal entities

Consumers of outcomes in health care have found multiple applications for the information generated by this approach to care including:

- Individual patient progress evaluation
- Disease management program evaluation

Treatment evaluation
Technology assessment
Provider evaluations, credentialing, contracting
Continuous quality improvement
Report cards, marketing, sales
Clinical support systems, guidelines and pathway
development
Payment decisions

DEFINING THE OUTCOMES OF INTEREST

What specifically are the outcomes of interest to the consumers of this information? There are three main categories under which outcomes of interest fall in health care in general, and radiation therapy in particular: clinical, humanistic, and economic. An outcomes-based management model of patient care incorporating these major outcomes is presented in Figure 1–2, the components of which are described as follows.

CLINICAL OUTCOMES

The PCS have historically assessed clinical outcomes using the model described by Donabedian, which focuses on structure, process, and outcome (Donabedian, 1966). Structure refers to the facility, equipment, personnel, and material used to provide care. For example, Hanks, Diamond, and Kramer (1985) were able to correlate facility characteristics and structure with outcomes after radiotherapy for Hodgkin's disease and prostate and cervical cancer through the PCS. Better outcomes were documented for improved technology with linear accelerators and higher photon energy than with less than 80-cm cobalt units. Monson et al. (1997) assessed outcomes of recurrence and morbidity for Stage I and II breast cancer with 4, 6, and 8 MV in women who received greater than or equal to 60 gray (Gy) to the tumor bed. They concluded that machine energy over the range of 4 to 8 MV did not significantly affect treatment outcome. Additional differences in outcomes have been reported in association with physician characteristics. For instance, physician specialty has been linked to variations in the use of breast-conserving surgery instead of mastectomy (Mandelblatt, Ganz, & Kahn, 1998).

Process refers to the activities of health care providers in evaluating, treating, and following patients (Owen, Sedransk, & Pajak,

Figure 1–2 An Outcomes-Based Management Model for Patient-Centered Care

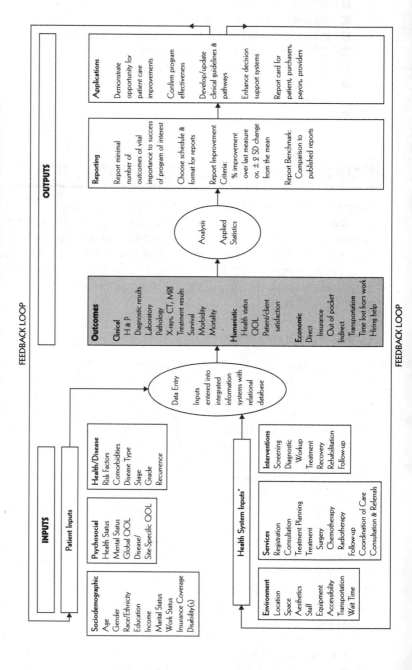

1997). New techniques may change the process of care, and outcomes should be evaluated with each change in process. For example, dose escalation with three-dimensional conformal radiation therapy (3D-CRT) has been associated with improved outcomes related to prostate cancer including PSA relapse-free survival (Hanks et al., 1998; Zelefsky et al., 1998).

Outcome in the Donabedian model refers to the changes in health status, which occur as a result of the process and within the structure of health care. Measurement of outcomes is at the heart of outcomes-based patient management, since improvements in outcome are the goal of providing quality clinical structure and process. There are numerous examples of the clinical outcomes of radiation therapy, many of which will be discussed in the site-specific sections of this book. Commonly, clinical outcomes have been reported in terms of morbidity and mortality. For example, early PCS surveys documented an increase from 3.5% to 7.0% of serious morbidity in terms of bowel and bladder toxicity when the prostate was treated with doses exceeding 70 Gy (Hanks, 1985). Over the past 20 years, significant improvements in survival outcomes have been documented through the PCS in the use of radiation therapy for stage III cervical cancer, all stages of Hodgkin's disease, and both survival and decreased morbidity of patients treated for seminoma (Lanciano, Thomas, & Eifel, 1997; Smitt, Buzydlowski, & Hoppe, 1997; Thomas, 1997).

HUMANISTIC OUTCOMES

Humanistic outcomes began with crude measures of health status like the Karnofsky Performance Status Scale (KPS) (Karnofsky & Burchenal, 1949). The KPS was meant to assess functional status of patients treated with chemotherapy. As clinical trials evolved, however, the KPS has been used to assess patients treated with surgery, radiotherapy, biologic response modifiers, and combined modality therapy. There are multiple measures of functional status besides the KPS, one example of which is the often cited Short Form-36 (Ware, 1995). The few studies of documented functional status during and after radiation therapy show fatigue to be one of the major symptoms interfering with activities of daily living (King, Nail, Kreamer, Strohl, & Johnson, 1985; Oberst, Change, & McCubbin, 1991). Fatigue has been shown to interfere with self-care, socialization, and functioning (Jensen & Given, 1991).

Although functional status is an important component of humanistic outcomes, it comprises only a portion of the concept

(Couch, 1997; Ganz, 1994). Two other components of humanistic outcomes include quality of life (QOL) and patient satisfaction. Research into QOL as a health care construct began in the 1960s (Jenkins, 1992). QOL is defined as a subjective, multidimensional construct measuring at the very least physical/functional status, emotional functioning, and social functioning (Aaronson et al., 1991; Ganz, 1994; Schipper, Clinch, & Powell, 1990). Other dimensions have been suggested such as spiritual, family well-being, and future orientation (Cella & Tulsky, 1990; Ferrans & Ferrell, 1990; Jenkins, 1992). The importance of QOL patient self-assessments in measuring outcomes has been well documented in radiation therapy. At least two studies involving radiation therapy have documented a 13% to 50% disagreement between the physician's assessment of QOL outcomes and the patient's own assessment of his or her QOL (Bruner et al., 1998; Bruner et al., 1995). Additional examples of QOL outcomes after radiation therapy will be presented in the site-specific sections.

Independent of health status, satisfaction with health care includes patient satisfaction with all of the components of health care including structure, process, and clinical/humanistic outcomes. Patient satisfaction is considered an important component and measure of the quality of health care (Fottler, Ford, & Bach, 1997). Patient satisfaction surveys have been used to improve care in a variety of settings (Levine, Plume, & Nelson, 1997; Seibert, 1996). Eleven factors that are thought to influence consumer satisfaction with health care delivery include:

- Caring, referring to how warm and interested the health care providers appear to be in the patient/family
- Tangibles, such as facility aesthetics
- Reliability, including dependable and consistent care
- Responsiveness, including timeliness of service
- Understanding, meaning that health care providers learn what the patient's and family's particular needs are and provide individualized care
- Access, including acceptance of the patient's insurance or noninsurance, distance to facility, telephone assistance, waiting time, and hours of operation
- Courtesy, including the politeness and tactfulness of the health care providers and ancillary staff (i.e., secretaries)
- Communication, referring to the ability of health care providers to explain treatment alternatives and expected side effects in layman's terms

■ Credibility, referring to the perceived trustworthiness and honesty of the staff

■ Security, including the freedom from unnecessary risk and confidentiality

■ Effects, that is, preventing death, increasing the life span, and/or relieving pain (Bowers, Swan, & Koehler, 1994; Carson, Carson, & Roe, 1998; Parasuraman, Zeithaml, & Berry, 1986)

Competence, referring to health care providers' knowledge and skills, has often been included in the preceding list, however it has been found that consumers are frequently unable to evaluate the technical components of health care (including provider competence) that lead to quality outcomes (Bowers et al., 1994). Therefore, it has been suggested that alternative paradigms of consumer satisfaction may be more appropriate. One such alternative comprises three levels of consumer satisfaction with health care:

1. Level One—implicit, referring to the ability of health care providers to fulfill basic functions that include minimum expectations of access, reliability, credibility, courtesy, competence, security, and effect

2. Level Two—explicit, referring to preferred functions that include access, understanding, communication, and caring

3. Level Three—latent, referring to unexpected functions such as appealing tangibles (i.e., aesthetically designed facilities, comfort measures such as pleasant music, beverages, and magazines) (Tenner & DeToro, 1992).

Meeting expectations at level one does not create satisfaction, since they are seen as basic requirements of health care functioning. On the other hand, if these basic expectations are not met, severe dissatisfaction will result. Evidence of this was documented by Zapka et al. (1995), who found a strong correlation between patients' reports of problems in systems performance (including access, coordination, and continuity of care) and dissatisfaction. Conversely, meeting the preferred expectations at level two will create satisfaction, but if these expectations are not met it will not create dissatisfaction because they are seen as optional functions. Meeting expectations at level three will more than satisfy patients, it will elate them, since these functions are unexpected. However, similar to level two, leaving these expectations unfulfilled will not affect satisfaction (Tenner & DeToro, 1992).

ECONOMIC OUTCOMES

As the percentage of the GDP devoted to healthcare increases over the next millennium, assessments of efficiency of resource allocation are being added to the historic clinical safety and efficacy assessments of therapeutic strategies. Hayman, Weeks, and Mauch (1996) encapsulated the basic methods used in assessing economic outcomes in radiation therapy, which are described in greater detail by Gold, Siegel, Russel, and Weinstein (1996). To assess the efficiency of resource allocation, clinical and humanistic outcomes are combined with measures of resource consumption to produce cost-effectiveness analyses. Cost-effectiveness assesses cost per unit of health outcome for the purpose of evaluating resources consumed in relation to benefits derived from a particular program, in comparison to other programs. With cost-effectiveness monetary units are presented in the numerator and natural units (i.e., life years saved, event averted, case detected) are presented in the denominator. Since the natural units may vary in each cost-effectiveness analysis, it makes comparison of different health care programs somewhat difficult. This has led to an interest in a common denominator that incorporates duration of health benefit and quality of health benefit. The result has been the development of the Quality-Adjusted Life Year (QALY) (Anderson, Bush, Chen, & Dolenc, 1985; Williams, 1985).

The QALY is a composite measure of health outcomes in which time in a health state is weighted by the quality of that health state. The weight is assigned a number between 1 (best possible health) and 0 (death or worst possible health). This weight is also called a utility or preference function. The theory behind QALY assessments assumes that individuals maximize a preference function (utility) for material consumption (including health care) and that this preference follows certain conditions of rationality and logical consistency. It also assumes that the overall welfare of society is the sum of these individual preference functions. Since the concern is for the best allocation of health care resources to society, preferences and utilities are best measured from a societal perspective (Gold et al., 1996).

There are three major categories of economic assessments:

- Direct costs (e.g., radiation therapy treatments, medications)
- Indirect costs (e.g., days of work lost, transportation to radiation therapy department)

■ Intangible costs (e.g., pain, decrements in QOL; accounted for in the denominator of $/QALY equations)

Most economic assessments of radiation therapy have focused on direct costs only (Best, 1993; Perez et al., 1993). Several of these studies have shown that the long-term benefits of radiotherapy far outweigh the high short-term capital costs of providing therapy (Barton, Gebski, Manderson, & Langlands, 1995; Glazebrook, 1992). Dale & Jones (1996) added an important caveat to the conclusions of previous discussions of the cost-benefit analysis of radiation therapy (Dale, Vijayakumar, Lawlor, & Merrell, 1996). Using standard radiobiological modeling based on the linear-quadratic model, they combined this with financial parameters to estimate the costs of different aspects of radiation therapy. Their results showed that *high-quality* radiotherapy (i.e., based on individual patterns of fractionation that are near optimal for particular subpopulations of tumors) was the key to effective therapy at the lowest global cost. One of their conclusions argued that their findings further stressed the need for guidelines for appropriate radiation therapy (Dale et al., 1996). As with clinical and humanistic outcomes studies, this illustrates the feedback loop that optimally arises from the measurement of outcomes to improve patient care.

As the discussion of outcomes suggests, the list of possible outcomes to be measured in health care seems overwhelming. How can the radiation oncology staff prioritize which outcomes to measure? As with CQI or TQM, it is best to choose outcomes related to either high volume or high-risk events. The key is to determine the minimal number of outcomes that are of vital importance to measuring the success of the treatment(s) of interest.

MEASURING OUTCOMES

How are outcomes data measured? Obtaining outcomes data that provide evidence of the effectiveness of an intervention in improving a patient's health status requires multiple factors. Among the factors to consider in designing an outcomes-based patient management program is selecting the right outcome variables; the right measures or instruments; the right methods and tools for data collection, storage, and analysis; and the right criteria or benchmarks for comparison, each of which will be discussed in turn.

SELECTING THE RIGHT OUTCOME VARIABLES

The types of outcomes—clinical, humanistic, and economic—that can be measured were listed previously. Choosing the outcome variables of interest (called indicators in CQI/TQM terminology) depends on your specific patient population. The chapters in this book focusing on specific sites describe expected outcomes by cancer site or type treated with radiation therapy. Initially, it would be most productive to focus on those sites or cancer types that account for your highest volume of patients or the patients that have the highest risk for poor clinical outcomes. There is no need to reinvent the wheel because these patients have most likely already been identified through many departments' CQI or TQM programs. An example of a successfully developed outcomes program in a radiation oncology department using CQI techniques has been published by Haas and Kuehn (1999).

SELECTING THE RIGHT OUTCOME MEASURES OR INSTRUMENTS

Evaluating the outcomes of interest requires measures that are accurate, involve minimum error, and are sensitive to change. Selected instruments should be, whenever possible, scientifically reliable and valid and also easy to use. In addition, they should include assessments of subpopulation variables of importance. These depend on the sociodemographic characteristics of a given department or institution (i.e., race, ethnicity, culture, income, education). For example, Meyerowitz and colleagues proposed a framework for the assessment of variables that link ethnicity with cancer outcomes (Meyerowitz, Richardson, Hudson, & Leedham, 1998).

In radiation therapy, a great deal of attention is given to the measure of radiation dose to a specific point, organ, or area of the body treated. These measures have been markedly improved as technology in dosimetry, treatment planning, and treatment machines and methods has advanced. Similarly, there are measures and instruments that accurately reflect the outcome to the patient receiving the radiation therapy. Examples of these measures include:

- ■ Clinical
  - Structure (e.g., PCS surveys)
  - Process (e.g., individual patient measures—history and physical, laboratory results, pathology reports; patient

population measures—time from initial phone registration to treatment by disease, wait time for daily treatments)
- Outcome (e.g., morbidity and mortality reports)
■ Humanistic
  - Health status (e.g., Short Form-36, Ware, 1995; KPS, Karnofsky & Burchenal, 1949) and treatment-related symptoms (e.g., The Symptom Distress Scale, McCorkle, 1987; Sickness Impact Profile, Bergner, Bobbitt, Carter, & Gilson, 1981)
  - Quality of life (e.g., Functional Assessment Chronic Illness-Therapy—FACIT, Cella & Webster, 1997; EORTC-QOL, Aaronson et al., 1993; Spitzer QL-Index, Spitzer, Dobson, Chesterman, & Levi, 1981)
  - Satisfaction with health care structure, process, and effects (e.g., patient surveys, interviews, SERVQUAL; Parasuraman et al., 1986)
■ Economic
  - Direct costs (e.g., utilization reports, cost accounting, billing)
  - Indirect costs (e.g., patient self-report)
  - Intangible (e.g., patient interview, self-report)

SELECTING THE RIGHT METHODS AND TOOLS FOR DATA COLLECTION, STORAGE, AND ANALYSIS

The selection of the measures and instruments that best reflect the outcomes of interest is just the beginning. The information must be documented accurately, collected consistently, and stored conveniently for easy access and analysis. There are two sources of documented outcomes data: nonelectronic and electronic. Nonelectronic data usually refer to the patient record including the history and physical, nurse's notes, follow-up notes, consultations, and referrals. Nonelectronic data require intensive labor to abstract and enter for analysis.

Electronic documentation includes claims data (e.g., ICD-O Topography and Morphology codes) and function-specific systems (e.g., laboratory, radiology), as well as clinical and humanistic data. The more data that can be documented electronically, the better. Radiation oncology specific electronic charting systems are available commercially through multiple sources such as Varian Medical Systems, Inc., Palo Alto, CA (http://www.varian.com); IMPAC Medical Systems, Inc., Mountain View, CA (http://www.impac.com); and Siemens

Medical Systems, Inc., Concord, CA (http://www.sms.siemens.com). These systems include a variety of industry-standard tools including AJCC Staging, the computerized version of the Oncology Nursing Society's Radiation Therapy Patient Record: A Tool for Documenting Nursing Care, the National Cancer Institute's Common Toxicity Criteria, and Registry Operations and Data Standards (ROADS). An electronic patient care record at point of service is ideal but available in few settings to date. It is inevitable that health care systems will implement these systems over the next decade or so, but for now abstracting data from nonelectronic records is an inconvenient necessity for outcomes management.

Outcomes data are collected and stored through integrated information systems that allow for data storage, retrieval, and analyses. Integrated information systems allow for the collection of varying combinations of data on clinical, humanistic, and economic information. These systems include generic programs such as the Health Plan Employer Data Information Set (HEDIS), developed by the National Committee for Quality Assurance to evaluate data on Health Maintenance Organizations (HMO) and used by the federal Health Care Financing Administration (HCFA) to evaluate data on Medicare and Medicaid participants. Radiation oncology specific information systems are also commercially available and include products such as ACCESS, an oncology management software program, and Précis™, a central registry data management system (IMPAC Medical Systems, Inc., Mountain View, CA, http://www.impac.com); Clinical Outcomes Management Analyses (COMA) system (Mountain Radiation Oncology, Asheville, NC); VARiS™ information management system (Varian Medical Systems, Inc., Palo Alto, CA, http://www.varian.com); and LANTIS™ oncology information management system (Siemens Medical Systems, Inc., Concord, CA, http://www.sms.siemens.com).

Improved outcomes using relational databases have been published (McCormack, 1998a, 1998b, 1998c). However, data quality is the major concern with these systems since they are subject to problems with systems and systems users. Problems with systems arise when the systems are incompatible with other inter- or intradepartmental systems. Problems with systems users arise when the data entries are incomplete or inaccurate. Periodic, routinely scheduled data monitoring is needed to ensure data quality.

In addition, specific methods of data collection enhance outcomes assessments. In particular, a method called process mapping, described in detail by Hunt (1996) has major implications for aiding in delimiting the exact activities and steps (including barriers or obstacles) involved in producing a specific outcome. For example, Kobeissi et al. (1998) have documented how process mapping can be used to determine physician resource utilization for the use of new technology in radiation therapy. Multiple commercial process mapping tools are available that include simple flowchart graphic software (Scitor Process™, Scitor Corporation, Sunnyvale, CA, http://www.scitor.com); iGrafx Process, Micrografx Inc., Allen, TX, http://www.micrografx.com); process mapping products (Varian Medical Systems, Inc., Palo Alto, CA, http://www.varian.com); and process simulation products (MedModel Optimization Suite™, PROMODEL Corporation, Orem, UT, http://www.promodel.com).

Once the outcomes data are collected and stored they need to be evaluated. Who collects, measures, analyzes, and reports outcomes? The skill mix is similar to that of CQI with the caveat that you already have a computer system, relational database, programmers, and staff that do data entry. There is an additional skill set required for outcomes analysts that optimally includes:

- Familiarity with the types of data, the format, and the quality of the data
- In-depth knowledge of applied statistics and data manipulation
- Understanding of the health care delivery system and its relational components
- Ability to communicate the analytic results in verbal, tabular, graphical, and numerical formats (Couch, 1997).

Outcomes data can be reported using reporting mechanisms similar to those used for CQI or TQM. The following factors need to be considered in reporting outcomes:

- Customer (e.g., department, institution, accrediting agency, consumer report)
- Purpose (e.g., CQI/TQM, internal audit, accounting)
- Schedule (e.g., which outcomes are to be measured at what time points)
- Format (e.g., verbal, tabular, graphical, and numerical)
- Context (e.g., comparative reporting to previous performance—two standard deviations from the mean, or percentage improvement; comparative reporting to norms or standards; benchmarking against best practices) (Couch, 1997).

SELECTING THE RIGHT CRITERIA OR BENCHMARKS

The concept of comparative reporting and benchmarking is particularly important in an outcomes-based management model of patient care. Comparative reporting refers to comparisons to an individual's, department's, or institution's prior outcomes. This is acceptable when there is little or no national, regional, or local data on outcomes for a particular disease, process, or program. For example, academic institutions testing new technology may have to use outcome comparisons to their own prior performance at specifically scheduled intervals to assess outcomes improvements. When new technology is introduced there is always a lag time before national outcomes can be measured and reported. On the other hand, when there are nationally recognized guidelines and published outcomes, they should be used for benchmarking. An example of this was presented in one recent study that assessed compliance with standards of care for early-stage breast cancer in women treated in two states. The authors collected data from medical records, patients, and their surgeons. Compliance with four indicators of evidence-based quality of care were assessed: radiation therapy after breast-conserving surgery, axillary lymph node dissection, chemotherapy for premenopausal women with positive lymph nodes, and hormonal therapy for postmenopausal women with positive lymph nodes and positive estrogen receptor status. Results from the two states studied indicated that practice appears to be consistent with the results of national consensus conferences and clinical trials regarding the treatment of early-stage breast cancer for three of the four indicators. Only the use of hormonal therapy for postmenopausal women was low (< 64%). Still, 90% of postmenopausal women received either chemotherapy or hormonal therapy (Guadagnoli et al., 1998).

Fortunately for practitioners in radiation oncology, the PCS provide regularly updated benchmarks for at least the clinical outcomes of most disease sites. One of the latest PCS surveys established the national benchmarks for the evaluation and treatment of patients with esophageal cancer. Clinical and functional status outcomes were collected from 61 institutions concerning 400 patients with squamous cell or adenocarcinoma of the thoracic esophagus who received radiation therapy as part of definitive or adjuvant management of their disease. Results indicated that 75% of all patients received chemotherapy and radiation therapy and 62.5% received concurrent chemotherapy and radiation therapy as part of their treatment. The median total dose of radiation therapy was 50.4 Gy and the median dose per fraction was 1.8 Gy. Karnofsky performance status was greater than or equal to 80 (on a 0, dead to 100, no decrement in functional ability scale) for over 85% of patients (Coia et al., 1999). As clinically useful as these studies are, much research is still needed to benchmark the humanistic and economic outcomes of interest in radiation therapy.

IMPROVING OUTCOMES

The purpose of all of this meticulous work is to improve patient outcomes. Outcomes are improved in two ways: through systems improvements or behavioral change. Systems improvements include changes in structure and process. The PCS have documented multiple improvements in both structure and process. For example, in early PCS, problems documented with high recurrence rates of several disease sites using cobalt-60 machines versus linear accelerators or betatrons changed the standard of equipment use (structure) in radiation therapy (Hanks et al., 1985). Improvements in process were documented after a 1974 PCS survey showed higher local-regional recurrence for stage III larynx cancer when treated with radiation alone versus surgery and radiation (Lustig, MacLean, Hanks, & Kramer, 1984). A second PCS survey was conducted in 1978 to assess the impact of changes in treatment process on outcome since the earlier report. Over that period, the use of surgery in conjunction with radiation of stage III larynx cancers increased from less than 30% to more than 60% with a concomitant decrease in the local recurrence rate (Lustig et al., 1991).

Behavioral change refers to change in either the health care provider or the patient. This is a complex and multitask process that begins with evidence-based guidelines. It has been well documented that the publication and distribution of guidelines alone do not improve patient care. For example, an expert consensus statement accepting the use of breast-conserving surgery and radiation therapy in selected patients with early-stage breast cancer was published in 1985. However, by 1990 the rates of breast-conserving surgery and radiation therapy had not noticeably increased nationally (14% in 1985 vs. 15% in 1990) (Nattinger et al., 1996). A similar lack of compliance with nationally developed and extensively publicized pain management guidelines developed by the Agency for Health

Care Policy and Research, has been documented (Kalua, 1998; Payne, 1998).

In addition to guidelines, ongoing education and monitoring of compliance are required. Physician support systems have been developed by a variety of sources and are offered (usually for a fee) as software packages or through Internet access. Some examples include Oncology KnowledgeBASE, developed by New Medicine, Inc., Lake Forest, CA (http://www.newmedinc.com), which includes information on drugs, drug targets and enabling technologies, and drug complications; and a disease outcomes database developed by MEDTAP™ Systems, Bethesda, MD (http://www.medtap.com). These support systems are helpful in both clinical decision making and research, but, like the publication of guidelines, they are not by themselves capable of behavioral change. An important factor required for behavioral change to occur is the individual feedback to practitioners of how their outcomes compare to local, regional, and/or national outcomes for specific diseases and aspects of patient care. In other words, individual report cards of performance provide some of the best-known incentives for outcomes improvements.

Patient change centers on self-care activities, which in reality usually involve the family. The increasing utilization of outpatient care has forced family members to become primary caregivers despite reports of their feelings of inadequacy in fulfilling the role (Freudenhein & Tarini, 1996; Given, 1995). There are several models for assessing self-care. One that has been extensively tested is Orem's self-care model. Orem defines self-care as the performance of activities that mature persons perform on their own behalf in order to maintain life, healthful functioning, personal development, and well-being (Orem, 1995). The factors associated with a person's health that make demands on self-care, their ability to perform self-care, conditions that would create self-care deficits, and the environment including home and health systems required to promote self-care are discussed at length elsewhere (Dodd & Dibble, 1993; Orem, 1995). Outcomes improvement have been reported after interventions to promote self-care in terms of increased patient satisfaction (Dodd & Dibble, 1993) and improved clinical outcomes (Dodd et al., 1996). In one self-care study, 46 women beginning a six-week program of radiation therapy for early-stage breast cancer were randomly assigned to an exercise or control group. Subjects in the exercise group maintained an individualized, self-paced, home-based walking exercise program throughout treatment. The control group received usual care. Outcomes were measured prior to and at the end of radiation therapy. The exercise group scored significantly higher than the usual care control group on physical functioning and symptom intensity, particularly fatigue, anxiety, and difficulty sleeping (Mock et al., 1997).

Behavioral change, whether it is directed at patients and families or health care professionals, is a challenging task and one that will require extensive research to determine successful methods to improve outcomes.

In summary, outcomes-based management is a method of measuring, evaluating, and improving patient care. The outcomes of interest in radiation oncology are clinical, humanistic, and economic. Issues and resources for measuring outcomes have been discussed in detail including selecting the outcome variables, the instruments, the methods, and tools for data collection; storage, and analysis; and the criteria or benchmarks for comparison. However, once the outcomes and measures of interest are chosen, it takes a multidisciplinary team to implement, evaluate, and improve an outcomes-based management model of patient care. Chapter 2 discusses the role of the radiation oncology team in providing quality patient outcomes.

REFERENCES

Aaronson, N., Ahmedzai, S., Bergman, B., Bullinger, M., Cull, A., Duez, A., Filberti, A., Fletchner, H., Fleishman, S. B., de Haes, J. C., Kaasa, S., Klee, M., Osoba, D., Razavi, D., Rofe, B. P., Shraub, S., Sneeuw, K., Sullivan, M., & Takeda, F. (1993). The European Organization for Research and Treatment of Cancer QLQ-C30; a quality-of-life instrument for use in international clinical trials in oncology. *Journal of the National Cancer Institute*, 85, 365–376.

Aaronson, N. K., Meyeritz, B. E., Bard, M., Bloom, J. R., Fawzy, F. I., Feldstein, M., Fink, D., Holland, J. C., Johnson, J. E., Lowman, J. T., Patterson, W. B., & Ware J. E., Jr., (1991). Quality of life research in oncology: Past achievements and future priorities. *Cancer*, 67, 839–843.

Anderson, J., Bush, J., Chen, M., & Dolenc, D. (1985). Policy space areas and properties of benefit-cost/utility analysis. *Journal of the American Medical Association*, 255(6), 794–795.

Barton, M. B., Gebski, V., Manderson, C., & Langlands, A. O. (1995). Radiation therapy: Are we getting value for money? *Clinical Oncology*, 7(5), 287–292.

Bergner, M., Bobbitt, R. A., Carter, W. B., & Gilson, B. S. (1981). The Sickness Impact Profile: Development and final version of a health status measure. *Medical Care*, 19, 787–805.

Bowers, M. R., Swan, J. E., & Koehler, W. F. (1994). What attributes determine quality and satisfaction with health care? *Health Care Management Review*, 19, 49–55.

Braden, B. R., Conlan, C. A., Lazenby, H. C., Martin, A. B., McDonnell, P. A., Sensenig, A. L., Stiller, J. M., Whittle, L. S., Donhan, C. S., Long, A. M., & Stewart, M. W. (1977), National health expenditures. *Health Care Financing Review*, 20(1), 83–126.

Bruner, D. W., Bucholtz, J., Iwamoto, R., & Strohl, R. (1998). *Manual for radiation oncology nursing practice and education* (2nd ed.). Pittsburgh, PA: Oncology Nursing Press.

Bruner, D. W., Scott, C., Lawton, C., DelRowe, J., Rotman, M., Buswell, L., Beard, C., & Cella, D. (1995). RTOG's first quality of life study—RTOG 90-20: A phase II trial of external beam radiation with etanidazole for locally advanced prostate cancer. *International Journal of Radiation Oncology, Biology, Physics*, 33(4), 901–906.

Burner, S. T., & Waldo, D. R. (1995). National health expenditure projections, 1994–2005. *Health Care Financing Review*, 16(4), 221–42.

Carson, P. O., Carson, K., & Roe, C. W. (1998). Toward understanding the patient's perception of quality. *Health Care Supervisor*, 16(3), 36–42.

Cella, D. F., & Tulsky, D. S. (1990). Measuring quality of life today: Methodological aspects. *Oncology*, 4(5), 29–38.

Cella, D., & Webster, K. (1997). Linking outcomes management to quality-of-life issues. *Oncology*, 11 (11A), 232–235.

Coia, L. R., Minsky, B. D., John, M. J., Haller, D. G., Landry, J., Pisansky, T. M., Willett, C. G., Hoffman, J. P., Berkey, B. A., Owen, J. B., & Hanks, G. E. (1999). The evaluation and treatment of patients receiving radiation therapy for carcinoma of the esophagus: Results of the 1992–1994 Patterns of Care Study. *Cancer*, 85(12), 2499–2505.

Couch, J. (1997). *The physician's guide to disease management.* Gaithersburg, MD: Aspen Publishers.

Dale, G. R., & Jones, B. (1996). Radiobiologically based assessments of the net costs of fractionated radiotherapy. *International Journal of Radiation Oncology Biology Physics*, 36(3), 739–746.

Dale, W., Vijayakumar, S., Lawlor, E., & Merrell, K. (1996). Prostate cancer, race, and socioeconomic status: Inadequate adjustment for social factors in assessing racial differences. *The Prostate*, 29, 271–281.

Dodd, M., & Dibble, S. (1993). Predictors of self-care: A test of Orem's model. *Oncology Nursing Forum*, 20, 895–901.

Dodd, M. J., Larson, P. J., Dibble, S. L., Miaskowski, C., Greenspan, D., MacPhail, L., Hauck, W. W., Paul, S. M., Ignoffo, R., & Shiba, G. (1996). Randomized clinical trial of chlorhexidine versus placebo of oral mucositis in patients receiving chemotherapy. *Oncology Nursing Forum*, 23(6), 921–927.

Domenighetti, G., Grilli, R., & Liberati, A. (1998). Promoting consumers' demand for evidence-based medicine. *International Journal of Technology Assessment in Health Care*, 14(1), 97–105.

Donabedian, A. (1966). Evaluating the quality of medical care. *Milbank Memorial Fund Quarterly*, 44(3), 166–206.

Ferrans, C. E., & Ferrell, B. R. (1990). Development of a quality of life index for patients with cancer. *Oncology Nursing Forum*, 17(Suppl. 3), 15–21.

Fottler, M. D., Ford, R. C., & Bach, S. A. (1997). Measuring patient satisfaction in health care organizations: Qualitative and quantitative approaches. *Best Practices and Benchmarking in Healthcare*, 2(6), 227–239.

Freudenhein, E., & Tarini, P. (1996). Chronic care in America: The health system that isn't. *Advances: The Quarterly Newsletter of the Robert Wood Johnson Foundation*, 4(1), 9–10.

Ganz, P. A. (1994). Quality of life and the patient with cancer: Individual and policy implications. *Cancer Supplement*, 74(4), 1445–1452.

Given, B. (1995). Believing and dreaming to improve cancer care. *Oncology Nursing Forum*, 22(6), 929–940.

Glazebrook, G. A. (1992). Radiation therapy: A long term cost benefit analysis in a North American region. *Clinical Oncology*, 4(5), 302–305.

Gold, M. R., Siegel, J. E., Russel, L. B., & Weinstein, M. C. (1996). *Cost-effectiveness in health and medicine*. New York: Oxford University Press.

Guadagnoli, E., Shapiro, C. L., Weeks, J. C., Gurwitz, J. H., Borbas, C., & Soumerai, S. B. (1998). The quality of care for treatment of early stage breast carcinoma: Is it consistant with national guidelines? *Cancer*, 83(2), 302–309.

Guidry, J. J., Aday, L. A., Zhang, D., & Winn, R. J. (1998). Cost considerations as potential barriers to cancer treatment. *Cancer Practice*, 6(3), 182–187.

Haas, M. L., & Kuehn, E. F. (1999). Outcomes measurements: Designing, implementing, and evaluating the process. *Group Practice Journal*, 48(5), 19–21.

Hanks, G. (1985). Optimizing the radiation treatment and outcome of prostate cancer. *International Journal of Radiation Oncology, Biology, Physics*, 11, 1235–1245.

Hanks, G., Coia, L., & Curry, J. (1997). Patterns of care studies: Past, present, and future. *Seminars in Radiation Oncology*, 7(2), 97–100.

Hanks, G., Diamond, J., & Kramer, S. (1985). The need for complex technology in radiation oncology: Correlations of facility characteristics and structure with outcome. *Cancer*, 55(Suppl. 9), 2198–2201.

Hanks, G. E., Hanlon, A. L., Schultheiss, T. E., Pinover, W. H., Movsas, B., Epstein, B. E., & Hunt, M. A. (1998). Dose-escalation with 3D conformal treatment: Five year outcomes, treatment optimization, and future directions. *International Journal of Radiation Oncology, Biology, Physics*, 41(3), 501–510.

Harlan, L., Brawley, O., Pommerenke, F., Wali, P., & Kramer, B. (1995). Geographic, age, and racial variation in the treatment of local/regional carcinoma of the prostate. *Journal of Clinical Oncology*, 13, 91–105.

Hayman, J., Weeks, J., & Mauch, P. (1996). Economic analyses in health care: An introduction to the methodology with an emphasis on radiation therapy. *International Journal of Radiation Oncology, Biology, Physics*, 35(4), 827–841.

Hillner, B. E. (1996). Economic and cost-effectiveness issues in breast cancer treatment. *Seminars in Oncology*, 23(1) (Suppl. 2).

Hunt, V. D. (1996). *Process mapping—How to reengineer your business processes.* New York: John Wiley & Sons.

Jenkins, C. (1992). Assessment of outcomes of health intervention. *Social Science in Medicine,* 35(4), 367–375.

Jensen, S., & Given, B. A. (1991). Fatigue affecting family caregivers of cancer patients. *Cancer Nursing,* 14, 181–187.

Kalua, P. M. (1998). Cancer pain guidelines: Are they being used? Results of a multi-site study conducted by the Hawaii Cancer Pain Initiative. *Hawaii Medicine Journal,* 57(10), 655–660.

Karnofsky, D. A., & Burchenal, J. H. (1949). The clinical evaluation of chemotherapeutic agents in cancer. In C. M. Maclead (Ed.), *Evaluation of chemotherapeutic agents* (pp. 199–205). New York: Columbia University Press.

King, K. B., Nail, L. M., Kreamer, K., Strohl, R. A., & Johnson, J. E. (1985). Patients' description for the experience of receiving radiation therapy. *Oncology Nursing Forum,* 12(4), 55–61.

Kobeissi, B. J., Gupta, M., Perez, C. A., Dopuch, N., Michaliski, J. M., Van Antwerp, G., Gerber, R., & Wasserman, T. H. (1998). Physician resource utilization in radiation oncology: A model based on management of carcinoma of the prostate. *International Journal of Radiation Oncology, Biology, Physics,* 40(3), 593–603.

Lanciano, R., Thomas, G., & Eifel, P. (1997). Over 20 years of progress in radiation oncology: Cervical cancer. *Seminars in Radiation Oncology,* 7(2), 122–126.

Lee-Feldstein, A., Anton-Culver, H., & Feldstein, P. J. (1994). Treatment differences and other prognostic factors related to breast cancer and survival: Delivery systems and medical outcomes. *Journal of the American Medical Association,* 271(15), 1163–1168.

Levine, A. S., Plume, S. K., & Nelson, E. C. (1997). Transforming patient feedback into strategic action plans. *Quality Management in Health Care,* 5(3), 28–40.

Lustig, R., Krall, J., Curran, W., MacLean, C., Hanks, G., & Kramer, S. (1991). Improvements observed in care and outcome in carcinoma of the larynx. *International Journal of Radiation Oncology, Biology, Physics,* 20, 101–104.

Lustig, R., MacLean, C., Hanks, G., & Kramer, S. (1984). PCS outcome studies: Results of the national practice in cancer of the larynx. *International Journal of Radiation Oncology, Biology, Physics,* 10, 2357–2362.

Mandelblatt, J. S., Ganz, P., & Kahn, K. L. (1999). Proposed agenda for the measurement of quality-of-care outcomes in oncology practice. *Journal of Clinical Oncology* 17(8): 2614–22.

McCorkle, R. (1987). The measurement of symptom distress. *Seminars in Oncology Nursing,* 3, 248–256.

McCormack, J. (1998a). Electronic records: Key to HCFA compliance? *Health Data Management,* 6(6), 40–42, 44.

McCormack, J. (1998b). Getting the most out of HEDIS reporting. *Health Data Management,* 6(4), 110–111.

McCormack, J. (1998c). Managed care. Database aids fight against cancer. *Health Data Management, 6*(3), 82, 84, 86.

Meyerowitz, B. E., Richardson, J., Hudson, S., & Leedham, B. (1998). Ethnicity and cancer outcomes: Behavioral and psychosocial considerations. *Psychological Bulletin, 123*(1), 47–70.

Mock, V., Dow, K. H., Meares, C. J., Grimm, P. M., Dienemann, J. A., Haisfield-Wolfe, M. E., Quitasol, W., Mitchell, S., Chakravarthy, A., & Gage, I. (1997). Effects of exercise on fatigue, physical functioning, and emotional distress during radiation therapy for breast cancer. *Oncology Nursing Forum, 24*(6), 991–1000.

Monson, J., Chin, L., Nixon, A., Gage, I., Silver, B., Recht, A., & Harris, J. (1997). Is machine energy (4–8 MV) associated with outcome for stage I-II breast cancer patients? *International Journal of Radiation Oncology, Biology, Physics, 37*(5), 1095–1100.

Nattinger, A. B., Gottlieb, M. S., Hoffman, R. G., Walker, A. P., & Goodwin, J. S., (1996). Minimal increase in use of breast-conserving treatment for breast cancer. *New England Journal of Medicine, 326*, 1102–1127.

Nattinger, A. B., Gottlieb, M. S., Veum, J., Yahnke, D., & Goodwin, J. S. (1992). Geographic variation in the use of breast-conserving treatment for breast cancer. *New England Journal of Medicine, 326*(17), 1102–1127.

Newschaffer, C. J., Penberthy, L., Desch, C. E., Retchin, S. M., & Whittemore, M. (1996). The effect of age and comorbidity in the treatment of elderly women with nonmetastatic breast cancer. *Archives of Internal Medicine, 156*, 85–90.

Oberst, M. T., Change, A. S., & McCubbin, M. A. (1991). Self-care burden, stress appraisal, and mood among persons receiving radiotherapy. *Cancer Nursing, 14*(2), 71–78.

Orem, D. E. (1995). *Nursing. Concepts of practice* (5th ed.). St. Louis: Mosby—Year Book.

Owen, J. B., Sedransk, J., & Pajak, T. F. (1997). National averages for process and outcome in radiation oncology: Methodology of the patterns of care study. *Seminars in Radiation Oncology, 7*(2), 101–107.

Parasuraman, A., Zeithaml, V. A., & Berry, L. L. (1986). SERVQUAL: A *multiple item scale for measuring customer perceptions of service quality.* Cambridge, MA: Marketing Science Institute.

Payne, R. (1998). Practice guidelines for cancer pain therapy: Issues pertinent to the revision of national guidelines. *Oncology, 12*(11A), 169–175.

PCS Consensus Committees. (1997). 1996 decision trees and management guidelines. *Seminars on Radiation Oncology, 7*(2), 163–181.

Perez, C. A., Kobeissi, B., Smith, B. D., Fox, S., Grigsby, P. W., Purdy, J. A., Procter, H. D., & Wasserman, T. H. (1993). Cost accounting in radiation oncology: A computer-based model for reimbursement. *International Journal Radiation Oncology, Biology, Physics, 25*(5), 895–906.

Schipper, H., Clinch, J., & Powell, V. (1990). Definitions and conceptual issues. In B. Spilker (Ed.), *Quality of life assessments in clinical trials* (pp. 11–24). New York: Raven Press.

Seibert, J. H. (1996). Patient focus with an eye on the bottom line. *Caring, 15*(10), 26, 29, 31–37.

Sidani, S., & Broden, C. J. (1998). *Evaluating nursing instructions—A theory.* Sage. Evaluating nursing intervention: A theory driven approach. Thousand Oaks, CA: Sage.

Smith, T. J., Penberthy, L., Desch, C. E., Whittemore, M., Newschaffer, C., Hillner, B. E., McClish, D., & Retchin, S. M. (1995). Differences in initial treatment patterns and outcomes of lung cancer in the elderly. *Lung Cancer, 13,* 235–252.

Smitt, M. C., Buzydlowski, J., & Hoppe, R. T. (1997). Over 20 years of progress in radiation oncology: Hodgkin's Disease. *Seminars in Radiation Oncology, 7*(2), 127–134.

Spitzer, W. O., Dobson, A. J., Chesterman, E., & Levi, J. (1981). Measuring the quality of life of cancer patients: A concise QL-index for use by physicians. *Journal of Chronic Diseases, 34,* 585–597.

Tenner, A. R., & DeToro, I. J. (1992). *Total quality management: Three steps to continuous improvement.* Reading, MA: Addison-Wesley.

Thomas, G. (1997). Over 20 years of progress in radiation oncology: Seminoma. *Seminars in Radiation Oncology, 7*(2), 135–145.

Ware, J. E., Jr., (1995). The status of health assessment 1994. *Annual Review of Public Health, 16,* 327–354.

Weeks, J. (1998). Overview of outcomes research and management and its role in oncology practice. *Oncology, 12*(3) (Suppl. 4), 11–13.

Williams, A. (1985). Economics of coronary artery bypass grafting. *British Medical Journal, 291,* 326–329.

Winn, R. J., Botnick, W., & Dozier, N. (1996). The NCCN guideline development program. *Oncology, 10*(5), 23–28.

Zapka, J. G., Palmer, R. H., Hargraves, J. L., Nerenz, D., Frazier, H. S., & Warner, C. K. (1995). Relationships of patient satisfaction with experience of system performance and health status. *Journal of Ambulatory Care Management, 18*(1), 73–83.

Zelefsky, M. J., Leibel, S. A., Gaudin, P. B., Kutcher, G. J., Fleshner, N. E., Venkatramen, E. S., Reuter, V. E., Fair, W. R., Ling, C. C., & Fuks, Z. (1998). Dose-escalation with three-dimensional conformal radiation therapy affects the outcome in prostate cancer. *International Journal of Radiation Oncology, Biology, Physics, 41*(3), 491–500.

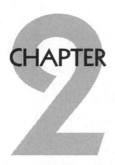

CHAPTER 2

ROLE OF THE MULTIDISCIPLINARY TEAM IN RADIATION THERAPY

Deborah Watkins Bruner
Benjamin Movsas

Improved technology and changing trends in health care are helping people live longer and are decreasing mortality and morbidity from the number-one killer in the United States: heart disease. This has led to predictions that cancer care will be the leading reason for inpatient and outpatient hospital visits, making cancer the dominant specialty in the United States in the twenty-first century (Fountain, 1993). Because cancer is both a multisystem event and a chronic disease, it requires a multidisciplinary team approach to provide the best outcomes. The multidisciplinary team can be defined as a functioning unit comprised of health care professionals from varying disciplines and specialties who coordinate their activities to provide services to well clients, patients, and families (Ducanis & Golin, 1979). Several health care organizations have stressed the importance of the multidisciplinary team approach to patient care including the Association of Cancer Care Centers, The American College of Surgeons, and the Joint Commission on Accreditation of Healthcare Organizations (Enck, 1987; Phillips, 1997).

Role delineation is an important aspect in the organization and effective collaboration of a multidisciplinary team. Ambiguous expectations among health care professionals, and between them and patients, can result in reduced quality of care. Conversely, clear role delineation has generally benefited overall health care system flexibility and responsiveness (Taylor, 1996). It is also recognized that dysfunctional teams exist where roles are blurred and the uniqueness of each discipline is stifled, where roles are so rigidly defined that spontaneity and creative problem solving are discouraged, or where individual accountability is lost and no one feels responsible (Hermann & Hilderely, 1993).

To promote the effective collaboration of a multidisciplinary team, several authors have suggested methods to enhance the effort including listening to and appreciating others; thinking across disciplines and roles; sharing ideas and linking those shared ideas to the implementation of change; appreciating systems and interdependencies; using research to improve evidence-based practices; using methods, skills, and techniques as facilitators of collaboration; and working across organizational boundaries (Batalden, Bronenwett, Brown, Moffatt, & Serrell, 1998). An outcome measure of teamwork, which assesses health care team attitudes toward Quality of Care/Process and Physician Centrality, has been developed. The Quality of Care/Process subscale measures team members' perceptions of the quality of care delivered by health care teams. The Physician Centrality subscale measures team members' attitudes toward physicians' authority in teams and their control over patient information (Heinemann, Schmitt, Farrell, & Brallier, 1999).

THE RADIATION THERAPY TEAM

Approximately 60% of patients with cancer are treated with radiation therapy. Therapeutic radiation can be curative in intent or it can provide palliative relief to patients with incurable cancer. "The success of radiation therapy depends on the delivery of an adequate dose to the entire tumor volume with acceptable morbidity in the surrounding normal tissues. The goals are to attain the highest probability of local and regional tumor control with the lowest achievable incidence of side effects and to prolong the life of the patient with the best possible quality of life" (Perez & Purdy, 1998). The achievement of these goals requires a multidisciplinary team. The core members of the radiation therapy team include the radiation oncologist, the radiation oncology nurse, the radiation therapist, medical physicist, and dosimetrist. Although there is occasional role overlap, each member has distinct responsibilities and accountabilities that together are aimed at providing the optimal outcome for the patient receiving radiation therapy. The core members of the team guide the patient and family through the process of radiation therapy, which has been described as:

- Clinical evaluation
- ■ Therapeutic decision making
- Target volume localization
- Treatment planning
- Simulation
- Fabrication of treatment aids
- Treatment
- Patient evaluation during treatment
- ■ Follow-up (American College of Radiology, 1991)

Each member of the team devotes and is responsible for varying amounts of time and activity at each point in the process.

THE RADIATION ONCOLOGIST

Although the field of therapeutic radiation began in the nineteenth century with the work of Roentgen, Becquerel, and the Curies, it did not develop into a medical specialty until the 1960s. Radiation oncology is now a recognized medical specialty that employs therapeutic ionizing radiation for the treatment of tumors. The Inter-Society Council for Radiation Oncology, comprised of 9 radiation-focused organizations, defines the radiation oncologist as a physician with special interest, training, and competence in managing patients with cancer and holding certification by the American Board of Radiology (American College of Radiology, 1991). The radiation oncologist is involved in every step of the process outlined previously and is ultimately responsible for the care delivered to the patient receiving radiation therapy. The responsibility for critical judgment and execution of the planning, treatment, and follow-up of radiation therapy rests with the radiation oncologist (Perez & Purdy, 1998). To treat patients effectively, the radiation oncologist must have sufficient training to define the target volume and critical structures, to interpret treatment planning information, and to guide the physicist or dosimetrist in achieving the best dose distribution; have sufficient knowledge to select the best possible combination of dose and fractionation for a given site and volume; be competent to judge the quality of the dose distribution and the technical feasibility and accuracy of the proposed plan; and understand the capabilities and limitations of the staff and computer systems involved in the radiation treatment planning process (Perez & Purdy, 1998).

MEDICAL PHYSICIST

The medical physicist is usually a Ph.D. with a background in diagnostic and radiologic physics and certified by the American Board of Radiology (American College of Radiology, 1991). The medical physicist must be well versed in the complexities of clinical treatment planning including the beam directions, the influence of beam geometry on the treatment planning volume, correction factors, computation of dose distribution, the determination of dose/time/volume relationships, verification of treatment accuracy, and continual assessment of equipment performance. The medical physicist must also be knowledgeable with regard to the sophisticated treatment planning systems that have been developed, particularly the three-dimensional (3D) treatment planning systems, intensity-modulated radiation therapy (IMRT), and delivery techniques.

DOSIMETRIST

The dosimetrist is usually responsible for the calculation of radiation dose distributions under the direction of the medical physicist and radiation oncologist (American College of Radiology, 1991). They are frequently master's prepared and familiar with the radiation treatment machines, equipment, and sources. The dosimetrist plays a major role in treatment planning, verification, and record keeping.

THE RADIATION THERAPIST

The radiation therapist is trained in the implementation of the treatment plan generated by the collaboration of the radiation oncologist, medical physicist, and dosimetrist. They are directly involved in the simulation process, including setting up the patient for measurement, radiographic documentation of the treatment ports, and construction and application of patient immobilization devices and custom blocks. The radiation therapist is responsible for the actual delivery of the ionizing radiation and must be meticulous about verification of treatment accuracy and documentation. During the treatment phase of radiation therapy, the radiation therapist is often the first to assess therapy-related symptoms and direct the patient to the radiation oncology nurse or physician for symptom management.

THE RADIATION ONCOLOGY NURSE

The role of the nurse in radiation oncology has been clearly delineated and includes as minimum priorities patient/family education and the promotion and/or maintenance of quality of life (Bruner, 1990a, 1990b, 1993, 1996; Bruner, Bucholtz, Iwamoto, & Strohl, 1998a). Patient and family education focuses on the treatment experience, potential treatment-related symptoms, and self-care activities. The nurse works with the radiation therapy team to promote good quality of life outcomes through assessment and management of symptoms, listening and responding promptly and appropriately to telephone calls, coordinating patient care, and assisting patients and families to cope with the diagnosis and treatment.

Additional roles for the radiation oncology nurse are emerging as more departments add nurse practitioners to their teams. In addition to the previously noted functions, nurse practitioners may extend the work of the medical team through participating in diagnosis and treatment decisions as prescribed by their state regulations.

Successful examples of nurse-physician collaborative practice in radiation oncology have been published (Hilderley, 1991). Nurses' success in improving medical outcomes for a host of different chronic diseases, including cancer, have been well documented (Johnson, Fieler, Wlasowicz, Mitchell, & Jones, 1997; Joint Commission on Accreditation of Health Care Organizations, 1999; Naylor et al., 1999).

Suggested minimum qualifications of the radiation oncology nurse have been published and include a baccalaureate degree in nursing, two years' experience in medical-surgical nursing, and one year of oncology experience (American College of Radiology, 1991; Bruner, 1990b).

MEDICAL AND SURGICAL ONCOLOGISTS

Radiation oncologists must work in close collaboration with their medical and surgical colleagues to achieve optimal patient and treatment outcomes. In recognition of the need for collaboration, specialty groups have published recommendations for multidisciplinary cancer care. For example, the International Working Group in Colorectal Cancer (IWGCC), a multidisciplinary group that encompasses expertise from a range of disciplines, has advocated a multidisciplinary approach to the treatment of advanced colorectal cancer. The IWGCC states that a multidisciplinary approach is likely to deliver the best possible outcomes (i.e., survival, objective response, and palliation) and safety. The authors suggest that to achieve this a broader, patient-centered evaluation of cancer treatment is required that acknowledges the views, experience, and perspectives of all specialties [and disciplines] involved in the treatment process (Minsky, 1998).

The achievement of successful outcomes with multidisciplinary teams has been documented. For example, one study evaluated the effectiveness of a multidisciplinary approach to spinal cord compression (SCC) in patients treated by radiation therapy. Patients with SCC were examined and treated by a multidisciplinary team consisting of a radiation oncologist, medical oncologist, neurologist, neurosurgeon, and orthopedic surgeon. Seventy-nine patients received radiation and a course of high dose dexamethasone. The primary treatment outcome was ambulation capabilities. Results indicated that 72% of patients were already nonambulatory at diagnosis and/or 33% had motor deficiency or pain. Pretreatment ambulation ability was the main prognostic indicator of treatment outcome; 90% of patients who were ambulatory before treatment remained so while 33% of the nonambulatory patients regained their ability to walk. Overall, 51% of the study group were ambulatory after radiation therapy. The ambulatory state after treatment was also the main predictor for survival. The authors indicated that it was the close cooperation of a multidisciplinary team in diagnosis and treatment that led to the achievement of good results with radiation treatment in SCC (Kovner et al., 1999).

FAMILY PHYSICIAN

Besides being a source of referral, the family physician often plays an important role in the follow-up of the patient. However, they are all too often left out of the communication loop. One study explored the oncologists' perspectives on the process of cancer patient follow-up. Oncologists described roles for themselves in reassuring patients, detecting recurrence, monitoring toxicity of treatment, and gathering data for clinical trials. Oncologists stated a desire for collaboration with family physicians, yet identified variable and unpredictable interest and poor communication with family physicians as a barrier. Oncologists themselves perceived the cancer system structure as a "black box" within which multidisciplinary teams worked well, but seldom included family physicians. The authors concluded that communication barriers, patient preferences, and misperceptions between groups must be addressed before collaboration in the follow-up period of cancer care can be improved (Wood & McWilliam, 1996).

PATHOLOGIST

Improvements in technology have increased the demand for greater input from pathologists. Pathologists provide morphological assessment, classification and grading of tumors necessary for treatment decision making, and the measure of outcomes. In addition, pathologists are in a position to make clinical use of the wealth of knowledge emerging from molecular biological analyses. It is the pathologist who can establish tissue banks for the provision of optimally preserved material, which is vital to facilitate molecular biological analysis. For example, recent developments in molecular biology have revealed that several oncogenes, suppressor genes, and adhesion molecules are involved in the development of esophageal cancer, and that combination analysis using molecular biological factors may be useful for the prediction of patient survival and recurrence after radiotherapy (Shimada et al., 1999).

Additionally, pathologists may oversee the analysis of fresh or archival material that can provide a source of DNA, which enables genetic abnormalities to be identified (Lalani, Stubb, & Stamp, 1997). For example, it has been suggested that the investigation of the interrelationship between p53 gene alterations and MDR1 gene expression from fine-needle samplings of breast cancer patients may identify a small subset of patients who may be resistant to radiation therapy or who should pursue an aggressive course of therapy (Chevillard et al., 1997).

RADIATION SAFETY OFFICER

The radiation safety officer assists the radiation team in keeping current with and monitoring Nuclear Regulatory Commission regulations and safety guidelines. For instance, the Nuclear Regulatory Commission regulations for the release of patients who were administered radioactive material have recently been revised to include dose-based or activity-based criteria. Patients may now be released if the total effective dose equivalent to another individual from exposure to a released patient is < 500 mrem. The radiation safety officer assists with incorporating the guidelines into policy and procedure and monitoring and documenting compliance. The radiation safety officer demonstrates compliance with this dose limit by using a default table for activity or dose rate provided in the Nuclear Regulatory Guide, by performing a patient-specific dose calculation, or by basing patient release on the patient-specific measured dose rate at 1 meter (Siegel, 1998).

Depending on the type of institution or radiation therapy facility, additional disciplines may be part of the radiation therapy team and contribute to improved patient outcomes. For example, in university or academic-based settings a radiobiologist or molecular biologist/geneticist may be part of the team.

RADIOBIOLOGIST

The radiobiologist helps improve outcomes through research into methods that enhance understanding of the radiosensitivity of tumors while maintaining normal tissue tolerance. For example, a recent study modeled increases in local tumor control without increasing normal tissue complications by prescribing a patient's radiation dose based on cellular radiosensitivity. Cellular radiosensitivity was measured using an assay that provided distributions of fibroblast radiosensitivity. The model showed that improvements in tumor control rates might be achievable through the individualization of radiotherapy dose prescriptions of cancer patients based on the variability in radiosensitivity (Mackay & Hendry, 1999).

MOLECULAR BIOLOGIST/GENETICIST

The relative explosion of new knowledge produced by the unprecedented efforts of the Human Genome Project affects most aspects of medical care including the practice of radiation oncology. It has already been stated that the advances in molecular biology and genetics will directly impact the role of radiation oncologists in the not-to-distant future (Coleman, 1996). One such example is the study of p53, which plays a central role in the cellular response to DNA-damaging agents, including ionizing radiation. Molecular biologists have documented the transcriptional responses associated with ionizing radiation-induced apoptosis. They have also documented that the responses of some genes to ionizing radiation and other DNA-damaging agents vary widely in cell lines from different tissues of origin and different genetic backgrounds. Several authors suggest that differences in gene responsiveness may be employed as molecular markers with prognostic value using a combination of informatics and genetic approaches (Fornace et al., 1999).

Although the preceding list of disciplines involved in the multidisciplinary care of the patient receiving radiation therapy is comprehensive, it is not exhaustive. In addition, varying disciplines and ancillary staff play essential roles in producing the best outcomes for patients treated with radiation therapy including but not limited to: secretarial staff, social workers, dieticians, pharmacists, pain team, psychologists, sex therapists, rehabilitation team, hospice team, and clergy. An enduring respect for the skills of each discipline and open communication among disciplines is required to achieve optimal patient outcomes before, during, and after radiation therapy.

It is important to note that for all of the team labor dedicated to improving outcomes for the patient treated with radiation therapy, from the patient's perspective it is generally only the direct clinical services that matter. Patients are generally unaware of all of the steps that go into delivering therapeutic radiation, since much of the work, like treatment planning, is conducted behind the scenes. The same is true for some of the members of the multidisciplinary team like, where available, the research staff who are vital to evaluating new technologies and interventions for improving outcomes, but who conduct their work in laboratories unseen by the patient.

CLINICAL SERVICES

From the patient's point of view there are three basic clinical services that the radiation therapy team provides: consultation, treatment, and follow-up.

CONSULTATION

The traditional radiation therapy consultation is comprised of the history, physical examination, and review of the previous tests and procedures that led the patient to consult with the radiation oncologist. The consultation usually includes an explanation to the patient/family of diagnosis and management. However, the literature is sparse on how to base recommendations for effective communication in the cancer consultation. One study identified a slightly different structure in some consultations, which they categorized as more "patient-centered." In the patient-centered consultation doctors or nurses introduce explanation and education into the early history-taking stage. This strategy is contrasted with the traditional approach in which the doctor elicits only information during the history and gives an explanation at subsequent visits. The authors suggest that the "early feedback" strategy may result in patients with chronic illnesses achieving greater understanding of their symptoms (Hak & Campion, 1999).

Active participation in the medical consultation has been demonstrated to benefit aspects of patients' subsequent psychological well-being (Brown, Utow, Boyer, & Tattersall, 1999). One study investigated the relationship between doctor-patient behavior during consultation and patient outcomes. One hundred and forty-two cancer patients attending their first consultation with a cancer specialist were audiotaped and the tapes were analyzed by computer for doctor-patient interaction. Baseline measures of patient anxiety and information and involvement preferences were taken prior to the consultation. Outcomes included recall of information, patient satisfaction with the consultation, and psychological adjustment to cancer. Doctor behavior was shown to vary significantly according to the age, gender, involvement preferences, and inpatient or outpatient status of the patient. Satisfaction with communication was related to a higher ratio of doctor-to-patient talk. However, better psychological adjustment at follow-up was related to the frequency with which patients' questions were answered. The results suggest that patient-centered consultations lead to improved satisfaction and psychological adjustment (Butow, Dunn, Tattersall, & Jones, 1995).

In an effort to improve outcomes through patient-centered consultations, Frederikson developed an information-exchange model of medical consultation. In a study to explore the association between information-exchange process variables and a range of other outcomes, it was demonstrated that the way the physician performed information-exchange was a significant predictor of patient satisfaction. In addition, the study indicated that the immediate outcome measures of patient understanding, the doctor-patient relationship, the patient's view of the appropriateness of treatment, and the perceptions of the doctor's response were each related to a particular subset of information-exchange activities. Frederikson concluded that attending to the perceptions and views of the patient offered a more effective strategy for consultation than focusing on providing large amounts of standardized information (Frederikson, 1995).

Most health care professionals focus on improved outcomes in the treatment and follow-up phases of radiation therapy. The consultation phase has to date received little attention. However, the maximization of optimal outcomes should start at the beginning. Collectively the studies just described provide a framework for improved outcomes through the initiation of the patient-centered consultation (Brown et al., 1999; Butow et al., 1995; Frederikson, 1995).

TREATMENT

Once the radiation oncologist and patient decide through the consultation process that radiation therapy is appropriate and desired, the patient enters the treatment phase. Treatment begins with informed consent/decision making.

Informed Consent/Decision Making

The old paradigm of informed consent in which the physician delivers a unidirectional monologue of treatment risks, benefits, and alternatives is giving way to an enlightened view that involves the sharing of decision making with the patient (Braddock, 1998; Lidz, Appelbaum, & Meisel, 1988). The need to improve the process of informed consent/decision making was highlighted in a recent article that assessed 1,057 audiotapes of patient-physician outpatient encounters. Patients were recruited from 59 primary physicians' and 65 general and orthopedic surgeons' practices. Alarmingly, only 9% of decisions met the authors' criteria of informed decision making (Braddock, Edwards, Hasenberg, Laidley, & Levinson, 1999).

The informed consent process varies widely by institution but at minimum should include at least a verbal explanation of the following:

■ Purpose and efficacy of treatment (cure, control, or palliation)
■ Option to participate in or to refuse appropriate clinical trials
■ Risks versus benefits of treatment
■ Uncertainties of treatment
■ Potential side effects
■ Treatment planning experience including the time it will take, the positioning required (if it tends to be uncomfortable), and the fitting of immobilization devices
■ Treatment experience (including sights, sounds, sensations, duration, and department logistics such as hours of operation, who to call during and after normal operating hours, etc.)
■ Alternative therapies
■ Recommended follow-up (Bruner et al., 1998a)

To move informed consent to the higher level of informed decision making, the following variables need to be included:

■ Active patient participation in decision making
■ Assessment of the patient's understanding of the information required for a decision
■ Exploration of the patient's preferences (Braddock et al., 1999)

Education

As discussed previously, education should optimally begin in the consultation phase of the patient encounter with the radiation therapy team and continue throughout the treatment and follow-up phases. However, the majority of the education occurs during the informed consent process and treatment phase. Multiple factors have been recommended for consideration in assessing the patient's learning needs and learning capability as follows:

- ■ Sociodemographic information that may influence learning including gender, age, socioeconomic status, education level, literacy level, cultural/ethnic background, and language barriers
- ■ Diagnosis, previous treatments, treatment expectations, misconceptions, fears and concerns, concomitant medical/psychiatric problems (e.g., pain, fatigue, anxiety), and medications

It has been well documented that concrete, objective information (verbal and written) improves comprehension, coping, and self-care outcomes of education (Fieler, Wlasowicz, Mitchell, Jones, & Johnson, 1996; Hinds, Streater, & Mood, 1995). Conversely a negative correlation has been documented between ambiguous information and patient comprehension (Patterson, Lipsett, Michel, & Archambeau, 1981). Besides providing concrete, objective information, other factors should be considered in the education process including providing an atmosphere conducive to enhancing respect, trust, and protecting confidentiality as well as attention to both verbal and nonverbal cues from the patient and family.

Several methods of providing information and education to patients receiving radiation therapy have been tested with mixed results.

- ■ A study undertaken to develop and test the effects of informational audiotapes on knowledge and self-care management of side effects in subjects undergoing radiation therapy randomized 75 patients (with a mean age of 53 years) into control and experimental groups. The control group received the facility's standard care, while the experimental group received the standard care and also listened to informational audiotapes. Outcome variables included number and severity of side effects, self-care measures used to manage the side effects, and helpfulness of these measures. Results indicated that patients in the experimental group were more knowledgeable about radiation therapy and its side effects, used more self-care measures, and practiced more helpful self-care behaviors than control group subjects. The use of audiotapes allowed the patients to receive the information they needed at times and places that were convenient to them. This led the author to conclude that audiotapes are an effective strategy for teaching self-care practices to patients undergoing radiation therapy and they provide patients with the knowledge necessary to become active participants in their own care (Hagopian, 1996).

■ A similar study was undertaken to assess the same self-care outcome variables with a weekly newsletter instead of audiotapes. Although the subjects who read the newsletter scored significantly higher on the knowledge test, there were no significant differences in the number of self-care behaviors or in the severity of side effects as compared to those who did not receive the newsletter. However, the author suggested that patient education in the form of a newsletter may provide benefits to patients other than knowledge (e.g., reduced anxiety) that may be just as important as the relief of side effects (Hagopian, 1991). Comparable results were found with a weekly telephone intervention (Hagopian & Rubenstein, 1990).

Understanding successful methods of educating patients undergoing radiation therapy as previously presented is as important as the content of the education. Basic content was previously outlined under informed consent, but in addition the teaching of self-care activities has been shown to improve patient outcomes. It may be that self-care activities help to engage the patient and family in the treatment process, giving them ownership and empowerment that cannot be conferred by passive education alone.

Successful programs that teach patients self-care abilities to prevent symptoms or to reduce symptom severity and duration associated with disease and treatment during radiation therapy and chemotherapy have been demonstrated (Larson, Dodd, & Aksamit, 1998). A good example of a successfully implemented nurse-prescribed and -monitored self-care exercise program was reported for women treated with radiation therapy for breast cancer. The self-paced, home-walking exercise program was found to help manage symptoms and improve physical functioning during radiation therapy. The authors concluded that the exercise program was an effective, convenient, and low-cost self-care activity that reduced symptoms and facilitated adaptation to breast cancer diagnosis and treatment in the study population (Mock et al., 1997).

Symptom Management

Managing the side effects of radiation and multimodality therapy is, next to survival, the primary outcome of concern for the patient. Specific strategies for intervention are described in detail throughout this book. It is important to remember that these side effects are not simply uncomfortable inconveniences to be tolerated for the sake of survival. Radiation therapy and combined modality therapy have been documented to cause major decrements in site-specific aspects of quality of life. In addition, studies have reported sizable cohorts of subjects willing to trade off significant amounts of survival to avoid specific symptoms, such as loss of speech or loss of potency, to maintain quality of life (McNeil, Weichselbaum, & Pauker, 1981; Singer et al., 1991). Yet, reports of the less-than-optimal levels of physician awareness of patient self-reported symptoms are consistent throughout the literature (Ford, Fallowfield, & Lewis, 1994).

■ Two Radiation Therapy Oncology Group (RTOG) reports highlight discrepancies between patient self-report and physician rating of the patient's symptoms. In RTOG 90-20, a phase II trial of external beam radiation therapy with etanidazole for locally advanced prostate cancer, patients were asked to self-report the level of symptoms on several quality of life instruments. In comparing these reports to physician ratings of the same symptoms using the RTOG acute toxicity rating scales, significant discrepancies were noted. For example, 25% to 44% of physician ratings were in moderate to low agreement in rating patient self-reported dysuria and diarrhea, respectively (13% of which was low agreement for both symptoms). (Bruner et al., 1995).

■ In an RTOG validation study of the Sexual Adjustment Questionnaire in 733 patients treated on two RTOG clinical trials for prostate cancer, it was found that physician and patient assessments of the patient's ability to have an erection differed in 47% of cases (Bruner et al., 1998b).

■ A corroborating report came from a more recent study that assessed physical symptoms and perceived needs among 204 patients visiting an outpatient oncology department. Participating patients and their medical oncologists completed a survey in which they indicated their perception of each patient's level of symptoms and needs for health information, provider care and support, psychological intervention, assistance with physical functioning and daily living, and improved interpersonal communication with the physician. The oncologists' and patients' symptom responses were most congruent (80%) for hair loss. Physician awareness of patient self-reported major physical symptoms of fatigue, nausea, vomiting, and diarrhea were congruent 58% to 52% of the time. However, for all other physical symptoms, including sore mouth, constipation, appetite loss, and skin rash, physician awareness was less than 50% and as low as 15%. Although physicians uniformly underestimated patient self-reported symptoms, they tended to overestimate levels of patients' perceived needs with the oncologists' and patients' responses congruent 34% to 49% of the time (Newell, Sanson-Fisher, Girgis, & Bonaventura, 1998).

Over the past decade, patient self-report symptom and quality of life assessments have increasingly been included in clinical trials, but their use in clinical practice is still uncommon. One recent pilot study investigated the feasibility of introducing individual quality of life assessments into the daily routine of an outpatient oncology clinic, and the potential impact of such assessments on doctor-patient communication. Participating patients completed the EORTC QLQ-C30, a standardized cancer-specific quality of life questionnaire, as a baseline measurement and at two subsequent visits. The patients' responses were computer-scored and transformed into a graphic summary. The summary included current scores as well as those elicited at the previous visit, and were given to both the physicians and the patients just prior to the medical consultation. Completing, scoring, and printing the quality of life data were done during waiting room time and did not lengthen the average consultation time. Although a small increase was noted in the average number of quality of life issues discussed per consultation, the most notable trend was the increased responsibility taken by the physicians in raising specific quality of life issues for discussion. When the quality of life summary was available, the physicians raised three times as many topics than was the case prior to its use. All participating physicians and the majority of patients believed that the quality of life summary facilitated communication and expressed interest in continued use of the procedure (Detmar & Aaronson, 1998).

Coordination/Communication

Symptom management as previously outlined may require referrals to surgeons, gynecologists, or urologists. Patients also need to be referred to appropriate medical professionals such as social workers, psychologists, psychiatrists, or sex therapists. Through education and experiences, nurses are well suited for the role of patient care coordinator within the radiation oncology department or through institution-employed nurse case managers. The coordination of patient services focuses on the networking, organization, and synchronization of patient care services across multidisciplinary providers and various care settings. The targeted outcomes of good coordination and communication are improved continuity of care, increased adherence to the treatment care plan, and enhanced patient satisfaction. This requires a commitment to effective team communication to overcome traditional barriers to information exchange such as time constraints and territorialism.

Documentation

Comprehensive documentation of sociodemographic data, diagnostic data, treatment data, and acute and chronic treatment sequelae is a decisive precondition for the appropriate evaluation of the treatment quality of any cancer therapy. Essential minimum requirements for inclusion in a radiation oncology treatment chart are as follows:

- General patient-related parameters such as sociodemographic data including gender, age, socioeconomic status, education level, literacy level, cultural/ethnic background, and language barriers
- Diagnostic data including diagnosis, TNM staging, previous treatments, concomitant medical/psychiatric problems, and medications
- Pretreatment patient education and informed consent/decision making
- Treatment data including planning, simulation, and delivery (site, dose, frequency, etc.) documentation
- The kind and the degree of acute radiation-related side effects (documented at least weekly)
- On-treatment patient education
- Tumor response to treatment
- The kind and the degree of chronic radiation-related side effects
- Impact of treatment on quality of life
- Recommendations and compliance with follow-up
- Recurrence, survival with or without disease, and date and cause of death

Interdisciplinary national and international efforts have resulted in a new consensus for the consistent documentation of treatment sequelae in oncology clinical trials. It is suggested that their use in clinical practice would greatly enhance comprehensive and consistent documentation required for the evaluation of outcomes. Acute treatment side effects (day 1 to 90 days after treatment) are recommended to be documented and evaluated using the Common Toxicity Criteria (CTC). Chronic treatment side effects (day 91 and thereafter) are recommended to be documented and evaluated using the Late Effect Normal Tissue (LENT) criteria. LENT allows for the differentiation between the Subjective, Objective, Management, and Analytic (SOMA) toxicity aspects of treatment. Both classification systems can be implemented not only for clinical applications using radiation therapy or chemotherapy alone but also for combined modality therapy. This would allow for comparative outcomes analysis and benchmarking between different treatments, different regions, different institutions, different insurers, and different health care practitioners (National Institutes of Health/National Cancer Institute, 1998; Rubin, Constine, Fajardo, Phillips, & Wasserman, 1995; Seegenschmiedt, 1998).

In a fast-paced outpatient clinic like radiation therapy, documentation is usually made easier and more comprehensive when standardized forms and checklists are used. Several clinical documentation tools have been published for use in radiation therapy (Blackman & Bull-Hurst, 1994; Bruner, Iwamoto, Keane, & Strohl, 1992; Bruner & Slivjak, 1994).

Electronic databases enable a fast and systematic recording and evaluation of outcomes documented by the multidisciplinary team in the radiation therapy patient care record. These databases are best designed as integrated delivery systems, the technology of which allows for networked infrastructure of health care information systems that can facilitate information exchange and sharing among multiple health care providers (Leonard, Tan, & Pink, 1998; Niehoff, Galalae, Zimmermann, & Kimmig, 1998).

FOLLOW-UP

Evidence-based guidelines for the follow-up of numerous cancers including prostate, colorectal, and head and neck have been proposed by a number of professional medical organizations such as The American Society of Therapeutic Radiology and Oncology (ASTRO) (American Society for Therapeutic Radiology and Oncology, 1999) the American Society of Clinical Oncology (ASCO) (Desch et al., 1999), the American Society for Head and Neck Surgery (ASHNS), and the Society of Head and Neck Surgery (SHNS) (Paniello, Virgo, Johnson,

Clemente, & Johnson, 1999) as well as the National Comprehensive Cancer Network (NCCN) (Winn, Botnick, & Dozier, 1996). In general, patients are seen more frequently in the first year of follow-up (i.e., at 1 month posttreatment then every 3 to 6 months) depending on the diagnosis, stage, and site treated, followed by decreasing frequency until follow-up is annual.

Two additional activities have increasingly become important to the efforts of the multidisciplinary team in managing and improving outcomes after radiation therapy: continuous quality improvement and cost containment.

QUALITY IMPROVEMENT

The multidisciplinary Quality Improvement (QI) Committee is vital to setting the QI process in motion. The committee chooses or develops the outcome standards for the department, educates staff, measures and reports outcomes, and devises a plan as well as oversees the implementation of department-wide activities to improve outcomes. The QI Committee should minimally include the radiation oncologists, radiation oncology nurses, medical physicists, dosimetrists, and radiation therapists (Purdy & Perez, 1996). Outcome measures should include the framework developed by Donabedian, which includes structure, process, and outcome (described in detail in Chapter 1) (Donabedian, 1986, 1992).

Historically, quality assurance in radiation oncology has aimed to evaluate and improve the consistent, safe, and optimal delivery of ionizing radiation to treat disease. A hierarchy of dosimetry, planning, and machine performance checks and evaluations of clinical outcomes have been widely used in radiation therapy. Procedures and guidelines for practice are readily available on the technical aspects of radiation therapy treatments, maintenance of which is achieved by quality control checks within a quality assurance program (Kehoe & Rugg, 1999). For example, a Task Group of the Radiation Therapy Committee of the American Association of Physicists in Medicine has developed the following comprehensive set of quality assurance guidelines that can be applied to clinical treatment planning:

- Image-based definition of patient anatomy
- 3D beam descriptions for complex beams including multileaf collimator apertures

- 3D dose calculation algorithms
- Complex plan evaluation tools including dose volume histograms for treatment planning (Fraass et al., 1998)

One radiation therapy quality improvement study analyzed error frequency and patterns, possible causes, and possible prevention strategies in treatment delivery. Treatment information, self-reported error documentation, and electronic treatment verification transcripts for approximately 2,000 consecutive patients treated with over 90,000 radiotherapy fields were reviewed and analyzed. The authors reported a total of 59 errors that affected 168 treatment fields. This was calculated as a crude radiation delivery error rate of 0.18%, which, the authors state, compares favorably with reported error rates for pharmaceutical administration in large tertiary care hospitals. All 59 errors were judged to be minor (defined as having a negligible chance of adverse medical outcome). The most common error category detected was treatment field block misplacements. An electronic record-and-verify linear accelerator interlock system seemed to have prevented the occurrence of many additional errors. However, even these automated error-minimization methods are not foolproof, since nine of the errors were directly related to the use of this system and involved the transposition of similar numbers within a series of treatment coordinate data sets (Macklis, Meier, & Weinhous, 1998). This highlights the need for multiple checks and balances, both human and automated, as well as good documentation systems. Implementation of a block bar-coding system may be helpful in further reducing errors related to block misplacements.

Electronic integrated documentation systems provide the infrastructure for good quality improvement programs. These systems make measurement and statistical reporting of outcomes realistic and manageable.

Most importantly, to ensure that patients receive the highest quality of radiation therapy, individual institutions need to develop and implement strict quality improvement standards based on national guidelines as well as their own needs (workshops on quality assurance, 1999; Bruner, 1990a; Bruner, 1992; Levitt & Khan, 1994). However, as described in Chapter 1 of this book, quality improvement and the measure of outcomes must go beyond the technical aspects of the delivery of ionizing radiation. The radiation therapy multidisciplinary team must seek continuous improvements in symptom management, quality of life, and patient satisfaction.

A step-by-step example of a multidisciplinary quality improvement project in radiation therapy, which describes the process of selecting, measuring, reporting, analyzing, and correcting patient care deficiencies has been reported in detail elsewhere (Bruner et al., 1998a). However, it should be stressed that the quality improvement process is not an end in itself. It is the identification of opportunities to improve the outcomes of radiation therapy that is the ultimate goal of the multidisciplinary radiation therapy team and continuous quality improvement activities.

COST CONTAINMENT

Finally, in a health care environment strongly concerned with cost containment, the radiation therapy team must incorporate cost-consciousness into their roles as never before. Several studies of the cost-benefit analysis of the use of radiation therapy in treating high-volume diseases such as breast and prostate cancers have found radiation therapy to be cost-effective relative to other therapies (Hayman, Hillner, Harris, & Weeks, 1998; Marks, Hardenbergh, Winer, & Prosnitz, 1999; Perez et al., 1997). For some cancers cost-effective radiotherapeutic treatment can be demonstrated in only subsets of patients. For example, one study found that although the median survival of selected patients with single-brain metastases treated with whole-brain irradiation and resection or radiosurgery is comparable, radiosurgery appears to be the more cost-effective procedure (Mehta et al., 1997). Or, depending on the radiotherapeutic technology used, cost-effective treatment may be patient volume depen-dent. For instance, radiosurgical treatment can be carried out by means of a gamma knife or a linear accelerator. The linear accelerator may be either a single-purpose appliance, exclusively employed in radiosurgery, or an adapted appliance that is used primarily for external beam radiation therapy and additionally for radiosurgical purposes. A cost comparison revealed that the adapted linear accelerator was the most favorable alternative when small numbers of patients were treated annually. However with larger numbers of patients, the gamma knife may be the equipment of choice from a cost-accounting perspective (Konigsmaier, de Pauli-Ferch, Hackl, & Pendl, 1998).

Nevertheless, the incremental gains in improved outcomes from new technologies may not always be cost-effective. For example, one study used activity-based cost accounting, a method widely recommended for estimating and managing the costs of specific activities, to estimate the comparative cost of physician time in treating patients with localized prostate cancer, using two-dimensional (2D) versus three-dimensional (3D) conformal irradiation techniques. Results indicated that patients treated with 3D conformal radiation therapy consumed about 50% more physician time than patients receiving 2D conventional radiation therapy. Yet, the average professional reimbursement for the 3D is only about 26% more than for the 2D treatment (Kobeissi et al., 1998). On the other hand, a recent study suggests that 3D conformal radiation for prostate cancer is cost-effective (Horwitz, Hanlon, Pinover, Hanks, 1999). In light of the rapidly evolving changes in managed care, this important issue continues to be debated in the literature (Perez, Michalski, Ballard et al., 1997).

- ■ Another method of assessing productivity for cost analysis is linear accelerator workload analysis (e.g., patients per hour or fields per hour). However, critics assert that this method fails to take into account the variations in complexity of different treatment techniques (Delaney et al., 1997).

- ■ To account for this complexity factor, a multidisciplinary team developed the Basic Treatment Equivalent (BTE) model of radiation therapy productivity and cost assessment. The authors report that when compared with patients per hour and fields per hour there was less variability of BTE per patient per hour. The study results indicated that radiation therapy departments that were able to treat a high number of patients or fields per hour were able to do so because they used less complicated techniques or had a less complicated case-mix of patients. This method may be useful for resource utilization comparisons, patient time allocations, waiting list estimates, and cost-benefit analysis (Delaney et al., 1997).

In this era of cost containment, it is imperative that health care professionals including the multidisciplinary radiation therapy team be fiscally aware in order to make prudent decisions. The present environment necessitates a critical appraisal of both established and new radiotherapeutic modalities, drug regimens, and symptom interventions.

In summary, to achieve the best patient outcomes in radiation therapy, a broad, patient-centered approach is required that acknowledges the views, experience, skills, and perspectives of all health care professionals involved in the treatment process (Minsky, 1998).

REFERENCES

Workshop on quality assurance of treatment planning systems and 5th biennial European Society for Therapeutic Radiology and Oncology (ESTRO) meeting on physics for clinical radiotherapy (1999). [Abstract]. *Radiotherapy and Oncology*, 51 (Suppl. 1), 21–27.

American College of Radiology. (1991). *Report of the Inter-Society Council for Radiation Oncology. Radiation oncology in integrated cancer management.* Reston, VA: American College of Radiology.

American Society for Therapeutic Radiology and Oncology. (1999). Consensus statements on radiation therapy of prostate cancer: Guidelines for prostate rebiopsy after radiation and for radiation therapy with rising prostate-specific antigen levels after radical prostatectomy. *Journal of Clinical Oncology*, 17(4), 1155.

Batalden, P. B., Bronenwett, L. R., Brown, L. L., Moffatt, C., & Serrell, N. P. (1998). Collaboration in improving care for patients: How can we find out what we haven't been able to figure out yet? *Joint Commission Journal on Quality Improvement*, 24(10), 609–618.

Blackman, A., & Bull-Hurst, T. (1994). *Radiation therapy patient care record: A tool for documenting nursing care.* Pittsburgh, PA: Oncology Nursing Society.

Braddock, C. H. (1998). Advancing the cause of informed consent: From disclosure to understanding. *American Journal of Medicine*, 105, 354–355.

Braddock, C. H., Edwards, K. A., Hasenberg, N. M., Laidley, T. L., & Levinson, W. (1999). Informed decision making in outpatient practice: Time to get back to basics. *Journal of the American Medical Association*, 282(24), 2313–2320.

Brown, R., Utow, P. N., Boyer, M. J., & Tattersall, M. H. (1999). Promoting patient participation in the cancer consultation: Evaluation of a prompt sheet and coaching in question-asking. *British Journal of Cancer*, 80(1–2), 242–248.

Bruner, D. W. (1990a). Model Quality Assurance Program. In radiation oncology nursing. *Cancer Nursing*, 13(6), 335–338.

Bruner, D. W. (1990b). Report of the Radiation Oncology Nursing Subcommittee of the American College of Radiology Task Force on Standards Development. *Oncology*, 4(8), 80–81.

Bruner, D. W. (1992). *Quality assurance in nursing care in radiation oncology.* Philadelphia: W. B. Saunders.

Bruner, D. W. (1993). The nurse in radiation oncology: Staffing patterns and role development. *Oncology Nursing Forum*, 20(4), 651–659.

Bruner, D. W. (1996). Managing a managed care contract in radiation oncology. *Oncology Nursing Forum*, 23(3), 451–455.

Bruner, D. W., Bucholtz, J., Iwamoto, R., & Strohl, R. (1998a). *Manual for radiation oncology nursing practice and education* (2nd ed.). Pittsburgh, PA: Oncology Nursing Press.

Bruner, D. W., Iwamoto, R., Keane, K., & Strohl, R. (1992). *Manual for radiation oncology nursing practice and education.* Pittsburgh, PA: Oncology Nursing Society.

Bruner, D. W., Scott, C., Lawton, C., DelRowe, J., Rotman, M., Buswell, L., Beard, C., & Cella, D. (1995). RTOG's first quality of life study—RTOG 90-20: A phase II trial of external beam radiation with etanidazole for locally advanced prostate cancer. *International Journal of Radiation Oncology, Biology, Physics*, 33(4), 901–906.

Bruner, D. W., Scott, C. B., McGowan, D., Lawton, C., Hanks, G., Prestidge, B., Han, S., Gore, E., & Asbell, S. (1998b). The RTOG modified sexual adjustment questionnaire: Psychometric testing in the prostate cancer population [Abstract]. *International Journal of Radiation Oncology, Biology, Physics*, 42(1), 202.

Bruner, D. W., & Slivjak, A. (1994). *Documentation manual for radiation oncology nursing*. Philadelphia: Fox Chase Cancer Center.

Butow, P. N., Dunn, S. M., Tattersall, M. H., & Jones, Q. J. (1995). Computer-based interaction analysis of the cancer consultation. *British Journal of Cancer*, 71(5), 1115–1121.

Chevillard, S., Lebeau, J., Pouillart, P., deToma, C., Beldjord, C., Asselain, B., Klijanienko, J., Fourquet, A., Magdelenat, H., & Vielh, P. (1997). Biological and clinical significance of concurrent p53 gene alterations, MDR1 gene expression, and S-phase fraction analyses in breast cancer patients treated with primary chemotherapy or radiotherapy. *Clinical Cancer Research*, 3(12 (Part 1)), 2471–2478.

Coleman, N. (1996). Biologic basis for radiation oncology. *Oncology*, 10(3), 399–406.

Delaney, G. P., Gebski, V., Lunn, A. D., Lunn, M., Rus, M., Manderson, C., & Langlands, A. O. (1997). An assessment of the basic treatment equivalent (BTE) model as measure of radiotherapy workload. *Clinical Oncology (Royal College of Radiologists)*, 9(4), 240–244.

Desch, C. E., Benson, A. B., III, Smith, T. J., Flynn, P. J., Krause, C., Loprinzi, C. L., Minsky, B. D., Petrelli, N. J., Pfister, D. G., & Somerfield, M. R. (1999). Recommended colorectal cancer surveillance guidelines by the American Society of Clinical Oncology. *Journal of Clinical Oncology*, 17(4), 1312.

Detmar, S. B., & Aaronson, N. K. (1998). Quality of life assessment in daily clinical oncology practice: A feasibility study. *European Journal of Cancer*, 34(8), 1181–1186.

Donabedian, A. (1986). Quality assurance in our health care system. *Quality Assurance Utilization Review*, 1(1), 6–12.

Donabedian, A. (1992). Quality assurance: Structure, process and outcome. *Nursing Standards*, 8 Vol. 7 No. II Supplement on Quality Assurance 7(11 Suppl. QA), 4–5.

Ducanis, A. J., & Golin, A. K. (1979). *The interdisciplinary health care team, a handbook*. Germantown, MD: Aspen Systems.

Enck, R. (1987). ACCC standards: Past, present and future. *Journal of Cancer Program Management*, 2, 11–20.

Fieler, V. K., Wlasowicz, G. S., Mitchell, M. L., Jones, L. S., & Johnson, J. E. (1996). Information preferences of patients undergoing radiation therapy. *Oncology Nursing Forum*, 23, 1603–1608.

Ford, S., Fallowfield, L., & Lewis, S. (1994). Can oncologists detect distress in their outpatients and how satisfied are they with their performance during bad news consultations. *British Journal of Cancer, 70,* 767–770.

Fornace, A. J., Jr., Amundson, S. A., Bittner, M., Myers, T. G., Meltzer, P., Weinsten, J. N., & Trent, J. (1999). The complexity of radiation stress responses: Analysis by informatics and functional genomics approaches. *Gene Express, 7*(4–6), 387–400.

Fountain, M. J. (1993). Key roles and issues of the multidisciplinary team. *Seminars in Oncology Nursing, 9*(1), 25–31.

Fraass, B., Doppke, K., Hunt, M., Kutcher, G., Starkschall, G., Stern, R., & Van Dyke, J. (1998). American association of physicists in medicine radiation therapy committee task group 53: Quality assurance for clinical radiotherapy treatment planning. *Medical Physics, 25*(10), 1773–1829.

Frederikson, L. G. (1995). Exploring information-exchange in consultation: The patients' view of performance and outcomes. *Patient Education and Counseling, 25*(3), 237–246.

Hagopian, G. A. (1991). The effects of a weekly radiation therapy newsletter on patients. *Oncology Nursing Forum, 18*(7), 1199–1203.

Hagopian, G. A. (1996). The effects of informational audiotapes on knowledge and self-care behaviors of patients undergoing radiation therapy. *Oncology Nursing Forum, 23*(4), 697–700.

Hagopian, G. A., & Rubenstein, J. H. (1990). Effects of telephone call interventions on patients' well-being in a radiation therapy department. *Cancer Nursing, 13*(6), 339–344.

Hak, T., & Campion, P. (1999). Achieving a patient-centered consultation by giving feedback in its early phases. *Postgraduate Medicine, 75*(885), 405–409.

Hayman, J. A., Hillner, B. E., Harris, J. R., & Weeks, J. C. (1998). Cost-effectiveness of routine radiation therapy following conservative surgery for early-stage breast cancer. *Journal of Clinical Oncology, 16*(3), 1022–1029.

Heinemann, G. D., Schmitt, M. H., Farrell, M. P., & Brallier, S. A. (1999). Development of an attitude toward health care teams scale. *Evaluation of Health Professionals, 22*(1), 123–142.

Hermann, J. F., & Hilderely, L. J. (1993). Teamwork: A blessing or a burden? *Cancer Practice, 1*(4), 329–330.

Hilderely, L. J. (1991). Nurse-physician collaborative practice: The clinical nurse specialist in a radiation oncology private practice. *Oncology Nursing Forum, 18*(3), 585–591.

Hinds, D., Streater, A., & Mood, D. (1995). Functions and preferred methods of receiving information related to radiotherapy: Perceptions of patients with cancer. *Cancer Nursing, 18,* 374–384.

Horwitz, E. M., Hanlon, A. L., Pinover, W. H., Hanks, G. E. (1999). The cost-effectiveness of 3D conformal radiation therapy compared with conventional techniques for patients with clinically localized prostate cancer. *International Journal Radiation Oncology Biology Physics*, 45(5): 1219–1225.

Johnson, J. E., Fieler, V. K., Wlasowicz, G. S., Mitchell, M. L., & Jones, L. S. (1997). The effects of nursing care guides by self-regulation theory on coping with radiation therapy. *Oncology Nursing Forum*, 24(6), 1041–1050.

Joint Commission on Accreditation of Health Care Organizations. (1999). *Florence Nightingale: Measuring hospital care outcomes.* Oakbrook Terrace, IL, JCAHO.

Kehoe, T., & Rugg, L. J. (1999). From technical quality assurance of radiotherapy to a comprehensive quality of service management system. *Radiotherapy and Oncology*, 51(3), 281–290.

Kobeissi, B. J., Gupta, M., Perez, C. A., Dopuch, N., Michaliski, J. M., Van Antwerp, G., Gerber, R., & Wasserman, T. H. (1998). Physician resource utilization in radiation oncology: A model based on management of carcinoma of the prostate. *International Journal of Radiation Oncology, Biology, Physics*, 40(3), 593–603.

Konigsmaier, H., de Pauli-Ferch, G., Hackl, A., & Pendl, G. (1998). The costs of radiosurgical treatment: Comparison between gamma knife and linear accelerator. *Acta Neurochirurgica Supplementum (Wien)*, 140(11), 1101–1110.

Kovner, F., Spigel, S., Rider, I., Otremsky, I., Ron, I., Shohat, E., Rabey, J. M., Avram, J., Merimsky, O., Wigler, N., Chaitchik, S., & Inbar, M. (1999). Radiation therapy of metastatic spinal cord compression. Multidisciplinary team diagnosis and treatment. *Journal of Neuro-Oncology*, 42(1), 85–92.

Lalani, E. N., Stubb, A., & Stamp, G. W. (1997). Prostate cancer; the interface between pathology and basic scientific research. *Seminar in Cancer Biology*, 8(1), 53–59.

Larson, P. J., Dodd, M. J., & Aksamit, I. A. (1998). Symptom-management program for patients undergoing cancer treatment: The pro-self program. *Journal of Cancer Education*, 13(4), 248–252.

Leonard, K., Tan, J. K., & Pink, G. (1998). Designing health care information systems for integrated delivery systems: Where we are and where we need to be. *Top Health Information Management*, 19(1), 19–30.

Levitt, S. H., & Khan, F. (1994). Quality assurance in radiation oncology. *Cancer*, 74 (Suppl. 9), 2642–2646.

Lidz, C., Appelbaum, P., & Meisel, A. (1988). Two models of informed consent. *Archives of Internal Medicine*, 148, 1385–1389.

Mackay, R. I., & Hendry, J. H. (1999). The modeled benefits of individualizing radiotherapy patients' dose using cellular radiosensitivity assays with inherent variability. *Radiotherapy and Oncology*, 50(1), 67–75.

Macklis, R. M., Meier, T., & Weinhous, M. S. (1998). Error rates in clinical radiotherapy. *Journal of Clinical Oncology*, 16(2), 551–556.

Marks, L. B., Hardenbergh, P. H., Winer, E. T., & Prosnitz, L. R. (1999). Assessing the cost-effectiveness of postmastectomy radiation therapy. *International Journal of Radiation Oncology, Biology, Physics*, 44(1), 91–98.

McNeil, B., Weichselbaum, R., & Pauker, S. (1981). Speech and survival. Trade-offs between quality and quantity of life in laryngeal cancer. *New England Journal of Medicine*, 305, 982–987.

Mehta, M., Noyes, W., Craig, B., Lamond, J., Auchter, R., French, M., Johnson, M., Levin, A., Robbins, I., & Kinsella, T. A. (1997). Cost-effectiveness and cost-utility analysis of radiosurgery vs. resection for single-brain metastases. *International Journal of Radiation Oncology, Biology, Physics*, 39(2), 445–454.

Minsky, B. D. (1998). Multidisciplinary case teams: An approach to the future management of advanced colorectal cancer. *British Journal of Cancer*, 77(Suppl. 2), 1–4.

Mock, V., Dow, K. H., Meares, C. J., Grimm, P. M., Dienemann, J. A., Haisfield-Wolfe, M. E., Quitasol, W., Mitchell, S., Chakravarthy, A., & Gage, I. (1997). Effects of exercise on fatigue, physical functioning, and emotional distress during radiation therapy for breast cancer. *Oncology Nursing Forum*, 24(6), 991–1000.

National Institutes of Health/National Cancer Institute. (1998). *Common toxicity criteria index*. Bethesda, MD: National Institutes of Health.

Naylor, M. D., Brooten, D., Campbell, R., Jacobsen, B. S., Mezey, M. D., Pauly, M. V., & Schwartz, J. S. (1999). Comprehensive discharge planning and home follow-up of hospitalized elders: A randomized clinical trial. *JAMA*, 281(7), 613–620.

Newell, S., Sanson-Fisher, R. W., Girgis, A., & Bonaventura, A. (1998). How well do medical oncologists' perceptions reflect their patients' reported physical and psychosocial problems. *Cancer*, 83(8), 1640–1651.

Niehoff, P., Galalae, R., Zimmermann, J. S., & Kimmig, B. (1998). Electronical recording and evaluation of acute radiation morbidity. *Strahlentherapie und Onkologie*, 174(Suppl. 3), 37–39.

Paniello, R. C., Virgo, K. S., Johnson, M. H., Clemente, M. F., & Johnson, F. E. (1999). Practice patterns and clinical guidelines for posttreatment follow-up of head and neck cancers: A comparison of 2 professional societies. *Archives of Otolaryngology—Head and Neck Surgery*, 125(3), 309–313.

Patterson, M. P., Lipsett, J. A., Michel, M., & Archambeau, J. O. (1981). Cancer patients and informed consent: A study of relationship between comprehension of information, perceived ambiguity and stress during radiotherapy [Abstract]. *International Journal of Radiation Oncology, Biology, Physics*, 7(Suppl.), 108.

Perez, C. A., Michalski, J., Ballard, S., Drzymala, R., Kobeissi, B. J., Lockett, M. A., & Wasserman, T. H. (1997). Cost benefit of emerging technology in localized carcinoma of the prostate. *International Journal of Radiation Oncology, Biology, Physics*, 39(4), 875–883.

Perez, C. A., & Purdy, J. A. (1998). Treatment planning in radiation oncology and impact on outcome of therapy. *Rays*, 23(3), 385–426.

Phillips, K. M. (1997). *The power of health care teams: Strategies for success*. Oakbrook Terrace, IL: Joint Commission on Accreditation of Health Care Organizations.

Purdy, J. A., & Perez, C. A. (1996). Quality assurance in radiation oncology in the United States. *Rays*, 21(4), 505–540.

Rubin, P., Constine, L. S., Fajardo, L. F., Phillips, T. L., & Wasserman, T. H. (1995). Late effects of normal tissues (LENT) consensus conference. *International Journal of Radiation Oncology, Biology, Physics*, 31(5), 1037–1360.

Seegenschmiedt, M. H. (1998). Interdisciplinary documentation of treatment side effects in oncology. Present status and perspectives. *Strahlentherapie und Onkologie*, 174 (Suppl. 3), 25–29.

Shimada, Y., Imamura, M., Watanabe, G., Uchida, S., Harada, H., Makino, T., & Kano, M. (1999). Prognostic factors of esophageal squamous cell carcinoma from the perspective of molecular biology. *British Journal of Cancer*, 80(8), 1281–1282.

Siegel, J. A. (1998). Revised nuclear regulatory commission regulations for release of patients administered radioactive materials: Outpatient iodine-131 anti-B1 therapy. *Journal of Nuclear Medicine*, 39 (Suppl. 8), 28S–33S.

Singer, P. A., Tasch, E. S., Stocking, C., Rubin, S., Siegler, M., & Weichselbaum, R. (1991). Sex or survival: Trade-offs between quality and quantity of life. *Journal of Clinical Oncology*, 9(2), 328–334.

Taylor, J. C. (1996). Systems thinking, boundaries, and role clarity. *Clinical Performance and Quality Health Care*, 4(4), 198–199.

Winn, R. J., Botnick, W., & Dozier, N. (1996). The NCCN guideline development program. *Oncology*, 10(5), 23–28.

Wood, M. L., & McWilliam, C. L. (1996). Cancer in remission. Challenge in collaboration for family physicians and oncologist. *Canadian Family Physician*, 42, 899–904, 907–910.

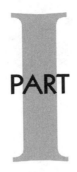

PART

MODALITY RELATED OUTCOMES

CHAPTER 3

TELETHERAPY: EXTERNAL RADIATION THERAPY

Marilyn L. Haas, PhD, ANP-C
Eric F. Kuehn, MD

PURPOSE

Management of patients with cancer requires a multidisciplinary approach with various treatment modalities. Method selection for radiation therapy (external beam, intracavitary, interstitial implant, stereotactic irradiation, conformal radiotherapy) depends on the location, size, and type of tumor. Whatever the selection type, radiation therapy uses high-energy ionizing radiation to kill cancer cells. The intent of radiation therapy should be clearly defined at the onset of therapeutic intervention. The purpose of radiation therapy is to:

> Deliver a precisely measured dose of radiation to a defined tumor volume, with minimal damage to surrounding healthy tissue, that results in eradication of the tumor, a high quality of life, prolongation of survival at competitive cost, and effective palliation or prevention of symptoms of cancer, including pain and restoring luminal patency, skeletal integrity, and organ function with minimal morbidity. (Chao, Perez, & Brady, 1999)

Radiation may be utilized in a variety of clinical settings for different purposes. These include the following:

- ■ Definitive—Radiation therapy is used as the primary treatment modality, with or without chemotherapy, for the treatment of cancer. Examples include cancer of the head and neck, lung, prostate, bladder, esophagus, anal, and Hodgkin's disease.

■ Neoadjuvant—Radiation therapy is used prior to definitive treatment, usually surgery, to improve the chance of successful resection.

■ Adjuvant—Radiation therapy is used after definitive treatment (either surgery or chemotherapy) to improve chances of local control.

■ Prophylaxis—Radiation therapy treats asymptomatic, but high-risk, areas to prevent growth of cancer cells. Examples may include treating the central nervous system to prevent relapse of certain forms of leukemia or lung cancer in the brain.

■ Control—When total tumor irradiation is not realistic, radiation therapy can limit the growth of cancer cells, which can extend the symptom-free interval for the patient. Examples may include pancreatic or lung cancers.

■ Palliation—Radiation therapy is used to manage symptoms (pain, bleeding, neurological compromise, or obstruction), improve quality of life, or alleviate life-threatening problems in noncurable cancers. Palliative examples are bone metastases, spinal cord compression, or blockage of organs causing various symptoms of pneumonia, jaundice, bowel or bladder obstruction, and spinal cord or brain dysfunction.

EXPECTED OUTCOMES

External beam radiation therapy, also known as teletherapy, is the most common delivery method. Teletherapy is the utilization of a radiation source that is placed at some distance from the target site (usually 80–100 cm). While the intent is to destroy the cancer cells, careful treatment planning is done to minimize effects on the normal surrounding tissues. Tissue tolerance to therapeutic irradiation has been established so that treatment planning can minimize the risk of possible complications or permanent damage (Table 3–1). The minimal tolerance dose, $TD_{5/5}$, refers to the dose of radiation that could cause no more than a 5% severe complication rate within 5 years after treatment (Emami et al., 1991). The maximal tolerance dose, $TD_{50/5}$, refers to the dose of radiation that could cause no more than a 50% severe complication rate within 5 years after treatment

TABLE 3–1 NORMAL TISSUE TOLERANCE TO IRRADIATION

Organ	TD$_{5/5}$	TD$_{50/5}$	Selected Clinical Outcome Endpoints
Bladder	6500	800	Symptomatic bladder contracture and volume loss
Bone:			
Femoral head I and II	5200	6500	Necrosis
TM joint: mandible	6000	7200	Marked limited joint function
Rib cage	5000	6500	Pathological fractures
Brain	4500	6000	Necrosis, infarction
Brain Stem	5000	6500	Necrosis, infarction
Colon	4500	5500	Obstruction, perforation, fistula
Ear: Middle/External	3000	4000	Acute serous otitis
Esophagus	5500	6800	Chronic stricture, perforation
Eye:			
Lens	1000	1800	Cataract requiring intervention
Retina	4500	6500	Blindness
Heart	4000	5000	Pericarditis
Kidney	2300	2800	Clinical nephritis
Larynx	7000	8000	Cartilage necrosis
Liver	3000	4000	Liver failure
Lung	1750	2450	Pneumonitis
Optic Nerve/Chiasm	5000	6500	Blindness
Parotid	3200	4600	Xerostomia
Rectum	6000	8000	Severe proctitis, necrosis, fistula, stenosis
Skin	5500	7000	Telangiectasia, necrosis, ulceration
Small Intestine	4000	5500	Obstruction, perforation, fistula
Spinal Cord	4700 (20 cm)	7000 (10 cm)	Myelitis necrosis
Stomach	5000	6500	Ulceration, perforation

Adapted from B. Emami et al. (1991). Tolerance of Normal Tissue to Therapeutic Radiation. *International Journal of Radiation Oncology, Biology, Physics*, 21(1), 109–122.

(Emami et al., 1991). However, combining other treatment modalities, such as surgery or chemotherapy, frequently modifies the tolerance dose and requires adjustments in the planning and dose prescription.

Understanding the principles of radiobiology is extremely important when caring for patients undergoing external beam radiation therapy and in achieving excellent clinical outcomes. Radiation kills cancer cells by permanently damaging their DNA (Murphy, Lawrence, & Lenhard, 1995). It does this either by creating electrons that damage the chromosomes or by causing nuclear free radicals that "indirectly" damage the DNA. This DNA damage results in misreading of the DNA, production of inactive proteins, reproductive cell death, and programmed cell death. While radiation has its effects at the cellular level, there are consequences to the surrounding tissues, organs, and the entire body. Factors that influence radiation sensitivity are determined by the four Rs in radiobiology:

- Repair of sublethal damage—Repair of a portion of the radiation damage in cells occurs between each treatment. Typically, if smaller doses per fraction are used the normal cells are better able to repair the damage than are cancer cells. Therefore, by fractionation of treatment (increased number of fractions for same dose) normal tissues are able to be preferentially spared and tumor cells preferentially damaged.
- Reoxygenation—Oxygen is needed for maximal tumoricidal effect of radiation. Since many tumors have poor blood supplies to portions of the lesion, parts of the tumor may be quite radioresistant. Fractionating the dose allows the tumor to slowly shrink, allowing gradual improvement in circulation to these hypoxic areas thus increasing radiosensitivity.
- Reassortment or redistribution—Parts of the cell cycle are more radiosensitive than others. Cells in the M (mitosis) and G_2 phases are more sensitive to radiation, and the cells in the G_1 phase and the late DNA synthetic phase (S phase) are more resistant to radiation. Thus, fractionating the radiation results in the killing of large numbers of cancer cells in the M/G_2 phases. Between fractions the remaining surviving cells again reassort in the cell cycle, effectively moving more tumor cells into the sensitive M/G_2 phases.
- Repopulation—Tumors grow over time, and in fact, the growth rate increases once cell killing with radiation begins. Therefore, protracting the overall number of weeks required to complete a course of treatment better allows the tumor to replace the cells being killed. This ultimately results in lower local control rates.

Complications from radiation therapy are divided into three categories according to timing of presentation:

- Acute Effects—occur during or shortly after treatment. These typically result from a depletion of rapidly proliferating, radiosensitive stem cells such as those in the skin, mucosa of the aerodigestive tract, or bone marrow. The extent of these effects tends to mimic the extent of tumor kill (Smith & Hoppe, 1999).

■ Subacute Effects—usually occur one to six months after completion of treatments and resolve over the next few months. Examples include Lhermitte's sign (tingling, numbness, shock-like sensation extending into arms or legs when the neck is flexed, resulting from spinal cord radiation therapy), pneumonitis, or rib fractures.

■ Late Effects—occur months or years after treatment and are typically permanent. These outcomes are the consequences of damage caused to slower-growing cells resulting in permanent decrease in functional elements (renal tubules, neural cells, etc.), damage to the microcirculation, and development of fibrosis (Smith & Hoppe, 1999). High dose per fraction has the potential for more severe effects later.

Overall, common symptoms that patients experience when receiving external beam radiation include the following:

■ Fatigue—Patients often begin to experience fatigue within two weeks of the initiation of treatments. Fatigue typically lasts throughout treatments and gradually improves over several weeks to months after completion. The mechanism is poorly understood, but fatigue may result from the release of toxic waste products from the tumor eradication into the bloodstream, direct effect of radiation on the circulating blood cells, or other unknown mechanisms.

■ Skin Reaction—Since all teletherapy is delivered through the skin, some type of skin reaction is to be expected. Two weeks into therapy, patients generally begin to develop erythema and tenderness. The severity of this skin reaction is variable, but may progress to dry or moist desquamation in the worst cases. The effect is temporary and will heal quickly after treatments are completed over a two- to four-week period. Patients can also expect a possible change in pigmentation.

Depending on the area being treated, patients can expect to develop other site-related disturbances. These may include:

■ Alimentary Tract Distress—Mucosal denudation of the upper aerodigestive tract can manifest within two to three weeks of initiation of radiation treatments. Confluent mucositis can develop on any of the mucosal surfaces in the treatment field and results in pain predominantly. Radiation can dull the sense of taste because of the decreased saliva flow. Also secretion can become thick and rope-like, thus inhibiting nutritional intake. Patients presenting with esophagitis report pain on swallowing, a lump in their throat, or substernal burning sensation. These symptoms can be managed with a variety of analgesics, topical anesthetics, aloe or sucralfate, and dietary modifications. Gastric irritation presents as nausea and/or vomiting, dyspepsia, epigastric burning pain, or anorexia. Antiemetics or antacids are helpful and can be utilized prophylactically. Acute effects on the small and large bowel can include nausea, vomiting, and diarrhea. These symptoms can be managed with antiemetics, antidiarrheal medications, and low-residue diet. Possible medications to alleviate gastric irritation and distress are included in Table 3–2.

■ Urinary Distress—Acute bladder or urethral symptoms may begin two to three weeks after the initiation of treatments. Dysuria, frequency, and/or urgency can be managed with bladder antispasmodics (flavoxate HCl) and urinary analgesics (phenazopyridine HCl).

■ Bone Marrow Depletion—Suppression usually occurs when treating large volumes of bone (e.g., ilia, vertebrae, metaphyses of long bones, skull, or sternum). Early effects of radiation result in progressive depopulation of white blood cells, thrombocytes, and erythrocytes in the circulating blood.

These complications can have an impact on quality of life, employment status, need for treatment interruptions, and/or the need for additional medical or surgical interventions or hospitalization.

Outcomes Measures

After obtaining a thorough history and physical, the workup is focused on identifying the tumor type, its extent, and if the cancer has spread to the lymph nodes or other parts of the body. This is accomplished through biopsies, laboratory studies, and diagnostic radiological studies. Pertinent information and studies include:

■ Operation Report—provides the surgeon's description of tumor size and extent.

TABLE 3–2   PHARMACOLOGICAL INTERVENTIONS FOR GASTRIC
IRRITATION AND DISTRESS

Classification	Medication
Aloe	RadioCare Oral Wound Rinse®
Analgesics	Codeine/Codeine with acetaminophen (Tylenol #3®)
	Hydrocodone (Hycodan®) with acetaminophen (Lortab®)
	Hydromorphone (Dilaudid®)
	Morphine (MS Contin®)
	Oxycodone (Roxicodone®) with acetaminophen (Percocet®)
Anesthetics	Miracle Mouthwash
	Viscous Lidocaine/Maalox
	Hurricaine®
Antacids	Prescription and over-the-counter doses:
	Cimetidine (Tagamet®)
	Famotidine (Pepcid®)
	Ranitidine (Zantac®)
Antidiarrheals	Attapulgite (Kaopectate®)
	Diphenoxylate/atropine (Lomotil®)
	Loperamide (Imodium®)
Antiemetics	Dexamethasone (Decadron®)
	Granisetron (Kytril®)
	Hydroxyzine (Atarax®)
	Lorazepam (Ativan®)
	Ondansetron (Zofran®)
	Prochlorperazine (Compazine®)
	Promethazine (Phenergan®)

Please note this table is not inclusive of all available medications. Refer to pharmaceutical companies' prescribing recommendations.

■ Pathology Report—includes the primary tumor's gross, microscopic, and nuclear findings. If applicable, the hormonal receptor status and regional lymph node findings are specified. Important information includes:

Gross findings: tumor size, location, and extent

Microscopic findings: histopathological type and grade, degree of invasion, and surgical margins

Nuclear findings (flow cytometry): DNA index, S-phase fraction, and ploidy

Hormone receptors (if applicable): estrogen and progesterone

Gene testing: HER-2/neu receptor

Nodal report: number of nodes sampled, size, any fixation, and degree of involvement by cancer

■ Laboratory Studies—complete blood count and chemistry profile, liver function tests, and site-specific tumor markers.

■ Diagnostic Radiological Studies—baseline imaging studies that may be conducted to assess the extent of the tumor and presence of any metastases. These studies include chest x-ray, bone scans, mammograms, computerized tomography (CAT) scans, magnetic resonance imaging (MRI), gallium scans, and position emission tomography (PET) scans.

After the results are obtained from the preceding information, the patient is staged according to the American Joint Committee on Cancer's clinical and pathological findings (**T**umor, Lymph **N**ode, **M**etastasis or TNM). The AJCC *Cancer Staging Handbook* (American Joint Committee on Cancer, 1998) has all the staging criteria for the different anatomical locations. Once the patient is staged, other risk factors should be taken into consideration. Factors that can impact a patient's site-specific prognosis, health status, and potential for radiation toxicity are as follows:

■ Smoking—Cocarcinogens found in cigarettes can affect the risk of radiation-induced malignancies. Irritants in cigarette smoke also tend to increase the acute reaction to radiation therapy in the upper aerodigestive tract.

■ Comorbidity—Presence of other diseases can affect clinical outcomes by increasing the risk of severe complications. For example, patients with lupus-like collagen-vascular disease have a 20% to 30% higher risk of developing complications (Smith & Hoppe, 1999). More general indicators, such as weight loss and Karnofsky Performance Score, also tend to be prognostic for many tumor sites.

■ Surgical Procedures—Surgical procedures can increase the risk of complications prior to or after radiation. For example, with head and neck cancers, tooth extraction can lead to mandibular osteoradionecrosis after mandible irradiation.

■ Chemotherapy—Numerous chemotherapy agents are available and have been utilized in conjunction with radiation treatments. The type, timing, and method of administration influence the risk of adverse interactions.

■ Infections—When the immune system is compromised through chemotherapy and/or radiation therapy, susceptibility to infections increases.

Other considerations such as quality of life issues are important for patients undergoing radiation treatments. Today, cancer management is looking beyond survival and raising the question of quality of life issues. Health-related quality of life refers to the extent of one's usual or expected physical, emotional, and social well-being as affected by a medical condition or its treatment. Numerous quality of life evaluations are available to ascertain the patient's functional status as perceived by the patient and are discussed in detail throughout this book. One generic instrument that measures quality of life is the Medical Outcomes Short Form 36, commonly referred to as SF-36 (Ware, 1993). This highly recognized instrument is easily administered and yields eight subscale health profiles. The eight concepts included in the Short Form Health Status Scale are:

1. **Physical Functioning:** assesses levels and kinds of limitations (lifting, carrying groceries, climbing stairs, bending, kneeling, stooping, walking moderate distances)
2. **Role Limitations Due to Physical Health Problems:** covers an array of role limitations (limitations in kind of work or other usual activities, reducing the amount of time spent in work or other usual activities, difficulty performing work or other usual activities)
3. **Bodily Pain:** questions the intensity of bodily pain and the extent to which it interferes with normal activities
4. **General Health:** overall general perception of health (poor to excellent)
5. **Vitality:** assesses energy level and fatigue
6. **Social Functioning:** captures the quantity and quality of social activities
7. **Role Limitations Due to Emotional Functioning:** identifies the impact of emotional problems on social activities
8. **Mental Health, Psychological Distress, and Psychological Well-Being:** measures four major mental health dimensions—anxiety, depression, loss of behavioral/emotional control, and psychological well-being

OUTCOMES MANAGEMENT

Radiation therapy uses high-energy x-rays to destroy tumor cells while trying to spare normal cells. During the treatment planning stage, decisions are made in regard to:

■ Dose is expressed in centigray (cGy) or gray (Gy). Doses prescribed depend on the size of the tumor, radiosensitivity of the tumor type, timing of treatments with other modalities (e.g., pre-operative, post-operative concurrent chemotherapy), and tolerance of surrounding normal tissues. Computerized dosimetry will be performed to maximize homogeneity of dose within the target tissues while minimizing dose to surrounding normal tissues.

- Time—The overall time to deliver a specified dose is stated. Typically, treatment is continuous five days a week, with treatment interruptions kept to a minimum. Shorter treatment times are associated with more aggressive tumor kill and more acute radiation therapy toxicity. Prolongation of treatment time allows less toxicity, but may result in tumor cell "repopulation."
- Fractionation is the amount of dose given per each fraction. In general, the more fractions per total dose, the more protection of normal tissues.
- Volume—Targets for the radiation could include the tumor +/− at-risk tissues (e.g., lymph nodes) or the "tumor bed" postoperatively. Typically, a shrinking fielding technique is used with larger initial volumes followed by smaller boost volumes taken to higher doses. Simulation films and port films identify and document treatment volumes.

Radiation safety measures are extremely important for the patient and those who participate in direct patient care. One of the most important considerations is ALARA—as low as reasonably achievable (Bruner, Bucholtz, Iwamoto, & Strohl, 1998). ALARA minimizes exposure to radiation personnel. Other important patient information that should be addressed includes the following:

- Treatment Planning—Preradiation treatment simulation and computerized dosimetry are often done to determine optimal energies and angles to minimize exposure to normal tissues. Immobilization aides are utilized to be sure that only the target area is treated each day and that the other tissues are shielded. Various types are utilized to achieve the highest level of accuracy including molds, masks, and bite blocks.
- Shielding—Cerrobend blocks are used to conform the beam to the target area and to protect vital body organs and tissues. These blocks are secured to plastic trays that are attached to the head of the treatment machine between the beam source and the patient. For young males, additional testicular shields are required to try to reduce scatter dose to the testes from abdominopelvic treatment. Special shields may also be used for the mouth or lens of the eye.
- Pregnancy—If treating a premenopausal woman, pregnancy can be an issue. Radiation treatments can have devastating

effects on the fetus. Counseling is extremely important for these women and they should be advised not to become pregnant during radiation treatment. It is advisable to perform serum pregnancy testing prior to beginning any course of radiation treatments. On rare occasions, a patient may become pregnant during radiation therapy.

■ Radioactivity Information—Reassure the patient receiving external beam therapy that he or she is not radioactive during a course of radiation treatments.

■ Cardiac Pacemakers—Linear accelerators can cause pacemakers and implantable defibrillators to malfunction even if they are not directly in the treatment field. Contacting the pacemaker manufacturer is always required prior to initiating any radiation. The American Association of Physicists in Medicine advises the following recommendations for patients with pacemakers (Marbach, Sontang, Van Dyk, & Wolbarst, 1994):

1. Patients should be evaluated by a cardiologist prior to the initiation of treatments.
2. If possible, pacemakers should always be kept outside the machine-collimated radiation beam during treatments and when taking portal films.
3. Permanent pacemakers (implanted) should never be treated with a betatron-type machine.
4. Patients must be monitored during the first treatment to verify that no transient malfunctions are occurring with the pacemaker.
5. The scattered dose must be estimated and recorded. The total accumulation dose should not exceed 2 Gy.

Limiting exposure to ionizing radiation is very important for radiation therapy personnel. The following are general guidelines:

■ Film badges are required to monitor exposure quantitatively. External beam radiation (x-rays, gamma rays, electrons, protons, neutrons) typically presents little risk to personnel because treatment is given remotely by therapists to patients in a shielded room. Some exposure is potentially received when fluoroscopy is used in treatment planning or when brachytherapy is being performed.

■ Protective shielding devices such as lead aprons should be worn whenever there is a likelihood of radiation exposure to low energy x-rays (fluoroscopy). Exposure to ionizing radiation has genetic effects (changes in the reproductive cells) and may result in abnormal offspring (Bruner, Bucholtz, Iwamoto, and Strohl, 1998).

■ Radiation monitors are placed in various places in the radiation department to alert personnel to areas where there is potential for high exposure.

■ Quality Assurance Program—Radiation standards have become more rigorous over the years, requiring more safety checks and monitoring systems. The National Council on Radiation Protection and Measurements (1993) has instituted radiation dose limit recommendations to protect radiation personnel and the general public. Both institutional committees and regulatory agencies have guidelines with which radiation departments must comply. They include the U.S. Nuclear Regulatory Commission, U.S. Food and Drug Administration, and various state commissions.

REFERENCES

American Joint Committee on Cancer. (1998). AJCC cancer staging handbook. Philadelphia: Lippincott-Raven.

Bruner, D., Bucholtz, J., Iwamoto, R., & Strohl, R. (1998). Manual for radiation oncology nursing practice and education (2nd ed.). Pittsburgh, PA: Oncology Nursing Press.

Chao, K., Perez, C., & Brady, L. (1999). Radiation oncology: Management decisions. Philadelphia: Lippincott-Raven.

Emami, B., Lyman, J., Brown, A., Coia, L., Goitein, M., Munzenrider, J., Shank, B., Solin,L., & Wesson, M. (1991). Tolerance of normal tissue to therapeutic radiation. International Journal of Radiation Oncology, Biology, Physics, 21 (1), 109–122.

Marbach, J., Sontag, M., Van Dyk, J., & Wolbarst, A. (1994). Management of radiation oncology patients with implanted cardiac pacemakers: Report of AAPM Task Group No. 34. Medical Physics, 21, 85–90.

Murphy, G., Lawrence, W., & Lenhard, R. (1995). American Cancer Society textbook of clinical oncology. Washington, DC: American Cancer Society.

National Council on Radiation Protection and Measurements. (1993). Limitation of exposure to ionizing radiation (NCRP Report No. 116). Bethesda, MD.

Smith, M. & Hoppe, R. (1999). Complications of radiation therapy. In J. Foley, J. Vose, & J. Armitage (Eds.), Current therapy in cancer. Philadelphia: W. B. Saunders.

Ware, J. (1993). SF-36 health survey manual and interpretation guide. Boston: New England Medical Center, The Health Institute.

CHAPTER 4

BRACHYTHERAPY

Marilyn L. Haas, PhD, ANP-C
Eric F. Kuehn, MD

PURPOSE

In general, radiation therapy is administered in one of two ways: externally (teletherapy) or internally (brachytherapy). In brachytherapy a radiation-producing source is implanted inside or placed very close to the target tissue, enabling delivery of a very high local dose to the tumor, but with a rapid falloff dose that helps protect the other surrounding normal tissues. These implanted radioactive sources can be temporarily or permanently placed. Temporary treatments utilize sealed radioactive sources that are removed after a calculated prescribed dose is delivered to the targets. Permanent treatments are sealed sources that are left in the body permanently and give off radiation to the tumor as the source decays. Frequently, brachytherapy is combined with teletherapy and used as a "boost" procedure.

Brachytherapy sources can be placed directly into the tumor or placed adjacent to the tumor. Various implantation techniques are utilized depending on the tumor size and location. These techniques include:

■ Interstitial—The sealed radioactive sources are surgically implanted directly into tissue or tumor. The sources are encapsulated and may be in the form of needles, seeds, wires, or catheters. For example, radioactive ^{125}I seeds may be placed directly and permanently into the prostate to treat localized prostate cancer. Another example is a temporary iridium-192 implant for oral tongue cancer.

■ Intracavitary—The radioactive source is placed temporarily into a body cavity to get the source in close proximity to the target. The source is then left in place for a prescribed amount of time to deliver a certain amount of dose. A common example is the insertion of after-loading intrauterine and vaginal ovoids for treatment of cervical cancer. Another example is treatment of lung or esophageal cancers with sources placed in catheters that are positioned endoscopically.

■ Surface (sometimes called plesiocurie or mold therapy) is designed to deliver a uniform dose distribution to the skin or mucosal surface. This consists of an applicator that sits on the target surface and holds an array of radioactive sources (Chao, Perez, & Brady, 1999). It has been used with iridium-192 for tumors of the eyeball, maxillary sinuses, and other natural cavities.

Various sources of radiation can be used for brachytherapy. These are typically isotopes that give off radioactivity as they decay. Examples include cesium-137, iridium-192, iodine-125, and others. The rates at which the radiation is given off vary. In general, implants are divided into high dose rate (HDR) and low dose rate (LDR). With HDR, doses of 0.2 Gy/min are delivered with a treatment time of a few minutes as compared with LDR treatments that typically give approximately 0.4–2 Gy/hr, requiring treatment times of 24 to 144 hours (Chao, Perez, & Brady, 1999). LDR brachytherapy has the advantage of being radiobiologically more sound, allowing curative doses to tumors, but sparing normal tissues better. HDR brachytherapy's advantage is that the dose is delivered quickly resulting in improved patient comfort, more reliable positioning of the source, less dose to ancillary personnel, and ability to perform the procedure as an outpatient.

To summarize, the aim of brachytherapy is to deliver a concentrated dose to a specific area while minimizing the exposure to surrounding normal tissues. The purposes for brachytherapy are the same for teletherapy: to cure, control, or palliate.

Expected Outcomes

When brachytherapy is administered, different tissue responses occur because of the continuous nature of administration instead of the daily fractionated treatments of teletherapy. Therefore, the basic principles of radiobiology change in brachytherapy. Recalling the four R's discussed in Chapter 3 (repair of sublethal damage, reoxygenation, reassortment, repopulation), cellular repair is typically completed within a few hours after receiving external beam radiation. However, when brachytherapy is combined with teletherapy, the malignant cells have less of a chance to undergo repair. During reoxygenation with fractionated therapy, there is a redistribution of oxygen to the cancer cells making the hypoxic tumor cells more sensitive to radiation. However, cells can be damaged with less dependence on oxygen effect. Therefore, brachytherapy seems to be more effective with anoxic tumor cells (Perez, Garcia, Grigsby, & Williamson, 1992). There is a reassortment or redistribution of cells during the cell cycle after receiving external beam radiation. Two phases in the cell cycle, mitosis and G_2, are more sensitive to radiation. During brachytherapy, there is a greater number of cells going through the G_2 phase, thus increasing the radiation effect. Finally, repopulation of normal and malignant cells occurs when the cells can finish multiplying after receiving radiation. Repopulation occurs at different times for different tissues. With continuous dosing there is a decrease in the ability of the malignant cells to reproduce.

Patients can expect similar outcomes with brachytherapy as with teletherapy. The ultimate goal is to kill tumor cells with the radiation while protecting normal cells. In general, expected outcomes for brachytherapy include:

- Improves local control of the disease by allowing delivery of higher doses of radiation over a shorter period.
- Preserve vital organ function by better concentrating radiation dose next to or in the tumor while sparing adjacent normal tissues (through rapid fall-off of dose).
- Provide palliation for those patients with recurrence after previous radiation therapy (because of better sparing of previously irradiated tissue).

In some cases, HDR may improve the prognosis of patients with unresectable tumors. Researchers (Iwasa et al., 1998) have found that HDR intraluminal brachytherapy for unresectable esophageal cancer was significantly effective on patients and improved their clinical outcomes. The adaptation of ultrasound and computerized tomography has led to a resurgence in the use and effectiveness of prostate seed implants (iodine-125) (Ramos, Carvalhal, Smith, Mager, & Catalona, 1999).

OUTCOMES MEASURES

The same considerations apply for brachytherapy as for teletherapy. Tissue histology needs to be confirmed to make the diagnosis prior to initiating radiotherapy. Staging the disease with appropriate clinical, surgical, radiographic, and laboratory procedures is essential in order to make the appropriate treatment decisions. Additional factors are taken into consideration when planning brachytherapy (age, current health status, comorbidities, size and location of tumor, prior surgical procedures, and need for teletherapy). All the treatment options and toxicities should be presented to the patient at the initial consult. The patient clinical outcomes are similar to teletherapy. Assessment includes:

- Direct Clinical Outcomes—A Priori versus actual patient outcomes (cause-specific mortality rates, survival rates, in-field recurrences, side effects).
- Patient Satisfaction—Focusing on clinical care questions (i.e., how well did the treatments relieve pain, did the physicians respond to any problems patients experienced during treatment, and the family members' perceptions of care/treatment responses).
- Quality of Life—The same quality of life studies for teletherapy can be applied to patients receiving brachytherapy (see Chapter 3). Functional status, pain scales using a visual analog scale, Short Form 36 Health Status (Ware, 1993), symptoms performance measures, and comparison of Karnofsky scores can be utilized for this population.

OUTCOMES MANAGEMENT

Strict, well-regulated guidelines have developed over the years in regard to the safe use and handling of radioactive isotopes. Although procedural care varies depending on the type of radioactive source utilized, there are some general principles that should govern care by attending personnel (Bruner, Bucholtz, Iwamoto, & Strohl, 1998). These guidelines are:

- Time—The amount of radiation exposure is directly related to the time spent near the radioactive source. Thus, the shorter the time spent around the patient with the radioactive source, the less exposure to radiation one receives. Therefore, careful planning and organization are required to minimize exposure while caring for a patient receiving brachytherapy.

■ Distance—Distance dramatically affects the amount of radiation exposure. The intensity of radiation varies inversely as the square of the distance from the source increases (inverse square law). For example, by doubling the distance from the radioactive source, the exposure is deceased by a factor of four. Therefore, personnel should limit their distance from the source by avoiding close proximity to the implant whenever possible.

■ Shielding—Determining the type and amount of shielding depends on the specific energy of ionizing radiation given off by the source. Most brachytherapy sources give off fairly low energy photons, which are easily shielded by lead or concrete (Dow, Bucholtz, Iwamoto, Fieler, & Hilderley, 1997). Implants must be done in specially shielded isolated rooms. Inside patient rooms, portable lead shields may be utilized to help minimize exposure to personnel and patient families. Doses beyond the walls and shields must be accurately measured by trained physics personnel.

Other special precautions include:

■ Knowledge of Radionuclide Type—The patient is not radioactive with temporary sealed sources, only the source is radioactive. Once the implanted source is removed, the patient no longer needs to be treated with any special precautions. The patient's bodily fluids and wastes are not radioactive. Temporary implants themselves should never be handled directly by hand. Time, distance from the patient, and shielding are always necessary precautions. Patients undergoing radiation treatments with unsealed sources, such as iodine-131 treatment for thyroid disorders, have radioactive bodily fluids (blood, sweat, saliva, urine, feces). Special precautions should be employed to avoid contamination in these situations. Patients are radioactive when sources are permanent, such as ^{125}I seed implants for the prostate.

■ Reproductivity Status of Personnel—Generally speaking, individuals under 18 years of age or pregnant individuals should not be working with brachytherapy patients. The threshold for damage to fetuses or young people from radiation is lower than for adults, and exposure in these cases should be avoided.

■ Trained Experienced Radiation Safety Officer (RSO)—This person oversees the implementation and monitoring of radiation exposure. His or her responsibilities include:
- Monitoring radiation exposure from patients who are undergoing brachytherapy
- Ensuring that policies and procedures are in place for spills, dislodgement, and contamination
- Training and supervising personnel in the radiation-protection practices of the institution
- Serving as a primary resource person in regard to radiation safety issues

REFERENCES

Bruner, D., Bucholtz, J., Iwamoto, R., & Strohl, R. (1998). *Manual for radiation oncology nursing practice and education* (2nd ed.). Pittsburgh, PA: Oncology Nursing Press.

Chao, K., Perez, C., & Brady, L. (1999). *Radiation oncology: Management decisions.* Philadelphia: Lippincott-Raven.

Dow, K., Bucholtz, J., Iwamoto, R., Fieler, V., & Hilderley, L. (1997). *Nursing care in radiation oncology.* Philadelphia: W. B. Saunders.

Iwasa, M., Ohmori, Y., Iwasa, Y., Yamamoto, A., Inoue, A., Maeda, H., Kume, M., Ogoshi, S., Nishioka, A., Ogawa, Y., & Yoshida, S. (1998). Effect of multidisciplinary treatment with high dose rate intraluminal brachytherapy on survival in patients with unresectable esophageal cancer. *Digestive Surgery, 15*(3), 227–235.

Perez, C., Garcia, D., Grigsby, P., & Williamson, J. (1992). Clinical applications of brachytherapy. In C. Perez & L. Brady (Eds.), *Principles and practice of radiation oncology.* Philadelphia: J. B. Lippincott.

Ramos, C., Carvalhal, G., Smith, D., Mager, D., and Catalona, W. (1999). Retrospective comparison of radical retropubic prostatectomy and 125-Iodine brachytherapy for localized prostate cancer. *Journal of Urology, 161*(4), 1212–1215.

Ware, J. (1993). *SF-36 health survey manual and interpretation guide.* Boston: New England Medical Center, The Health Institute.

CHAPTER 5

TOTAL BODY IRRADIATION

Giselle J. Moore-Higgs, ARNP, MSN
Robert B. Marcus, Jr., MD

PROBLEM

Total body irradiation (TBI) is a form of systemic therapy that has been used in a variety of cancers since the early 1900s. It involves the use of external radiation sources that produce penetrating rays of energy to deliver a relatively uniform amount of radiation to the entire body. By the 1940s, TBI was recognized as an acceptable treatment for certain radiosensitive cancers that are widely disseminated throughout the body, such as leukemia and lymphoma. Until the availability of mechanisms for bone marrow rescue, the usefulness of TBI was limited by the median lethal dose to humans of 3 Gy in a single fraction. Currently, there are three main applications of TBI: immunosuppression (lymphocyte kill) to allow engraftment of donor marrow; eradication of malignant cells (leukemias, lymphomas, and some solid tumors); and eradication of cell populations with genetic disorders, such as Fanconi's anemia and thalassemia major (Shank, 1998).

LYMPHOPOIETIC DISEASE

- Since the late 1950s TBI and total lymphatic irradiation (TLI) have been used in conditioning regimens for bone marrow transplantation (BMT) for radiosensitive cancers and non-malignant disease. These treatment approaches are currently used in a number of clinical protocols and cooperative group trials involving bone marrow transplantation for the treatment of lymphopoietic disease. The objective of TBI is the eradication of malignant cells throughout the body and suppression of the immune response to permit survival of the engrafted stem cell. TLI has been used only when immunosuppression is needed (for example, aplastic anemia).

MYCOSIS FUNGOIDES

■ Mycosis fungoides (MF) is a T-cell lymphoma that predominantly affects the skin. Systemic treatment of mycoses fungoides may include topical measures, oral agents, interferon, and photophoresis. Radiation therapy plays an efficacious role in the treatment of cutaneous lymphomas using total skin electron (TSE) therapy for patients with limited and superficial forms of the disease. TSE therapy provides treatment to the body surface while sparing the deeper tissues.

PALLIATIVE THERAPY

■ Hemibody radiotherapy can be used to palliate symptomatic diffuse metastatic disease, especially in patients with bone metastasis (prostate and breast cancer).This approach allows the patient an option for treating a large volume of disease in a relatively short period of time. The most effective hemibody doses found by an RTOG study were 6 Gy for upper hemibody irradiation and 8 Gy for lower and middle hemibody (Salazar et al., 1986).

ASSESSMENT

TOTAL BODY IRRADIATION

■ Before initiation of TBI as part of the conditioning regimen for BMT, the patient is evaluated to determine extent of disease, current physical performance status, and emotional well-being. The studies selected to evaluate extent of disease are individualized to the age of the patient, specific disease, stage of disease, and previous treatment. Of importance in assessing the patient for TBI is the patient's current physical status. The following studies should be included in the evaluation process:

- Pulmonary function studies—Pulmonary function abnormalities in total lung volume, diffusing capacity, or oxygenation before BMT have been shown to increase the risk of mortality among patients with cancer whereas airflow obstruction does not. Abnormal pulmonary function studies probably modify the risks associated with age, relapse, and GVHD. In the absence of other factors, abnormal pulmonary function studies rarely represent sufficient risk to contraindicate BMT (Crawford, 1994).
- Complete cardiac evaluation including stress testing and echocardiography should be performed if there is a history of angina, anthracycline administration, or other cardiovascular disease.
- Baseline ophthalmology exam.
- Dental evaluation to repair or remove any teeth that increase the risk of oral cavity infections during and after transplant.

TOTAL LYMPHATIC IRRADIATION

■ The assessment for TLI is the same as for TBI with the exception of the baseline ophthalmology exam, which is not necessary.

TOTAL SKIN ELECTRON THERAPY

■ The evaluation of the patient with mycosis fungoides should include the following:
- Thorough physical examination of the skin including the scalp, perineum, feet, and nails.
- Thorough physical examination of all nodal areas.
- Photographs and diagrams should be obtained that carefully describe all of the lesions.
- The thickest lesions should be measured for depth, which will influence choice of electron energy.
- Review of pathology from biopsy of skin lesion.
- Laboratory studies should include complete blood count, routine chemistry, and liver function studies.
- CT scans of neck, chest, abdomen, and pelvis should be performed to evaluate for evidence of nodal disease.

- If there is evidence of nodal disease, a bone marrow biopsy should be performed before initiating further treatment.

HEMIBODY RADIATION

■ Patient assessment before hemibody radiotherapy for palliation should include the following:
  - Complete blood count: patients with widely metastatic bone disease may have associated neutropenia, anemia, and thrombocytopenia, which may increase the morbidity associated with hemibody radiotherapy
  - Radiographic evidence of widely metastatic disease

EXPECTED OUTCOMES

TOTAL BODY IRRADIATION / TOTAL LYMPHATIC IRRADIATION

■ Specific survival outcomes are difficult to assess in patients who receive TBI or TLI as part of the conditioning treatment for BMT. Survival is affected by numerous BMT factors including age, patient performance status, type of disease, stage of disease, previous treatment, type of transplant, response to transplantation, and complications of treatment. With the introduction of autologous transplants, the potential for improved survival has increased as the potential complications decrease, and as new pharmaceutical products and technology are available to manage potentially life-threatening complications.

■ Quality of life (QOL) has been evaluated extensively in BMT patients, particularly adults. With the number of different disease sites and transplant procedures performed, the lack of homogeneity of this data makes it difficult to interpret. In addition, many of the studies have failed to define QOL before measuring the concept, have measured only one domain of QOL, have been retrospective, have been focused on a specific time period rather than longitudinal, and have used tools that do not specifically address issues related to transplant (Eilers & King, 1998).

■ Survivorship has been associated with a highly rated quality of life, but is accompanied by a number of psychosocial difficulties that negatively affect patients (Neitzert Ritvo, Dancey, Weiser, Murray, Avery, 1998). Fatigue, psychological distress, mood disturbances such as anxiety and depression, interruption in sexual activity, and increased sexual difficulty have all been reported. McQuellon and colleagues (1998) found a recovery trajectory with three distinct trends (during the first year after BMT) that had affected quality of life. The trajectory for distress was linear and improved over time with approximately 20% of patients continuing to have psychological distress at 1 year. The trend for overall quality of life was parabolic—worsening at discharge then improving at 100 days and at 1 year. However, there were individual areas of deficit at follow-up, even while overall quality of life mean scores improved. Finally, the trend for patient concerns over time was linear and worsening.

TOTAL SKIN ELECTRON THERAPY

■ Almost all patients treated with TSE for mycosis fungoides have a partial or complete response. The response is related to the type and extent of disease. The most advanced stages are not controlled by TSE; however the treatment offers good palliation (Kirova et al., 1999). The most favorable responses are seen in the early stage of disease, particularly the plaque phase (Meyler & Purser, 1998). Hoppe (1991) in the Stanford experience found the following responses: plaque, 98%; generalized plaque, 71%; tumor, 35%; and erythroderma, 64%. Unfortunately, despite the high response rates, most patients go on to relapse. In the Stanford series, long-term freedom from relapse was 50% for patients with limited plaque and 20% in patients with generalized plaque (Hoppe, 1991). Similar findings were reported by Jones, Rosenthal, and Wilson (1999). The rate of cutaneous remission was 74% with 27% remaining progression-free at 10 years using a more intense method of treatment (32–40 Gy). Another study evaluated TSE with or without adjuvant topical nitrogen mustard or nitrogen mustard alone as initial treatment in T2 and T3 disease (Chinn, Chow, Kim, & Hoppe, 1999). TSE with or without nitrogen mustard yielded significantly higher complete response rates than nitrogen mustard alone (76% vs. 39% in T2, 44% vs. 8% in T3). In T2 disease, treatment with nitrogen mustard was associated with longer freedom from relapse when compared to observation after TSE.

■ Currently there are no QOL studies that have been conducted in patients who have received TSE.

Hemibody Radiation

■ Hemibody radiation is given for palliation of symptomatic diffuse disease. Therefore outcome results depend on type of disease and extent of disease.

■ In prospective randomized trials by the Radiation Therapy Oncology Group (RTOG), single high-dose hemibody radiation therapy was found to be as effective as conventional fractionated irradiation in achieving pain control for patients with multiple metastases (Salazar et al., 1986).

■ No QOL studies are available on this patient population. However, pain relief is a quality of life issue and good pain relief has been documented in certain diseases.

Outcomes Measures

Total Body Irradiation/Total Lymphatic Irradiation

■ Follow-up evaluation of the patient treated with TBI or TLI with BMT depends on the disease site and type of transplant procedure. In most instances, these patients are cared for by the BMT team where they are enrolled and follow an evaluation process that is directed by specific treatment protocol or cooperative group trial enrollment.

■ Quality of life evaluation in patients treated with TBI or TLI with BMT may include one of the following instruments:

1. Functional Assessment of Cancer Therapy: Bone Marrow Transplant Scale (FACT-BMT)(McQuellon et al., 1997): A 12-item bone marrow transplant subscale that is combined with the general FACT measure. In the validation study, coefficients of reliability and validity ranged from 0.86 to 0.89 for the entire FACT-BMT and 0.54 to 0.63 for

the BMT scale. The BMT scale was able to discriminate patients on the basis of performance status rating and also demonstrated sensitivity to change over time.

2. Quality of Life Scale: Bone Marrow Transplant (Grant, Ferrell, Schmidt, Fonbuena, Neland and Forman, 1992): City of Hope 84-item questionnaire developed to assess quality of life of adults after BMT.

3. The Bush Bone Marrow Transplant Symptom Inventory (Bush, 1994): An addendum to the European Organization for Research and Treatment of Cancer (EORTC) QLQ-C30 quality of life questionnaire to assess the symptomatology of long-term recovery from BMT over time in adults. Has undergone reliability and validity studies, but is still under development.

TOTAL SKIN ELECTRON THERAPY

■ Follow-up evaluation of the patient treated with TSE should include:
  • Careful physical examination of all skin surfaces for evidence of new plaques of disease
  • Careful physical examination of all nodal bearing areas for evidence of new or progressive adenopathy
  • Radiographic evaluation for indicated physical findings including new plaques of disease or palpable adenopathy

■ Currently, there are no QOL instruments that specifically measure QOL in this patient population. General QOL instruments including FACT (Cella et al. 1993) and EORTC QLQ-C30 (Aaronson, 1993) would be appropriate to use.

HEMIBODY IRRADIATION

■ Follow-up should consist of complete blood counts obtained 7 to 10 days after treatment and repeated on a weekly basis until they return to pretreatment levels (usually 4–6 weeks).

■ Quality of life instruments related to palliation of symptoms are appropriate to document treatment outcomes. These may include:

1. Hospice Quality of Life Index (HQLI) (McMillan & Weitzner, 1998): A 28-item self-report instrument that includes three subscales: psychophysiological well-being,

functional well-being, and social/spiritual well-being. Allows patients the opportunity to express beliefs about quality of life issues and to maintain direction over a critical aspect of their care.

2. Missoula-VITAS Quality of Life Index (MVQOLI) (Byock & Merriman, 1998): developed to provide a measure of quality of life of terminally ill patients.

OUTCOMES MANAGEMENT

■ The NCI Common Toxicity Criteria (CTC) Version 2 instrument with the Radiation Therapy Oncology Group (RTOG) and European Organization for Research and Treatment of Cancer (EORTC) Acute Effects Criteria provides a scale for many different organ systems and some symptoms (National Cancer Institute, 1999). It is a very useful tool for grading severity of acute effects of radiation therapy in all sites.

TOTAL BODY IRRADIATION/TOTAL LYMPHATIC IRRADIATION

■ A number of serious, and potentially life-threatening, complications are associated with BMT. These complications can affect every organ system and are usually multifactorial. However, there are several toxicities associated with TBI that can be divided into acute and late effects. The acute toxicities can occur within hours of the initial fraction of treatment and anytime during the first 4 weeks after BMT. The late effects may occur 60 days or more after treatment. The use of fractionated regimen TBI instead of single-dose regimen TBI has decreased the severity of many of these toxicities.

Acute Toxicities

1. Nausea and vomiting: TBI has the most emetogenic potential followed by radiotherapy to the abdomen. Patients are usually on a conditioning chemotherapy regimen during this time that should include adequate doses of antiemetics to control this side effect. Studies of TBI with both fractionated and high-dose single treatments have clearly demonstrated the value of 5-HT3-receptor antagonist antiemetics with a response between 60% and 97%. There has been no significant

difference identified in the efficacy of the different 5-HT3-antagonists (Feyer, Zimmerman, Titlbach, Buchali, Hinkelbein, & Budach, 1998).

2. Oral mucositis and transient xerostomia will usually occur within the first 48 to 72 hours after initiation of treatment for most patients. Those who receive TBI and chemotherapy in combination are more likely to experience a severely compromised oral cavity. Patients who are older, have poorer oral cavity status, and have decreased renal function are also at increased risk for the development of severe mucositis (Berger & Eilers, 1998). For evaluation methods and treatment options see Chapter 21.

3. Pulmonary disease develops in 40% to 60% of patients at some time after BMT, and up to 40% require intensive care (Crawford, 1994). The incidence of pulmonary complications depends on transplant characteristics, such as degree of human leukocyte antigen (HLA) disparity and donor source, specific conditioning regimen agents and doses, underlying disease, and age of the patient (Crawford, 1994). These complications can be caused by pulmonary edema, airway obstruction, hemorrhage, graft-versus-host disease (GVHD) and commonly by interstitial pneumonitis (IP). IP is an inflammatory process involving the intraalveolar lining of the lung. Its origin may be infectious (66%) or idiopathic (23%) (Wilke, 1991). Although idiopathic IP is most likely attributable to irradiation, other factors may have a role, such as chemotherapy and GVHD. Furthermore, although infectious IP may not be directly attributable to irradiation, TBI may have a role in terms of side effects that increase opportunity for systemic infection (oral mucositis, gastritis, diarrhea). Median time to diagnosis of IP is about 2 months (Chao, Perez, & Brady, 1999). Patients who received prior radiation therapy to the chest (such as for lymphoma or breast cancer) may have an increased risk of developing pneumonitis. Current research is investigating the use of MnSOD plasmid/liposome gene therapy as a method of preventing irradiation-induced lung damage and improving survival (Epperly, Travis, Sikora, & Greenberger, 1999). Treatment of these pulmonary complications requires critical intensive care.

4. Fatigue occurs in almost all patients undergoing BMT and increases with subsequent radiotherapy during the course of

the conditioning regimen. Evaluation and treatment approaches may be found in Chapter 20.

5. Parotitis may occur after the first day of treatment and subsides in 24 to 48 hours.

6. Mild skin erythema may occur within several days of treatment, with reversible alopecia developing approximately 14 days after treatment. Some patients may experience significant erythema on hands, feet, and scrotum. Occasionally, moist desquamation may occur.

7. Ocular symptoms including decreased lacrimation, dryness, photophobia, and conjunctival edema may occur during the first 5 to 10 days after treatment. Ophthalmic moisturizers may be prescribed to reduce symptoms and improve comfort.

Latent Toxicities

1. Graft-versus-host disease (GVHD) is a syndrome caused by donor immunocompetent-lymphocytes recognizing and mounting an immune attack against host cells, which differ by histocompatibility antigens (Graze & Gale, 1979). It is a major contributing factor in the morbidity and mortality associated with allogeneic BMT. The disease may manifest as an isolated organ system or present as a multifocal system syndrome. Evaluation and treatment depend on signs and symptoms at presentation and the patient may require hospitalization.

2. Cataracts: the eye cannot be adequately shielded during TBI resulting in an increased risk of posterior capsulated cataracts. The peak onset is 3 years after TBI, with a range of 1 to 5 years (Deeg et al., 1984). Approximately 20% of patients treated with fractionated TBI develop cataracts (Deeg, 1992). High-dose rate and STBI are the main risk factors for cataract development and the need for surgery. The administration of heparin may have a protective role in cataractogenesis during TBI (Belkacemi et al., 1998).

3. Hepatic dysfunction including GVHD; chronic hepatitis; viral, fungal, and bacterial infections; drug reactions; and vascular occlusive disease (VOD) of the liver may occur after BMT. VOD is the result of deposits of fibrotic materials that subsequently obstruct small venules in the liver. It may occur 1 to 3 weeks after transplantation. Approximately 40% to 50% of patients die of this complication. Chemotherapy and TBI are considered to be the principal causes of VOD, but the exact

etiology is multifactorial. Evaluation and treatment depend on signs and symptoms at presentation and the patient usually requires intensive critical care.

4. Renal insufficiency may be experienced by 50% to 64% of patients 9 months or more after BMT as a result of radiation nephritis. This is manifested by increased serum creatinine levels, decreased creatinine clearance, increased BUN, decreased glomular filtration rate, anemia, hypertension, peripheral edema, and elevated levels of lactate dehydrogenase. It is a frequent sequelae in children. Its etiology is multifactorial and evaluation and treatment depend on the severity of manifestations.

5. Endocrine complications can affect the patient's level of functioning and performance status. Functional impairments of the hypothalamus-pituitary-gonad/thyroid axis are common while disturbances in growth hormone, adrenal and prolactin occur less often. Typically, the target organ is more commonly affected than the hypothalamus-pituitary axis (Kauppila, Koskinen, Irjala, Remes, and Viikari, 1998).

   a. TBI may result in hypothyroidism in 30% to 60% of patients treated with single-dose and 15% to 25% in patients given fractionated therapy (Deeg, 1992). Evaluation includes a serum thyroid panel indicating an increased thyroid stimulating hormone level > 5.0. Treatment is oral thyroid replacement medication daily. Patients should have careful follow-up with repeat thyroid panels to determine response and appropriate dosage.

   b. TBI is also a determinant of gonadal failure in men and women after BMT.
      • In men, the germinal epithelium is very sensitive to radiation-induced damage with changes to spermatogonia occurring after as little as 0.1 Gy and permanent infertility after fractionated doses of 2 Gy and above. Irradiation to prepubertal testes results in damage to the testicular germinal epithelium that does not become apparent until after puberty. A hormonal profile reflects normal testosterone levels, slightly elevated LH, and significantly elevated FSH levels. Azoospermia is evident on semen analysis. In terms of future reproduction, sperm banking remains the only proven method in men, although hormonal manipulation to enhance the recovery of spermatogenesis

and cryopreservation of testicular germ cells are possibilities for the future (Howell & Shalet, 1998).

- The return of ovarian function in females who receive TBI depends on age and total dose. Women older than 40 years require doses of only 6 Gy to result in permanent ovarian function, whereas up to 50% of the younger women will recover gonadal function with doses up to 20.0 Gy (Kay & Mattison, 1985). Ovarian failure is characterized by the cessation of menses, elevated levels of gonadatropins, and decreased levels of estradiol. Current research is focused on cryopreservation of ovarian tissue resected before BMT for use in in vitro fertilization procedures at a later date. Otherwise, patients are evaluated and treated for menopausal symptoms with hormone replacement therapy.

- Patients exposed to 10.0 to 15.75 Gy TBI have a 10% to 15% chance of affecting germ cells, which may induce mutations that could result in congenital abnormalities. Some clinical studies have shown no increase in abnormalities or spontaneous abortions (Saunders & Seattle Marrow Transplant Team, 1992).

- Patients who would like to consider cryopreservation of sperm or ova should be referred to a reproductive endocrinologist for evaluation before TBI. Patients who develop gonadal dysfunction after TBI should also be referred to an endocrinologist for hormone replacement therapy.

6. Sexual dysfunction: sexual dysfunction was found in 80% of female and 29% of male survivors of BMT at 1 and 3 years posttransplantation (Syrjala, Roth-Roemer, & Abrams, 1998). A lack of hormone replacement therapy at 1 year after transplant was an important variable in female sexual dissatisfaction. Even when HRT was given, it did not ensure sexual quality of life. Vaginal stenosis after allogeneic bone marrow transplantation has been reported (DeLord, Treleaven, Shepherd, Saso, & Powles, 1999). It is thought to be a manifestation of chronic GVHD. Women who develop GVHD should be instructed to use a method of vaginal dilatation 3 to 4 times a week (sexual intercourse or vaginal dilator) with a vaginal lubricant to prevent stenosis.

7. Secondary cancer development is multifactorial. Its etiology is associated with TBI, immunosuppression, chronic immune stimulation, viral infection, and genetic predisposition. The median incidence is approximately 1 year. Common secondary malignancies include lymphoproliferative disorders, chronic or acute leukemia, and solid tumors.

TOTAL SKIN ELECTRON THERAPY

The nature and severity of acute and chronic radiation effects are a function of technique, fractionation, total dose, concomitant use of topical or systemic cytotoxic drugs, previous treatments, and the condition of the skin before irradiation (Chao et al, 1999).

Acute Toxicities

a. Skin: mild erythema, dry desquamation, and hyperpigmentation usually occur. At doses > 25 Gy, patients may develop transient edema of the hands and ankles, and occasionally may develop areas of moist desquamation. Alopecia and loss of fingernails and toenails may occur if shielding is not provided. The nails usually regenerate in 4 to 6 months (Chao et al., 1999). See Chapter 21 for treatment options.
b. Gynecomastia may also develop; the mechanism for this is unknown (Chao et al., 1999).

Latent Toxicities

a. Skin changes may include atrophy, wrinkling, telangiectasias, xerosis, uneven pigmentation, frank poikiloderma, permanent alopecia, skin fragility, and subcutaneous fibrosis (Chao et al., 1999). See chapter 21 for treatment options.

HEMIBODY IRRADIATION

Acute Toxicities

a. Nausea and vomiting usually occur within 30 to 60 minutes of treatment. Prophylactic use of antiemetics 1 hour before treatment may prevent this. Patients should be kept NPO at least 1 hour prior to treatment.
b. Bone marrow depression usually occurs within 7 to 10 days and returns to pretreatment levels 4 to 6 weeks after treatment.
c. Interstitial pneumonitis may occur if upper hemibody irradiation exceeds 6 Gy (Chao et al., 1999).

Latent Toxicities

Because treatment with hemibody irradiation is usually for palliation of metastatic disease, latent toxicities are uncommon. Patients usually succumb to their disease before such toxicities could occur.

REFERENCES

Aaronson, N. K., Ahmedzai, S., Bergman, B. , Bullinger, M., Cull, A., Duez, N. J., Filiberti, A., Flechtner, H., Fleishman, S. B., de Haes, J. C. J. M., Kaasa, S., Klee, M., Osoba, D., Razavi, D., Rofe, P. B., Schraub, S., Sneeuw, K., Sullivan, M., & Takeda, F. (1993). The European Organization for Research and Treatment of Cancer QLQ-C: A quality-of-life instrument for use in international clinical trials in oncology. *Journal of the National Cancer Institute*, 85(5), 365–376.

Belkacemi,Y., Labopin, M., Vernant, J.P., Prentice, H. G., Tichelli, A., Schattenberg, A., Boogaerts, M. A., Ernst, P., Della-Volpe, A., Goldstone, A. H., Jouet, J. P., Verdonck, L. F., Locasciulli, A., Rio, B., Ozahin, M., & Gorin, N.C. (1998). Cataracts after total body irradiation and bone marrow transplantation in patients with acute leukemia in complete remission: A study of the European Group for Blood and Marrow Transplantation. *International Journal of Radiation Oncology, Biology, & Physics*, 41(3), 659–668.

Berger, A. M., & Eilers, J. (1998). Factors influencing oral cavity status during high-dose antineoplastic therapy: A secondary data analysis. *Oncology Nursing Forum*, 25(9), 1623–1626.

Bush, Nigel (1994). Bush Bone Marrow Transplant Symptom Inventory. Fred Hutchinson Cancer Research Center. Mail Stop M0224, 1124 Columbia Street, Seattle, WA 98014-2092.

Byock, I. R., & Merriman, M. P. (1998). Measuring quality of life for patients with terminal illness: The Missoula-VITAS quality of life index. *Palliative Medicine*, 12(4), 231–244.

Cella, D., Tulsky, D.S., Gray, G. Sarafin, B., Linn, E., Bonomi, A., Silberman, M., Yellen, S. B., Winicour, P., Brannon, J., Eckberg, K., Lloyd, S., Purl, S., Blendowski, C., Goodman, M., Barnicle, M., Stewart, I., McHale, M., Bonomi, P., Kaplan, E., Taylor, S. IV., Thomas, C. R. Jr., & Harris, J. (1993). The Functional Assessment of Cancer Therapy scale: Development and validation of the general measure. *Journal of Clinical Oncology*, 11(3), 570–579.

Chao, K. S. C., Perez, C. A., & Brady, L. W. (1999). *Radiation oncology management decisions* (pp. 53–56, 121–126). Philadelphia: Lippincott-Raven.

Chinn, D. M., Chow, S., Kim, Y. H., & Hoppe, R. T. (1999). Total skin electron beam therapy with or without adjuvant topical nitrogen mustard or nitrogen mustard alone as initial treatment of T2 and T3 mycosis fungoides. *International Journal of Radiation Oncology, Biology, Physics*, 43(5), 951–958.

Crawford, S. W. (1994). Critical care and respiratory failure. In S. J. Forman, K. G. Blume, & E. D. Thomas (Eds.), *Bone marrow transplantation*. Boston: Blackwell Scientific Publications.

Deeg, H. J. (1992). Delayed complications of marrow transplantation. *Marrow Transplantation Review*, 2(1), 10–13.

Deeg, H. J., Flournoy, N., Sullivan, K. M. , Sheehan, K., Bucker, C. D., Sanders, J. E., Storb, R., Witherspoon, R. P., & Thomas, E. D. (1984). Cataracts after total body irradiation and bone marrow transplantation: A sparing effect of dose fractionation. *International Journal of Radiation Oncology, Biology, Physics*, 10(7), 957–964.

DeLord, C., Treleaven, J., Shepherd, J., Saso, R., & Powles, R. L (1999). Vaginal stenosis following allogeneic bone marrow transplantation for acute myeloid leukemia. *Bone Marrow Transplantation*, 23(5), 523–552.

Eilers, J. G., & King, C. R. (1998). Quality of life: Issues related to marrow transplantation. In C. R. King & P. S. Hinds (Eds.), *Quality of life from nursing and patient perspectives* (pp. 204–230). Boston: Jones & Bartlett.

Epperly, M. W., Travis, E. L., Sikora, C., & Greenberger, J. S. (1999). Magnesium superoxide dismutase (MnSOD) plasmid/liposome pulmonary radioprotective gene therapy: Modulation of irradiation-induced mRNA for IL-I, TNF-alpha, and TGF-beta correlates with delay of organizing alveolitis/fibrosis. *Biology of Blood Marrow Transplantation*, 5(4), 204–214.

Feyer, P., Zimmermann, J. S., Titlbach, O.J., Buchali, A., Hinkelbein, M., Budach, V., (1998). Radiotherapy-induced emesis. An overview. *Strahlenther-Onkologie*, 174 (Suppl. 3), 56–61.

Grant, M., Ferrell, B., Schmidt, G. M., Fonbuena, P., Niland, J. C., & Forman, S. J. (1992). Measurement of quality of life in bone marrow transplantation survivors. *Quality of Life Research*, 1(6), 375–384.

Graze, P., & Gale, R. (1979). Chronic graft-versus-host disease: A syndrome of disordered immunity. *American Journal of Medicine*, 66(4), 611–620.

Hoppe, R. (1991). The management of mycosis fungoides at Stanford. Standard and innovative treatment programs. *Leukemia*, 5(Suppl. 1), 46.

Howell, S. & Shalet, S. (1998).Gonadal damage from chemotherapy and radiotherapy. *Endocrinology and Metabolism Clinics of North America*, 27(4), 927–943.

Jones, G. W., Rosenthal, D., & Wilson, L. D. (1999). Total skin electron radiation for patients with erythrodermic cutaneous T-cell lymphoma (mycosis fungoides and the Sezary syndrome). *Cancer*, 85(9), 1985–1995.

Kauppila, M., Koskinen, P., Irjala, K., Remes, K., & Viikari, J. (1998). Long-term effects of allogeneic bone marrow transplantation (BMT) on pituitary, gonad, thyroid and adrenal function in adults. *Bone Marrow Transplantation*, 22(4), 331–337.

Kay, H., & Mattison, D. (1985). How radiation and chemotherapy affect gonadal function. *Contemporary Obstetrics and Gynecology*, 109, 106–115.

Kirova, Y. M., Piedbois, Y., Haddad, E., Levy, E., Calitchi, E., Marinello, G., & Le-Bourgeois, J. P. (1999). Radiotherapy in the management of mycosis fungoides: Indications, results, prognosis. Twenty years experience. *Radiotherapy and Oncology*, 51(2), 147–151.

McMillan, S. C., & Weitzner, M. (1998). Quality of life in cancer patients: Use of a revised hospice index. *Cancer Practice*, 6(5), 282–288.

McQuellon, R. P., Russell, G. B., Cella, D. F., Craven, B. L., Brady, M., Bonomi, A., Hurd, D. D. (1997). Quality of life measurement in bone marrow transplantation: Development of the Functional Assessment of Cancer Therapy-Bone Marrow Transplant (FACT-BMT) scale. *Bone Marrow Transplantation*, 19(4), 357–368.

McQuellon, R. P., Russell, G. B., Rambo, T.D., Craven, B. L., Radford, J., Perry, J. J., Cruz, J., & Hurd, D. D. (1998). Quality of life and psychological distress of bone marrow transplant recipients: The "time trajectory" to recovery over the first year. *Bone Marrow Transplantation*, 21(5), 477–486.

Meyler, T. S., & Purser, P. (1998). Mycosis fungoides. In S. A. Leibel & T. L. Phillips (Eds.), *Textbook of radiation oncology* (pp. 1115–1129). Philadelphia: W.B. Saunders.

National Cancer Institute. (1999). *Common toxicity criteria, version 2.0 with RTOG and EORTC acute effects criteria.* Bethesda, MD: National Cancer Institute.

Neitzert, C. S., Ritvo, P., Dancey, J., Weiser, K., Murray, C., & Avery, J. (1998). The psychosocial impact of bone marrow transplantation: A review of the literature. *Bone Marrow Transplantation*, 22(5), 409–422.

Salazar, O. M., Rubin, P., Hendrickson, F. R., Komaki, R., Poulter, C., Newall, J., Asbell, S. O., Mohiuddin, M., & Van-Ess, J. (1986). Single-dose half-body irradiation for the palliation of multiple bone metastasis from solid tumors: A preliminary report. *Cancer*, 58(1), 29–32.

Saunders, J. E., & Seattle Marrow Transplant Team (1992). Effect of bone marrow transplant on reproductive function. In D. M. Green & G. J. D'Angio (Eds.), *Late effects of treatment for childhood cancer.* New York: John Wiley and Sons.

Shank, B. (1998). Total body irradiation. In S. A. Leibel & T. L. Phillips (Eds.), *Textbook of radiation oncology* (pp. 253–275). Philadelphia: W.B. Saunders.

Syrjala, K. L., Roth-Roemer, S. L., & Abrams, J. R. (1998). Prevalence and predictors of sexual dysfunction in long-term survivors of marrow transplantation. *Journal of Clinical Oncology*, 16(9), 3148–3157.

Wilke, T. J. (1991). Pulmonary and cardiac complications of bone marrow transplantation. In M. B. Whedon (Ed.), *Bone marrow transplantation: Principles, practice, and nursing insights.* Boston: Jones & Bartlett.

CHAPTER 6

STEREOTACTIC RADIOSURGERY AND RADIOTHERAPY

Giselle J. Moore-Higgs, ARNP, MSN
William M. Mendenhall, MD

PROBLEM

STEREOTACTIC RADIOSURGERY (SRS)

■ Stereotactic radiosurgery is an external irradiation technique in which multiple collimated beams of radiation are stereotactically aimed at a radiographically discrete target volume to deliver a single high dose of radiation to a small volume of tissue (Leksell, 1951). The procedure is aimed at defining a small, three-dimensional target volume, delivering a clinically significant dose of radiation while delivering a much smaller, consequently less effective, dose to surrounding tissue. The radiobiologic effects of this focal dose distribution may include thrombosis of small blood vessels, reproductive death, or both of these consequences (Larson, Shrieve, & Loeffler, 1998). There are three delivery systems used for SRS: (1) the modified linear accelerator, (2) the gamma knife, and (3) the charged particle beam produced by a cyclotron or synchrotron.

■ SRS is indicated for patients with small tumors or arteriovenous malformations (AVM) when surgical resection is not possible, or the risk of embolization is too great (Flickinger,

Loeffler, & Larson, 1994). Currently, it is commonly used to treat AVMs and benign intracranial tumors including acoustic schwannomas, meningiomas, and pituitary adenomas. In addition, it may be used in selected patients with brain metastasis or primary brain tumors to boost residual disease or small recurrent disease sites after conventional radiotherapy.

■ SRS has been incorporated into staged treatment protocols, together with embolization, surgery, and radiation; and it is being used as immediate adjuvant therapy to prevent recurrence in gliomas and other primary brain tumors in preference to observation followed by treatment at recurrence (Larson et al., 1998).

■ Ideal target volumes for SRS are nearly spherical and small (≤ 3 cm in maximum dimension). Irregular volumes may require treatment to multiple isocenters to shape a selected isodose surface to conform to the target volume (Chao, Perez, & Brady, 1999).

■ The use of SRS techniques to treat extracranial sites is currently under evaluation in a number of institutions. Procedures include bone screw fixation, contour mold fixation, and frameless stereotaxis to treat spinal cord neoplasms and other extraaxial targets (Takacs & Hamilton, 1999).

STEREOTACTIC RADIOTHERAPY (SRT)

■ Stereotactic radiotherapy (SRT) is the delivery of fractionated radiation therapy to brain tumors using a planning and delivery system similar to that of SRS.

■ SRT is used to treat brain tumors that are small and well defined or may be inoperable due to their location in the brain. In addition, SRT may be used to treat small recurrent tumors in previously irradiated areas. These tumors include meningiomas, craniopharyngiomas, pituitary adenomas, low-grade astrocytomas, optic pathway gliomas, retinoblastomas, and acoustic schwannomas.

ASSESSMENT

In most clinical settings, a multidisciplinary team of radiation oncologists, neurosurgeons, and physicists participate in the assessment of patients referred for SRS and SRT. Most institutions enter patients on specific institution protocols or cooperative group trials with specific eligibility criteria. The following is a general evaluation process:

- Detailed medical history including previous surgery, conventional radiation therapy, or SRS.
- Comprehensive neurologic exam to document evidence of neurologic deficit. Complications from conventional surgery or radiosurgery are more likely to develop in patients with preexisting neurologic deficits (Friedman, Buatti, Bova & Mendenhall, 1998).
- Pathology review may be conducted to confirm diagnosis if patient has had a biopsy or resection of the primary site performed prior to referral for treatment.
- Radiology studies including detailed MRI and CT scan of the brain. These studies are carefully reviewed to determine location and size of the lesion(s), number of lesions, and proximity to adjacent critical structures. Optic nerves are very radiosensitive and do not tolerate a single fraction dose of > 7.5 Gy (Friedman et al., 1998). The facial nerve, trigeminal nerve, cochlear nerve, motor cranial nerves that travel through the cavernous sinus and the jugular foramen are relatively radiosensitive also.
- Angiography in patients with AVMs.
- Evaluation of performance status is commonly performed using the Karnofsky Performance Status Scale. Most protocols require a KPS score of at least 70 prior to treatment with SRS or SRT.

SELECTION CRITERIA

In each of the following indications for stereotactic radiosurgery, a number of variables have been associated with an improved outcome.

Benign Tumors

Acoustic Schwannomas

- At one time, SRS was primarily limited to patients with tumors that were recurrent after primary surgery and those occurring in patients who were elderly or infirm and thought to be high risk for surgery. However, the cure rates following SRS are similar to those observed after conventional surgery and the morbidity is less so that it is currently an excellent alternative to surgery for patients with small operable tumors. The dose must be lowered in patients with large lesions (≥ 3 cm diameter) so that the risks of late complications are not unacceptably high. The reduced dose may eventually result in an increased risk of local recurrence so that many patients with larger lesions are managed surgically. Another option for patients with larger tumors who are medically high risk is SRT.

Meningiomas

- Most patients with benign meningiomas are treated surgically. Patients with relatively small, well-defined or incompletely resected meningiomas have a high rate of cure following SRS. Patients with tumors located adjacent to dose-limiting radiosensitive structures, such as the optic nerve, and those that are larger and less well defined are better treated with SRT.

  A small subset of patients have atypical or malignant meningiomas that are very aggressive and have a high likelihood of recurrence following surgery alone. These patients may be best managed by surgery (if feasible) followed by fractionated irradiation followed by a SRS boost to areas of gross disease.

Pituitary Adenomas

- Small tumors are managed surgically via transphenoid hypophysectomy. Large, incompletely resectable tumors are subtotally resected to relieve symptoms caused by the tumor, such as optic nerve compromise, followed by irradiation. Because most of these tumors are adjacent to the optic nerves and/or optic chiasm, they are usually treated with SRT rather than SRS to minimize the risks of optic neuropathy.

AVMs

■ Patients with AVMs that are amenable to surgical management are usually managed with surgery. One advantage of surgery is that the AVM is obliterated immediately so that the risk of hemorrhage following the procedure is nil. Patients who have lesions that are not amenable to surgery usually because of the location of the AVM, may either be treated with SRS or closely followed. Patients who are elderly with a limited life expectancy may be closely followed.

The remaining patients are treated with SRS unless the lesion is thought to be too large. Resolution of the AVM may require 2 to 3 years following SRS, and until it has resolved completely the patient remains at risk for a hemorrhage. The patient should be evaluated 3 years after SRS and, if resolution is incomplete, offered retreatment.

Brain Metastases and colleagues

■ Cho and colleagues found that larger tumor size, multiplicity of metastases, and infratentorial location of metastases were significant variables in predicting a worse prognosis in patients treated with SRS for brain metastases (Cho, Hall, Gerbi, Higgins, Bohen & Clark, 1998). They determined that patients who meet the following three criteria would most likely benefit from the increased local control in the brain achieved by SRS:

1. Absence of extracranial disease
2. KPS ≥ 70
3. Single intracranial metastasis

Similar findings were found by Lagerwaard and colleagues in a review of 1,292 patients with brain metastases. In addition to the preceding criteria, they found that site of primary tumor, age, response to steroid treatment, systemic tumor activity, and serum lactate dehydrogenase were important prognostic factors that should be considered (Lagerwaard, Levendag, & Nowak, 1999).

Primary Brain Tumors

■ Larson et al. (1996) found five variables associated with decreased survival in patients with malignant glioma treated with the gamma knife: (1) higher pathologic tumor grade, (2) older age of the patient, (3) lower KPS score, (4) large tumor volume, and (5) multifocal versus unifocal tumor. Patients with unfavorable constellations of these variables are unlikely to benefit from radiosurgery. Most formal institutional protocols for radiosurgical treatment of glioblastoma require that patients meet the following criteria (Larson et al., 1998):

1. KPS score of at least 70
2. Unifocal, well-demarcated tumor that enhances on CT or MRI imaging
3. Target no greater than 3 to 4 cm in largest diameter
4. Complete a course of conventional external beam irradiation to approximately 60 Gy prior to SRS

EXPECTED OUTCOMES

BENIGN TUMORS

■ The goal of treatment for benign tumors is to halt the tumor's growth permanently, and in the case of hormonally active pituitary tumors, to ablate abnormal hormone production permanently (Larson et al., 1998). Two additional goals are the maintenance of neurologic function and prevention of new neurologic deficits. Loeffler and colleagues compiled the following data reporting results of SRS for benign tumors: (Loeffler, Flickinger, Shrieve & Larson, 1995):

• Acoustic Schwannomas—local control rate of 85% to 100% (≥ 2 years follow-up)

• Meningiomas—local control rate of 95% to 100% (≥ 2 years follow-up)

• Pituitary Adenomas—normalization of hormone levels in 85% to 95% of patients (> 5 years follow-up)

■ In an analysis of the cost of treating acoustic schwannomas with microsurgery versus radiosurgery, van Roijen and colleagues found that treating patients with an extrameatal tumor diameter of less than 3 cm with radiosurgery was more cost-effective than microsurgery and the general health rating was better (van Roijen, Nijs, & Avezaat, 1997).

AVMs

■ Radiosurgery induces a progressive thickening of the vascular wall and luminal thrombosis, which takes months to years to complete. In most series, the obliteration rates at 2 years after radiosurgical treatment of small AVMs are higher (90–100%) than those for larger AVMs (50–70%) (Loeffler et al., 1995).

BRAIN METASTASES

■ Brain metastases are usually relatively small (< 30 mm) when diagnosed, and they are often nearly spherical and radiographically distinct. They are minimally invasive, and they displace normal brain parenchyma circumferentially beyond the target volume, which reduces the risk of radiation injury to normal tissue. These characteristics make most brain metastases optimally suited for radiosurgery (Larson et al., 1998).

■ Results in >2,000 treated patients have been published during the past 8 years. These results indicate that permanent local control can be obtained in >80% of treated lesions with complications in fewer than 10% of patients. Success was independent of the histology of the treated lesion or number of lesions treated (Loeffler, Barker, & Chapman, 1999).

■ Patients who receive whole brain radiotherapy in addition to radiosurgery experience a better local control than those who undergo radiosurgery alone (Loeffler & Alexander, 1993).

PRIMARY BRAIN TUMORS

■ For a small group of highly selected patients with glioblastoma multiforme, radiosurgery may provide improved survival following conventional fractionated radiation therapy (Larson et al., 1996). Shrieve and colleagues (1999) reported on 78 patients treated with SRS as part of their initial treatment for glioblastoma multiforme. All patients had received conventional radiotherapy prior to SRS. The median length of actuarial survival for all patients was 19.9 months. Twelve- and 24-month survival rates were 88.5% and 35.9%, respectively. Thirty-nine patients (50%) underwent reoperation for symptomatic necrosis or recurrent tumor. The rate of reoperation at 24 months following SRS was 54.8%. The addition of the radiosurgery boost did appear to confer a survival advantage to selected patients, specifically those patients who fall into RTOG class III.

OUTCOMES MEASURES

■ Benign Tumors—Patients with acoustic schwannomas and meningiomas should be evaluated every 12 months with a clinical exam and MRI for a minimum of 5 years of radiographic follow-up. At that point, follow-up is maintained on a yearly basis with imaging dictated by clinical symptoms (Friedman, Buatti, Bova, & Mendenhall, 1998).

- AVM patients should have follow-up clinical exams along with MRI/MRA scans at 12-month intervals until the AVM resolves. An angiogram should be performed at 3 years to confirm thrombosis. Angiograms are necessary because MRI/MRA results are relatively unreliable as the nidus shrinks to less than 1 cm in size. If no nidus is present on MRI/MRA, a repeat angiogram should be scheduled at 3 years (Friedman et al., 1998).

- Malignant tumors including both metastases and gliomas require more frequent follow up with CT or MRI and clinical exam. For metastases, a scan to assess the response of the lesion should be made 3 months after radiosurgery and then every 6 months thereafter for a minimum of 3 years. Patients with malignant gliomas should have a scan every 3 months for the first 2 years and then every 6 months. Scan frequency is often dictated by clinical symptoms and the availability of effective salvage treatment in the event of recurrent disease (Friedman et al., 1998).

- Evaluation of the cost-effectiveness and cost-utility of SRS versus resection for single-brain metastases has shown that both resection and SRS yield superior survival and functional independence compared to whole brain radiotherapy alone. Resection resulted in a 1.8-fold increase in cost compared to SRS. The latter modality yielded superior cost outcomes on all measures (Mehta et al., 1997). Rutligliano et al. (1995) found that SRS had a lower uncomplicated procedure cost, lower average complication cost per case, lower total cost per procedure, and was more cost-effective and had a better incremental cost-effectiveness than resection.

- Specific functional outcomes can be measured using the National Cancer Institute Common Toxicity Criteria Version 2.0 that includes the Radiation Therapy Oncology Group (RTOG) and European Organization for Research and Treatment of Cancer (EORTC) acute effects criteria (NCI, 1999).

- Quality of life evaluations of patients receiving SRS and SRT have been limited to the use of KPS and documentation of acute and long-term physical sequelae. For example, Gerosa, Nicolato, and Severi (1996) in an evaluation of patients using SRS for intracranial metastases found the KPS and neurological performance scores were consistently high for most of the follow-up period in this group of patients. Several additional instruments are available that would be appropriate and expand the value of this evaluation:

1. EORTC QLQ-C30 version 2.0 (Aaronson et al., 1993). An integrated system for assessing QOL of cancer patients participating in international clinical trials. The current version is a 30-item instrument that has been extensively used.
2. FACT-Brain (Weitzner, Meyer, Gelke, Byrne, Cella & Levin, 1995). A subscale specifically designed for patients with brain tumors has been added to the FACT-General scale. The validity and reliability coefficients are high for both scales. The brain subscale tests substantially different QOL issues than the core instrument.

Outcomes Management

Werner-Wasik et al. (1999) reported on the immediate side effects of patients treated with SRS or SRT using a dedicated linear accelerator. Any side effects occurring during and up to 2 weeks after the treatment were included. The incidence of symptoms was higher for the diagnosis of acoustic schwannomas (50%), gliomas (46%), and AVMs (36%), and lowest for meningiomas (33%) and brain metastases (21%).

Acute Effects

- Discomfort from the invasive, fixated head frame
- Infection at the head frame pin sites
- Vertigo—common and unique for patients with acoustic schwannomas (33%)
- Nausea/vomiting—may occur after head frame placement and during the first 12 to 24 hours following treatment
- Cerebral edema—occurs as an acute reaction of the tumor to the radiation or as a result of radiation necrosis. Edema causes increased intracranial pressure (ICP) with associated symptoms of increased frequency of seizures and focal neurologic deficits, most notably motor weakness. Cerebral edema may be treated with corticosteroid administration.
- Seizures—approximately 20% to 30% of patients with primary brain tumors or metastatic lesions present with seizures that are usually focal in nature. Seizures that occur in the first 24 to 48 hours after SRS or SRT are more common in patients who present with seizures at diagnosis.

LATENT EFFECTS

- Persistent headaches may occur more commonly in patients for whom headaches were a presenting symptom.
- Cerebral radionecrosis is the major, dose-limiting complication of brain irradiation and occurs in two forms, focal and diffuse, which differ significantly in clinical and radiologic features. Focal and diffuse injuries both include a wide spectrum of abnormalities from subclinical changes detectable only by MRI imaging to overt brain necrosis. Asymptomatic focal edema is commonly seen on CT and MRI following focal or large-volume irradiation.
  - Focal necrosis has the CT and MRI characteristics of a mass lesion with clinical evidence of focal neurologic abnormality and raised intracranial pressure. Microscopically, the lesion shows characteristic vascular changes and white matter pathology ranging from demyelination to coagulative necrosis.
  - Diffuse radiation injury is characterized by periventricular decrease in attenuation of CT and increased signal on proton-density and T2-weighted MRI images. Most patients are asymptomatic. When clinical manifestations occur, impairment of mental function is the most prominent feature. Pathologic findings in focal and diffuse radiation necrosis are similar.
  - Late radiation injury of large arteries is an occasional cause of postradiation cerebral injury, and cerebral atrophy and mineralizing microangiopathy are common radiologic findings of uncertain clinical significance. Functional imaging by PET scan can differentiate recurrent tumors from focal radiation necrosis with positive and negative predictive values for tumors of 80% to 90% (Valk & Dillon, 1991).
  - Symptoms develop related to radiation therapy injury between 3 to 18 months after treatment and usually resolve in 6 to 12 months in 50% of patients (Hall, 1995). Administration of corticosteroids is usually the first line of treatment. Another approach is the use of hyperbaric oxygen therapy (HBO) therapy. It has been beneficial in the treatment of radiation-induced bone and soft tissue necrosis. HBO raises the tissue pO_2 and initiates a cellular and vascular repair mechanism. Leber and colleagues treated two patients with gamma knife radiosurgery induced cerebral

radionecrosis with HBO (Leber, Eder, Kovac, Anegg & Pendl, 1998). Both responded well to HBO, one lesion disappeared and the other was reduced significantly in size.

■ Cranial nerve deficits may occur depending on the location and size of the tumor and the SRS dose. The nerves at risk for acoustic schwannoma patients are the trigeminal (V) and facial (VII) nerves. The risk is primarily related to the dose delivered to the brainstem with very low probability of injury ($\leq$ 5%) using optimal SRS treatment techniques.

■ Hemorrhage occurs in 3% to 5% of patients treated with SRS for AVM within the first 2 years after treatment. Significant risk factors for hemorrhage appear to correlate with increasing AVM volume (Friedman et al., 1996).

■ Cyst formation may occur after the tumor resolves or in response to radiation necrosis.

■ Changes in cognitive ability are not well understood. However, the size, location, histology, radiation fields, and total dose are considered important factors.

REFERENCES

Aaronson, N. K., Ahmedzai, S., Bergman, B., B., Bullinger, M., Cull, A., Duez, N. J., Filiberti, A., Flechtner, H., Fleishman, S. B., de Haes, J. C. J. M., Kaasa, S., Klee, M., Osoba, D., Razavi, D., Rofe, P. B., Schraub, S., Sneeuw, K., Sullivan, M., & Takeda, F. (1993). The European Organization for Research and Treatment of Cancer QLQ-C30: A quality-of-life instrument for use in international clinical trials in oncology. *Journal of the National Cancer Institute, 85*(5), 365–376.

Chao, K. S. C., Perez, C. A., & Brady, L. W. (1999). *Radiation oncology: Management decisions* (pp. 73–77). Philadelphia: Lippincott-Raven.

Cho, K. H., Hall, W. A., Gerbi, B. J., Higgins, P. D., Bohen, M., Clark, H. B. (1998). Patient selection criteria for the treatment of brain metastases with stereotactic radiosurgery. *Journal of Neuro-oncology, 40*(1), 73–86.

Flickinger, J. C., Loeffler, J. S., & Larson, D. A. (1994). Stereotactic radiosurgery for intracranial malignancies. *Oncology, 8*(1), 81–84.

Friedman, W. A., Blatt, D. L., Bova, F. J., Buatti, J. M., Mendenhall, W. M., & Kubilis, P. S. (1996). The risk of hemorrhage after radiosurgery for arteriovenous malformations. *Journal of Neurosurgery, 84*(6), 912–919.

Friedman, W. A., Buatti, J. M., Bova, F. J., & Mendenhall, W. M. (1998). *Linac radiosurgery. A practical guide* (pp. 122–124). New York: Springer.

Gerosa, M., Nicolato, A., & Severi, F. (1996). Gamma Knife radiosurgery for intracranial metastases: From local tumor control to increased survival. *Stereotactic and Functional Neurosurgery, 66*(Suppl. 1), 184–192.

Hall, W. A. (1995). Stereotactic radiosurgery in perspective. In A. R. Cohen & S. J. Haines (Eds.), *Neurosurgery: Minimal invasive techniques in neurosurgery*. Baltimore: Williams & Wilkins.

Lagerwaard, F. J., Levendag, P. C., Nowak, P. J. (1999). Identification of prognostic factors in patients with brain metastases: A review of 1292 patients. *International Journal of Radiation Oncology, Biology, Physics*, 43(4), 795–803.

Larson, D. A., Gutin, P. H., McDermott, M. , Lamborn, K., Sneed, P. K., Wara, W. M., Flickinger, J. C., Kondziolka, D., Lunsford, L. D., Hudgins, W. R., Friehs, G. M., Haselsberger, K., Leber, K., Pendl, G., Chung, S. S., Coffey, R. J., Dinapoli, R., Shaw, E. G., Vermeulen, S., Young, R. F., Hirato, M., Inoue, H. K., Ohye, C., & Shibazaki, T. (1996). Gamma knife for glioma: Selection factors and survival. International Journal of Rediation Oncology, Biology, 36(5): 1045–53.

Larson, D. A., Shrieve, D. C., & Loeffler, J. S. (1998). Radiosurgery. In S. A. Leibel & T. L. Phillips (Eds.), *Textbook of radiation oncology* (pp. 383–399). Philadelphia: W.B. Saunders.

Leber, K. A., Eder, H.G., Kovac, H., Anegg, U., & Pendl, G. (1998). Treatment of cerebral radionecrosis by hyperbaric oxygen therapy. *Stereotactic and Functional Neurosurgery*, 70(Suppl. 1), 229–236.

Leksell, L. (1951). The stereotaxic method and radiosurgery of the brain. *Acta Chirurgica Scandinavica*, 102: 316.

Loeffler, J. S., & Alexander, E. I., III. (1993). Radiosurgery for the treatment of intracranial metastases. In E. I. Alexander, III, J. S. Loeffler, & L. D. Lunsford (Eds.), *Stereotactic radiosurgery* (pp. 197–198). New York: McGraw-Hill.

Loeffler, J. S., Barker, F. G., & Chapman, P. H. (1999). Role of radiosurgery in the management of central nervous system metastases. *Cancer Chemotherapy and Pharmacology*, 43(Suppl): S11–S14.

Loeffler, J. S., Flickinger, J. C., Shrieve, D. C., & Larson, D. A. (1995). Radiosurgery for the treatment of intracranial lesions. In V. T. DeVita, S. Hellman, & S. A. Rosenberg (Eds.), *Important advances in oncology* (p. 141). Philadelphia: J.B. Lippincott.

Mehta, M., Noyes, W., Craig, B., Lamond, J., Auchter, R., French, M., Johnson, M., Levin, A., Badie, B., Robbins, I., & Kinsella, T. (1997). A cost-effectiveness and cost-utility analysis of radiosurgery versus resection for single-brain metastases. *International Journal of Radiation Oncology, Biology, Physics*, 39(2), 445–454.

National Cancer Institute. (1999). *Common toxicity criteria, Version 2.0 with EORTC and RTOG acute effects criteria*. Bethesda, MD: National Cancer Institute.

Rutligliano, M. J., Lunsford, L. D., Kondziolka, D., Strauss, M. J., Khanna, V., & Green, M. (1995). The cost effectiveness of stereotactic radiosurgery versus surgical resection in the treatment of solitary metastatic brain tumors. *Neurosurgery*, 37(3), 445–453.

Shrieve, D. C., Alexander, E., III, Black, P. M., Wen, P. Y., Fine, H. A., Kooy, H. M., & Loeffler, J. S. (1999). Treatment of patients with primary glioblastoma multiforme with standard postoperative radiotherapy and radiosurgical boost: Prognostic factors and long-term outcome. *Journal of Neurosurgery*, 90(1), 72–77.

Takacs, I., & Hamilton, A. J. (1999). Extracranial stereotactic radiosurgery: Applications for the spine and beyond. *Neurosurgery Clinics of North America*, 10(2), 257–270.

Valk, P. E. & Dillon, W. P. (1991). Radiation injury of the brain. *American Journal of Neuroradiology*, 12(1), 45–62.

van Roijen, L., Nijs, H. G., Avezaat, C. J. (1997). Costs and effects of microsurgery versus radiosurgery in treating acoustic neuroma. *Acta Neurochirurgica Supplementum (Wien)*, 139(10), 972–978.

Weitzner, M. A., Meyers, C. A., Gelke, C. K, Byrne, K. S., Cella, D. F., & Levin, V. A. (1995). The Functional Assessment of Cancer Therapy (FACT) scale. Development of a brain subscale and revalidation of the general version (FACT-G) in patients with primary brain tumors. *Cancer*, 75(5), 1151–1161.

Werner-Wasik, M., Rudoler, S., Preston, P. E., Hauck, W. W., Downes, B. M., Leeper, D., Andrews, D., Corn, B. W., & Curran, W. J. Jr.(1999). Immediate side effects of stereotactic radiotherapy and radiosurgery. *International Journal of Radiation Oncology, Biology, Physics*, 43(2), 299–304.

CHAPTER 7

RADIATION MODIFIERS CHEMICAL AND THERMAL

Cynthia W. Martin, ANP, MSN, RN, CS, AOCN
Thomas Whitehead, MD

PURPOSE OF RADIATION MODIFIERS

Both normal cells and cancer cells are vulnerable to the effects of radiation and may be injured or destroyed by radiation therapy. Cells vary in sensitivity to radiation with rapidly dividing cells, both normal and malignant, generally more sensitive to the effects of radiation therapy than those cells that grow more slowly. These cells are referred to as radiosensitive. Nondividing or more slowly dividing cells are referred to as radioresistant (Sitton, 1998). Well-oxygenated cells are more radiosensitive than hypoxic cells, which require about three times the radiation dose to achieve the same degree of cytotoxicity (Rowkinsky, 1999). The goal of chemical modification is to achieve a therapeutic gain, that is, to increase tumor cell death while sparing the surrounding normal tissue from similar injury (Curran, 1998). The term *chemical modifier* has generally been used for agents that are nontherapeutic by themselves, but that enhance or mitigate the action of another effective therapy and, therefore, are usually used in combination with other therapies (Noll & Riese, 1997).

The outcome of radiation therapy can be affected by multiple factors that contribute to the radioresistance of a cell:

- Intrinsic radiosensitivity of the cell
- Degree of tumor hypoxia
- The rate of repopulation of tumor cells; The radiosensitivity of the surrounding normal cells also determines the dose of radiation that can safely be administered (Begg, 1998).

Though the exact mechanism is not well understood, it has been hypothesized that the presence of oxygen during radiation favors the production and persistence of chemically unstable particles called *free radicals*. The effect of free radicals on the outcome of radiation therapy includes:

- Free radicals then may interact with DNA resulting in tissue damage.
- The presence of oxygen in the tumor cell also decreases the likelihood of damaged DNA repair, further resulting in increased cell damage (Noll & Riese, 1997).
- Drug compounds have been developed that modify the initial radiochemical event by increasing the availability of oxygen to the cell. In addition, physiologic modifications such as hyperbaric oxygen and hyperthermia can also modify radiation response.

Radiosensitizers and *radioprotectors* are chemical compounds that modify the effect of radiation on cells and tissues as follows:

- Radiosensitizing agents have been broadly classified as hypoxic cell sensitizers or nonhypoxic cell sensitizers or both. Rationale for their use is based on the knowledge that many tumors have areas that are highly radioresistant due to tissue hypoxia. These chemical radiosensitizers replace oxygen in the chemical reactions following irradiation, thereby enhancing the radiation effectiveness (Scofield, Leibman, & Popkin, 1991). The exact mechanism of nonhypoxic radiosensitizers is not well understood.
- Radioprotectors are agents that must be selectively taken up by the healthy tissue in order to obtain the desired result of tumor lethality with normal tissue protection.

HYPOXIC CELL SENSITIZERS

METRONIDAZOLE

In 1974, metronidazole, a 5-nitroimidazole, became the first compound to be investigated as a possible agent that when used in conjunction with radiation therapy increased tumorcidal activity.

- ■ In its Phase I trial, metronidazole produced significant nausea and vomiting, which proved to be its dose-limiting toxicity. Additionally, later studies showed that neurologic toxicity, specifically central neuropathy, with somnolence, confusion, and transient coma may occur (Hilderley, 1993).
- ■ A Canadian study tested metronidazole in conjunction with radiation therapy and concomitant cisplatin and mitomycin C in patients with malignant gliomas and poor prognosis anaplastic astrocytomas. Central nervous system toxicity, ranging from drowsiness to loss of consciousness, was frequent and gastrointestinal toxicity while substantial was mild to moderate in severity. Three of eleven patients evaluable for response achieved a partial remission with treatment, with a median survival of 26 weeks for all patients from the time of initial diagnosis. The study was terminated prematurely because of significant toxicity (in this study as well as in parallel concurrent studies of similar design in other tumor types) and apparent lack of benefit (Stewart, Dahrouge, Agboola, & Girard, 1997).
- ■ Currently, this drug is not being used clinically, but further studies are pending.

MISONIDAZOLE

Misonidazole (RO-07-0582) began clinical evaluation in 1977 and Phase III trials were completed 7 years later. Misonidazole exhibited the same gastrointestinal and neurologic side effects as metronidazole, but demonstrated increased efficacy as a hypoxic cell sensitizer.

From 1979 though 1983, 268 patients with unresectable locally advanced non-small-cell lung cancer were randomized to radiation therapy alone (50 Gy large field and 10 Gy boost) or combined with misonidazole (400 mg/m^2 2 to 4 hours prior to radiation therapy daily to a maximum dose of 12 g/m^2 or until tumor progression). At the time of analysis, 95% of the patients had died with a median survival of 8 months. Seventy percent in the radiation alone group and 77% of the radiation and misonidazole group died of progressive disease. There was no significant improvement in response rates, local control, or survival in patients who received the misonidazole arm as compared to the radiation alone arm (Simpson et al., 1989). During this same time, RTOG 7916 studied the use of misonidazole used in combination with whole brain irradiation in brain metastases from either lung or breast cancer, and randomized patients to either receive radiation therapy alone (in either 3.0 Gy × 10 fractions or 5.0 Gy × 6 fractions) or given in combination with misonidazole (1 g/m^2 to a total of 10 mg/m^2 or 2 g/m^2 to a total of 12 mg/m^2). Median survival was 3.9 months with no statistical difference seen in any treatment arm. Because up to one-third of the patients in this study died from uncontrolled brain metastases, local control with a minimum of toxicity was an important goal. Due to previously mentioned toxicities, the addition of misonidazole did not add therapeutic benefit and should not be considered a reasonable addition to radiation for brain metastases (Komarnicky et al., 1991).

In an evaluation of studies from RTOG (RTOG 76-11 and RTOG 79-18) and ECOG (ECOG 74-01) of long-term survival in patients with anaplastic astrocytomas who were treated with either radiation therapy alone, radiation plus chemotherapy, or radiation therapy plus chemotherapy plus misonidazole with adjustments made in prognostic factors, the patients treated with misonidazole had a significantly worse overall outcome. Median survival for patients in the radiation alone arm was 3.0 years with a 5-year survival of 35%, chemotherapy and radiation therapy was 2.3 years with a 5-year survival of 29%, and the chemotherapy plus radiation plus misonidazole was 1.2 years with a 5-year survival of 24% (Fischbach et al., 1991).

- Peripheral neuropathies, which were debilitating and long-lasting, occurred in 40% to 50% of patients at the maximum tolerated dose of 10 to 12 g/m^2. The neuropathies were decreased with addition of phenytoin (Dilantin®) and dexamethasone (Phillips, 1981).
- Confusion and ototoxicity with mild hearing loss occurred in 10% of the patients. The drug penetrated well into the tumors with drug concentrations at the center of the tumor at 70% to 80% of plasma level (Wasserman, Chapman, Coleman, & Kligerman, 1998).

A trial for patients with head and neck cancer showed a slight trend toward higher duration of complete response, but no difference in overall survival (Wasserman et al., 1998). Stage IIIB and IVA carcinomas of the cervix also showed no statistically significant differences in pelvic response, disease-free survival, patterns of failure, or toxicity in the radiation alone arm versus the radiation and misonidazole arm (Grigsby et al., 1999). Patients with T_2 and T_3 bladder cancers were randomized to receive either radiation alone (40 Gy in 2 Gy fractions 5 times/week) or radiation (12 Gy in 6 Gy fractions 1 time/week) plus misonidazole orally (3.0 mg/m^2) and intravesically (1.0 g in 35 ml of solvent). As in the previously mentioned studies, no statistical significance was seen in disease-free survival or bladder preservation, but patients in the misonidazole arm may have experienced increased bowel morbidity and subsequently underwent cystectomy, perhaps due to the unconventional radiation fraction schedule (Abratt, Craighead, Reddi, & Sarembock, 1991).

Due to lack of therapeutic benefit and substantial toxicity, misonidazole is not currently used in clinical practice, but it continues to be studied.

ETANIDAZOLE

Etanidazole (SR-2508), an analog of misonidazole, underwent RTOG Phase II and III studies on patients with unresectable stage III and IV head and neck cancers comparing conventional radiation therapy (66 to 74 Gy at 2 Gy per fraction, 5 fractions/week) alone to the same dose of radiation with the addition of etanidazole (2 g/m^2 3 times/week for a total of 17 doses). Toxicities included only transient peripheral sensory neuropathy (18% Grade I and 5% Grade II), no central neuropathy, nausea, and vomiting (27%), and reversible neutropenia (15%) (Lee et al., 1995).

- A Phase III study in head and neck tumors (RTOG 85-27) showed an increase in the 2-year local control in N_0 and N_1 disease with 55% in the etanidazole arm and 37% in the radiation alone arm showing local control (Lee et al., 1995).
- A similar study of head and neck patients in France failed to find any evidence of therapeutic benefit in using etanidazole in early-stage disease (Eschwege et al., 1997).
- In a Phase I study, patients with glioblastoma multiforme failed to demonstrate any improvement in survival over conventional radiation therapy when etanidazole was added to their treatment regimen, although treatment associated toxicity was equivalent (Chang et al., 1998).

■ In a Phase II trial, patients with locally advanced adenocarcinoma of the prostate received external beam radiation therapy and etanidazole and showed similar outcomes to historical controls of patients who received radiation therapy alone (Beard et al., 1994). In an additional study, patients with locally advanced (T_{2b}, T_3, and T_4 tumors) adenocarcinoma of the prostate who received standard four-field whole pelvis external beam radiation therapy at 45 to 50 Gy followed by a cone down with a minimal dose of 66 Gy to the prostate were randomized to either receive standard therapy or to add etanidazole at 1.8 g/m^2 3 times per week. PSA response levels were similar in both groups, and although there was no significant toxicity from the etanidazole, there appeared to be no clinical indication to adding this drug in the treatment of prostate cancer (Lawton et al., 1996).

NIMORAZOLE

Nimorazole is in the same structural class as metronidazole, and although less potent and with dose-limiting toxicities of nausea and vomiting, has significantly less cumulative neurotoxicity than either misonidazole or etanidazole. In a multicenter randomized, balanced, double-blinded Phase III trial of nimorazole versus placebo in patients with squamous cell cancers of the supraglottic larynx and pharynx, patients received nimorazole as a hypoxic cell radiosensitizer versus placebo in conjunction with primary radiation therapy at 62 to 68 Gy at 2 Gy per fraction, 5 fractions per week. Patients receiving nimorazole realized a statistically significant difference (49% vs. 33% at 5 years) in improvement of locoregional control over the placebo group. Drug-related side effects were minor and tolerable with transient nausea and vomiting the most reported side effect (Overgaard et al., 1998).

Currently, this drug is not used clinically, however further studies are underway in various disease sites.

NONHYPOXIC CELL SENSITIZERS

The halogenated pyrimidines, bromodeoxyuridine (BrdUrd) and IUdR, are compounds that are rapidly taken up by actively dividing cells and are incorporated into the DNA of the cycling cells, making them more sensitive to radiation damage (Noll & Riese, 1997). The mechanism of action is not well understood, but it is thought to influence radiation-induced DNA strand breaks and repair. Early studies in Japan involving brain tumors appeared promising, but there were significant problems concerning normal tissue toxicity with the dose-limiting toxicity being myelosuppression, particularly thrombocytopenia. Phase II trials in sarcomas, gliomas, and liver metastases show promising preliminary results (Wasserman et al., 1998).

In a RTOG (89-05) study of radiation therapy with and without the addition of BrdUrd in patients with brain metastases (primary disease breast, lung, or other), BrdUrd did not enhance the efficacy of the radiotherapy regimen tested. Patients were randomized to receive 37.5 Gy in 15 fractions of 2.5 Gy each alone, or at the same dose with BrdUrd $0.8g/m^2$ per day for 4 days of each of the 3 weeks. Patients in the radiotherapy alone group had a median survival of 6.12 months while patients in the BrdUrd group had a survival of 4.3 months. BrdUrd caused significant Grade 4 and 5 hematological toxicity in five of the patients.

BIOREDUCTIVE AND HYPOXIC CELL CYTOTOXIC AGENTS

TIRAPAZAMINE

Tirapazamine is a bioreductive agent that is preferentially cytotoxic to hypoxic cells in vitro. Many hypoxic cell sensitizers enhance tissue response of hypoxic tissue to standard radiation generally by mimicking the effects of oxygen, which induces the formation of toxic free radicals that may interact with the DNA (Rowkinsky, 1999). This agent differs from oxygen-mimetic sensitizers in that it requires metabolic activation, and enhancement is seen when given prior to or after radiation therapy.

In a Phase II study of head and neck patients (oropharynx, supraglottic larynx, and hypopharynx), tirapazamine was given at $159 \, mg/m^2$ 3 times per week for 12 doses in conjunction with conventional radiation therapy of 70 Gy over 7 weeks. Compliance was 82% with a median follow-up of 13 months while the 1- and 2-year local control rates were 64% and 52%, respectively. Tirapazamine was well tolerated with muscle cramps (77%) and nausea and vomiting (62%) with usually Grade 1 or 2 overall reported (Lee, Trotti, Spencer et al., 1998).

■ Phase I studies of tirapazamine demonstrated muscle cramping as the most common side effect of the drug. In doses from 18 mg/m^2 to 293 mg/m^2, there was no reported dose-dependent variation in the severity of muscle cramps and no consistent abnormality in clinical laboratory values found (Doherty et al., 1994).

Glutathione Depletion

Glutathione (GSH) is found in high concentrations in both normal cells and tumor cells and provides a wide range of protective functions for the cell. GSH is a major intracellular non-protein-bound sulfhydryl that plays an important role in the intrinsic radioresistance of the cell by scavenging free radicals, and thereby protecting the cell from chemical damage. Some studies show that depletion of this important thiol compound sensitizes hypoxic cells to radiation without affecting the sensitivity of aerobic cells, while others note varying degrees of aerobic sensitization (Wasserman et al., 1998). GSH depletion can enhance the efficacy of misonidazole and etanidazole and may also be useful in increasing the cell sensitivity to tirapazamine.

■ A group of women ($n = 30$) with invasive cervical cancer were studied and were found to have lower levels of GSH than the age-matched normal control group (Mukundan et al., 1999).

■ In studies of breast cancer patients, results were mixed in identifying risk for disease recurrence in patients whose tumors expressed or did not express glutathione S-transferase-pi. One study showed higher risk at 6 years for local recurrence for the group who expressed the enzyme and received surgery alone. Conversely, in the review of patients given conservative surgery followed by radiotherapy, there was no difference in local recurrence between patients whose tumors did or did not express the enzyme.

■ In a separate study of 45 patients with squamous cell carcinoma of the cervix (FIGO stages IIB and IIIB) who received external radiation therapy of 35 Gy in 16 fractions over 4 weeks or at 45 Gy in 20 fractions over 5 weeks respectively, the glutathione levels in both blood and tumor showed a significant decrease, even after just 1 fraction of radiation therapy. There was good correlation between the extent of GSH decrease and tumor response, with those patients who had a complete response showing a $\geq$ 70% decrease in both blood and tumor GSH (Jadhav et al., 1998).

The measurement of GSH may be beneficial in determining tumor response to therapy and may help in identifying radioresistance in a select number of patients.

CHEMOSENSITIZATION

The use of hypoxic cell sensitizers with chemotherapeutic agents, mainly alkylating agents, in addition to radiation therapy, has been extensively studied. Melphalan and oral misonidazole have been used in patients with lung cancer with superior response rates to melphalan alone. Newer agents such as docetaxel (Taxotere®) show promise as well, with Taxotere® showing the greatest cytotoxic and radiosensitizing effect on the SW48 (p52wt) cell line (Creane, Seymour, Collucci, & Mothersill, 1999).

Paclitaxel (Taxol®) is an antimicrotubular agent that blocks the cells in the G_2/M phase of the cell cycle. Because of this mechanism it is presumed that this drug can be a potent radiation sensitizer (Preisler et al., 1998). Preliminary studies indicate that the drug is reasonably well tolerated in a variety of disease settings including non-small-cell lung cancer, laryngeal cancer, cervical cancer, gastric cancer, and pancreatic cancers with the dose-limiting toxicity being neutropenia (Herscher et al., 1998). Further studies are necessary to evaluate the effectiveness of this drug on long-term survival.

Topoisomerase I-targeting drugs exert their cytotoxic effect by producing enzyme catalytic activity. DNA topoisomerase I recently has been established as a biochemically mediated radiosensitizer in cultured mammalian cells. This sensitization appears to be schedule dependent, cell cycle phase-specific, cell line dependent, and not strictly dependent on cell cytotoxicity. Studies are ongoing to establish which disease types and which schedules produce maximum benefits (Chen, Choy, & Rothenberg, 1999).

Cisplatin, long known as a radiation sensitizer, has been studied in patients with ovarian carcinoma who also received either low-dose rate or high-dose rate irradiation. Given 1 hour prior to radiation therapy, the radiosensitization of the tumor was increased by a fraction of 1.6 to 5.8 (Raaphoorst, Wand, & Stewart, & Ng, 1996). Given in combination with etoposide (Vepesid®), cisplatin shows a 42% increased survival benefit at 2 years (Kalemkreian, 1999).

A potent radiosensitizer, 5 fluorouracil (5FU), has been used extensively in patients with rectal and anal cancers. Simultaneous delivery of large doses of 5FU with irradiation is associated with improved survival compared with radiation alone, but with significantly increased tissue toxicity (Rich, 1999). Severe, dose-limiting toxicities include mucositis, diarrhea, and desquamation, which are much worse than when either therapy is given alone. Current treatment regimens using continuous infusion 5FU seem to produce less local and systemic toxicity than when the drug is given by bolus.

ENHANCING OXYGEN EFFECT

HYPERBARIC OXYGEN

Since it is known that well-oxygenated cells are more radiosensitive than hypoxic cells, hyperbaric oxygen was the first radiation sensitizer to be clinically tested. The breathing of pure oxygen, carbogen, or oxygen at increased pressure results in increased oxygen concentration in the blood and, therefore, its deeper infusion into the tumor (Wasserman et al., 1998).

- Randomized clinical trials in patients with head and neck cancers and cancer of the cervix showed positive results, but the treatment was complicated by the cumbersome nature of hyperbaric oxygen and some patients demonstrated increased normal-tissue injury
- More recent trials in patients with cancer of the larynx failed to show any therapeutic benefit in patients who received hypofractionated radiation therapy in conjunction with hyperbaric oxygen as compared to those patients who received standard protracted radiation therapy with and without chemotherapy (Haffty, Hurley, & Peters, 1999).
- Clinically, hyperbaric oxygen is used to enhance healing in patients with radiation therapy-associated tissue necrosis.

HYPERTHERMIA

The use of heat in combination with radiation and cytotoxic drugs has received varying levels of interest over the years, but definite clinical benefit has yet to be determined. Heat may be more damaging to malignant tissues for the following reasons:

- Chronically hypoxic cells may have an increased sensitivity to heat.
- Cells with a low pH ($<$ 6.8) that are metabolically deprived (such as tumor cells) are more heat sensitive.
- Heat affects cells in the S phase, which are known to be more resistant to irradiation.

The differential heat sensitivity of tumors is a consequence of tumor physiology, with nutrient deprivation and lower pH being the main contributing factors to the increased sensitivity of tumors and not a consequence of the intrinsic state of malignancy of the cells (Myerson, Moros, & Roti Roti, 1997).

The physical agents used for power deposition in clinical hyperthermia include electromagnetic (EM) fields at very high microwave frequencies, low-frequency microwaves, radiofrequencies, and ultrasound, all of which may be delivered superficially or interstitially (Myerson et al., 1997). Temperatures vary from 41° to 43°C depending on the area to be treated, the amount and schedule of radiotherapy to be administered, and the absence or inclusion of radiosensitizing agents.

The most important factor in the use of hyperthermia remains the radiation dose. Hyperthermia enhances the effect of radiation through an additive and synergistic effect, with the most therapeutic benefit attained when the irradiation is followed by hyperthermia. Smaller tumors ($<$ 3 cm) demonstrate a better therapeutic outcome than larger tumors. Also, anatomic sites such as the chest wall, which can be heated with current hypothermic technology, have demonstrated better therapeutic outcomes than sites such as the head and neck regions, which are more difficult to heat due to complex contours of the anatomy (Myerson et al., 1997).

RADIOPROTECTORS

A major goal of radiation therapy is to achieve maximum injury and cell death to tumor cells while sparing the surrounding normal tissues. One strategy to increase the efficacy of radiation is to use compounds that protect the normal tissues in the radiation field, but do not spare the tumor of the cytotoxic effect of the therapy. Some examples follow:

- As a primary example, Vitamin A, Vitamin E, Vitamin C, and beta-carotene protect cellular membranes from the action of the radiation-produced peroxy radicals by scavenging these radicals (Wasserman et al., 1997; Narra, Harapanhalli, Howell, Sastry , & Roa, 1994; and Harapanhalli et al., 1994).

■ Sulfhydryl compounds are known to protect cells from radiation damage by scavenging the products of irradiated water (free radicals) and by repairing radiation-damaged molecules to their active form.

Amifostine (Ethyol®) was originally developed to protect military personnel from the effects of nuclear radiation and was given a clinical indication through its ability to protect renal cells in patients receiving cisplatin chemotherapy (Viele & Holmes, 1998). Originally studied in the late 1980s, amifostine was found to be a safe and effective radioprotector of bone marrow function with side effects of emesis, malaise, and hypotension at 340 mg/m^2 (Constine, Zagars, Rubin, & Kligerman, 1986; Kligerman et al., 1988).

Xerostomia is the most common toxicity associated with standard fractionated radiation therapy to the head and neck region. Whereas acute xerostomia from radiation is due to an inflammatory reaction, late xerostomia, which includes xerostomia occurring one year after treatment, reflects fibrosis of the salivary gland and is usually permanent. Xerostomia results in dry mouth, affecting a person's ability to eat or speak, and increases the risk for dental caries, oral infections, and osteonecrosis. Newer research has shown Amifostine (Ethyol®) reduces the incidence of postradiation xerostomia in patients receiving postoperative radiation therapy to the head and neck area where a substantial volume of salivary glands is included in the radiation field (Hensley et al., 1999).

■ The American Society of Clinical Oncology (ASCO), in its Clinical Practice Guidelines, notes that the use of amifostine may be considered to decrease the incidence of acute and late xerostomia in certain patients undergoing fractionated radiation therapy of the head and neck region, although present data are insufficient to recommend the use of amifostine to prevent radiation therapy-associated mucositis (Hensley et al., 1999).

■ The results of a Phase II randomized trial of amifostine in patients with squamous cell carcinoma of the head and neck region who receive Carboplatin® (paraplatin) and radiation therapy suggest that amifostine may protect against radiation-induced toxicities. In this study, 86% of the patients who received radiation therapy (up to a total of 60 Gy) and

Carboplatin® (70 mg/m^2) experienced Grade 3 or 4 mucositis, whereas the group who received the same radiation and chemotherapy with the addition of amifostine had no patients who experienced mucositis. In addition, 17% of the patients who were pretreated with amifostine experienced Grade 2 xerostomia, whereas in the group without the amifostine 55% experienced xerostomia (Hensley et al., 1999).

■ A German study of patients receiving high-dose radioiodine shows amifostine reduces the damage to salivary glands and improves quality of life in patients with differentiated thyroid cancer, with 9 out of 25 patients in the control group reporting Grade I or II xerostomia versus 0 out of 25 patients in the amifostine group (Bohuslavizki et al., 1999).

Concern that amifostine could affect tumor response led to several studies.

■ In a rat study of marrow ablative chemotherapy for leukemia, cure rates were similar (10 out of 25 in the amifostine group versus 8 out of 11 in the control group) with an increase in protection against treatment-related mortality. In the control group, 9 out of 40 animals died of treatment-associated toxicity compared to none in the amifostine group (Martens & Hagenbeek, 1999).

■ Amifostine appears to reduce the incidence of radiation-induced esophagitis in patients receiving radiation therapy for lung cancer without affecting treatment efficacy. In a Phase II trial evaluating 25 stage IIIA and IIIB non-small-cell lung cancer patients, patients received amifostine (740 or 910 mg/m^2), followed by high-dose cisplatin (120 mg/m^2) on days 1 and 29, and vinblastine without amifostine weekly for five weeks. Following chemotherapy, patients received large-field thoracic irradiation to 60 Gy, preceded by amifostine at either 340 mg/m^2 or 200 mg/m^2 (Tannehill et al., 1997). No patient experienced Grade 3 or 4 esophagitis or required discontinuation of therapy because of hypotension. There was a 60% response rate with 1-, 2-, and 3-year response rates at 55%, 23%, and 23%, respectively (Mehta, 1998).

Several studies are currently underway to further assess amifostine's role in the prevention of radiation esophagitis (RTOG 95-03) and to assess its benefit in the reduction of mucositis in patients receiving chemotherapy and radiation therapy in rectal cancers.

OUTCOMES MEASURES

Follow-up measures for patients receiving radiosensitizing or radioprotective agents will be dependent on the disease state and the anatomic site to be treated, and should conform to standard follow-up for that clinical location. Quality of life measures that can be used to document the impact of radiosensitizers and radioprotectors are discussed in the individual site chapters.

OUTCOMES MANAGEMENT

Initially, amifostine, a radioprotector, was administered at higher doses (900 mg/m^2) to patients receiving cisplatin who required renal protection. These doses resulted in significant nausea and vomiting. When used concomitantly with radiation therapy, amifostine should be administered at 200 mg/m^2 in 10 ml normal saline by a 3-minute IV push infusion in a running IV, resulting in less-documented emesis and hypotension (Wagner, Radmard, & Schonekaes, 1999).

- Patients receiving either amifostine or a radiosensitizing agent should be treated with antiemetics such as HT3 receptor agonists (Kytril®, Zofran®) prior to administration.
- Amifostine may also cause significant hypotension.
- Hydrate patient prior to its administration with patient receiving the drug in a supine position. Blood pressure should be monitored immediately before the infusion and immediately afterward with continued monitoring at 15-minute intervals if clinically indicated.
- Radiosensitizers, such as metronidazole, also have significant emetogenic potential with metronidazole producing severe nausea, vomiting, and hypotension when administered to patients who consume alcohol.
- The use of radiosensitizers may also result in significant side effects of peripheral and central neuropathy. Phenytoin (Dilantin®) and dexamethasone may alleviate these symptoms.

Patients receiving hyperthermia must undergo careful evaluation prior to the procedure.

- No metal objects should be in the area to be heated (surgical clips, prosthesis, shrapnel, foreign bodies) because this will cause excessive heat and tissue injury.

- Pacemakers are also a contraindication for hyperthermia (Wojtas & Smith, 1997).
- The duration of a hyperthermic procedure can range from 60 to 90 minutes, so patient comfort must be assured. Vital signs must be monitored every 15 minutes.

The patient should be educated in side effects management:

- Meticulous skin care is an absolute must.
- In patients receiving whole-body hyperthermia, nausea and vomiting can occur for approximately 12 hours following treatment.
- Fever, cardiac arrhythmias, seizures, and disseminated intravascular coagulation (DIC) rarely occur, but have been reported.
- Liver damage in patients receiving hyperthermia at temperatures greater than 42°C has been reported.
- In patients receiving hyperthermia to the head and neck region, cataract development may occur due to inadvertent heating of the eye.

While the use of radiosensitizers has not gained favor in everyday clinical practice, research continues with these compounds in hopes that higher doses of therapy can safely be delivered with a minimum of toxicity. The use of chemotherapeutic agents as radiation sensitizers is more commonly seen in clinical practice and is addressed in Chapter 8, "Combined Modality Treatments." It is anticipated that radioprotectors such as amifostine will gain greater clinical acceptance as better side effects management is developed and increased clinical use is discovered.

REFERENCES

Abratt, R. P., Craighead, P., Reddi, V. B., & Sarembock, L. A. (1991). A prospective randomized trial of radiation with or without oral and extravesical misonidazole for bladder cancer. *British Journal of Cancer,* 64 (5), 968–970.

Beard, C., Buswell, L. Rose, M. A., Noll, L., Johnson, D., & Coleman, C. N. (1994). Phase II trial of external beam radiation with etanidazole (SR 2508) of the treatment of locally advanced prostate cancer. *International Journal of Radiation Oncology, Biology, and Physics,* 29 (3), 611–616.

Begg, A. C. (1998). Prediction of radiation response. In S. Leibel & T. Phillips (Eds.), *Textbook of radiation oncology* (pp. 55–68). Philadelphia: W. B. Saunders.

Bohuslavizki, K. H., Klutmann, S., Brenner, W., Mester, J., Henze, E., Clausen, M. (1998). Salivary gland protection by amifostine in high-dose radioiodine treatment: results of a double blind placebo controlled study. *Journal of Clinical Oncology*, 16 (11), 3542–3549.

Chang, E. L., Loeffler, J. S., Riese, N. E., Wen, P. Y., Alexander, E., III, Black, P. M., & Coleman, C. N. (1998). Survival results from a phase I study of etanidazole (SR2508) and radiotherapy in patients with malignant glioma. *International Journal of Radiation Oncology, Biology, and Physics*, 40 (1), 65–70.

Chen, A. Y., Choy, H., & Rothenberg, M. L. (1999). DNA topoisomerase I-targeting drugs as radiation sensitizers. *Oncology*, 13 (10), 39–46.

Constine, L. S., Zagars, G., Rubin, P., & Kligerman, M. (1986). Protection by WR-2721 of human bone marrow function following irradiation. *International Journal of Radiation Oncology, Biology, and Physics*, 12 (8), 1505–1508.

Creane, M., Seymour, C. B., Collucci, S., & Mothersill, C. (1999). Radiobiological effects of docetaxel (Taxotere®): A potential radiation sensitizer. *International Journal of Radiation Biology*, 75 (6), 731–737.

Curran, W. J. (1998). Radiation-induced toxicities: The role of radioprotectants. *Seminars in Radiation Oncology*, 8 (Suppl. 4), 2–4.

Doherty, N., Hancock, S. L., Kaye, S., Coleman, C. N., Shulman, L., Marquez, C., Mariscal, C., Rampling, R., Senan, S., & Roemeling, R. V. (1994). Muscle cramping in phase I clinical trials of tirapazamine (SR 4233) with and without radiation. *International Journal of Radiation Oncology, Biology, and Physics*, 29 (2), 379–382.

Eschwege, F., Sancho-Garnier, H., Chassagne, D., Brisgand, D., Guerra, M., Malaise, E. P., Bey, P., Busutti, L., Cionin, L., N'Guyen, T., Romanini, A., Chavaudra, J., & Hill, C. (1997). Results of a European randomized trial of Etanidazole combined with radiotherapy in head and neck carcinomas. *International Journal of Radiation Oncology, Biology, and Physics*, 39 (2), 275–281.

Fenton, B. M., Lord, E. M., Paoni, S. F., (2000). Enhancement of tumor perfusion and oxygenation by carbogen and nicotinamide during single and multifractionated irradiation. *Radiation Research*, 153 (1), 75–83.

Fischbach, A. J., Martz, K. L., Nelson, J. S., Griffin, T. W., Chang, C. H., Horton, J., & Nelson, D. F. (1991). Long-term survival in treated anaplastic astrocytomas. A report of combined RTOG/ECOG studies. *American Journal of Clinical Oncology*, 14 (5), 365–370.

Grigsby, P. W., Winter, K., Wasserman, T. H., Marcial, V., Rotman, M., Cooper, J., Keys, H., Asbell, S. O., & Phillips, T. L. (1999). Irradiation with or without misonidazole for patients with stage IIIB and IVA carcinoma of the cervix: Final results of RTOG 80-05. Radiation Therapy Oncology Group. *International Journal of Radiation Oncology, Biology, and Physics*, 44 (3), 513–517.

Haffty, B. G., Hurley, R. A., & Peters, L. G. (1999). Carcinoma of the larynx treated with hypofractionated radiation and hyperbaric oxygen: Long-term tumor control and complications. *International Journal of Radiation Oncology, Biology, and Physics*, 45 (1), 13–20.

Harapanhalli, R. S., Narra, V. R., Yaghmai, V., Azure, M. T., Goddu, S. M., Howell, R. W., Rao, D. V. (1994). Vitamins as radioprotectors in vivo. II. Protection by vitamin A and soybean oil against radiation damage caused by radionuclides. *Radiation Research*, 139 (1), 115–122.

Hensley, M. L., Schuter, L. M., Lindley, C., Meropol, N. J., Cohen, G. I., Broder, G., Gradisher, W. J., Green, D. M., Langdon, R. J., Jr., Mitchell, R. B., Negrin, R., Szatrowski, T. P., Thigpen, J. T., Von Hoff, D., Wasserman, T. H., Winer, E. P., & Pfister, D. G. (1999). American Society of Clinical Oncology clinical practice guideline for the use of chemotherapy and radiotherapy protectants. *Journal of Clinical Oncology*, 17 (10), 3333–3355.

Herscher, L. L., Hahn, S. M., Kroog, G., Pass, H., Temeck, B., Goldspiel, B., Cook, J., Mitchell, J. B., & Leibman, J. (1998). Phase I study of paclitaxel as a radiation sensitizer in the treatment of mesothelioma and non-small-cell lung cancer. *Journal of Clinical Oncology*, 16 (2), 635–641.

Jadhav, G. K., Bhanumathi, P., Uma Devi, P., Seetharamaiah, T., Vidyasagar, M. S., Rao, K. K., Hospet, C. S., & Solomon, J. G. (1998). Possible role of glutathione in predicting radiotherapy response of cervical cancer. *International Journal of Radiation Oncology, Biology, and Physics*, 41 (1), 3–5.

Kligerman, M. M., Turrisi, A. T., Urtasun, R. C., Norfleet, A. L., Phillips, T. L., Barkley, T., & Rubin, P. (1988). Final report on phase I trial of WR-2721 before protracted fractionated radiation therapy. *International Journal of Radiation Oncology, Biology, and Physics*, 14 (6), 1119–1122.

Komarnicky, L. T., Phillips, T. L., Martz, K., Asbell, S., Isaacson, S., & Urtasun, R. (1991). A randomized phase III protocol for the evaluation of misonidazole combined radiation in the treatment of patients with brain metastases (RTOG-7916). *International Journal of Radiation Oncology, Biology, and Physics*, 20 (1), 53–58.

Lawton, C. A., Coleman, C. N., Buzydlowski, J. W., Forman, J. D., Marcial, V. A., DelRowe, J. D., & Rotman, M. (1996). Results of a phase II trial external beam radiation with etanidazole (SR 2508) for the treatment of locally advanced prostate cancer (RTOG Protocol 90-20). *International Journal of Radiation Oncology, Biology, and Physics*, 36 (3), 673–680.

Lee, D. J., Cosmatos, D., Marcial, V. A., Fu, K. K., Rotman, M., Cooper, J. S., Ortiz, H. G., Beitler, J. J., Abrams, R. A., Curran, W. J., Coleman, C. N., & Wasserman, T. (1995). Results of an RTOG phase III trial (RTOG 85-27) comparing radiotherapy plus etanidazole with radiotherapy alone for locally advanced head and neck carcinomas. *International Journal of Radiation Oncology, Biology, and Physics*, 32 (3), 567–576.

Martens, A. C., & Hagenbeek, A. (1999). Amifostine (WR 2721) for dose escalation in marrow-ablative treatment of leukaemia. *European Journal of Cancer*, 35 (4), 634–640.

Mehta, M. P. (1998). Protection of normal tissues from the cytoxic effects of radiation therapy: Focus on amifostine. *Seminars in Radiation Oncology*, 8 (4 Suppl. 1), 14–16.

Mukundan, H. Bahadur, A. K., Kumar, A., Sardana, S., Naik, S. L., Ray, A., & Sharma, B. K. (1999). Glutathione level and its relation to radiation therapy in patients with cancer of the uterine cervix. *International Journal of Radiation Oncology, Biology, and Physics*, 37 (9), 859–864.

Myerson, R., Moros, E., & Roti Roti, J. (1997). Hyperthermia. In C. Perez & L. Brady (Eds.), *Principles and practice of radiation oncology*, (3rd ed., pp. 637–683). Philadelphia: Lippincott-Raven.

Narra, V. R., Harapanhalli, R. S., Howell, R. W., Sastry, K. S., & Rao, D. V. (1994). Vitamins as radioprotectors in vivo. I. Protection by vitamin C against internal radionuclides in mouse testes: Implications to the mechanisms of damage caused by the Auger effect. *Radiation Research*, 147 (3), 394–399.

Noll, L. & Riese, N. (1997). Chemical modifiers of radiation therapy. In K. Dow, J. Bucholtz, R. Iwamoto, V. Fieler, & L. Hilderley (Eds.), *Nursing care in radiation oncology* (2nd ed., pp. 47–56). Philadelphia: W. B. Saunders.

Overgaard, J., Hansen, H. S., Overgaard, M., Bastholt, L., Berthelsen, A., Specht, L., Lindelov, B., & Jorgensen, K. (1998). A randomized double-blind phase III study of nimorazole as hypoxic radiosensitizer of primary radiotherapy in supraglottic larynx and pharynx carcinoma. Results of the Danish Head and Neck Cancer Study (DAHANCA) Protocol 5-85. *Radiotherapeutic Oncology*, 46 (2), 135–146.

Phillips, T. L., Wasserman, T. H., Johnson, R. J. (1981). Final report on the United States phase I clinical trials of the hypoxic cell radiosensitizer misonidazole (RO-07-0582 NSC #261037). *Cancer*, 48, p. 1697.

Preisler, V. K., Stopper, H., Schindler, D. Friedl, R., Pfreundner, L., Hoppe, F., & Hagen, R. (1998). Cytotoxic and genotoxic effects of paclitaxel (Taxol®) and radiation in a squamous cell carcinoma cell line of the larynx. *Otolaryngology*, 118 (4), 600–605.

Raaphoorst, G. P., Wand, G., Stewart, D., & Ng, C. E. (1996). Concomitant low-dose rate irradiation and cisplatin treatment in ovarian carcinomas cell lines sensitive and resistant to cisplatin treatment. *International Journal of Radiation Biology*, 69 (5), 623–631.

Rich, T. A. (1999). Infusional chemoradiation for rectal and anal cancers. *Oncology*, 13 (10), 131–134.

Riese, N. E., Buswell, L., Noll, L., Pajak, T. F., Stetz, J., Lee, D. J., & Coleman, C. N. (1997). Pharmacokinetic monitoring and dose modification of etanidazole in the RTOG 85-27 phase III head and neck trial. *International Journal of Radiation Oncology, Biology, and Physics*, 39 (4), 855–858.

Rowkinsky, E. K. (1999). Novel radiation sensitizers targeting tissue hypoxia. *Oncology*, 13 (10), 61–70.

Scofield, R., Leibman, M., & Popkin, J. (1991). Multimodal therapy. In S. Baird, R. McCorkle, & M. Grant (Eds.), *Cancer nursing—A comprehensive textbook* (pp. 344–354). Philadelphia: W. B. Saunders.

Simpson, J. R., Bauer, M., Perez, C. A., Wasserman, T. H., Emami, B., Doggett, R. L., Byhardt, R. W., Phillips, T. L., & Mowry, P. A. (1989). Radiation therapy alone or combined with misonidazole in the treatment of locally advanced non-oat-cell lung cancer: Report of an RTOG prospective randomized trial. *International Journal of Radiation Oncology, Biology, and Physics*, 16 (6), 1483–1491.

Sitton, E. (1998). Nursing implications of radiation therapy. In J. Itano & K. Taoka (Eds.), *Core curriculum in oncology nursing* (pp. 616–629). Philadelphia: W. B. Saunders.

Stewart, D. J., Dahrouge, S., Agboola, O., & Girard, A. (1997). Cranial radiation and concomitant cisplatin and mitomycin-C plus resistance modulators for malignant gliomas. *Journal of Neuro-oncology*, 32 (2), 161–168.

Tannehill, S. P., Mehta, M. P., Larson, M., Storer, B., Pellet, J., Kinsella, T. J., & Schiller, J. H. (1997). Effect of amifostine on toxicities associated with sequential chemotherapy and radiation therapy for unresectable non-small-cell lung cancer: Results of a phase II trial. *Journal of Clinical Oncology*, 15 (8), 2850–2857.

Viele, C. S., & Holmes, B. C. (1998). Amifostine: Drug profile and nursing implications of the first pancytoprotectant. *Oncology Nursing Forum*, 25 (3), 515–523.

Wagner, W., Prott, F. J., Schonekas, K. (1998). Amifostine: a radioprotector in locally advanced head and neck tumors. *Oncology Reports*, 5, 1255–1257.

Wagner, W., Radmard, A., & Schonekaes, K. G. (1999). A newer administration schedule for amifostine as a radioprotector in cancer therapy. *Anticancer Research*, 3B, 2281–2283.

Wasserman, T., Chapman, J. D., Coleman, C. N., & Kligerman, M. (1998). Chemical modifiers of radiation. In C. Perez & L. Brady (Eds.), *Principles and practice of radiation oncology* (3rd ed., pp. 685–704). Philadelphia: Lippincott-Raven.

Wojtas, F., & Smith, R. (1997). Hyperthermia and intraoperative radiation therapy. In K. Dow, J. Bucholtz, R. Iwamoto, V. Fieler, & L. Hilderley (Eds.), *Nursing care in radiation oncology* (2nd ed., pp. 36–46). Philadelphia: W. B. Saunders.

CHAPTER 8

COMBINED MODALITY TREATMENTS

Cynthia W. Martin, ANP, MSN, RN, CS, AOCN
Thomas Whitehead, MD

PURPOSE OF COMBINED MODALITY TREATMENTS

Combined modality treatments have been the standard of care for many cancers for years. Modern chemoradiation began in the 1950s with the belief that the combination of local and systemic therapies enhances the potential of local control and long-term survival. The use of one of these early agents, 5-fluorouracil (5-FU), in combination with radiation therapy continues today, and as a combined modality treatment it remains a standard of care for many anal and rectal cancers when used in combination with surgery (Rich, 1999). One of the first Radiation Therapy Oncology Group (RTOG) studies was a randomized study comparing radiotherapy alone versus radiotherapy and methotrexate in the treatment of head and neck cancers (John, 1998). Increasing efforts for organ preservation and a decrease in normal tissue toxicity (breast, anus, head and neck, esophagus) have also driven the need for combined modality treatment, with combined therapies showing improved or similar cure rates as compared to single modality treatments such as large surgical resection (John, 1998).

Tumors may be resistant to chemotherapy or radiation therapy alone for a variety of reasons as follows:

- Inability of the treatment to reach the tumor cells can be a significant problem in cancer therapy. This could be the result of poor blood supply to the tumor, poorly vascularized areas, tumor cells in "sanctuary sites" of the body where cytotoxic drugs may not reach them, such as the central nervous system (CNS), or tumors next to vital structures, which limits the ability to remove them surgically or to deliver high enough doses to control them with radiation.

- Solid tumors are likely to develop hypoxic areas that are more resistant to radiation, which may be secondary to a large tumor volume, prior surgical intervention, or necrosis. The poor vascular access that made these cells hypoxic may also mean that they are less likely to be affected by cytotoxic drugs in circulation. Reduction in the tumor mass by chemotherapy and/or fractionated radiation therapy may improve blood supply and lead to reoxygenation of the cells, making them more sensitive (Rotman, Aziz, & Wasserman, 1997).

- The presence of subclinical tumor cells outside the confines of the surgical margin or radiation field means that the malignant cells cannot be affected by these local therapies and chemotherapy is relied on to destroy the malignant cells in this setting. Surgery and radiation do not affect cells that are outside the surgical area or the radiation field. These are often microscopic foci and chemotherapy is relied upon to destroy the malignant cells in this setting.

Within a given tumor, a wide variety of response and resistance to therapy occurs. Metastatic phenotypes in the tumor have been experimentally shown to occur over time.

- The Goldie-Coleman hypothesis assumes that drug-resistant and radioresistant populations of cells arise spontaneously according to the number of clonogenic cells present and the frequency of mutations and that the early eradication of these resistant cells with a second modality may actually cause reduction of clonogenic cells and the eventual number of mutations (Rotman et al., 1997).

- However, cross-resistance to chemotherapy and radiation therapy is common. This potential insensitivity of the cells to the therapy mandates the use of a variety of treatment modalities for best results.

■ Spatial cooperation occurs when one treatment modality is able to treat disease at one site while at another site, disease is eradicated by a second modality of treatment with improved overall results. In spatial cooperation, there is *no* interaction between the two modalities (Rotman et al., 1997).

Radiation therapy and chemotherapy kill tumor cells in an exponential fashion. Larger tumors are more difficult to completely eradicate than smaller ones, a relationship occurring between the volume of tumor and amount of treatment needed to destroy the tumor.

■ Combined modality therapy is the treatment of choice in many large, locally advanced tumors. Hyperfractionation (multiple smaller fractions of radiation therapy) has been one way to deliver radiation therapy in bulky lesions. It results in killing a portion of the tumor cells with each dose and allowing reoxygenation to increase sensitivity for the next dose, but not allowing tumor regrowth between doses.

Increased toxicity caused by the dose of therapy needed to eradicate tumor cells as well as host intolerance to the therapy often hampers the ability to deliver doses high enough to cause tumor cell death without unacceptable side effects.

■ Combined modality treatment may shorten treatment time or reduce the dose for either or both the chemotherapy and the radiation therapy, thus potentially reducing treatment-associated toxicity.

■ The use of supportive measures during treatment, such as growth factors, antibiotics, IV, or enteral alimentation and hydration, greatly reduces the toxicities experienced under treatment.

As in all therapies, the treatment goals for combined modality therapy in any stage of disease may be cure, local control, or palliation.

■ In patients who cannot tolerate the rigors of cancer therapy, the goal is one of supportive care only.

■ Radiation and chemotherapy given in subtoxic doses may act as palliative agents to reduce pain, diminish disfigurement, and lessen symptoms without the intensive regimens reserved for the goal of cure.

Timing of Combined Modality Therapy

Many current chemotherapy medications function as radiosensitizers as well as cytotoxic agents. The timing of the administration of the chemotherapy medication and radiation therapy depends on the drug used and the disease to be treated and may be termed sequential, concurrent, or alternating. In choosing the timing of the treatment, care is taken to reduce the toxicity of therapy while increasing its therapeutic benefit. The rationale for the differing administration schedules includes additive killing, whereby the drug kills tumor cells not otherwise killed by radiation or synergistic killing; thus more tumor cells are killed by the combination than by any of the agents alone.

- ■ Neoadjuvant therapy is the use of treatment, generally chemotherapy, prior to definitive treatment such as surgery. It is used to allow a higher systemic dose up front to decrease possible metastases or to downstage the tumor making it easier to remove. Examples of neoadjuvant therapy include up front chemotherapy in inflammatory breast cancer and radiation prior to surgery in rectal cancer.

- ■ Adjuvant therapy is given to "help" the main treatment, generally surgery. It is also given to eradicate microscopic local-regional or distant disease and decrease the risk of later recurrence.

- ■ Sequential Therapy—The goal of treatment is to administer full-dose radiation therapy and a full course of chemotherapy. With sequential therapy, a full course of chemotherapy and a full course of radiation therapy are administered in time, usually one following the other. The toxicity of the treatment is limited by giving the modalities separately and the intensity of the treatment is reduced.

- ■ Simultaneous/Concomitant Therapy—Combined radiation therapy and chemotherapy has been studied extensively in an effort to improve control and survival rates of solid tumors (Colin, 1994). Although the increased toxicity of simultaneous therapy is its greatest disadvantage, the simultaneous delivery of chemotherapy and radiation therapy has its advantages. With this delivery schedule, both modalities can be given with greater intensity over a shorter period of time and the development of cross-resistant cells is minimized, since there is zero time interval between modalities.

- Cisplatin, 5-FU, mitomycin C, etoposide, and hydroxyurea are particularly efficient in sensitizing radiation treatment in order to obtain supraadditive effect (Colin, 1994).

■ Alternating Therapies—With this treatment schedule, chemotherapy is given intermittently every 3 to 4 weeks with radiation therapy given between successive courses of chemotherapy. Toxicity is reduced by the temporal separation.

■ Circadian Therapy—Selective environmental pressure to keep 24-hour time (circadian rhythm) seems to affect various biologic functions. Coordination of cancer therapies is being studied with respect to response and outcome (Wood & Hrushesky, 1995).

- Scheduling of the dosing of biotherapies may affect tumor cure probabilities, although further research is needed (Jones & Dale, 1999).

- The toxicities of bolus 5-FU versus infusional 5-FU in patients with advanced rectal cancer receiving concurrent radiation therapy were studied, with patients receiving infusional 5-FU being able to withstand twice the dose intensity as those receiving bolus therapy. In the infusional group, hematological and gastrointestinal (frequency and severity of diarrhea and weight loss) toxicities were less, with skin reactions the same in both groups. Local recurrence rates of 3.8% and distant recurrence frequency of 34.6% were comparable in both groups (Thrall, Wood, King, Rivera, & Hrushesky, 2000).

- Camptothecins (CPTs) are potent radiosensitizers in vivo, but the optimal schedule of administration is unknown. In mouse studies with mammary and gastrointestinal cancers, the effects of radiation therapy combined with 9-aminocamptothecin (9-AC) was studied. Given in single doses, the radiation therapy and 9-AC resulted in little radiosensitization compared to the repeated 9-AC schedule combined with fractionated radiation (tumor regrowth in 7.1 days vs. 6.6 days, respectively). Toxicity was comparable in both groups and appeared to be time dependent regardless of whether the drug was delivered in one dose or several (Kirichenko & Rich, 1999). Further study on the timing of these agents is needed in human trials.

NEW CHEMOTHERAPY AND OTHER AGENTS

New methods of administration including intrahepatic artery infusion pumps, 24-hour delivery systems, and encapsulating drugs in li-
posomes (Doxil®) are new delivery systems aimed at increasing delivery of the drug to the tissue while limiting normal tissue toxicity.

■ In Phase I dose escalation trials, Doxil® (liposomal doxorubicin) was administered concurrently with conventionally
fractionated radiation therapy to patients with non-small-cell
lung cancer and head and neck cancer. Oral/pharyngeal mucositis was the dose-limiting toxicity for the head and neck
patients while in-field skin toxicity was slightly increased in
both patient groups. Hematologic toxicity was minimal. Complete response rate was 21% in the lung cancer group and 75%
in the head and neck cancer group (p = 0.049) (Koukourakis,
Koukourakis, Giatromanolaki, et al., 1999).

While currently not given in conjunction with radiation therapy,
monoclonal antibodies such as Rituxan® and Herceptin® target specific tumor proteins while sparing normal cells.

■ Rituxan® (rituximab), a chimeric mouse/human im-
munoglobulin IGI kappa anti-CD 20 antibody, is currently
indicated for single-agent treatment of relapsed or refractory CD-20 positive, B-cell, low-grade or follicular non-
Hodgkin's lymphoma.
■ The recommended dose is 375 mg/m^2 administered weekly
times 4 by intravenous infusion.
■ Treatment is usually well tolerated and is administered on
an outpatient basis. Common side effects include fevers,
chills, and hypotension and they are usually Grade I or II.
■ In a Phase II single-agent clinical trial, overall response rate
was 50% with a median time to progression in responders of
10.2 months. In a larger multicenter trial, the overall response rate was 48% with a median time to progression of
13.2 months. Combination studies have been performed
with interferon, CHOP combination (cyclophosphamide,
doxorubicin, vincristine, and prednisone), and radioim-
munotherapy (Grillo-Lopez et al., 1999).

HER2/neu proto-oncogene is overexpressed by 25% to 30% of
patients with breast cancer. Herceptin® (trastuzumab) is currently
indicated in the treatment of metastatic breast cancer in women who

express the HER2/neu (human epidermal growth factor receptor 2) protein on the surface of the breast cancer cell.

■ Phase II single-agent studies showed an 11.6% increase in overall response rate in women with widespread metastatic disease (Baselga et al., 1999). When combined with pacli- taxel (Taxol®), response rates increased to 44% (Peyrot, 1999). Herceptin is also indicated in second and third line therapy when given in combination with doxorubicin and cy- clophosphamide with a higher response rate reported than with chemotherapy given alone (Lebwolhl & Canetta, 1999).

■ Reported toxicities are mild in chemotherapy naïve patients and include fever and chills, especially in the first infusion, which resolved easily with diphenhydramine and acetamin- ophen, slight to moderate nausea, mild diarrhea, mild hair loss, mouth sores, neutropenia, and thrombocytopenia (Peyrot, 1999). In early clinical studies, cardiomyopathy was reported and may be worse in patients who have received previous or concurrent anthracyclines (Ewer, Gibbs, Swaf- ford, & Benjamin, 1999).

■ Herceptin alone has shown clinical activity in androgen- dependent prostate cancers and has at least an additive effect on growth in combination with paclitaxel (Taxol®) in both androgen-dependent and androgen-independent tumors, although response to Herceptin® did not correlate to PSA levels (Agus et al., 1999).

Obliteration of tumor vasculature is an effective means of achieving tumor regression. Combined with radiation therapy, an- tiangiogenic agents are now entering clinical trials.

■ Ionizing radiation activates the inflammatory cascade and increases the procoagulative state within blood vessels of both tumors and normal tissues. Proinflammatory and pro- thrombotic biologic response modifiers given concurrently with radiation therapy are known to induce vascular obliter- ation and necrosis of tumors. Further study is needed to as- sess the effects of radiation therapy on tumors (Hallahan, Chen, Teng, & Cmelak, 1999).

Newer radiosensitizing agents, along with enhanced radiation therapy techniques such as three-dimensional radiotherapy plan- ning and conformal radiotherapy treatment, offer hope for the future that even more patients can benefit from combined modality ther- apy with acceptable toxicity (Rich, 1999).

EXPECTED OUTCOMES

The goals of combined modality treatments will depend on the stage of the disease. Patients with advanced disease may obtain palliation of side effects of the disease, whereas patients with early-stage disease may obtain good cancer control or cure. With careful monitoring of treatment toxicities, enhancement of the tumor's response to treatment may be obtained with tolerable side effects. In downstaging of the tumor, preservation of organ function may be possible with less radical surgery being necessary for the same outcome. The main goal is increased overall survival and enhanced quality of life (Table 8–1).

TABLE 8–1   EXPECTED OUTCOMES WITH COMBINED TREATMENT MODALITIES—RADIATION AND CHEMOTHERAPY

Modality	Outcomes	Barriers
Preoperative Radiation	Decreasing the tumor size, thus increasing the possibility of resectability.	May interfere with normal tissue healing.
	Decreasing the number of viable cells within the operative field, thus lessening tumor implantation/metastases.	
Postoperative Radiation	Eliminating residual tumor cells.	Delay in the initiation of radiation treatments.
		Vascular changes may impede radiation effects by decreasing oxygen supply.
Chemotherapy	Adjuvant chemotherapy destroys cells during radiation, often enhancing the effects of radiation.	Can potentiate side effects.
	Neoadjuvant chemotherapy destroys cells before irradiation, thus reducing the number of cancer cells needing to be eliminated.	

OUTCOMES MEASURES

Toxicity assessment of patients undergoing combined modality therapies is crucial. Normal tissue responses may be enhanced, particularly in concomitant regimens, and local toxicities and fatigue are often greatly exaggerated. Assessments such as monitoring the complete blood count and weight need to be performed more frequently, since acute toxicities may occur earlier in the course of treatment and may be more severe in nature. When to evaluate the efficacy of treatment and what type of diagnostic test is required is dependent on the disease site treated and the chemotherapeutic agents used. Side effects management of chemotherapy agents is a multidisciplinary task (Table 8–2).

OUTCOMES MANAGEMENT

The management of patients undergoing combined modality treatment is often a complex and multidisciplinary process. The medical oncology team, while primarily responsible for chemotherapy-associated toxicities, depends on the watchful eyes of the radiation team to assess for side effects as well. From a radiation oncology perspective, toxicity management is dependent on the antineoplastic agents used and the body sites under treatment, the treatment volume, dose rate, and overall total dose of radiation given. As a general rule, fatigue will be magnified in patients receiving chemotherapy with their radiation. Other side effects and their management are listed in Table 8–2.

Drug delivery must be designed for the particular tumor site and must be tailored to the individual patient to limit toxicity.

Combined modality treatments with chemotherapy and radiation therapy are important treatment strategies for cancer patients in all phases of their illness. Toxicities are increased, but therapeutic benefit should be increased also if the treatment is to be worthwhile. Many drug combinations are under study with newer ones being developed constantly. New drug delivery systems including continuous infusion pumps, liposomal encapsulation, and monoclonal antibodies are the wave of the future in enhancing therapeutic benefit while decreasing treatment-related toxicity.

TABLE 8–2 COMBINED MODALITY TOXICITY MANAGEMENT

Chemotherapy Agents Commonly Used in Combination with Radiation Therapy	Common Disease Sites for Which These Agents Are Used	Side Effects Associated with the Use of These Agents	Management of the Side Effects Associated with the Use of These Agents
Carboplatin (Paraplatin®)	Small cell and non-small-cell lung, ovarian nasopharynx	Nausea and vomiting, cytopenia	Antiemetics (usually requires HT-3 antagonists), careful hematologic monitoring
Cisplatin (Platinol®)	Small cell and non-small-cell lung, esophageal	Nausea and vomiting (severe), cytopenia, renal dysfunction	Antiemetics (usually requires HT-3 antagonists), careful hematologic and renal function monitoring (patients may benefit by growth factors)
Docetaxel (Taxotere®)	Head and neck, non-small-cell lung, breast	Hypersensitivity (requires premeditation with steroids), cytopenia, liver failure, fluid retention, asthenia, nail changes, myalgia, stomatitis, nausea and vomiting, diarrhea	Antiemetics (usually requires HT-3 antagonists), careful monitoring of blood counts and liver profile (patients may benefit by growth factors), meticulous oral care and local measures for comfort, analgesics
Doxorubicin (Adriamycin®, Doxil®)	Breast	Nausea and vomiting, alopecia, cytopenia, extravasation necrosis, radiation recall, intensified skin reaction, cardiomyopathy	Antiemetics (usually requires HT-3 antagonists), careful hematologic monitoring, meticulous skin care
Etoposide (VP16, Vepesid®)	Small cell lung	Nausea and vomiting, cytopenia	Antiemetics, careful hematologic monitoring

Drug	Uses	Side Effects	Nursing Considerations
5-Fluorouracil (5-FU)	Anal, rectal, pancreas	Nausea and vomiting, increased skin sensitivity and reaction, vein darkening over the site of infusion, mild alopecia, oral mucositis, stomatitis, esophagitis, cytopenia, diarrhea	Maintain adequate hydration, antiemetics (HT-3 antagonists rarely necessary), meticulous skin care in the treatment area, local measures for oral care, analgesics, monitor blood counts, antidiarrheals such as Immodium®
Hydroxyurea (Hydrea®)	Cervix, head and neck	Cytopenia	Careful hematologic monitoring
Irinotecan (Camptosar®)	Head and neck, colon	Diarrhea, nausea and vomiting, alopecia, cytopenia, asthenia, anorexia	Antidiarrheals (Immodium®), antiemetics, careful hematologic monitoring, maintain hydration, frequent weights, nutritional monitoring
Paclitaxel (Taxol®)	Lung (small cell and non-small-cell), esophageal, ovarian, unknown primary, head and neck, breast, astrocytoma, melanoma, thyroid	Alopecia, nausea and vomiting, cytopenia, peripheral neuropathy (may be severe), arthralgias, hypersensitivity (requires premedication with steroids)	Antiemetics (usually requires HT-3 antagonists), careful monitoring of blood counts (patients may benefit by growth factors), antihistamines for arthralgias

REFERENCES

Agus, D. B., Scher, H. I., Higgins, B., Fox, W. D., Heller, G. Fazzari, M., Cordon-Cardo, C., & Golde, D. W. (1999). Response of prostate cancer to anti-Her2neu antibody in androgen-dependent and independent human xenograft models. *Cancer Research*, 59 (19), 4761–4764.

Baselga, J., Tripathy, D., Mendelsohn, J., Baughman, S., Benz, C. C., Dantis, L., Sklarin, N. T., Seidman, A. D., Hudis, C. A., Moore, J., Rosen, P. P., Twaddell, T., Henderson, I. C., & Norton, L. (1999). Phase II study of weekly intravenous trastuzumab (Herceptin) in patients with HER2/neu-overexpressing metastatic breast cancer. *Seminars in Oncology*, 26 (4) (Suppl. 12), 78–83.

Colin, P. H. (1994). Concomitant chemotherapy and radiotherapy: Theoretical basis and clinical experience. *Anticancer Research*, 14 (6A), 2357–2361.

Ewer, M. S., Gibbs, H. R., Swafford, J., & Benjamin, R. S. (1999). Cardiotoxicity in patients receiving trastuzumab (Herceptin): Primary toxicity, synergistic or sequential stress or surveillance artifact? *Seminars in Oncology*, 26 (4) (Suppl. 12), 96–101.

Grillo-Lopez, A. J., White, C. A., Varns, C., Shen, D., Wei, A., McClure, A., & Dallaire, B. K. (1999). Overview of the clinical development of rituximab: First monoclonal antibody approved for the treatment of lymphoma. *Seminars in Oncology*, 26 (5) (Suppl. 14), 66–73.

Hallahan, D. E., Chen, A. Y., Teng, M., & Cmelak, A. J. (1999). Drug-radiation interactions in tumor blood vessels. *Oncology (Huntington)*, 13 (10) (Suppl. 5), 71–77.

John, M. (1998). Radiotherapy and chemotherapy. In S. Leibel & T. Phillips (Eds.), *Textbook of radiation oncology* (pp. 69–89). Philadelphia: W. B. Saunders.

Jones, B., & Dale, R. G. (1999). Inclusion of molecular biotherapies with radical radiotherapy: Modeling of combined modality treatment schedules. *International Journal of Radiation Oncology, Biology, Physics*, 45 (4), 1025–1034.

Kirichenko, A. V., & Rich, T. A. (1999). Radiation enhancement by 9-aminocamptothecin: The effect of fractionation and timing of administration. *International Journal of Radiation Oncology, Biology, Physics*, 44 (3), 659–664.

Koukourakis, M. I., Koukouraki, S., Giatromanolaki, A., Archimandritis, S. C., Skarlatos, J., Beroukas, K., Bizakis, J. G., Retalis, G., Karkavitasas, N., & Helidonis, E. S. (1999). Liposomal doxorubicin and conventionally fractionated radiotherapy in the treatment of locally advanced non-small-cell lung cancer and head and neck cancer. *Journal of Clinical Oncology*, 17 (11), 3512–3521.

Lebwolhl, D. E., & Canetta, R. (1999). New developments in chemotherapy of advanced breast cancer. *Annals of Oncology*, 10 (Suppl. 6), 139–146.

Perry, M. (Ed.) 1997. *The Chemotherapy Source Book 2nd Edition*. Baltimore: Williams & Wilkins.

Peyrot, J. (1999). Herceptin. *Oncology Nursing Forum*, 26 (3), 515–516.

Rich, T. A. (1999). Infusional chemoradiation for rectal and anal cancers. *Oncology*, 13 (10), 131–134.

Rotman, M., Aziz, H., & Wasserman, T. (1997). Chemotherapy and irradiation. In C. Perez & L. Brady (Eds.), *Principles and practice of radiation oncology* (3rd ed., pp. 705–722). Philadelphia: Lippincott-Raven.

Thrall, M. M., Wood, P., King, V., Rivera, W., & Hrushesky, W. (2000). Investigation of the comparative toxicity of 5FU bolus versus 5FU continuous infusion circadian chemotherapy with concurrent radiation therapy in locally advanced rectal cancer. *International Journal of Radiation Oncology, Biology, Physics*, 46 (4), 873–881.

Wood, P. A., & Hrushesky, W. J. (1995). Biological perspectives of circadian cancer therapy. *Journal of Infusional Chemotherapy*, 5 (4), 182–190.

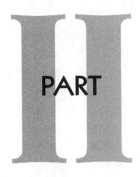

PART

TREATMENT RELATED OUTCOMES

CHAPTER 9

BRAIN MALIGNANCIES

Terri Armstrong, RN, MS, ANP, CS
Mark R. Gilbert, MD
Benjain Movsas, MD

PROBLEM

- Approximately 114,000 people were diagnosed with a primary or metastatic brain or spinal cord tumor in 1997. Of these, 80,000 were metastatic tumors and 34,000 were primary brain tumors (Central Brain Tumor Registry of the United States, 1998; Laws, 1993).
- The annual incidence rate in the United States for all primary brain tumors is 11.5 per 100,000 population (Central Brain Tumor Registry of the United States, 1998).
- The male to female ratio is 1:1 for all primary brain tumors.
- Brain tumors are the second most common cause of cancer death in people ages 15 to 34, the fourth most common cause of cancer death in males ages 35 to 54, and the ninth leading cause of cancer death in all White Americans (Cancer Statistics, 1998).

PRIMARY BENIGN BRAIN TUMORS

- Benign tumors of the brain constitute about 40% of all primary brain neoplasms. This is an annual incidence rate of 4.6 per 100,000 population.

- Benign tumors are composed of slow-growing cells and rarely spread. A tumor that is composed of slow-growing cells but located in vital areas can be life-threatening.
- Benign tumors of the brain include meningiomas, acoustic neuromas, and low-grade forms of tumors primarily thought of as malignant including astrocytomas, ependymomas, and oligodendrogliomas.

PRIMARY MALIGNANT BRAIN TUMORS

- Primary malignant tumors of the brain represent 1.4% of all cancers diagnosed in the United States.
- Primary malignant brain tumors cause 2.4% or 13,300 of the deaths due to cancer in the United States each year.
- Primary malignant tumors are usually invasive and composed of rapidly proliferating cells.
- Primary tumors rarely spread outside of the central nervous system.
- The most common type of primary malignant tumor in adults is the glioblastoma multiforme.

METASTATIC BRAIN TUMORS

- Metastatic brain tumors begin growing elsewhere in the body and then travel to the brain.
- Metastatic tumors are by far the most common cause of brain cancer, having an incidence rate higher than all types of primary brain tumors combined.
- The most common types of tumors that metastasize to the brain are lung, breast, renal, melanoma, and colon cancer.
- Certain cancers, such as sarcoma, ovarian, prostate, and bladder primaries, seldom metastasize to the brain.

ASSESSMENT

RISK FACTORS

- Approximately 15% of patients with tumors of the central nervous system have a family history of cancer (Mahaley, Mettlin, Natarajan, Laws, & Peace, 1989).
- Certain hereditary and congenital diseases are known to carry an increased risk for CNS tumors. These include neu-

rofibromatosis (Blatt, Jaffe, Deutsch, & Adkins, 1986), ataxia telangiectasia (Swift et al., 1986), Gorlin syndrome and Turcot syndrome (Bolande, 1989), and Li-Fraumeni tumor syndrome (Lynch et al., 1989).

■ Exposure to ionizing radiation has been implicated in the development of central nervous system tumors. This exposure has been seen in utero (Bithell & Stewart, 1975), low-dose delivery in children (Ron et al., 1988), and adults (Martin, Yu, Henderson, & Benton, 1983).

■ Risk factors commonly associated with other cancer sites, such as dietary factors, ingestion of alcohol, or smoking cigarettes, have not shown to be related to the development of primary brain tumors.

■ Certain occupational groups carry a higher risk of developing primary malignant gliomas. These include farming and farm residence, electrical worker, oil refining, rubber manufacturing, airplane manufacturing, machining, and chemical or pharmaceutical industries. Exposure to benzenes and other chemical compounds are thought to be the offending agents (Thomas et al., 1987).

■ Exposure to loud noise has been shown to be a risk factor for acoustic neroma (Preston-Martin, Thomas, Henderson, Bernstein, & Wright, 1989).

■ Less information is known about metastatic brain tumors. One study showed that metastases were more common in men than women (9.7 for men vs. 7.1 for women per 100,000) (Walker, Robins, & Weinfeld, 1985).

PREVENTION, SCREENING, PRESENTING SYMPTOMS, AND DIAGNOSTIC TESTS

Primary Benign and Malignant Brain Tumors

■ Currently there are no recommended guidelines for screening for primary tumors of the brain.

■ Initial evaluation should include the following:
  • Complete history and physical examination.
  • Karnofsky Performance Status (KPS)—an individual's performance status should be evaluated when determining the method of evaluation and treatment.
  • Neuroimaging studies: typically, a CAT scan with and without contrast is initially performed to reveal the lesion. This is often followed by Magnetic Resonance Imaging (MRI) of the brain with and without gadolinium. This

allows for better visualization of the brain parenchyma and delineation of the tumor's borders.

■ Additional diagnostic studies should be undertaken if:
- The lesion has characteristics typical of metastatic disease (i.e., round in appearance, increased edema, location at the gray-white junction).
- The lesion is in an area where surgical intervention would carry a significant risk.
- The lesion has the appearance of other neurologic diseases (i.e., multiple sclerosis, Lyme disease, or sarcoidosis).

■ These studies include Lyme titer, sedimentation rate, immunoelectrophoresis and cerebrospinal fluid to rule out Lyme disease, connective tissue disease such as lupus, or multiple sclerosis, respectively.

■ Specific criteria for presentation and diagnosis of particular tumors follow:

Gliomas

Low-Grade Astrocytoma

- Low-grade astrocytomas constitute approximately 15% of brain tumors in adults (Guthrie & Laws, 1990).
- The median age of patients with low-grade astrocytomas is 35 (Morantz, 1997).
- The frontal lobe is the most common location (Zulch, 1986).
- Headache, lethargy, and personality change are the most common symptoms.
- The CT scan typically reveals a nonenhancing lesion. MRI is thought to be more sensitive than CT and usually reveals a low intensity area on the T_1 images, rarely showing contrast-enhancement (Morantz, 1997).
- Histopathologic features include increased number of astrocytes with no mitotic figures seen.

Malignant Astrocytoma

- Glioblastomas comprise approximately 27.7% of all cases of primary brain tumors and anaplastic astrocytomas comprise 26.6% (Mahaley et al., 1989).
- The mean age of patients diagnosed with glioblastoma is 62, whereas the mean age of patients diagnosed with anaplastic astrocytoma is a full decade younger (Mahaley et al., 1989).

- Both glioblastoma and anaplastic astrocytoma are more common in men (with a ratio of 1.6:1), and more frequently diagnosed in Whites than in Blacks (Ohaegbula, Saddeqi, & Ikerionwu, 1980).
- Patients with a strong family cancer syndrome (Li & Fraumeni, 1982), Turcot syndrome (Todd et al., 1981), tuberous sclerosis, and neurofibromatosis (Schoenberg, 1977) are at higher risk.
- Environmental risk factors such as childhood cranial radiation and extensive exposure to petrochemical plants have been reported (Schoenberg, 1991).
- Malignant astrocytomas can occur in any part of the brain or spinal cord, and often straddle more than one functional area (Salcman, 1997).
- Symptoms depend on the location of the tumor within the brain. Both generalized signs of increased intracranial pressure and focal neurologic deficits may occur. Only one-third of patients present with the classic triad of headache, seizure, and hemiparesis (Salcman, 1997).
- Only 20% have a history of symptoms longer than 1 month and 10% have symptoms for longer than 1 year (Roth & Elvidge, 1960).
- Of patients admitted for a stroke, 3% are later found to have a tumor (Salcman, 1997). CT or gadolinium-enhanced MRI may be used to determine location and anatomical boundaries. The glioblastoma often has a classic "ring-enhancing lesion" pattern.
- There are no specific blood or CSF tests that can be performed to make the diagnosis. Tissue sampling is necessary to make a definitive diagnosis.

Oligodendroglioma
- Oligodendrogliomas represent 4% to 7% of all primary intracranial gliomas (Mork, Halvorsen, Lindegaard, & Eide, 1985), although with recent advances in neuropathology they are being recognized more frequently.
- They are reported equally among the sexes (Rubinstein, 1972).
- They most frequently occur in the fourth and fifth decades of life.
- Tumors are classified as oligodendroglioma (low grade) or anaplastic oligodendroglioma (Couldewell & Hinton, 1997).

- Tumors can have mixed cytology (i.e., oligoastrocytoma).
- Patients with anaplastic oligodendrogliomas have a longer median survival time than those with glioblastoma, anaplastic astrocytoma, or anaplastic mixed glioma (Winger, Macdonald, & Cairncross, 1989).
- Several studies have related survival to several grading characteristics including number of mitoses and degree of necrosis (Burger et al., 1987), and endothelial proliferation, necrosis, maximal nuclear/cytoplasmic ratios, maximal cell density, and pleomorphism in another study (Smith et al., 1983).
- These tumors most often occur in the cerebral hemispheres, with the frontal lobes being most common (Couldwell & Hinton, 1997).
- Cranial radiation therapy for other primary tumors is a risk factor for development of an oligodendroglioma (Huang, Chiou, & Ho, 1987).
- One-half of patients present with seizures (Wilkinson, Anderson, & Holmes, 1987).
- On CT imaging, 60% of these tumors show calcification (Segall et al., 1990).

Ependymoma
- Ependymomas represent 1.9% to 7.8% of all intracranial tumors, with one-half occurring in the first two decades of life (Duncan & Hoffman, 1997).
- There is no sex predilection or known risk factors.
- Tumors are classified either as benign or anaplastic (malignant).
- Compared to other low grade tumors, ependymomas have the lowest incidence of cranial nerve signs (25%), the lowest incidence of invasion (22.2%), and the highest rate for gross total resection (71%) of all noninvasive tumors.
- Common presenting signs include increased intracranial pressure and brain stem compression (infratentorial location), and headache, seizures, or other focal neurologic signs (supratentorial)(Duncan & Hoffman, 1997).
- There is no characteristic neuroimaging finding.
- Once the diagnosis is established, neuroimaging is necessary of the entire neuroaxis to rule out spinal fluid seeding.

Choroid Plexus Tumors

- Incidence is reported to be between 0.4% and 0.6% of all intracranial neoplasms (Scott & Knightly, 1997). It is more common in childhood.
- From 20% to 30% are choroid plexus carcinoma, while the rest are papillomas (Allen et al., 1992).
- Sex, age in adulthood, race, or nationality does not play a factor in occurrence (Scott & Knightly, 1997).
- Almost all choroid plexus papillomas reported in adults occur in the posterior fossa (Russell & Rubinstein, 1989).
- Headaches are the most common symptom along with cranial nerve dysfunction (McGirr et al., 1988).
- Diagnostic tests include plain film of the skull (20% show a calcified mass), CT of the brain (up to 80% show a calcified mass), and MRI.
- Of choroid plexus carcinomas, 44% have seeding throughout the craniospinal axis, with extraneural metastasis extremely rare (St. Clair et al., 1991).

Medulloblastoma and PNET Tumors

- These tumors account for 7% to 8% of all intracranial tumors, being much more common in children.
- The average age of the adult patient is 34, and it is slightly more common in the Caucasian adult than in Blacks (Bunin, 1987).
- Medulloblastomas may accompany other hereditary syndromes, such as Gorlin's syndrome, blue nevus syndrome, Turcot syndrome, and Li-Fraumeni syndrome (Berger, Magrassi, & Geyer, 1997).
- In adults, tumors above the tentorium are termed PNET; medulloblastomas are below the tentorium.
- Most studies report that symptoms are more common in children. The studies usually show signs of increased intracranial pressure, including nausea, impaired upgaze, headache, and vomiting as the most common symptoms.
- Diagnosis is made by MRI of the brain as well as evaluation of the spinal cord and spinal fluid with cytologic analysis.
- Systemic metastasis (bone marrow, lymph nodes, and liver) have been reported in 5% to 15% of children with medulloblastoma (Amador, 1983).

Nerve Sheath Tumors

Acoustic Neuroma

- Account for approximately 6% to 8% of all intracranial tumors (Macfarlane & King, 1997).
- Tumors occur bilaterally in 5% of cases.
- Postmortem studies suggest the condition remains underdiagnosed and asymptomatic (Brackmann & Kwartler, 1990).
- Malignant acoustic neurinomas are extremely rare with only a few cases ever reported (Macfarlane & King, 1997).
- Patients with neurofibromatosis are at increased risk, and the incidence occurs at younger ages (third decade of life). It is reported that 96% of cases are sporadic and not related to any hereditary conditions (Macfarlane & King, 1997).
- It is estimated that in 78% of cases, the lesion size will increase at a rate of less than 2 mm per year (Nedzelski et al., 1992).
- Tumors occur more commonly in women than men (57% vs. 43% of cases) and in the fifth or sixth decade of life (50%) (Evans et al., 1992).
- From 50% to 60% of tumors arise from the superior vestibular nerve, 40% from the inferior vestibular nerve, and less than 10% from the cochlear nerve (Clemis et al., 1986).
- Common symptoms include unilateral hearing loss (96%), unsteadiness (77%), tinnitus (71%), mastoid pain (28%), headache (29%), facial numbness (7%), and diplopia (7%)(Hardy et al., 1989).
- MRI is the imaging study of choice. In addition, audiometry, speech discrimination scoring, and caloric testing are useful to document and track effects on hearing.

Meningeal Tumors

Meningioma

- The mean incidence of meningiomas is approximately 20% (DeMonte & Al-Mefty, 1997).
- There are numerous histologic variants of meningioma, none of which have any prognostic significance with the exception of malignant meningioma.
- Malignant meningioma is characterized by brain invasion, distant metastasis (lungs, pleura, liver, lymph nodes, or bone), papillary pattern, or necrosis (Stoller et al., 1987).

- The ratio of men to women incidences ranges from 1:1.4 to 1:2.8 (DeMonte & Al-Mefty, 1997).
- In the African American population, there are equal male to female ratios (Fan & Pezeshkpour, 1992).
- The incidence increases with increasing age (Sutherland et al., 1987).
- Head trauma has not been shown to be a risk factor for meningioma (DeMonte & Al-Mefty, 1997).
- It is reported that 70% of meningiomas have monosomy of chromosome 22 (Zanki & Zang, 1980). This is common in patients with neurofibromatosis Type 2.
- Meningiomas have been reported in patients who receive radiation to the head or brain including low levels of irradiation (1,000 Gy, Modan, Baodatz, & Mart, 1974); high doses (5,500–7,500 Gy, Mack & Wilson, 1993); and intermediate doses of radiation (Waga & Handa, 1976).
- Common presenting symptoms include headache (36%) and paresis (30%) (Rohinger et al., 1989).
- CT or MRI imaging may be used to identify meningiomas, with contrast-enhanced MRI providing the highest level of detection (Zimmerman, 1991).
- MRI scans show a lesion with homogeneous enhancement.

Meningeal Hemangiopericytoma

- Meningeal hemangiopericytomas are rare, comprising less than 1% of intracranial neoplasms (Guthrie, Ebersold, Scheithauer, & Shaw, 1989).
- From 56% to 75% of incidences occur in men between the ages of 38 to 42 (Guthrie et al., 1989).
- Of these, 15% are located in the posterior fossa and 15% are located in the spine (Guthrie et al., 1989).
- Meningeal hemangiopericytomas can metastasize outside of the central nervous system. The most common sites are bone, lung, and liver (Guthrie, et al., 1989).
- The probability of metastasis at 5 years is 13% (Guthrie et al., 1989).
- In a detailed review, Guthrie et al. (1989) found age, sex, or mitotic activity of the tumor to be unrelated to prognosis.
- Presenting symptoms are related to tumor location, and 16% of patients present with seizures (Guthrie et al., 1989).

- CT imaging or MRI can be used to identify lesions, but cannot distinguish these tumors from meningiomas (Guthrie, 1997).

Meningeal Sarcoma
- Incidence has been reported from 0.1% to 1.2% of all intracranial tumors (Russell & Rubinstein, 1989; Paulus, Slowik, & Jellinger, 1991).
- Meningeal sarcomas occur in any age (child to elderly) and have no gender predisposition (Paulus et al., 1991).
- No preferential site of occurrence exists (Russell & Rubinstein, 1989).
- Higher incidence is reported in those with neurofibromatosis, those with monosomy 22, in those who received prior brain irradiation, and after known trauma (Haddad & Al-Mefty, 1997).
- Symptoms include seizures, hydrocephalus, or spinal cord pathology (Haddad & Al-Mefty, 1997).
- CT and MRI imaging assist in locating lesions, but there is no pathognomonic radiologic picture (Haddad & Al-Mefty, 1997).
- Dissemination along the dura is common.

Pineal Region Tumors

Pineal and Germ Cell Tumors
- Actual data on incidence is difficult because of several factors including referral patterns of specific institution's influence data on incidence, pathologic classification has changed, and the fact that in the past tumors were treated empirically without histologic diagnosis (Bruce, Connolly, & Stein, 1997).
- Germ cell tumors have a reported total incidence of 0.2 per 100,000 population, with 52% germinomas, 19% teratomas, and 16% mixed cell tumors (Jennings, Gelman, & Hochberg, 1985).
- Pineal cell tumors have a reported total incidence of 0.1 per 100,000 population with 42% pineocytomas, 32% pinealblastomas, and 26% mixed cell tumors (Bruce et al., 1997).
- It has been reported that 70% occur between the ages of 10 and 21 and 95% occur before age 33 (Jennings et al., 1985).

- Germ cell tumors occur more frequently in men (2.24 times more likely than in women), whereas pineal cell tumors have no gender preference (Bruce et al., 1997).
- The most common symptoms for tumors occurring above the sella are visual field defects and diabetes insipidus (Jennings et al., 1985).
- Pineal region tumors present with symptoms of increased intracranial pressure, cranial nerve dysfunction, or endocrine dysfunction (Sawaya et al., 1990).
- Workup for patients suspected of having a germ cell or pineal cell tumor should include:
  - High resolution MRI scan with gadolinium of the head
  - Measurement of AFP and b-HCG in the serum and CSF to detect malignant germ cell elements
  - Cytologic examination of CSF
  - Evaluation of pituitary function if endocrine abnormalities are suspected
  - Formal visual field examination for suprasellar tumors (Bruce et al., 1997)

Pituitary Tumors

- Account for 15% of all primary brain tumors (Cushing, 1912).
- Pituitary tumors have a reported incidence of 1 to 14 per 100,000 population (Annegers et al., 1978).
- Pituitary tumors are predominant in women, particularly during child-bearing age.
- Tumors are classified as adenomas or carcinoma's (rare).
- Adenomas are subclassified by size:micro-(< 10 mm) or macroadenoma.
- Adenomas are further classified by hormone production. These include somatotroph (growth hormone), lactotroph (prolactin), corticotroph (ACTH, MSH, POMC), gonadotroph (FSH, LH), thyrotroph (TSH), null cell (none).
- Genetic predisposition occurs in multiple endocrine neoplasia Type I syndrome.
- Patients present with one of three patterns: hormonal hypersecretion, hormonal hyposecretion, or neurologic dysfunction secondary to the sellar mass.
- Diagnosis is made by neuroimaging and endocrinologic workup.
- The distinction between a macro- and microadenoma is based on MRI measurements.

- Laboratory analysis should include measurement of the previously mentioned hormones.

Skull-Based Tumors

Chordoma and Chondrosarcoma of the Cranial Base

- Chordomas occur most commonly in the third to fifth decades of life and have a 2:1 male to female ratio (Kendall & Lee, 1977).
- Chondrosarcomas occur frequently in the second and third decades of life and are twice as likely to occur in men (Hassounah et al., 1985).
- Presenting symptoms are headaches (75%) and cranial nerve palsy, especially diplopia (60–90% of cases)(Gay, Sekhar, & Wright, 1997).
- Physical findings usually include sixth nerve palsy (50–90%) followed by visual field defect (Gay et al., 1997; Rich et al., 1985).
- Chondrosarcomas also usually present with hearing loss (86%)(Gay et al., 1997).
- CT and MRI are important for diagnosis, but there are no imaging features that allow for the accurate differentiation of the two, or to distinguish from other tumor types (Coltera et al., 1986).
- Cerebral angiography is performed prior to surgery to evaluate vascular encasement and displacement.

Glomus Jugulare Tumors

- Glomus tumors account for only 0.03% of all neoplasms of the brain (Boyle, Shimm, & Coulthard, 1990).
- Glomus tumors are the most common tumor of the middle ear.
- Bilateral tumors occur in 1% to 2% of all cases and multicentricity occurs in up to 10% (Olsen, 1994).
- Of bilateral or multiple tumors, 31.8% occur in familial disease (Van Der Mey et al., 1992). An autosomal trait localized to chromosome 11q23 has been implicated in some cases. Therefore, genetic counseling is recommended for persons with bilateral or multiple tumors (Ebersold, Morita, & Olsen, 1997).
- Tumors are classified as glomus tympanicum or glomus jugulare depending on location. Tumors are then subclassified from Type 1 to Type IV depending on invasiveness.

- Common presenting symptoms include conductive hearing loss, tinnitus, bleeding, vertigo, or seventh nerve weakness.
- Diagnosis is made by MRI imaging and angiography.

Primary Central Nervous System Lymphoma (PCNSL)

- Conservative estimates indicate that cerebral lymphoma comprises 8% to 10% of all intracranial tumors (Rosenthal & Green, 1997).
- Increased incidence has been related to acquired immune deficiency syndrome(AIDS) and increased use of immunosuppressive drugs (Rosenthal & Green, 1997). However, the incidence has also increased in the nonimmunosuppressed patient population.
- Primary cerebral lymphoma in immunocompetent patients usually arises in the sixth decade, whereas in the immunosuppressed it occurs at younger ages.
- Male to female ratio in immunocompetent patients is 1.5:1. In the immunosuppressed, the male to female ratio is 17:1 (DeAngelis et al., 1992).
- Factors that predispose patients to systemic lymphoma also predispose a person to developing PCNSL, such as congenital immunodeficiency syndromes, acquired immunodeficiency syndromes, immunosuppressive therapy, autoimmune disease, infectious mononucleosis, Epstein-Barr virus, and celiac disease (Rosenthal & Green, 1997). The categories of cerebral lymphoma are:
  - Non-Hodgkin's lymphoma
  - Secondary cerebral lymphoma
  - Primary cerebral lymphoma
  - Immunocompetent
  - Immunosuppressed
  - AIDS-related
  - Organ transplant-related
  - Congenital
  - Therapeutic
  - Hodgkin's disease
  - Ocular lymphoma
  - Mycosis fungoides
  - Lymphomatoid granulomatosis
  - Malignant angioendotheliosis
- Most tumors are solitary supratentorial (52.1%), but 33.5% are multifocal. The most common sites are frontal and temporal lobes (Murray, Kun, & Cox, 1986).

- Presenting symptoms include memory loss, headache, altered affect, and a 10% incidence of seizures (Hochberg & Miller, 1988).
- Presenting signs include motor and sensory deficits, altered visual acuity, papilledema, and confusion.
- CT or MRI are used to visualize the tumor, but cannot make a definitive diagnosis. Most lesions enhance. Necrotic regions are uncommon.
- At presentation, 10% of patients will have malignant cells detectable in the spinal fluid (Murray et al., 1986).
- Workup should include a formal ophthalmologic examination.

Metastatic Tumors

- Lung, breast, melanoma, renal, and colon cancers are the most common tumors causing brain metastasis (Sawaya & Bindal, 1997).
- The rate increased from 1 per 100,000 to > 30 per 100,000 in persons over 35. Among women, metastasis from breast cancer has an equal incidence to metastasis from lung cancer.
- Lung cancer is the most common cause of metastasis in males (Takakura, 1982).
- Sarcoma, ovarian, prostate, and bladder cancers rarely metastasize to the brain.
- Of metastases, 80% to 85% occur in the cerebrum (Delattre et al., 1988).
- Pelvic and gastrointestinal tumors may have a higher incidence in the posterior fossa (Delattre et al., 1988).
- Of colon cancer patients, 50% present with multiple tumors, and 85% of autopsy studies show multiple brain metastases from a variety of cancers (Delattre et al., 1988).
- It is estimated that one-third of all patients developing brain metastasis do not have a previous cancer history (Dhopesh & Yagnik, 1985).
- In 16% to 35% of patients with brain metastasis as the first sign of cancer, no systemic cancer is ever found (Dhopesh & Yagnik, 1985; Debevec, 1990; Rasmussen et al., 1991).
- Over two-thirds of lesions from unknown primaries are multiple (Delattre et al., 1988).
- Symptoms include signs of increased intracranial pressure or focal irritation, which is dependent on tumor location.

- MRI characteristics often include spherical lesions, which are well demarcated from brain tissue and located at the junction of the gray and white matter (Sawaya & Bindal, 1997).
- Of patients with solitary lesions on MRI and a history of cancer, 89% to 93% are found to have brain metastasis (Patchell et al., 1990).
- Approximately one-half of patients present with a solitary brain metastasis and one-half with more than one metastasis.

STAGING

- Because primary brain tumors tend not to metastasize outside of the central nervous system, the American Joint Committee on Cancer's TNM/UICC staging system does not apply and is rarely used in current clinical trials.
- Tumors are staged according to histopathologic evaluation. The WHO classification of brain tumors has been accepted by most groups participating in clinical trials as the staging system used for treatment decisions (Table 9-1).

EXPECTED OUTCOMES

GLIOMAS

Low-Grade Astrocytoma

- Adults with low-grade astrocytomas of the cerebral hemispheres have an expected survival of 3 to 7 years.
- It is estimated that a large portion of these tumors will dedifferentiate to a more malignant type (usually glioblastoma multiforme). Several studies have reported conflicting results with the incidence of dedifferentiation as two-thirds (Muller, Afra, & Schroder, 1977); 50% (Laws, Taylor, Clifton, & Okazaki, 1984), or over 95% (Vertosick, Selker, & Arena, 1991; McCormack, Miller, & Budzilovich, 1992). Prognostic indicators include age (83% 5-year survival vs. 12% 5-year survival if less than 20 years of age or greater than 50 years of age, respectively) (Laws et al., 1984), postoperative neurologic deficits, altered consciousness, type of surgery (extent of resection), and tumor site (frontal/temporal worse).

TABLE 9–1   WHO CLASSIFICATION OF BRAIN TUMORS

Tumors of Neuroepithelial Tissue

Astrocytic Tumors
Astrocytoma
Anaplastic astrocytoma
Glioblastoma
Pilocytic astrocytoma
Pleomorphic xanthroastrocytoma
Subependymal giant cell astrocytoma

Oligodendroglial Tumors
Oligodendroglioma
Anaplastic oligodendroglioma

Ependymal Tumors
Ependymoma
Anaplastic ependymoma
Myxopapillary ependymoma
Subependymoma

Mixed Gliomas
Mixed oligoastrocytoma
Anaplastic oligoastrocytoma
Others

Chorid Plexus Tumors
Choroid plexus papilloma
Choroid plexus carcinoma

Neuroepithelial Tumors of Uncertain Origin
Astroblastoma
Polar spongioblastoma
Gliomatosis cerebri

Neuronal and Mixed Neuronal-Glial Tumors
Gangliocytoma
Dysplastic gangliocytoma of cerebellum
Desmoplastic infantile ganglioglioma
Dysembryoplastic neuroepithelial tumor
Ganglioglioma
Anaplastic ganglioglioma
Central neurocytoma
Olfactory neuroblastoma

Pineal Tumors
Pineocytoma
Pineoblastoma
Mixed pineocytoma-pineoblastoma

Embryonal Tumors
Medulloepithelioma
Neuroblastoma
Ependymoblastoma
Retinoblastoma
Primitive neuroectodermal tumor

Tumors of Cranial and Spinal Nerves
Schwannoma
Neurofibroma
Malignant peripheral nerve sheath tumor

Tumors of the Meninges

Tumors of Meningothelial Cells
Meningioma
Atypical meningioma
Anaplastic meningioma

NonMeningothelial Tumors of the Meninges
Mesenchymal tumor
Hemangioblastoma

Hematopoietic Tumors
Primary malignant lymphoma
Plasmocytoma
Granulocytic sarcoma
Others

Germ Cell Tumors
Germinoma
Embryonal carcinoma
Yolk sac tumor
Choriocarcinoma
Teratoma
Mixed germ cell tumors

Malignant Astrocytoma

■ The median survival rate of glioblastoma multiforme after surgery and conventional radiation therapy and chemotherapy is 37 weeks (Salcman, 1980).

■ Curran and colleagues (1992) reported median survival rate of 49 months for patients with small (< 5 cm) anaplastic astrocytomas occurring in the frontal lobes versus 25 months for tumors in other locations within the brain.

■ In addition, Donahue and colleagues (1997) found a median survival rate of 7.3 years in patients with anaplastic astrocytomas with an oligodendroglial component versus 3 years in patients with anaplastic astrocytomas.

■ The best survival rate (median survival 17 months) for patients with glioblastoma multiforme was associated with the occurrence of at least three of the following characteristics: < 40 years of age, high KPS, frontal tumors, and total resection (Simpson et al., 1993).

■ The addition of postoperative radiation to surgery is associated with a significant improvement in median survival from approximately 4 to 9 months (Walker et al., 1978).

■ It has been reported that 10% to 20% of patients will live 18 to 24 months after diagnosis of a glioblastoma and less than 5% will live 3 years or longer (Salcman, 1997).

■ A recent review of patients with both anaplastic astrocytoma and glioblastoma at recurrence found the median progression-free survival to be 13 weeks and 9 weeks, respectively (Wong et al., 1999).

Oligodendroglioma

■ Median survival of patients with anaplastic oligodendroglioma has been reported as 278 weeks (Winger et al., 1989).

■ Less than 50% of patients undergoing surgical treatment for oligodendroglioma fail to survive longer than 5 years postoperatively.

Ependymoma

■ The 5-year survival rate is approximately 50% for all ependymomas (Lyons & Kelly, 1991).

■ Malignant ependymomas have a 12% 5-year survival rate versus 70% for low-grade tumors (Nazar et al., 1990).

■ The median time to recurrence is considered to be 22 to 24 months, with recurrence infrequent after 36 months and rare past 62 months (Hendrick & Raffel, 1989; Nazar et al., 1990).

■ The addition of postoperative radiotherapy to incompletely resected ependymomas resulted in a 5-year survival rate of 40% to 87% in patients receiving doses of 45 Gy or higher (Leibel & Sheline, 1987; Salazar, 1983).

Choroid Plexus Tumors

■ Choroid plexus papilloma has been reported to have 100% 5-year survival rates, and a recent report revealed a 0% operative mortality (Knierim, 1990).

■ Choroid plexus carcinoma has a 50% 5-year survival rate (Ellenbogen, Winston, & Kupsky, 1989).

Medulloblastoma and PNET Tumors

■ The incidence rate in adults is too low to accurately predict median survival.

■ In children, most of the tumors that relapse do so at a period equal to the age at diagnosis plus 9 months (Gerosa et al., 1981).

NERVE SHEATH TUMORS

Acoustic Neuroma

■ After complete excision, recurrence rates are less than 1% to 2%. Incomplete excision carries a 9% death rate at 5 years (Shea et al., 1985).

■ Radiosurgery has an 85% 2-year control rate.

MENINGEAL TUMORS

Meningioma

■ Mirimanoff et al. (1985) reported survival rates of 93% at 5 years, 80% at 10 years, and 68% at 15 years if meningiomas are able to be totally resected. The 5-, 10-, and 15-year survival dropped to 63%, 45%, and 9% if only partial resection was obtained.

Meningeal Hemangiopericytoma

■ Median survival after initial surgery is 60 months, with a 5-year survival rate of 67% (Guthrie, 1997).

Meningeal Sarcoma

■ Median survival is 32 months, with a 5-year postoperative survival rate of 16% (Guthrie & Laws, 1990).

■ A favorable outcome is most likely after radical excision of a better-differentiated, well-circumscribed tumor (Rubinstein, 1971).

PINEAL REGION TUMORS

Pineal and Germ Cell Tumors

■ Benign germ cell tumors such as dermoid, teratoma, and epidermoid tumors are associated with 100% 5- and 10-year survival rates with surgical resection alone (Stein & Bruce, 1992).

■ The 5-year survival rate for germinomas is reported to be 75% to 80% after surgical resection and radiation therapy (Bruce & Stein, 1993; Edwards et al., 1988).

■ Patients with malignant nongerminomatous germ cell tumors rarely survive beyond 2 years (Edwards et al., 1988; Jennings, Gelman, & Hochberg, 1985).

■ A worse prognosis is seen with the presence of elevated tumor markers in patients with malignant nongerminomatous germ cell tumors (Takakura, 1982).

■ Of pineocytomas, 16% are thought to be small and histologically benign and can be cured with surgical resection (Rubinstein, 1971).

Pituitary Tumors

■ Cure rates for macroadenomas are 53% and 28% if locally invasive (Randell et al., 1985).

■ Microadenomas have a 90% cure rate if completely resected (Salassa et al., 1978).

■ Radiation therapy is effective (75–80%) in controlling microadenomas, but the major drawback compared to surgery is the time to hormone normalization, which often takes greater than or equal to 1 year. Radiation is also utilized in nonsurgical candidates and those with recurrent tumors (Thapar & Laws, 1997).

■ Pituitary carcinoma is extremely rare, but almost all cases reported result in patient death from local invasion despite aggressive therapy.

SKULL-BASED TUMORS

Chordoma and Chondrosarcoma of the Cranial Base

■ Nontreated chordomas are reported to have an average survival time from 0.6 to 2 years (Eriksson, Gunterberg, & Kindblom, 1981; Heffelfinger et al., 1973).

■ Most studies report poor overall survival rates of 51% and 35% at 5 and 10 years, respectively after subtotal or partial surgery followed by radiation therapy (Forsyth et al., 1993; Cummings, Ian-Hodson, & Bush, 1983; Heffelginer et al., 1973). Better results have been achieved with charged particles (such as protons or helium) than with standard photon irradiation.

■ Tumor-free survival time for patients undergoing extensive surgical resection is 76% at 5 years (92% and 69% for chondrosarcomas and chordomas) (Gay, Sekhar, & Wright, 1997).

■ By classification, 5-year survival rates are 90%, 81%, and 43% for Grades I, II, and III lesions, respectively (Evans, Ayala, & Romodahl, 1977).

Glomus Jugulare Tumors

■ Due to advances in recent years, and the relative rarity of this tumor type, most patients who have undergone definitive surgery have not had time for extensive follow-up years. Therefore, comments on survival cannot be made (Ebersold et al , 1997). Radiation is typically recommended in symptomatic lesions that cannot be totally resected.

Primary Central Nervous System Lymphoma (PCNSL)

■ Median survival times have been reported between 14.5 and 40.8 months in those patients with PCNSL receiving cranial irradiation alone (Leibel & Sheline, 1987).

■ Prognosis in AIDS-related PCNSL is poor, with the median survival less than 3 months (Remick et al., 1990). Outcomes may be improved with concurrent treatment with effective antiretroviral therapies.

■ Survival in mycosis fungoides, secondary cerebral lymphoma and malignant angioendotheliosis is also poor, with no long-term survivors being reported (Liang et al., 1989; Smadja et al., 1991; Lindae, Lucy, Abel, & Kaplan, 1990).

■ Hodgkin's lymphoma of the brain and ocular lymphoma are rare occurrences, and clear definitions of survival are not reported (Clark, Callihan, Schwartzberg, & Fontanesi, 1992).

METASTATIC TUMORS

■ Recent studies examining heterogeneous groups of patients report survival times of 10 to 14 months with surgical excision (Sundaresan & Galicich, 1985; Ferrara et al., 1990; Patchell, et al., 1990; Bindal et al., 1993).

■ Bindal et al., (1993) found equivalent survival in patients with multiple metastases that were completely removed compared with those with solitary lesions.

■ Recursive partitioning analysis of prognostic factors in three Radiation Therapy Oncology Group (RTOG) brain metastasis trials revealed a median survival of 7.1 months in patients < 65 years of age with a Karnofsky Performance Status (KPS) of at least 70 and a controlled primary tumor with the brain being the only site of metastasis. The worst survival (median 2.3 months) was seen in patients with a KPS of less than 70 (Gaspar et al., 1997).

■ Improvement in local surgery has resulted in extent of systemic cancer being the most important prognostic factor.

OUTCOMES MEASURES

■ No standard for follow-up exists for any tumor type. Frequency will be determined on the basis of tumor histology, treatment type, participation in clinical trials, and patient symptoms. The more aggressive lesions require diligent patient management including frequent neuroimaging and symptom assessment.

■ Primary Benign Brain Tumors:
  • A follow-up evaluation should be performed 1 to 2 months after the completion of radiation therapy. Patients are then followed at least every 12 months for life. After 5 years, follow-up is maintained on a yearly basis with imaging dictated by clinical symptoms (Friedman et al., 1998). This evaluation should include:
    History and physical examination, including complete neurologic assessment
    Imaging study of the brain. Usually this is an MRI with and without gadolinium
    Additional laboratory and radiographic studies as clinically indicated

■ Primary Malignant Brain Tumors:
  • A follow-up evaluation should be performed 2 to 6 weeks after the completion of radiation therapy (National Comprehensive Cancer Network, 1997). Patients are then followed at least every 3 to 4 months for the first year, every

4 to 6 months for the second year and every 6 to 12 months for life (National Comprehensive Cancer Network, 1997). Evaluations may be more or less frequent depending on patient symptoms or participation in clinical trials. This evaluation should include:

History and physical examination including complete neurologic assessment

Imaging study of the brain. Usually this is an MRI with and without gadolinium. Patients with ependymomas should also undergo screening MRI of the spine (National Comprehensive Cancer Network, 1997)

Additional laboratory and radiographic studies as clinically indicated.

■ Metastatic Brain Tumors:

• A follow-up evaluation should be performed 1 to 3 months after surgery, radiation, or radiosurgery. Patients should then be followed at least every 3 months for the first year (National Comprehensive Cancer Network, 1997). Evaluations may be more or less frequent depending on patient symptoms or participation in clinical trials. This evaluation should include:

History and physical examination including complete neurologic assessment

Imaging study of the brain. Usually this is an MRI with and without gadolinium

Additional laboratory and radiographic studies as clinically indicated

QUALITY OF LIFE

■ Most studies on QOL in people with brain tumors have assessed this via the unidimensional measures of physical functioning, such as the KPS (Armstrong, 1999). These studies have shown that patients with malignant glioma tend to maintain a certain level of function then experience a rapid decline before death (Sachsenheimer, Piotrowski, & Bimmler, 1992). Sachsenheimer also reported that patients with astrocytomas maintained physical functioning, that patients with brain metastases reached their highest functional ability 3 weeks after radiation therapy then experienced a rapid decline, and that 35% of patients with meningiomas were unfit to work after treatment.

■ Patients with brain tumors have been shown to achieve daily functional gains similar to patients with traumatic brain injury when undergoing intensive inpatient rehabilitation (O'Dell et al., 1998).

■ Mackworth, Fobair, and Prados (1992) looked at KPS as well as a self-developed tool to measure quality of life. They found that KPS did not correlate well with quality of life scores in patients with GBM when the KPS score was greater than 90. This suggests that KPS is not as accurate a measure of quality of life as it is of functional ability.

■ Several instruments are available to measure quality of life in persons with brain tumors including the FACT-Brain (Weitzner et al., 1995), and the EORTC QLQ-C30 version 2.0 (Aaronson et al., 1993). Choucair and colleagues (1997) reported that utilizing quality of life and neuropsychological evaluation were more cost-effective than formal neuropsychological testing and provided accurate additional data on patients enrolled in clinical trials.

■ The literature reveals variable opinions on the effect of radiation therapy on quality of life in patients with low grade gliomas. Taphoorn and colleagues (1994) found no difference in quality of life and neurologic and functional status between those who had received radiation therapy and those who had not. The EORTC performed a Phase III trial looking at dose of radiation therapy and the effect on quality of life. This study showed that patients with low-grade cerebral gliomas who received high-dose radiotherapy (59.4 Gy in 6.5 weeks) reported lower levels of functioning and more symptom burden after radiation therapy than those receiving low-dose (45 Gy in 5 weeks) radiation therapy (Kiebert et al., 1998). There was no difference in survival between the two radiation doses.

■ Radiation therapy is associated with posttreatment fatigue. Faithful (1991) followed patients for 6 weeks postradiation therapy and described a somnolence syndrome that occurred during this period. It was associated with subjective complaints of sleepiness, sensory changes, and arm and leg weakness. Lovely and colleagues(1999) showed that this treatment-related fatigue is associated with decreases in almost all aspects of patients' quality of life.

■ Kleinberg, Wallner, and Malkin (1993) found that long-term glioma survivers (median 3.5 years) maintained a stable KPS after the completion of radiation therapy and did not experience progressive decline in neuropsychological function in the absence of recurrence.

SYMPTOM ASSESSMENT AND MANAGEMENT

Seizures

■ Patients with primary brain tumors that are supratentorial should be placed on prophylactic anticonvulsants.

■ Patients with metastatic tumors that present with a seizure or those whose primary cancer is melanoma, renal cell, or choriocarcinoma should be placed on anticonvulsants (Armstrong & Gilbert, 1995).

■ Prohibition of driving based on seizure activity varies from state to state. Most restrict driving for a period of 6 months to 1 year after last known seizure.

■ Most anticonvulsants require careful monitoring of serum drug levels as well as liver function and complete blood cell differential at least every 6 months.

■ Dilantin (phenytoin) is associated with a reported 20% to 30% risk of rash.

■ There is no standardized time criteria for whether anticonvulsants can be stopped after seizures with brain tumors. If considering stopping anticonvulsants, consider a formal neurologic consult with EEG testing.

Radiation Effect

■ The effect of radiation therapy on the brain can be divided into early-acute reactions, early-delayed reactions, and late-delayed reactions.

■ Early-acute reactions occur during radiation and include hair loss, fatigue, acute skin reactions, and transient worsening of neurologic effects due to brain edema.

■ Early-delayed reactions may occur several weeks or months after radiation. These include lethargy, nausea, vomiting, ataxia and worsening focal deficits. They are typically characterized by somnolence and felt to be caused by transient demyelinization.

■ Late-delayed reactions are reported to occur 6 months to 2 years after radiation therapy and can include focal necrosis, cognitive impairment, cranial nerve damage, cataract formation, and hearing loss. The risk for brain necrosis with fractionated radiation therapy is very low. The risk of damage to the optic chiasm (with associated blindness) typically is very low (~1–2%) and can be reduced by minimizing the total radiation dose to this structure. Using reduced daily fraction sizes of less than or equal to 200 cGy can also reduce the risk of damage and resultant blindness.

Hypercoagulability

■ Patients with primary brain tumors are known to have an increased risk for thromboembolic complications. Patients with glioblastoma multiforme are thought to be at highest risk, reported as 30% to 50% (Sawaya et al., 1992).

■ Often clinical signs of deep vein thrombosis (DVT) are masked due to corticosteroids. A painless cord can be palpated in the calf without associated erythema or edema (Armstrong & Gilbert, 1996).

■ Use of pneumatic pressure devices in the perioperative period and careful monitoring for signs/symptoms are indicated (Cerrato, Ariano, & Fiaccjiono, 1978).

■ The use of prophylactic anticoagulation has not been studied.

■ In patients diagnosed with a DVT, the use of anticoagulation has been found to be safe (Zeltzman et al., 1991).

OUTCOMES MANAGEMENT

GLIOMAS

Low-Grade Astrocytoma

■ Treatment often includes resection and/or radiation, but controversy exists as to when to treat patients.

Surgery

• Extent of resection as well as age at diagnosis has been found to affect outcome (Berger et al., 1994). In a series of 221 patients, Berger and colleagues found no recurrence at 54 months if low-grade astrocytomas were completely resected. Postoperative residual tumors of <10 cm^3 were associated with a 14.8% recurrence rate at 50 months. Larger residual tumors were associated with a 46% recurrence rate at 30 months.

Radiation Therapy

• The role of radiation therapy remains controversial. Many retrospective studies have been completed that show a survival benefit (Shaw et al., 1989; Winger et al., 1989), versus no benefit (Philippon et al., 1993). The results of an EORTC trial randomizing patients after surgery to observation versus radiation are not yet reported. For pilocytic astrocytomas, postoperative radiation therapy is not indicated following a complete or near-complete resection.

- If radiation therapy is utilized at initial diagnosis or at recurrence, local therapy administered to the tumor bed plus edema plus a 2-cm margin is the standard.
- A recent EORTC randomized trial showed no benefit to higher-dose (59.4 Gy) versus low dose (45 Gy) radiation (Kiebert et al., 1998).
- Potential side effects include damage to normal brain cells leading to cognitive difficulties, the occurrence of other tumors from radiation damage, and the potential for radiation necrosis.

Chemotherapy

- At the present time there is no proven beneficial effect of chemotherapy in the treatment of low-grade astrocytomas (Morantz, 1997).

Glioblastoma and Malignant Astrocytoma

■ Multimodality therapy is the standard of care for malignant gliomas. Components of this treatment plan are controversial, but typically include surgery (biopsy or resection), and radiation therapy, and sometimes chemotherapy (usually a nitrosurea).

■ No standard of care exists for malignant gliomas at recurrence.

Surgery

- The role of surgical resection remains controversial. Obtaining tissue for diagnosis is critical. The patient will usually undergo stereotactic biopsy, open biopsy, partial resection, or gross total resection. There has been no prospective randomized trial looking at type of surgery and affect on outcome. Most studies support maximal surgical resection when technically feasible.
- Three Radiation Therapy Oncology Group (RTOG) trials reviewed the relationship between extent of resection and survival for GBM (Simpson et al., 1993). Survival for those undergoing gross total resection was 11.3 months versus 6.6 months for those who underwent biopsy only.

Radiation Therapy

- Standard radiation therapy for patients with glioblastoma multiforme encompasses the area of tumor (or tumor bed if gross total resection was completed); plus edema plus a 2-centimeter margin. Total dose is usually 60 Gy in 30 to 36 fractions (National Comprehensive Cancer Network, 1997). A randomized RTOG trial showed no benefit to 60 Gy plus 6 Gy boost versus 60 Gy alone.

- The value of postoperative radiation therapy was established by the multicenter randomized trial of the Brain Tumor Study Group (Walker et al., 1978). Median survival was increased to 37.5 weeks for those patients treated with radiation therapy in addition to surgery. Those receiving surgery alone lived an average of 17 weeks.

- There is no clear benefit to the patient receiving whole brain irradiation versus focal irradiation to the tumor (Shapiro et al., 1989).

- Hyperfractionization or the addition of most radiosensitizers has not shown any survival advantage over conventional therapy in randomized trials (Deutsch et al., 1989). A recent retrospective review of patients treated in several Radiation Therapy Oncology Group (RTOG) and Northern California Oncology Group (NCOG) trials suggested a survival advantage for patients with glioblastoma multiforme treated with the radiosensitizer, BrdU (9.8–13 months median survival for the RTOG and NCOG groups, respectively) (Prados et al., 1998).

Brachytherapy

- The use of radioactive seeds allows high doses of radiation to be delivered to the tumor bed while sparing the rest of the brain. Usual doses are 50 to 75 Gy.

- Survival reports when brachytherapy was utilized at the time of recurrence have been between 37 to 54 weeks for GBM (Salcman et al., 1993; Leibel et al., 1989) and 81 weeks for anaplastic astrocytomas (Leibel et al., 1989).

- A randomized trial failed to show statistically significant improvement in survival in patients receiving brachytherapy (Gutin et al., 1987).

- Only 20% to 30% of patients are eligible for brachytherapy because of limitations of size or location. The tumor must be unifocal, less than 5 cm in greatest diameter, and susceptible to implantation by catheters, none of which require a trajectory through any major blood vessel or critical structure.

Radiosurgery

- The use of radiosurgery as an adjunct to other therapies remains controversial. Shrieve and colleagues (1999) reported median survival of 19.9 months for patients treated with radiosurgery in addition to standard radiation therapy. As with brachytherapy, selection bias may play a role in affecting a more positive outcome.
- Doses usually range between 10 to 20 Gy. Radiation necrosis may occur 3 to 5 months after the procedure is completed. In one study, reoperation was the major side effect of concern because of necrosis, and was required in 19% of treated patients at a median time of 5 months (Loeffler et al., 1992).

Chemotherapy

- The BTSG reported that surgery plus radiation therapy and BCNU chemotherapy significantly adds to the survival of patients with malignant gliomas as compared with surgery plus radiation therapy without chemotherapy (Green et al., 1983). While other randomized trials have been negative, a meta-analysis of chemotherapy in malignant gliomas demonstrated a 10% survival advantage at 1 year. This small difference in survival is controversial. Most consider chemotherapy in younger patients with a good KPS.
- The usual starting dose is 200 to 240 mg/m^2 given IV over 1 to 3 days and repeated every 6 to 8 weeks.
- Dose-limiting toxicities include pulmonary fibrosis and myelosuppression. Cumulative doses of BCNU above 1.2 to 1.5 g/m^2 expose the patient to the risk of pulmonary toxicity (Selker et al., 1980; O'Driscoll et al., 1990).
- Other agents or routes of administration have not shown a survival benefit over BCNU for patients with glioblastoma at diagnosis or recurrence (Mahaley, 1991; National Comprehensive Cancer Network, 1997).
- BCNU-containing wafers have been approved for the treatment of malignant gliomas at recurrence. These wafers are placed into the tumor bed after resection and

contain BCNU in a polymer matrix, which is slowly released into the tumor cavity. In a multicenter controlled trial, median survival of the 110 patients who received BCNU polymers was significantly longer than that of those who received placebo polymers (31 vs. 23 weeks) (Brem et al., 1993).

- The standard of care for patients with anaplastic astrocytomas has been the use of procarbazine, CCNU, and vincristine (PCV) combination chemotherapy either before or after radiation therapy. A recent retrospective review revealed equal efficacy of BCNU in this population (Prados et al., 1999). Therefore, either treatment is appropriate for this patient population.
- No standard exists for treatment of anaplastic tumors at recurrence.
- A Phase II RTOG trial reported all-trans-retinoic acid to have a response rate of 12% and a stabilization rate of 12% when utilized in patients with recurrent malignant astrocytomas (Phuphanich et al., 1997).
- Temozolomide (Temodar®) has recently been approved for use in this patient population. In a multicenter clinical trial, 22% of patients with refractory anaplastic astrocytoma had a partial or complete response (Shering Plough, 1999).

Oligodendroglioma
■ There remains controversy as to the optimum treatment.

Surgery
- The role of surgical resection in oligodendroglioma remains controversial, although most support maximal surgical debulking.
- Several series have shown a survival benefit with complete tumor resection including median survival of 12.6 years (Shaw et al., 1992); 7 years (Lindegaard et al., 1987); and 3.8 years (Mork et al., 1985). One study reported an 84% 5-year survival rate with complete tumor resection compared to 41% in those patients who underwent subtotal resection or biopsy only (Whitton & Bloom, 1990).

Radiation Therapy
- The role of radiation therapy has not been established for low grade oligodendrogliomas (Shaw, 1990).

- Current recommendations as delineated by Morantz (1987) include consideration of the use of radiation therapy in patients whose oligodendroglioma on pathologic examination exhibits poor prognostic features (such as regions of anaplasia) or is subtotally resected.

Chemotherapy

- Because of the rare occurrence of this class of tumors they have often been included in evaluations of chemotherapy regimens for malignant gliomas.
- Several small institutional trials indicate that these tumors may be more sensitive to chemotherapy than other glial neoplasms (Couldwell & Hinton, 1997).
- At this time it is unknown whether PCV, which has been used most frequently, is superior to other cytotoxic drugs (Brown et al., 1990; Cairncross & Macdonald, 1988).
- Adjunctive chemotherapy should be considered in those cases with residual or recurrent anaplastic oligodendroglioma, or in those tumors that behave clinically and radiographically in an aggressive manner (Couldwell & Hinton, 1997).
- Ongoing randomized trials will evaluate the role of combining chemotherapy with radiotherapy in low-grade and anaplastic oligodendrogliomas.

Ependymoma

Surgery

- Gross total resection (GTR) has been shown to be positively correlated with survival in infratentorial lesions. Healey and colleagues (1991) report a 75% 5-year survival rate after GTR versus no 5-year survivors if gross total resection was not possible.
- The effect of gross total resection on survival in supratentorial lesions has not been established.
- Operative morbidity is reported as 10% to 30%, whereas mortality is reported as less than 1% at specialized centers (Tomita et al., 1988).

Radiation Therapy

- Patients should be treated postoperatively typically to doses of greater than 50 Gy or higher (Leibel & Sheline, 1987; Salazar, 1983).

- It is not clear whether whole brain irradiation or craniospinal irradiation improves outcome compared with involved field irradiation (Hendrick & Raffel, 1989; Shaw et al., 1987; Kun et al., 1988). Craniospinal radiation typically is utilized for spinal fluid dissemination, intraoperative spillage, or if imaging studies show spinal spread.

Chemotherapy

- To date, no conclusive evidence support the use of any agent to treat either newly diagnosed or recurrent tumors (Tamura et al., 1990; Sutton et al., 1990; Goldwin et al., 1990; Bertolene et al., 1989).

Choroid Plexus Tumors

Surgery

- Primary modality of treatment for both choroid plexus papilloma and carcinoma (Scott & Knightly, 1997).
- No further treatment is necessary for papillomas, if a complete surgical resection is obtained.
- Even with surgical resection, staging of the entire neuroaxis is necessary for choroid plexus carcinoma.

Radiation

- Necessary postoperatively for residual choroid plexus carcinoma and occasionally for incompletely resected papilloma.
- Published reports have used regional external beam radiation therapy, the role of radiosurgery is unknown.
- Craniospinal radiation therapy is used in cases of spinal fluid dissemination (Scott and Knightly, 1997).

Chemotherapy

- Chemotherapy has been used in pediatric patients. There is limited experience in adults (Scott & Knightly, 1997).

Neuronal and Neuronal Precursor Tumors

Medulloblastoma and PNET tumors

Surgery

- The goals of surgery include obtaining tissue for histology, removal of tumor, and alleviation of obstructive hydrocephalus (in 40% of patients, shunt placement is required)(Berger et al., 1997).

- In children, removal of 90% of the tumor has been shown to statistically improve survival (Gerosa et al., 1981).

Radiation
- Radiation therapy is standard in treatment of children and has been shown to improve survival compared to surgery alone. Usually the area of tumor bed is treated to 54 Gy and the entire neuraxis is treated with 36 Gy (Berger et al., 1997). Gross spinal disease should be boosted to a higher dose than the rest of the neuroaxis. Very young children are often treated with chemotherapy and delayed radiation therapy.

Chemotherapy
- A variety of chemotherapy regimens have been utilized in children. High-risk tumors (large or with systemic metastasis) are indications for its use. No trial to date has been completed in the adult population.

NERVE SHEATH TUMORS

Acoustic Neuroma

Surgery
- Surgical resection is considered standard treatment.
- Improvements in operative technique have reduced mortality, allowing emphasis on hearing and facial nerve preservation.
- Complications of surgery include hemorrhage into the operative cavity (2%) (Macfarlane & King, 1997); cerebrospinal fluid leak (10–15%); meningitis (3–6%); and hearing loss.
- Facial weakness varies on size of tumor from 0% for small tumors to 21% for large tumors (House & Luetje, 1979).

External Beam RT and Radiosurgery
- Local control rate of 85% to 100% (> 2-year follow-up) (Loeffler & Alexander, 1993).
- May be treatment of choice for poor surgical candidates (confounding medical illness, elderly).
- Van Roijen, Nijs, and Avezaat (1997) reported that radiosurgery was more cost-effective than surgery for tumors smaller than 3 cm.

MENINGEAL TUMORS

Meningioma

Surgery

- Surgical excision is the mainstay of treatment for meningiomas.
- Surgical approach is determined by tumor location.
- Salazar (1988) performed a retrospective review and found a 58% recurrence rate following gross total resection and a 90% recurrence rate after subtotal resection of malignant meningiomas.

Radiation Therapy

- External beam radiotherapy has been reported to be effective following subtotal resection both at the primary operation and at the time of recurrence (Taylor et al., 1988; Mirabell et al., 1992) for malignant meningiomas.
- Less conclusive data exist for the use of external beam radiation therapy in meningiomas or meningiomas considered unresectable due to location, poor health of the patient, or refusal of surgery by the patient (Kennerdell et al., 1988; Forbes & Goldberg, 1984).
- Salazar (1988) found decreased recurrence rates of 36% following gross total resection and 41% following subtotal resection of malignant meningiomas when radiation therapy was administered postoperatively.
- The recommended radiation dose postoperatively is typically 54 Gy for benign, subtotally resected meningiomas and 60 Gy for atypical/malignant meningiomas (Busse, 1991).

Radiosurgery

- Radiosurgery can be used for patients with benign meningiomas that are relatively small, well defined, or incompletely resected.
- Loeffler, Barker, and Chapman (1999) reported local control rates of 95% to 100% for a 2-year follow-up period in patients with meningiomas, although this is a short follow-up for this slow-growing tumor.
- The usefulness of radiosurgery to treat malignant meningiomas is currently being studied.

Chemotherapy

- Little data exist for the use of traditional antineoplastic agents to treat either benign or malignant meningiomas.
- Antagonism of mitogenic hormones utilizing tamoxifen has been attempted with little response (Goodwin et al., 1993).
- Mifepristone (RU486) has also been studied with response seen in small studies (Grunberg et al., 1991; Lamberts et al., 1992). Phase III trials are currently underway.

Meningeal Hemangiopericytoma

■ Management includes surgery, radiation therapy, and diligent follow-up with chest x-ray and workup of bone pain if it occurs (Guthrie, 1997).

Surgery

- Extent of surgical resection has not been shown to affect recurrence rates. Guthrie and colleagues (1989) found an average survival of 109 months versus 65 months with partial resection.
- Aggressive surgical excision is still indicated. Often cauterization or embolization is required to prevent interoperative hemorrhage (Guthrie, 1997).

Radiation

- Radiation therapy has been found to be the treatment variable most strongly related to prognosis. Studies have indicated survival of 4.6 years versus less than 1 year (Chan & Thompson, 1985); and recurrence rates on average of 29 months versus 74 months if irradiated (Guthrie et al., 1989).
- Recommended radiaton doses are 50 to 55 Gy delivered to the site of tumor plus margin (Guthrie et al., 1989; Schroder, Firsching, & Kochanek, 1986).

Chemotherapy

- There is no proven role for chemotherapy either at initial diagnosis or recurrence.

Meningeal Sarcoma

Surgery

- Radical resection is the treatment of choice (Tomita & Gonzales-Crussi, 1984).

Radiation
- Radiation has uncertain benefit in these tumors.

Chemotherapy
- Chemotherapy also has uncertain benefit in these tumors, although the more malignant tumors may respond to sarcoma regimens (Raney, et al., 1987).

PINEAL REGION TUMORS

Pineal and Germ Cell Tumors

Surgery
- Aggressive surgical resection is usually recommended.
- With benign tumors, complete resection is usually curative (Stein & Bruce, 1992).
- With malignant tumors, complete resection is thought to improve response to adjunctive therapies (Stein & Bruce, 1992).
- Operative mortality is reported from 0% to 8% and permanent morbidity from 0% to 12% (Stein & Bruce, 1992; Herrmann, Winkler, & Westphal, 1992).

Radiation Therapy
- Patients with malignant germ cell or pineal cell tumors require radiation therapy, typically to doses of 50 to 55 Gy (Bruce et al., 1997).
- Germinomas are very radiosensitive and may be cured with radiation therapy.
- Long-term complications from radiation therapy occur in these patients, since long-term survival is often possible. Most series report nearly 100% incidence of mental slowing or mental retardation (Jenkin et al., 1990).

Chemotherapy
- Nongerminomatous malignant germ cell tumors are usually treated with chemotherapy prior to radiation therapy, but optimal timing of adjuvant therapy has not been conclusively determined (Bruce et al., 1997).
- A wide variety of chemotherapy regimens have been tried, most using some variation of the Einhorn regimen of cisplatin, vinblastine, and bleomycin (Sawaya et al., 1990; Bruce et al., 1997).

- Chemotherapy for germinomas is typically reserved until recurrence.
- Chemotherapy for pineal cell tumors has not been studied extensively. Currently, no treatment recommendations exist and no definitive response to treatment has been reported (Schild et al., 1993).

Pituitary Tumors

Surgery
- Definitive treatment for microadenoma and most macroadenomas. A transphenoidal surgical approach is used and is usually curative (Thapar & Laws, 1997).
- Surgery is associated with a 0.5% mortality and a 2% morbidity.

Radiation
- Radiation is used as a treatment for large unresectable or partially resectable macroadenomas that are refractory to pharmacologic treatment. Radiation therapy is also effective in treating microadenomas. However, correction of hormonal elevations is more gradual following radiation than surgery.

Radiosurgery
- Increasingly being used for pituitary tumors, the efficacy is uncertain (Thapar & Laws, 1997). In this location, fractionated stereotactic radiation therapy may be useful to protect adjacent normal structures.

Chemotherapy
- Conventional cytotoxic chemotherapy has not been used for pituitary tumors.
- Dopamine agonists such as bromocriptine are useful for prolactin secreting tumors.
- Somatostatin analogs are used for growth hormone secreting tumors.

SKULL-BASED TUMORS

Chordoma and Chondrosarcoma of the Cranial Base

Surgery
- New postoperative cranial nerve deficits are seen mostly during the early postoperative period.

- One-third to one-half of preoperative dysfunction completely resolve after surgery (Gay, 1997).

Radiation Therapy

- Radiation therapy is typically indicated as the tumor is usually not completely resected or a high-grade malignancy. The dose is greater than 50 Gy delivered to the tumor area plus edema (Amendola et al., 1986). Results with a charged particle (e.g., protons or helium) appear superior to those with conventional photon radiation therapy.
- Forsyth and colleagues (1993) reported a significant effect on prolonged disease-free survival, but no improvement in survival time with conventional postoperative radiation therapy.
- The use of hyperfractionation or radioactive sources have not demonstrated improved survival over standard radiation therapy (Kondziolka, Lunsford, & Flickinger, 1991; Kumar et al., 1988).

Radiosurgery

- Few reports on the use of radiosurgery for chordomas or chondrosarcomas are available, so the effect on outcome is unclear (Gay et al., 1997; Kondziolka et al., 1991).

Chemotherapy

- Effective chemotherapy is not available (Finn, Goeffert, & Batsakis, 1984; Fuller & Bloom, 1988; Gay et al., 1997).

Glomus Jugulare Tumors

Surgery

- Surgical resection is the mainstay of treatment for glomus tumors (Cece et al., 1987).

Radiation Therapy

- Radiation therapy is usually recommended for unresectable or incompletely resected tumors.
- 45 to 50 Gy has been recommended (Larner et al., 1992).

Radiosurgery

- Radiosurgery has been utilized for unresectable tumors (Ebersold et al., 1997).
- The number of patients treated thus far have been too small to comment on effectiveness (Ebersold et al., 1997).

Primary Central Nervous System Lymphoma (PCNSL)

■ Principles of management include obtaining a histologic diagnosis, ensuring that the disease is confined to the brain, excluding an underlying predisposing illness, and instituting definitive therapy (Rosenthal & Green, 1997).

■ If PCNSL is suspected, the institution of steroids should be delayed until definitive tissue diagnosis is obtained, unless herniation is imminent. Radiologic disappearance of the tumor can occur rapidly after the commencement of steroids (DeAngelis, 1990).

Surgery

• Surgical debulking does not improve median survival (Murray et al., 1986). Therefore, biopsy is usually performed (Sherman et al., 1991; Feiden, Bise, & Steude, 1990).

• The success rate in obtaining accurate tissue diagnosis with biopsy is > 95% (Sherman et al., 1991).

Radiation Therapy

• PCNSL is a radiosensitive tumor with response rates of up to 80% (Rosenthal & Green, 1997). However, the response duration is typically short.

• The dose and volume of irradiation required for disease control have not been clearly defined. In general, most centers irradiate the whole brain initially followed by a boost to the tumor site to a cumulative dose of greater than 50 Gy (Rosenthal & Green, 1997).

• Some have suggested that patients with poor performance status should receive 30 Gy over two weeks (Cooper, 1989).

Chemotherapy

• There are no studies that clearly define optimal chemotherapy for primary central nervous system lymphoma. Current multicenter clinical trials are underway.

• Recent data show higher response rates with high-dose methotrexate-based regimens and improved outcomes with chemotherapy and radiation therapy versus radiation alone. Median survival is approximately 20 months versus 40 months with combined therapy (DeAngelis, 1990).

Metastatic Tumors

■ Appropriate treatment has been a matter of debate for decades (Sawaya & Bindal, 1997).

■ Patients with < or = three lesions have been shown to have a statistically significant prolonged survival (albeit only 3 weeks) over those with four or more lesions (Swift et al., 1993).

Surgery

• Surgical excision of solitary brain metastasis should be attempted if the patient is deemed a good surgical candidate. Factors to consider include inaccessible location of the tumor, Karnofsky performance status, extent of neurologic deficits, length of time between the first diagnosis of cancer and the diagnosis of brain metastasis, disease status of the primary lesion, and type of primary tumor (Galicich et al., 1980; Burt et al., 1992; Yardeni, Reichenthal, & Zucker, 1984; White, Fleming, & Laws, 1981; Sundaresan & Galicich, 1985).

• A randomized study of whole brain radiation therapy (WBRT) versus surgery and WBRT for a solitary brain metastases showed a significant improvement in survival with the addition of surgery (Patchell et al., 1990).

• The presence of multiple lesions is typically a contraindication to surgery.

• Surgical morbidity after resection of brain metastasis, defined as increased postoperative neurologic deficits, has been reported as 5% or lower (Sundaresan & Galicich, 1985; Brega et al., 1990; Patchell et al., 1990; Bindal et al., 1993).

• Surgical complications can include thromboembolic complications (estimated 10% incidence)(Sawaya et al., 1992; Constantini et al., 1991), hematomas infection, and pseudomeningocele formation (estimated 8–9% incidence)(Bindal et al., 1993).

• Recurrence of tumors after surgery occurs locally in 5% to 15% of patients, distant recurrence occurs in 10% to 20%, and 5% to 10% have both local and distance recurrence (Sundaresan & Galicich, 1985; Patchell et al., 1990; Bindal et al., 1993).

Radiation therapy

• The use of postoperative whole brain radiation therapy (WBRT) has been associated with a significant improvement in local control and disease-free survival compared to surgery alone (Patchell, Tibbs, & Regina, 1998). Current guidelines recommend WBRT as initial treatment for those with lymphoma or small cell lung cancer and in conjunction with surgery for other metastatic tumors (National Comprehensive Cancer Network, 1997).

- According to the National Comprehensive Cancer Network guidelines(1997), either whole brain XRT or Focal XRT may be utilized in patients with melanoma, renal cell, or sarcoma, since these tumors are often not radiosensitive.

- For patients with multiple (> 2) metastatic lesions, treatment recommendations include WBRT (30–40 Gy in 10–20 fractions). The most common fractionation scheme in the United States is 30 Gy in 10 fractions. However, a prior RTOG randomized trial showed no difference in survival between this and other shorter or longer regimens. If the patient has poor performance status, a more rapid course can be utilized (National Comprehensive Cancer Network, 1997).

- Four retrospective studies have been completed reviewing the outcome of patients treated with WBRT. Three showed a reduced recurrence rate (Smalley et al., 1987; DeAngelis et al., 1989a; Hagen et al., 1990) and one indicated a significantly extended survival (Smalley et al., 1987).

- Wong and colleagues (1996) reported a median survival of 4 months for patients reirradiated for brain metastases with no significant toxicity.

- Hyperfractionation (Murray et al., 1997) and the use of radiosensitizers (Kormanicky et al., 1991; Phillips et al., 1995) have not shown a survival benefit.

Radiosurgery

- Radiosurgery has been found to have the best outcome in patients who meet the following criteria: absence of extracranial disease, KPS > 70, single intracranial metastasis (Cho et al., 1998), age less than 45, response to steroid treatment, and site of primary tumor (Lagerwaard, Levendag, & Nowak, 1999).

- Permanent local control can be obtained in > 80% of treated lesions with complications in fewer than 10% (Loeffler et al., 1999).

- Patients who receive WBRT in addition to radiosurgery have better local control (Loeffler & Alexander, 1993), such that radiosurgery alone is usually not advocated for treatment of brain metastases.
- Radiosurgery has shown superior cost outcomes on all measures compared to surgery (Mehta et al., 1997).
- Rutigliano et al. (1995) also found radiosurgery had lower average complication cost per case, lower total cost per procedure, lower uncomplicated procedure cost, and had a better incremental cost-effectiveness than resection (Rutigliano et al., 1995).
- RTOG trial 89-05 demonstrated a 0% to 7% incidence of acute toxicity in patients with recurrent, previously irradiated metastatic brain metastases less than or equal to 40 mm in maximum diameter (Shaw et al., 1996).

Chemotherapy

- The use of chemotherapy is undefined for metastatic tumors from sites other than germ cell or small cell lung cancer. Reports indicate that response rates for these two tumor types are similar to response rates seen for systemic cancer in these patients (Twelves et al., 1990; Boogerd et al., 1992, Lange, Scheef, & Hasse, 1990).

REFERENCES

Aaronson, N. K., Ahmedzai, S., Bergman, B., Bullinger, M., Cull A., Duez, N.J., Filiberti, A., Flechtner, H., Fleishman, S.B., & Haes, J.C. et al (1993). The European Organization for Research and Treatment of Cancer QLQ-C30: A quality of life instrument for use in international clinical trials in oncology. *Journal of the National Cancer Institute*, 85(5), 365–376.

Allen, J., Wisoff, J., Helson, L., Pearce, J., Arenson, E. (1992). Choroid Plexus Carcinoma-responses to chemotherapy alone in newly diagnosed young children. *Journal of Neuro-oncology*, 12; 69–74.

Amador, L. V. (1983). *Brain tumors in the young* (pp. 3–22). Springfield, IL: Charles C. Thomas.

Amendola, B. E., Amendola, M. A., Oliver, E., McClatchery, K. D. (1986). Chordoma: role of radiation therapy. *Radiology*, 158(3) 839–843.

Annegers, J. F., Coulam, C. B., Abboud, C. F., Laws, E. R. Jr., Kuland, L. T. et al., (1978). Pituitary adenoma in Olsted County, Minnesota, 1935–1977. *Mayo Clinic Proceedings*, 53, 641–643.

Armstrong, T. S. (1999). Harvesting hope in the autumn of life. *Clinical Journal of Oncology Nursing*, 3(1), 23–28.

Armstrong, T. S., & Gilbert, M. R. (1995). Management of seizures in the adult patient with cancer. *Cancer Practice*, 3(3), 143–149.

Armstrong, T. S., & Gilbert, M. R. (1996). Glial neoplasms: Classification, treatment, and pathways for the future. *Oncology Nursing Forum*, 23(4), 615–624.

Berger, M. S., Deliganis, A. V., Dobbins, J., Keles, G. E. (1994). The effect of extent of resection on recurrence in patients with low grade cerebral hemisphere gliomas. *Cancer*, 74, 1784–1791.

Berger, M. S., Magrassi, L., & Geyer, R. (1997). Medulloblastoma and primitive neuroectomermal tumors. In A. H. Kaye & E. R. Laws (Eds.), *Brain tumors*. New York: Churchill Livingstone.

Bertolene, S. J., Baum, E. S., Krivit, W., et al., (1989). A phase II study of cisplatin therapy in recurrent childhood brain tumors. A report from the Children's Cancer Study Group. *Journal of Neuro-oncology*, 7, 5–11.

Bindal, R., Sawaya, R., Leavens, M., Lee, J. J. (1993). Surgical treatment of multiple brain metastases. *Journal of Neurosurgery*, 79, 210–216.

Bithell, J. F., & Stewart, A. M. (1975). Pre-natal irradiation and childhood malignancy: A review of British data from the Oxford Survery. *British Journal of Cancer*, 31, 271–287.

Blatt, J., Jaffe, R., Deutsch, M., & Adkins, J. C. (1986). Neurofibromatosis and childhood cancers. *Cancer*, 57, 122–129.

Bolande, R. P. (1989). Teratogenesis and oncogenesis: A developmental spectrum. In H. T. Lynch, T. Hirayama (Eds.), *Genetic epidemiology of cancer* (pp. 55–68). Boca Raton, FL: CRC Press.

Boogerd, W., Dalesio, O., Bais, E., Van der Sande, J. J. (1992). Response of brain metastases from breast cancer to systemic chemotherapy. *Cancer*, 69, 972–980.

Boyle, J. O., Shimm, D. S., Coulthard, S. W. (1990). Radiation therapy for paragangliomas of the temporal bone. *Laryngoscope*, 100, 896–899.

Brackmann, D. E., & Kwartler, J. A. (1990). A review of acoustic tumors: 1983–1988. *American Journal of Otology*, 11, 216–232.

Brega, K., Robinson, W., Winston, K., & Wittenberg, W. (1990). Surgical treatment of brain metastases in malignant melanoma. *Cancer*, 66, 2105–2120.

Brem, H., Piantodose, S., Burger, P. C., Walker, M., Selker, R., Vick, N. A., Black, K., Sisti, M., Brem, S., Mohr, G. (1995). Placebo-controlled trial of safety and efficacy of intraoperative controlled delivery by biodegradable polymers of chemotherapy for recurrent gliomas. *Lancet*, 345, 1008–1012.

Brown, M., Cairncross, J. G., Vick, N. A., (1990). Differential response of recurrent oligodendroglioma versus astrocytoma to intravenous melphalan [Abstract]. *Neurology*, 40 (Suppl. 1), 397–398.

Bruce, J. N., Connolly, E. S., & Stein, B. M. (1997). Pineal cell and germ cell tumors. In A. H. Kaye, & E. R. Laws (Eds.), *Brain tumors*. New York: Churchill Livingstone.

Bruce, J. N., & Stein, B. M. (1993). Complications of surgery for pineal region tumors. In K. D. Post, E. D.Friedman, & P. C. McCormick (Eds.), *Postoperative complications in intracranial Neurosurgery* (pp. 74–86). New York: Thieme Medical Publishers.

Bunin, G. (1987). Racial patterns of childhood brain cancer by histologic type. *Journal of the National Cancer institute*, 78, 875–880.

Burger, P. C., Rawlings, C. E., Cox, E. B., Schold, S. C. Jr., Burger, P., & Halperin, E. C. (1987). Clinicopathological correlations in the oligodendroglioma. *Cancer*, 59, 1345–1352.

Burt, M., Wronski, M., Arbit, E., & Galicich, J. H. (1992). Resection of brain metastases from non-small-cell lung carcinoma. *Journal of Thoracic and Cardiovascular Surgery*, 103, 339–411.

Busse, P. M. (1991). Radiation therapy for meningiomas. In H. H. Schmidek (Ed.), *Meningiomas and their surgical management* (p. 506). Philadelphia: W. B. Saunders.

Cairncross, J. G., & Macdonald, D. R. (1988). Successful chemotherapy for recurrent malignant oligodendroglioma. *Annals of Neurology*, 23, 360–364.

Cece, J. A., Lawson, W., Eden, A. R., Parisler, S. C. (1987). Complications in the management of large glomus jugulare tumors. *Laryngoscope*, 97, 152–157.

Central Brain Tumor Registry of the United States. (1998). Manuscript in preparation.

Cerrato, D., Ariano, C., & Fiaccjiono, F. (1978). Deep vein thrombosis and low dose heparin prophylaxis in neurosurgical patients. *Journal of Neurosurgery*, 49, 378–381.

Chen, T. C., Gonzalez-Gomez, I., & McComb, J. G. (1997). Uncommon glial tumors. In A. H. Kaye, & E. R. Laws (Eds.), *Brain tumors*. New York: Churchill Livingstone.

Cho, K. H., Hall, W. A., Gerbi, B. J., Higgins, P. D., Bohan, M., Clark, H. B. (1998). Patient selection criteria for the treatment of brain metastases with stereotactic radiosurgery. *Journal of Neuro-oncology*, 40(1), 73–86.

Choucair, A. K., Scott, C., Urtasum, R., Nelson, D., Mousas, B., Curran, W. (1997). Quality of life and neuropsychological evaluation for patients with malignant astrocytomas: RTOG 91-14. Radiation Therapy Oncology Group. *International Journal of Radiation Oncology, Biology, Physics*, 38(1), 9–20.

Clark, W. C., Callihan, T., Schwartzberg, L., & Fontanesi, J. (1992). Primary intracranial Hodgkin's lymphoma without dural attachment. *Journal of Neurosurgery*, 76, 692–695.

Clemis, J. D., Ballad, W. J., Baggot, P. J., Lyon, S. T. (1986). Relative frequency of inferior vestibular schwannoma. *Archives of Otolaryngology Head and Neck Surgery*, 112, 190–194.

Coltrera, M. D., Googe, P. B., Harrist, T. J., Hyams, V. J., Schiller, A. L., Goodman, M. L. (1986). Chondrosarcoma of the temporal bone. Diagnosis and treatment of 13 cases and review of the literature. *Cancer*, 58, 2689–2696.

Constantini, S., Kornowski, R., Pomeranz, S., Rappaport, Z. H. (1991). Thromboembolic phenomena in neurosurgical patients operated upon for primary and metastatic brain tumors. *Acta Neurochirurgica (Wien)* 109, 93–97.

Cooper, J. S. (1989). Radiation therapy and the treatment of patients with AIDS. In *Radiation oncology: Rationale, techniques, results* (pp. 762–776). Baltimore: CV Mosby.

Couldewell, W. T., & Hinton, D. R. (1997). Oligodendroglioma. In A. H. Kaye & E. R. Laws,(Eds.), *Brain tumors*. New York: Churchill Livingstone.

Cummings, B. J., Ian Hodson, D., & Bush, R. S. (1983). Chordoma: The results of megavoltage radiation therapy. *International Journal of Radiation Oncology, Biology, Physics, 9*, 633–642.

Curran, W. J., Scott, C. B., Horton, J., Nelson, J. S., Weinstein, A. S., Nelson, D. F., Fischbach, A. J., Chang, C. H., Rotman, M., Asbell, S. O. (1992). Does extent of surgery influence outcome for astrocytoma with atypical or anaplastic foci (AAF)? A report from three Radiation Therapy Oncology Group (RTOG) trials. *Journal of Neuro-oncology, 12*(3), 219–227.

Cushing, H. (1912). The pituitary body and its disorder (p. 297). Philadelphia: J. B. Lippincott.

DeAngelis, L. M. (1990). Primary central nervous system lymphoma imitates multiple sclerosis. *Journal of Neuro-oncology, 9*, 177–181.

DeAngelis, L., Mandell, L., Thaler, H., Kimmel, D. W., Galicich, J. H., Fuks, Z., Posner, J. B. (1989). The role of postoperative radiotherapy after resection of single brain metastases. *Neurosurgery, 24*, 798–805.

DeAngelis, L. M., Wong, E. Rosenblum, M., (1992). Epstein-Barr virus in Acquired Immune Deficiency Syndrome (AIDS) and non-AIDS primary central nervous system lymphoma. *Cancer, 70*, 1607–1611.

Debevec, M. (1990). Management of patients with brain metastases of unknown origin. *Neoplasm, 37*, 601–606.

Delattre, J., Krol, G., Thaler, H., Posner, J. B. (1988). Distribution of brain metastases. *Archives of Neurology, 45*, 741–744.

DeMonte, F., & Al-Mefty, O. (1997). Meningiomas. In A. H. Kaye & E. R. Laws (Eds.), *Brain tumors*. New York: Churchill Livingstone.

Deutsch, M., Green, S. B., Strike, T. A., Burger, P. C., Robertson, J. T., Selker, R. G., Shapiro, W. R., Mealey, J., Jr., Ransahoff, J. 2nd, Padletti, P. (1989). Results of a randomized trial comparing BCNU plus radiotherapy, streptozotocin plus radiotherapy, BCNU plus hyperfractionated radiotherapy, and BCNU following misonidazole plus radiotherapy in the postoperative treatment of malignant glioma. *International Journal of Radiation Oncology, Biology, Physics, 16*, 1389–1396.

Dhopesh, V., & Yagnik, P. (1985). Brain metastasis: Analysis of patients without known cancer. *Southeran Medical Journal, 78*, 171–172.

Donahue, B., Scott, C. B., Nelson, J. S., Rotman, M., Murray, K. J., Nelsen, D. F., Banker, F. L., Earl, J. D., Fischbab, J. D., Asbell, S. O., Gaspar, L. E., Markoe, A. M., Curran, W. (1997). Influence of an oligodendroglial component on the survival of patients with anaplastic astrocytomas: A report of Radiation Therapy Oncology Group 83-02. *International Jouranl of Radiation Oncology, Biology, Physics, 38*(5), 911–914.

Duncan, J. A., & Hoffman, H. J. (1997). Intracranial ependymomas. In A. H. Kaye & E. R. Laws (Eds.), *Brain tumors*. New York: Churchill Livingstone.

Ebersold, M. J., Morita, A., & Olsen, K. D. (1997). Glomus jugulare tumors. In A. H. Kaye & E. R. Laws (Eds.), *Brain tumors*. New York: Churchill Livingstone.

Edwards, M. S. B., Hudgins, R. J., Wilson, C. B., Levin, V. A., Wara, W. M. (1988). Pineal region tumors in children. *Journal of Neurosurgery, 66,* 689–697.

Ellenbogen, R. G., Winston, K. R., & Kupsky, W. J. (1989). Tumors of the choroid plexus in children. *Neurosurgery, 25,* 327–335.

Eriksson, B., Gunterberg, B., & Kindblom, L. G. (1981). Chordoma, a clinicopathologic and prognostic study of a Swedish national series. *Acta Orthopaedica Scandinavica, 52,* 49–58.

Evans, D. G. R., Huson, S. M., Donnai, D., Neary, W., Blair, V., Newton, V., Strachan, T., Harris, R. (1992). A genetic study of type 2 neurofibromatosis in the United Kingdom. I. Prevalence, metation rate, fitness, and confirmation of maternal transmission effect on severity. *Journal of Medical Genetics, 29,* 841–846.

Evans, H. L., Ayala, A. G., Romsdahl, M. M. (1977). Prognostic factors in chondrosarcoma of bone. A clinicopathologic analysis with emphasis on histologic grading. *Cancer, 40,* 818–831.

Fan, K. J., & Pezeshkpoar, G. H. (1992). Ethnic distribution of primary central nervous stystem tumors in Washington, DC 1971–1985, *Journal of the National Medical Association, 84*(10)858–863.

Faithful, S. (1991). Patients' experiences following cranial radiotherapy: A study of the somnolence syndrome. *Journal of Advanced Nursing, 16*(8), 939–946.

Feiden, W., Bise, K., & Steude, U. (1990). Diagnosis of primary cerebral lymphoma with particular reference to CT-guided stereotactic biopsy. *Virchows Archives. A, Pathological Anatomy and Histopathology, 417,* 21–28.

Ferrara, M., Bizzozzero, F., Talamonti, G., D'Angelo, V. A. (1990). Surgical treatment of 100 single brain metastases. *Journal of Neurosurgical Science, 34,* 303–308.

Finn, D. G., Goeffert, H. G., & Batsakis, J. G. (1984). Chondrosarcoma of the head and neck. *Laryngoscope, 94,* 1539–1543.

Forbes, A. R., & Goldberg, I. D. (1984). Radiation therapy in the treatment of meningioma: The joint center for radiation therapy experience, 1970–1982. *Journal of Clinical Oncology, 2,* 1139–1143.

Forsyth, P. A., Cascino, T. L., Shaw, E. G., Scheithauer, B. W., O'Fallon, J. R., Dozia, J. C., Piepgias, D. G. (1993). Intracranial chordomas: A clinicopathological and prognostic study of 51 cases. *Journal of Neurosurgery, 78,* 741–747.

Friedman, W. A., Blatt, D. L., Bova, F. J. (1998). *Linac radiosurgery. A practical guide.* New York: Springer.

Fuller, D. B., & Bloom, J. G. (1988). Radiotherapy for chordoma. *International Journal of Radiation Oncology, Biology, Physics, 15,* 331–339.

Galicich, J., Sundaresan, N., Arbit, E., Passe, S. (1980). Surgical treatment of single brain metastasis: Factors associated with survival. *Cancer, 45,* 38–386.

Gaspar, L., Scott, C., Rotman, M., Asbell, S., Phillips, T., Wasserman, T., Mckenar, W. G., Byhardt, R. (1997). Recursive partitioning analysis (RPA) of prognostic factors in three Radiation Therapy Oncology Group (RTOG) brain metastases trials. *International Journal of Radiation Oncology, Biology, Physics,* 37(1), 745–751.

Gay, E., Sekhar, L. N., & Wright, D. C. (1997). Chordomas and chondrosarcomas of the cranial base. In A. H. Kaye & E. R. Laws (Eds.), *Brain tumors.* New York: Churchill Livingstone.

Gerosa, M. A., DeStefano, E., Olivi, A., Carteri, A. (1981). Multidisciplinary treatment of medulloblastoma: A 5-year experience with the SIOP trial. *Childs Brain,* 8, 107–118.

Goldwein, J. W., Glauser, T. A., Packer, R. J., Finlay, J. L., Sutton, L. N., Curran, W. J., Lachy, J. M., Rorke, L. B., Schut L., D'Anglo, G. J. (1990). Recurrent intracranial ependymomas in children. *Cancer,* 66, 557.

Goodwin, J. W., Crowley, J., Stafford, B., Jaeckle, K. A., Townsend, J. J. (1993). A phase II evaluation of tamoxifen in unresectable or refractory meningiomas: A southwest oncology group study. *Journal of Neuro-oncology,* 15, 75–77.

Green, S. B., Byar, D. P., Walker, M. D., Pistenmaa, D. A., Alexander, E., Jr., Batzdorf, V., Brooks, W. H., Hunt, W. E., Mealey, J. Jr., Odom, G. L., Paoletti, P., Ransohoff, J. Z, Robertson, J. T., Selker, R. G. Shapiro, W. R., Smith, K. R., Jr., Wilson, C. B., Strike, T A. (1983). Comparisons of carmustine, procarbazine and high-dose methylprednisolone as additions to surgery and radiotherapy for the treatment of malignant glioma. *Cancer Treatment Report,* 67, 121–132.

Grunberg, S. M., Weiss, M. H., Ahmadi, J., Sadun, A., Russell, C. A., Lucci, L., Stevenson, L. L., Spitz, I. M. (1991). Treatment of unresectable meningiomas with the antiprogesterone agent mifepristone. *Journal of Neurosurgery,* 74, 861–866.

Guthrie, B. L. (1997). Meningeal hemangiopericytoma. In A. H. Kaye & E. R. Laws (Eds.), *Brain tumors.* New York: Churchill Livingstone.

Guthrie, B. L., Ebersold, M. J., Scheithauer, B. W., & Shaw, E. G. (1989). Meningeal hemangiopericytoma: Histopathological features, treatment, and long-term follow-up of 44 cases. *Neurosurgery,* 25, 514–522.

Guthrie, B. L., & Laws, E. R. (1990). Supratentorial low grade gliomas. *Neurosurgery Clinics of North America,* 1, 37–48.

Gutin, P. H., Leibel, S. A., Wara, W. M., Choucair, A., Levin, V. A., Philips, T. L., Silver, P., Da Silva, V., Edwards, M. S., Davis, R. L. (1987). Recurrent malignant gliomas: Survival following interstitial brachytherapy with high-activity iodine-125 sources. *Journal of Neurosurgery,* 67, 864–973.

Haddad, G. F., & Al-Mefty, O. (1997). Meningeal sarcoma. In A. H., Kaye & E. R. Laws (Eds.), *Brain tumors.* New York: Churchill Livingstone.

Hagen, N., Cirrincione, C., Thaler, H., DeAngelis, L. M. (1990). The role of radiation therapy following resection of single brain metastasis from melanoma. *Neurology*, 40, 158–160.

Hardy, D. G., Macfarlane, R., Baguley, D., Moffat, D. A. (1989). Surgery for Acoustic neurinoma. An analysis of 100 translabyrinthine operations. *Journal of Neurosurgery*, 71, 799–804.

Hassouneh, M., Al-Mefty, O., Akhtar, M., et al. (1985). Primary cranial and intracranial chondrosarcoma. A survey. *Acta Neurochirurgicawien*, 78, 123–132.

Healey, E. A., Barnes, P. D., Kupsky, W. J., Scott, R. M., Sallan, S. E., Black, P. M., Tarbell, N. J. (1991). The prognostic significance of postoperative residual tumor in ependymoma. *Neurosurgery*, 28, 666–672.

Heffelfinger, M. J., Dahlin, D. C., MacCarty, C. S., Beabout, J. W. (1973). Chordomas and cartilaginous tumors at the skull base. *Cancer*, 32, 410–420.

Hendrick, E. B., & Raffel, C. (1989). Tumors of the fourth ventricle: Ependymomas, choroid plexus papillomas and dermoid cysts. In *Pediatric neurosurgery*, (pp. 366–371). Philadelphia: W. B. Saunders.

Herrmann, H. D., Winkler, D., & Westphal, M. (1992). Treatment of tumors of the pineal region and posterior part of the third ventricle. *Acta Neurochirurgica*, 116: 137–146.

Hochberg, F. C., & Miller, D. C. (1988). Primary central nervous system lymphoma. *Journal of Neurosurgery*, 68, 835–853.

House, W. F., & Luetje, C. E. (1979). Evaluation and preservation of facial function. In W. F. House & C. M. Luetje (Eds.), *Acoustic tumors* (pp. 89–94). Baltimore, MD: University Park Press.

Huang, C. I., Chiou, W. H., & Ho, D. M. (1987). Oligodendroglioma occurring after radiation therapy for pituitary adenoma. *Journal of Neurology, Neurosurgery and Psychiatry*, 50, 1619–1624.

Jenkin, D., Berry, M., Chan, H., Greenberg, M., Hendrick, B., Hoffman, H., Humphreys, R., Sonley, M., Weitzman, S. (1990). Pineal region germinomas in childhood treatment considerations. *International Journal of Radiation Oncology, Biology, Physics*, 18, 541–545.

Jennings, M. T., Gelman, R., & Hochberg, F. (1985). Intracranial germ-cell tumours: Natural history and pathogenesis. *Journal of Neurosurgery*, 63, 155–167.

Johnson, B. E., Patronas, N., Hayes, W., Grayson, J., Becker, B., Gnepp, D., Rowland, J., Anderson, A., Glatstein, E., Ihde, D. C. (1990). Neurologic, computed cranial tomographic, and magnetic resonance imaging abnormalities in patients with small-cell lung cancer. Further follow-up of 6- to 13-year survivors. *Journal of Clinical Oncology*, 8, 48–56.

Kendall, B. E., & Lee, B. C. P. (1977). Cranial chordomas. *British Journal of Radiology*, 50, 687–698.

Kennerdell, J. S., Maroon, J. C., Malton, M., Warren, F. A. (1988). The management of optic nerve sheath meningiomas. *American Journal of Ophthalmology*, 106, 450–457.

Kiebert, G. M., Curran, D., Aaronson, N. K. (1998). Quality of life after radiation therapy of cerebral low-grade gliomas of the adult: Results of a randomised phase III trial on dose response (EORTC trial 22844). EORTC Radiotherapy Co-operative Group. *European Journal of Cancer*, 34 (12), 1902–1909.

Kleinberg, L., Wallner, K., & Malkin, M. G. (1993). Good performance status of long-term disease-free survivors of intracranial gliomas. *International Journal of Radiation Oncology, Biology, Physics*, 26 (1), 563.

Knierim, D. S. (1990). Choroid plexus tumors in infants. *Pediatric Neurosurgery*, 16, 276–280.

Konziolka, D., Lunsford, L. D., & Flickinger, J. C. (1991). The role of radiosurgery in the management of chordoma and chondrosarcoma of the cranial base. *Neurosurgery*, 29, 38–46.

Komarnicky, L. T., Phillips, T. L., Martz, K., Asbell, S., Isaacson, S., Urtasun, R. (1991). A randomized phase III protocol for the evaluation of misonidazole combined with radiation in the treatment of patients with brain metastases (RTOG-7916). *International Journal of Radiation Oncology, Biology, Physics*, 20(1), 53–58.

Kumar, P. P., Good, R. R., Skultery, F. M., Leibrock, L. G. (1988). Local control of recurrent clival and sacral chordoma after interstitial irradiation with Iodine-125: New techniques for treatment of recurrent or unresectable chordomas. *Neurosurgery*, 22, 479–483.

Kun, L. E., Kovnar, E. H., Sanford, R. A. (1988). Ependymomas in children. *Pediatric Neuroscience*, 14, 57–63.

Lagerwaard, F. J., Levendag, P. C., & Nowak, P. J. (1999). Identification of prognostic factors in patients with brain metastases: A review of 1292 patients. *International Journal of Radiation Oncology, Biology, Physics*, 43 (4), 795–803.

Lamberts, S. W. J., Tanghe, H. L. J., Avezaat, C. J. J., Brackman, R., Wijngaarde, R., Koper, J. W., de Jong, H., et al. (1992). Mifepristone (RU486) treatment of meningiomas. *Journal of Neurology, Neurosurgery and Psychiatry*, 55, 486–490.

Lange, O., Scheef, W., & Haase, K. (1990). Palliative radiochemotherapy with ifosfamide and BCNU for breast cancer patients with cerebral metastases: A 5-year experience. *Cancer Chemotherapy and Pharmacology*, 26(Suppl.), 78–80.

Lardis, S. H., Murray, T., Boldev, S, Wingo, P. A. (1998). Cancer Statistics, 1998. *CA: Cancer Journal for Clinicians*, 48(1): 6–29.

Larner, J. M., Hahn, S. S., Spaulding, C. A., Constable, W. C. (1992). Glomus jugulare tumors. Long-term control by radiation therapy. *Cancer*, 69, 1813–1817.

Laws, E. R., & Kamat, M. (1993). Brain tumors. *CA: Cancer Journal for Clinicians*, 43, 263–265.

Laws, E. R., Taylor, W. F., Clifton, M., & Okazaki, H. (1984). Neurosurgical management of low-grade astrocytomas of the cerebral hemispheres. *Journal of Neurosurgery*, 61, 665–673.

Leibel, S. A., Gutin, P. H., Wara, W. M., Silver, P. S., Larson, D. A., Edwards, M. S., Lano, S. A., Hau, B., Weaver, K. A., Barnett, C. (1989). Survival and quality of life after interstitial implantation of removable high-activity iodine-125 sources for the treatment of patients with recurrent malignant gliomas. *International Journal of Radiation Oncology, Biology, Physics,* 17, 1129–1139.

Leibel, S. A., & Sheline, G. E. (1987). Radiation therapy of neoplasms of the brain. *Journal of Neurosurgery,* 66, 1–22.

Li, F. P., & Fraumeni, J. F. (1982). Prospective study of a family cancer syndrome. *Journal of the American Medical Association,* 247, 2692–2694.

Liang, R. H. S., Woo, E. K. W., Yu, Y., Todd, D., Chan, T. K., Ho, F. C., Tso, S. C., Shum, J. S. (1989). Central nervous system involvement in non-Hodgkin's lymphoma. *European Journal of Clinical Oncology,* 25, 703–710.

Lindae, M. L., Luy, J., Abel, E. A., Kaplan, R. (1990). Mycosis fungoides with CNS involvement: Neuropsychiatric manifestations and complications of treatment with intrathecal methotrexate and whole-brain irradiation. *Journal of Dermatology and Surgical Oncology,* 16, 550–553.

Lindegaard, K. F., Mork, S. J., Eide, G. E., Halvorsen, T. B., Hatlevoll, R., Solgaard, T., Dahl, O., Ganz, J. (1987). Statistical analysis of clinicopathological features, radiotherapy, and survival in 170 cases of oligodendroglioma. *Journal of Neurosurgery,* 67, 224–240.

Loeffler, J. S., & Alexander, E. I., III. (1993). Radiosurgery for the treatment of intracranial metastases. In E. I. Alexander, III, J. S. Loeffler, & L. D. Lunsford (Eds.), *Stereotactic radiosurgery* (pp. 197–198). New York: McGraw-Hill.

Loeffler, J. S., Alexander, E., Shea, W. M., Wen, P. Y., Fine, H. A., Kooyz, H. M., Black, P. M. (1992). Radiosurgery as part of the initial management of patients with malignant gliomas. *Journal of Clinical Oncology,* 10, 1379–1385.

Loeffler, J. S., Barker, F. G., & Chapman, P. H. (1999). Role of radiosurgery in the management of central nervous system metastases. *Cancer Chemotherapy and Pharmacology,* 43 (Suppl.), S11–S14.

Lovely, M. P., Miakowski, C., Dodd, M. (1999). Relationship between fatigue and quality of life in patients with glioblastoma multiforne. "Oncology Nursing Forum" 26(5) 921–925.

Lynch, H. T., Marcus, J. M., Watson, P., Conway, T., Fitzsimmons, M. L., Lynch, J. F. (1989). Genetic epidemiology of breast cancer. In H. T. Lynch, T. Hirayama (Eds.), *Genetic epidemiology of cancer* (pp. 289–232). Boca Raton, FL: CRC Press.

Lyons, M. K., & Kelly, P. J. (1991). Posterior fossa ephendymomas: Report of 30 cases and review of the literature. *Neurosurgery,* 28, 659–665.

Macfarlane, R., & King, T. T. (1997). Acoustic neurinoma. In A. H. Kaye & E. R. Laws (Eds.), *Brain tumors.* New York: Churchill Livingstone.

Mack, E. E., & Wilson, C. B. (1993). Meningiomas induced by high-dose cranial irradiation. *Journal of Neurosurgery,* 61, 136–142.

Mackworth, N., Fobair, P., & Prados, M. (1992). Quality of life self-reports from 200 brain tumor patients: Comparison with Karnofsky performance scores. *Journal of Neuro-oncology,* 14, 243–253.

Mahaley, M. S. (1991). Neuro-oncology index and review (adult primary brain tumors): Radiotherapy, chemotherapy, immunotherapy, photo-dynamic therapy. *Journal of Neuro-oncology, 11*, 85–147.

Mahaley, M. S., Mettlin, C., Natarajan, N., Laws, E. R., & Peace, B. B. (1989). National survery of patterns of care for brain-tumor patients. *Journal of Neurosurgery, 71*, 826–836.

McCormack, B. M., Miller, D. C., Budzilovich, G. N. (1992). Treatment and survival of low-grade astrocytomas in adults—1977–1988. *Neurosurgery, 31*, 636–642.

McGirr, S. J., Ebersold, M. J., Scheithauer, B. W., Quast, L. M., Shaw, E. G., (1988). Choroid plexus papillomas: Long-term follow-up results in a surgically treated series. *Journal of Neurosurgery, 69*, 843–849.

Mehta, M., Noyes, W., Craig, B., Lamond, J., Auchter, R., French, M., Johnson, M., Lenin, A., Bode, B., Robbins, I., Kinsella, T. (1997). A cost-effectiveness and cost-utility analysis of radiosurgery versus resection for single-brain metastases. *International Journal of Radiation Oncology, Biology, Physics, 39*(2), 445–454.

Miralbell, R., Linggood, R. M., de la Monte, S., Convery, K., Munzcurider, J. E. (1992). The role of radiotherapy in the treatment of subtotally re-sected menign meningiomas. *Journal of Neuro-oncology, 13*, 157–164.

Mirimanoff, R. O., Dosoretz, D. E., Linggood, R. M., Ojemann, R. G., Martuza, R. L. (1985). Meningioma: Analysis of recurrence and pro-gression following neurosurgical resection. *Journal of Neurosurgery, 62*, 18–24.

Modan, B., Baodatz, D., & Mart, H. (1974). Radiation-induced head and neck tumors. *Lancet, 1*, 277–279.

Morantz, R. A. (1987). Radiation therapy in the treatment of cerebral astro-cytomas. *Neurosurgery, 20*, 975–982.

Morantz, R. A. (1988). Editorial comment. *Neurosurgery, 22*, 890–891.

Morantz, R. A. (1997). Low grade astrocytomas. In A. H. Kaye & E. R. Laws (Eds.), *Brain tumors*. New York: Churchill Livingstone.

Mork, S. J., Halvorsen, T. B., Lindegaard, K. F., & Eide, G. E. (1985). Oligo-dendroglioma: Histological evaluation and prognosis. *Journal of Neuropathology and Experimental Neurology, 45*, 65–78.

Muller, W., Afra, D., & Schroder, R. (1977). Supratentorial recurrences of gliomas: Morphological studies in relation to time intervals with as-trocytomas. *Acta Neurochirurgica, 37*, 75–91.

Murray, K., Kun, L., & Cox, J. (1986). Primary malignant lymphoma of the central nervous system. Results of treatment of 11 cases and review of the literature. *Journal of Neurosurgery, 65*, 600–607.

Murray, K. J., Scott, C., Greenberg, H. M., Emami, B., Seider, M., Vora, N. L., Olson, C., Whilton, A., Mousas, B., Curran, W. (1997). A randomized phase III study of accelerated hyperfractionation versus standard in patients with unresected brain metastases: A report of the Radiation Therapy Oncology Group (RTOG) 9104. *International Journal of Radiation Oncology, Biology, Physics, 39*(3), 571–574.

Nagib, M. G., Haines, S. J., Erickson, D. L., Mastri, A. R. (1984). Tuberous sclerosis: A review for the neurosurgeon. *Neurosurgery, 14*, 93–98.

National Cancer Institute. (1999). *Common toxicity criteria, version 2.0 with EORTC and RTOG acute effects criteria.* Bethesda, MD: National Cancer Institute.

National Comprehensive Cancer Network. (1997). NCCN adult brain tumor practice guidelines. NCCN *Proceedings—Oncology,* 11(1), 237–277.

Nazar, G. B., Hoffman, H. J., Becker, L. E., Jenkin, D., Humphreys, R. P., Hendrick, E. B. (1990). Infratentorial ependymomas in childhood: Prognostic factors and treatment. *Journal of Neurosurgery,* 72, 408–417.

Nedzelski, J. M., Schessel, D. A., Pleiderer, A., Kassel, E. E. (1992). The natural history of growth of acoustic neuromas and its role in nonoperative management. In M. Tos & J. Thomsen (Eds.), *Acoustic neuroma,* (pp. 149–158). Amsterdam: Kugler.

O'Dell, M. W., Barr, K., Spanier, D., Warnick, R. E. (1998). Functional outcome of inpatient rehabilitation in persons with brain tumors. *Archives of Physical Medicine and Rehabilitation,* 79(12), 1530–1534.

O'Driscoll, B. R., Hasleton, P. S., Taylor, P. M., Poulter, L. W., Gattameneni, H. R., Woodcock, A. A. (1990). Active lung fibrosis up to 17 years after chemotherapy with carmustine (BCNU) in childhood. *New England Journal of Medicine,* 323, 378–382.

Ohaegbula, S. C., Saddeqi, N., & Ikerionwu, S. (1980). Intracranial tumors in Enugu, Nigeria. *Cancer,* 46, 2322–2324.

Olsen, K. D. (1994). Tumors and surgery of parapharyngeal space. *Laryngoscope,* 104, 1–28.

Patchell, R. A., Tibbs, P. A., Regina, W. R. (1998). Postoperative radiotherapy in the treatment of single brain metastases to the brain. JAMA, 280, 1485–1489.

Patchell, R., Tibbs, P., Walsh, J., Dempsey, R. J., Maruyama, Y., Kryscio, R. J., Markesbery, W. R., Macdonald, J. S., Young, B. (1990). A randomized trial of surgery in the treatment of single brain metastases. *New England Journal of Medicine,* 322, 494–545.

Paulus, W., & Peiffer, J. (1988). Does the pleomorphic xanthroastrocytoma exist? Problems in the application of immunological techniques to the classification of brain tumors. *Acta Neuropathologica,* 76, 245–252.

Paulus, W. F., Slowik, L., & Jellinger, K. (1991). Primary intracranial sarcomas: Histopathological features of 19 cases. *Histopathology,* 18, 395–402.

Philippon, J. H., Clemenceau, S. H., Fauchon, F. H., Foncin, J. F. (1993). Supratentorial low-grade astrocytomas in adults. *Neurosurgery,* 32, 554–559.

Phillips, T. L., Scott, C. B., Leibel, S. A., Rotman, M., Weigensberg, I. J. (1995). Results of a randomized comparison of radiotherapy and bromodeoxyuridine with radiotherapy alone for brain metastases: A report of RTOG trial 89-05. *International Journal of Radiation Oncology, Biology, Physics,* 33(2), 339–348.

Phupanich, S., Scott, C., Fischbach, A. J., Langer, C., Yung, W. K. (1997). All-trans-retinoic acid: A phase II Radiation Therapy Oncology Group study (RTOG 91-13) in patients with recurrent malignant astrocytoma. *Journal of Neuro-oncology,* 34(3), 193–200.

Prados, M. D., Scott, C., Curran, W. J., Nelson, D. F., Leibel, S., Kramer, S. (1999). Procarbazine, Lomustine, and Vincristine (PCV) chemotherapy for anaplastic astrocytoma: A retrospective review of radiation therapy oncology group protocols comparing survival with Carmustine or PCV adjuvant chemotherapy. *Journal of Clinical Oncology*, 17(1), 3389–3395.

Prados, M. D., Scott, C. B., Rotman, M., Rubin, P., Murray, K., Sause, W., Asbell, S., Comis, R., Curran, W., Nelson, J., Davis, R. L., Levin, V. A., Lamborn, K., Phillips, T. L. (1998). Influence of bromodeoxyuridine radiosensitization on malignant glioma patient survival: A retrospective comparison of survival data from the Northern California Oncology Group (NCOG) and Radiation Therapy Oncology Group (RTOG) trials for glioblastoma multiforme and anaplastic astrocytomas. *International Journal of Radiation Oncology, Biology, Physics*, 40(3), 653–659.

Preston-Martin, S., Thomas, D. C., Henderson, B. E., Bernstein, B. E., & Wright, W. E. (1989). Noise in the aitology of acoustic neuromas in men in Los Angeles County, 1978–1985. *British Journal of Cancer*, 59, 783–786.

Preston-Martin, B., Yu, M. C., Henderson, B. E., & Benton, B. (1983). Risk factors for meningiomas in men. *Journal of the National Cancer Institute*, 70, 863–866.

Randell, R. V., Scheithauer, B. W., Laws, E. R., Abbound, C. F., Ebersold, M. J., Kao, P. C. (1985). Pituitary adenomas associated with hyperprolactinemia: A clinical and immunohistochemical study of 97 patients operated on transsphenoidally. *Mayo Clinic Proceedings*, 60, 753–762.

Raney, R. B., Tefft, M., Newton, W. A., Ragab, A. H., Lawrence, W. Jr., Gehan, E. A., Maurer, H. M. (1987). Improved prognosis with intensive treatment of children with cranial soft tissue sarcomas arising in nonorbital parameningeal sites: A report from the intergroup rhabdomyosarcoma study. *Cancer*, 59, 147–155.

Rasmussen, H B., Teisner, B., Schroder, H., Yde-Andersen, & Andersen, J. A. (1991). Fetal antigen 2 in primary and secondary brain tumors. *Tumor Biology*, 12, 330–338.

Remick, S. C., Diamond, C., Migliozzi, J. A., Solis, O., Wagner, H. Jr., Haase, R. F., Ruckdeschel, J. C.(1990). Primary central nervous system lymphoma in patients with and without the Acquired Immune Deficiency Syndrome. A retrospective analysis and review of the literature. *Medicine*, 69, 345–360.

Rich, T. A., Schiller, A., Suit, H. D., Mankin, H. J. (1985). Clinical and pathologic review of 48 cases of chordoma. *Cancer*, 56, 182–187.

Rohinger, M., Sutherland, G. R., Louw, D. F., Sima, A. A. (1989). Incidence and clinicopathological features of meningioma. *Journal of Neurosurgery*, 7, 665–672.

Ron, E., Modan, B., Boice, J. D., Alfandary, E., Stovall, M., Chetrit, A., Katz, L. (1988). Tumors of the brain and central nervous system after radiotherapy in childhood. *New England Journal of Medicine*, 319, 1033–1039.

Rosenthal, M. A., & Green, M. D. (1997). Cerebral lymphoma. In A. H. Kaye & E. R. Laws (Eds.), *Brain tumors*. New York: Churchill Livingstone.

Roth, R. J., & Elvidge, A. R. (1960). Glioblastoma multiforme: A clinical survey. *Journal of Neurosurgery*, 17, 736–750.

Rubinstein, L. J. (1971). Sarcomas of the nervous system. In J. Minckler (Ed.), *Pathology of the nervous system* (Vol. 2, pp. 2144–2164). New York: McGraw-Hill.

Rubinstein, L. J. (1972). Oligodendrogliomas. In *Tumors of the central nervous system* (pp. 85–104). Washington, DC: Armed Forces Institute of Pathology.

Russell, D. S., & Rubinstein, L. J. (1989). *Pathology of tumours of the nervous system* (5th ed.). Baltimore: Williams & Wilkens.

Rutigliano, M. J., Lunsford, L. D., Kondziolka, D., Strauss, M. J., Khanna, V., Green, M. (1995). The cost-effectiveness of stereotactic radiosurgery versus surgical resection in the treatment of solitary metastatic brain tumors. *Neurosurgery*, 37(3), 445–453.

Sachsenheimer, W., Piotrowski, W., & Bimmler, T. (1992). Quality of life in patients with Intracranial tumors on the basis of Karnofsky's performance status. *Journal of Neuro-oncology*, 13(2), 177–181.

Salazar, O. M. (1983). A better understanding of CNS seeding and a brighter outlook of postoperatively irradiated patients with ependymomas. *International Journal of Radiation Oncology, Biology, Physics*, 9, 1231–1234.

Salazar, O. M. (1988). Ensuring local control in meningiomas. *International Journal of Radiation Oncology, Biology, Physics*, 15, 501–504.

Salcman, M. (1980). Survival in glioblastoma: Historical perspective. *Neurosurgery*, 7, 435–439.

Salcman, M., Scholtz, H., Kaplan, R. S., Kulik, S. (1993). Long term survival in patients with malignant astrocytoma. *Neurosurgery*, 34,(2), 219–220.

Salassa, R. M., Laws, E. R., Carpenter, P. C., Northcutt, R. C. (1978). Transphenoidal removal of pituitary microadenoma in Cushing's disease. *Mayo Clinic Proceedings*, 53, 24–28.

Sawaya, R., & Bindal, R. J. (1997). Metastatic brain tumors. In A. H. Kaye & E. R. Laws, (Eds.), *Brain tumors*. New York: Churchill Livingstone.

Sawaya, R., Hawley, D. K., Tobler, W. D. (1990). Pineal and third ventricular tumors. In J. Youmanns (Ed.), *Neurological surgery* (pp. 3171–3203). Philadelphia: W. B. Saunders.

Sawaya, R., Zuccarello, M., Elkalliny, M., Nishiyama, H. (1992). Postoperative venous thromboembolism and brain tumors: Part I. Clinical profile. *Journal of Neuro-oncology*, 14, 119–125.

Schild, S. E., Scheithauer, B. W., Schomberg, P. J., Hook, C. C., Kelly, P. J., Frick, J. L., Robinow, J. S., Buskirk, S. J. (1993). Pineal parenchymal tumors: Clinical, pathologic, and therapeutic aspects. *Cancer*, 72, 870–880.

Schoenberg, B. S. (1977). Multiple primary neoplasms and the nervous system. *Cancer*, 40, 1961–1967.

Schoenberg, B. S. (1991). Epidemiology of primary intracranial neoplasms: Disease distribution and risk factors. In M. Salcman (Ed.), *Neurobiology of brain tumors* (pp. 3–18). Baltimore: Williams & Wilkens.

Schroder, R., Firsching, R., & Kochanek, S. (1986). Hemangiopericytoma of the meninges. II. General and clinical data. *Zentralblatt fur Neurochirurgie*, 47, 191–199.

Scott, R. M., & Knightly, J. (1997). Choroid plexus papillomas. In A. H. Kaye & E. R. Laws (Eds.), *Brain tumors*. New York: Churchill Livingstone.

Segall, H. D., Destian, S., Nelson, M. D., Kirsch, D. L. (1990). CT and MRI imaging in malignant gliomas. In M. L. J. Apuzzo (Ed.), *Malignant cerebral glioma* (pp. 63–77). Park Ridge, IL: AANS Publications Committee.

Selker, R. G., Jacobs, S. A., Moore, P. B., Wald, M., Fisher, E. R., Cohen, M., Bellot, P. (1980). 1,3-Bis(20chloroethyl)-1-nitrosurea (BCNU)-induced pulmonary fibrosis. *Neurosurgery*, 7, 560–565.

Shapiro, W. R., Green, S. B., Burger, P. C., Mahaley, M. S. Jr., Selker, R. G., VanGilder, J. C., Robertson, J. T., Ransohoff, J., Mealey, J. Jr., Strike, T. A. (1989). Randomized trial of three chemotherapy regimens and two radiotherapy regimens in postoperative treatment of malignant glioma: Brain Tumor Cooperative Group Trial 8001. *Journal of Neurosurgery*, 71, 1–9.

Shapiro, W. R., & Rankin-Shapiro, J. (1998). Biology and treatment of malignant glioma. *Oncology*, 12, 233–240.

Shaw, E. G. (1990). Low-grade gliomas. To treat or not to treat? A radiation oncologist's viewpoint. *Archives of Neurology*, 47, 1138–1139.

Shaw, E. G., Daumas-Duport, C., Scheithauer, B. W., Gilbertson, D. T., O'Fallon, J. R., Earle, J. D., Laws, E. R. Jr., Arokki, H. (1989). Radiation therapy in the management of low-grade supratentorial astrocytomas. *Journal of Neurosurgery*, 24, 853–861.

Shaw, E. G., Evans, R. G., Scheithauer, B. W., Ilstrup, D. M., Earle, J. D. (1987). Postoperative radiotherapy of intracranial ependymoma in pediatric and adult patients. *International Journal of Radiation Oncology, Biology, Physics*, 13, 1457–1462.

Shaw, E. G., Scjeotjaier, B. W., O-Fallon, J. R., Tazelaar, H. D., Davis, D. H. (1992). Oligodendrogliomas: The Mayo Clinic experience. *Journal of Neurosurgery*, 76, 428–434.

Shaw, E., Scott, C., Souhami, L., Dinapoli, R., Bahary, J. D., Kline, R., Wharan, M., Schultz, C., Daley, P., Loeffler, J., DelRowe, J., Marks, L., Fisher, B., and Shiv, K. (1996). Radiosurgery for the treatment of previously irradiated recurrent primary brain tumors and brain metastases: Initial report of radiation therapy oncology group protocol (90-05). *International Journal of Radiation Oncology, Biology, Physics*, 34(3), 647–654.

Shea, J. J., Hitselberger, W. E., Benecke, J. E., Brackmann, D. E. (1985). Recurrence rate of partially resected acoustic tumors. *American Journal of Otology* (Suppl. 11), 107–109.

Shering Plough. (1999). *Temozolomide product information*. Shering Oncology Biotech. NJ: Kenilworth.

Sherman, M. E., Erozan, Y. S., Mann, R. B., Kumar, A. A., McArthur, J. C., Royal, W., Vematsus, Naota, H. J. (1991). Stereotactic brain biopsy in the diagnosis of malignant lymphoma. *American Journal of Clinical Pathology*, 95, 878–883.

Shrieve, D. C., Alexander, E., III, Black, P. M., Wen, P. Y., Fine, H. A., Kooy, H. M., Loeffla, J. S. (1999). Treatment of patients with primary glioblastoma multiforme with standard postoperative radiotherapy and radiosurgical boost: Prognostic facts and long-term outcome. *Journal of Neurosurgery,* 90(1), 72–77.

Simpson, J. R., Horton, J., Scott, C., Curran, W. J., Rubin, P., Fischbach, J., Isaacson, S., Rotman, M., Asbell, S. O., Nelson, J. S. (1993). Influence of location and extent of surgical resection on survival of patients with glioblastoma multiforme: Results of three consecutive Radiation Therapy Oncology Group (RTOG) clinical trials. *International Journal of Radiation Oncology, Biology, Physics,* 26, 239–244.

Smadja, D., Mas, J., Fallet-Bianco, C., Meyniard, O., Sicard, D., de Recordo, J., Rondot, P. (1991). Intravascular lymphomatosis of the central nervous system: Case report and literature review. *Journal of Neuro-oncology,* 11, 171–180.

Smalley, S., Schray, M., Laws, E., O'Fallon, J. R. (1987). Adjuvant radiation therapy after surgical resection of solitary brain metastasis: Association with pattern of failure and survival. *International Journal of Radiation Oncology, Biology, Physics,* 13, 1611–1616.

Smith, M. T., Ludwig, C. L., Godfrey, A. D., Armbrustmacher, V. W. (1983). Grading of oligodendrogliomas. *Cancer,* 52, 2107–2114.

St. Clair, S. K., Humphreys, R. P., Pillay, P. K., Hoffman, H. T., Blasa, S. I., Beeker, L. E. (1991). Current management of choroid plexus carcinoma in children. *Pediatric Neurosurgery,* 17, 225–233.

Stein, B. M., & Bruce, J. N. (1992). *Surgical management of pineal region tumors* (pp. 509–532). Baltimore: Williams & Wilkens.

Stoller, J. K., Kavuru, J., Mehta, A. C., Weinstein, C. E., Estes, M. L., Gephardt, G. N. (1987). Intracranial meningioma metastatic to the lung. *Cleveland Clinic Journal of Medicine,* 54, 521–527.

Sundaresan, N., & Galicich, J. (1985). Surgical treatment of brain metastases: Clinical and computerized tomography evaluation of the results of treatment. *Cancer,* 55, 1382–1388.

Sutherland, G. R., Florell, R., Louw, D., Choi, N. W., Sima, A. A. (1987). Epidemiology of primary intracranial neoplasms in Manitoba, Canada. *Canadian Journal of Neurological Sciences,* 14, 586–592.

Sutton, L. N., Goldwein, G., Perilongo, B., Lang, B., Schut, L., Rorke, L., Packer, R. (1990). Prognostic factors in childhood ependymomas. *Pediatric Neurosurgery,* 16, 57–65.

Swift, M., Morrell, D., Cromartie, E., Chambelin, A. B., Skolnick, M. H., Bishop D. T. (1986). The incidence and gene frequency of ataxia-telangiectasia in the United States. *American Journal of Human Genetics,* 39, 573–583.

Swift, P. S., Phillips, T., Martz, K., Wara, W., Mohiuddin, M., Chang, C. H., Asbell, S. U. (1993). CT characteristics of patients with brain metastases treated in RTOG study 79-16. *International Journal of Radiation Oncology, Biology, Physics,* 25(2), 209–214.

Takakura, K. (1982). Intracranial germ cell tumors. *Clinical Neurosurgery,* 32, 429–444.

Tamura, N., Ono, M., Kurihara, H., Ohye, C., Miyazaki, M. (1990). Adjunctive treatment for recurrent childhood ependymoma of the IV ventricle: Chemotherapy with CDDP and MCNU. *Childs Nervous System*, 6, 186.

Taphoorn, M. J., Schiphorst, A. K., Snoek, F. J., Lindeboom, J., Wolbers, J. G., Kamm, A. B., Huijgens, P. C., Helmans, J. J. (1994). Cognitive functions and quality of life in patients with low-grade gliomas: The impact of radiotherapy. *Annals of Neurology*, 36(1), 48–54.

Taylor, B. W., Marcus, R. B., Friedman, W. A., Ballinger, W. E. Jr., Million, R. R. (1988). The meningioma controversy: Postoperative radiation therapy. *International Journal of Radiation Oncology, Biology, Physics*, 15, 299–304.

Thapar, K., & Laws, E. (1997). Pituitary tumors. In A. H. Kaye & E. R. Laws (Eds.), *Brain Tumors*. New York: Churchill Livingstone.

Thomas, T. L., Steward, P. A., Stemhagen, A., Correa, P., Norman, S. A., Bleecker, M. L., Hoover, R. N. (1987). Risk of astrocytic brain tumours associated with occupational chemical exposures. *Scandinavian Journal of Work, Environment and Health*, 13, 417–423.

Todd, D. W., Christoferson, L. A., Leech, R. W., Rudolf, L. (1981). A family affected with intestinal polyposis and gliomas. *Annals of Neurology*, 10, 390–392.

Tomita, T., & Gonzales-Crussi, F. (1984). Intracranial primary nonlymphomatous sarcomas in children: Experience with eight cases and review of the literature. *Neurosurgery*, 14, 529–549.

Tomita, T., McLone, D. G., Das. L., Brand, W. N. (1988). Benign ependymomas of the posterior fossa in childhood. *Pediatric Neuroscience*, 14, 277–285.

Twelves, C., Souhami, R., Harper, P., Ash, C. M., Spiro, S. G., Earl, H. M., Tobias, J. S., Quinn, H., Geddes, D. M. (1990). The response of cerebral metastases in small cell lung cancer to systemic chemotherapy. *British Journal of Cancer*, 61, 147–150.

Van Der May, A. G. L., Frijns, J. H., Cornelisse, C. J., Brons, E. N., Terpstra, H. L., Schmidt, P. H., Van Dulken, H. (1992). Does intervention improve the natural course of glomus tumors? A series of 108 patients seen in a 32-year period. *Annals of Otology, Rhinology, and Laryngology*, 97, 613–620.

Van Roijen, L., Nijs, H. G., & Avezaat, C. J. (1997). Costs and effects of microsurgery versus radiosurgery in treating acoustic neuroma. *Acta Neurochirurgica (Wien)*, 139(10), 972–978.

Vertosick, F. T., Selker, R. G., & Arena, V. C. (1991). Survival of patients with well-differentiated cerebral astrocytomas in the adult. *Neurosurgery*, 28, 496–501.

Waga, S., & Handa, H. (1976). Radiation-induced meningioma with review of the literature. *Surgical Neurology*, 5, 215–219.

Walker, A. E., Robins, M., & Weinfeld, F. D. (1985). Epidemiology of brain tumors: The national survery of intracranial neoplasms. *Neurology*, 35, 219–226.

Walker, M. D., Alexander, E., Hunt, W. E., MacCarty, C. S., Mahaley, M. S. Jr., Mealey, J. Jr., Norrell, H. A., Owens, G., Ransahoff J., Wilson, C. B., Gehon, E. D., Strike, T. A. (1978). Evaluation of BCNU and/or radiotherapy in the treatment of anaplastic gliomas: A cooperative clinical trial. *Journal of Neurosurgery, 49,* 333–343.

Weitzner, M. A., Meyers, C. A., Gelke, C. K., Cella, D. F., & Levin, V. A. (1995). The Functional Assessment of Cancer Therapy (FACT) scale. Development of a brain subscale and revalidation of the general version (FACT-G) in patients with primary brain tumors. *Cancer, 75*(5), 1151–1161.

White, K., Fleming, T., & Laws, E. (1981). Single metastasis to the brain. Surgical treatment in 122 consecutive patients. *Mayo Clinic Proceedings, 56,* 424–428.

Whitton, A. C., & Bloom, H. J. G. (1990). Low grade glioma of the cerebral hemispheres in adults: A retrospective analysis of 88 cases. *International Journal of Radiation Oncology, Biology, Physics, 18,* 783–786.

Wilkinson, I. M. S., Anderson, J. R., & Holmes, A. E. (1987). Oligodendroglioma: An analysis of 42 cases. *Journal of Neurology, Neurosurgery, and Psychiatry, 50,* 304–312.

Winger, M. J., Macdonald, D. R., & Cairncross, J. G. (1989). Supratentorial anaplastic gliomas in adults: The prognostic importance of extent of resection and prior low-grade glioma. *Journal of Neurosurgery, 71,* 487–493.

Wong, E. T., Hess, K. R., Gleason, M. J., Jaeckle, K. A., Kyritsis, A. P., Prados, M. D., Levin, V. A., Yung W. K. (1999). Outcomes and prognostic factors in recurrent glioma patients enrolled onto phase II clinical trials. *Journal of Clinical Oncology, 17*(8), 2572–2578.

Wong, W. W., Schild, S. E., Sawyers, T. E., Shaw, E. G. (1996). Analysis of outcome in patients reirradiated for brain metastases. *International Journal of Radiation Oncology, Biology, Physics, 34*(3), 585–590.

Yardeni, D., Reichenthal, E., & Zucker, G. (1984). Neurosurgical management of single brain metastasis. *Surgical Neurology, 21,* 377–384.

Zanki, H., & Zang, K. D. (1980). Correlations between clinical and cytogenetical data in 180 human meningiomas. *Cancer Genetics and Cytogenetics, 1,* 351–356.

Zeltzman, M., Grossman, S. A., Sheidler, V. R., Baust, S., Braine, H. (1991). Favorable outcome despite high risks for intracranial bleeding (ICB) in patients with astrocytomas (AC) following intensive chemotherapy [Abstract]. *Proceedings of the American Society of Clinical Oncology, 10,* A378.

Zimmerman, R. D. (1991). MRI of intracranial meningiomas. In O. Al-Mefty (Ed.), *Meningiomas* (pp. 209–223). New York: Raven Press.

Zulch, K. J. (1986). *Brain tumors: Their biology and pathology* (3rd ed., pp. 210–213). Berlin: Springer-Verlag.

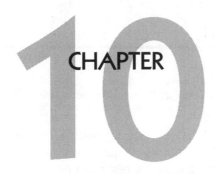

CHAPTER 10

HEAD AND NECK CANCERS

Marilyn L. Haas, PhD, ANP-C
Eric F. Kuehn, MD

PROBLEM

Head and neck cancers constitute approximately 5% of all newly diagnosed invasive malignancies in the United States (American
Cancer Society, 1999). This accounts for approximately 60,000 new
cases a year. According to the American Cancer Society's cancer
statistics, the highest rate of malignancies occurs in the oral cavity
(40%), followed by laryngeal cancer (25%), cancers of the oropharynx and hypopharynx (17%), salivary gland malignancies (7%), and
the rest in the remaining sites (13%) (Landis, Murray, Bolden, &
Wingo, 1998). In terms of demographics, the men to women incidence ratio for head and neck cancer is 3:1. The incidence of this
type of cancer increases with age. More than 90% of head and neck
cancers occur in patients over the age of 40, with half after age 65
(Landis et al., 1998). Also, there is a higher incidence of head and
neck cancers among the lower socioeconomic groups (Gale &
Charette, 1994).

ASSESSMENT

RISK FACTORS

Assessing the patient's risk factors is an extremely important element of the patient's history. Factors that can impact outcomes are:

- Tobacco—There is a strong relationship between the use of any tobacco products (cigarettes, cigars, pipes, and smokeless chewing tobacco) and head and neck cancers. In fact, 95% of squamous cell carcinomas of the head and neck are associated with the use of tobacco (Mood, 1997).

- Alcohol—Heavy alcohol consumption is considered another strong risk factor. Combining tobacco with alcohol has a synergistic effect that increases the risk by five times (Mood, 1997).

- Viral Infections—Exposure to herpes simplex and human papilloma viruses may increase the risk and has been implicated in the pathogenesis of oral, laryngeal, and nasopharyngeal carcinomas (Clayman, Lippman, Laramore, & Hong, 1997). Exposure to Epstein-Barr virus has been associated with nasopharyngeal carcinomas, especially in younger patients (Taylor, 1999).

- Vitamin A Deficiency—Cancers of the oral cavity and pharynx are seen in higher incidence in patients who are Vitamin A deficient (Shaha & Strong, 1995).

- Poor Oral Hygiene/Poor Dentition—Constant irritation from dental caries or ill-fitting dentures may increase risk over time (Bruner, Bucholtz, Iwamoto, & Strohl, 1998).

- Noxious Substance Exposure—Higher incidences have been observed in patients who have been exposed to wood dust, nickel compounds, nitrosamines, hydrocarbons, and asbestos. Also, workers dealing with leather, cotton, wool, and asphalt products can have higher risks (Taylor, 1999).

- Poor Nutritional Intake—Nutritional deficiencies leading to Plummer-Vinson syndrome (iron deficiency anemia) have shown strong correlations with the development of head and neck cancers.

- Genetic Predisposition—Cantonese people have the presence of a specific HLA antigen, which places them at a higher risk for nasopharyngeal cancers. Investigational studies of comparative genomic hybridization patterns of chromosomal imbalances may soon help to define the malignancy potential of head and neck squamous cell carcinomas (Bockmuhl et al., 1998).

PREVENTION/SCREENING AND PRESENTING SYMPTOMS

Since there is a strong correlation between the consumption of large quantities of alcohol and the use of tobacco products with the development of head and neck cancers, prevention and screening are essential. Prevention efforts include stop smoking programs, counseling for alcohol abuse, and public education about these risky behaviors. Patients are often ignorant of the symptoms of disease. The American Cancer Society has identified three warning signs that pertain to cancers of the head and neck: dysphagia, chronic ulcer, and/or a lump in the neck. Unfortunately, many patients ignore these warning signs and present with advanced disease. Also, tumors may go undiagnosed for long periods because symptoms can mimic bacterial infections, sinusitis, or allergic rhinitis. Screening for nasopharyngeal carcinomas is under investigation with the supplemental use of nasopharyngeal swab (polymerase chain reaction) being utilized with serologic screening of these cancers (Sheen et al., 1998).

The importance of early identification of premalignant or early malignant mucosal lesions in the head and neck cannot be overemphasized since early detection improves survival rates. A thorough physical assessment and recognition of signs and symptoms are essential. Most premalignant changes or in situ carcinomas of the oral mucosa occur as red (erythroplasia) or white patches (leukoplakia) that are easily visualized with direct examination. Common symptoms of oral cavity primaries include a painful ulceration, slurred speech, bleeding in the oral cavity, and/or an exophytic mass. In other areas where tumors are difficult to see, (hypopharynx or larynx) chronic hoarseness or other voice changes, chronic sore throat, otalgia, or dysphagia may be presenting symptoms. Palpation and visualization of the oral cavity, pharynx, and larynx are extremely important in the physical examination. The oral cavity, base of the tongue, and the tonsils should be palpated with a gloved finger. Indirect visualization via mirror or fiber-optic laryngoscopy provides the clinician with detailed information about the nasopharynx, hypopharynx, base of tongue, and larynx. Lesions that persist despite the treatment with antibiotics or removal of local irritants, or that may or may not have associated ulceration, induration, or a change in size should be biopsied. Other possible presenting symptoms include the following:

- Pain may or may not be present. Pain can be due to ulceration, involvement of bone, or tumor pressure. There can be referred pain to surrounding areas, particularly the ears (otalgia). Painful swallowing (odynophagia) can occur as well as voice changes that are secondary to pain, commonly referred to as "hot potato voice."
- Weight loss—Unintentional weight loss of 10 or more pounds within the last 6 months is potentially a correlate of cancer (DeWys et al., 1980).
- Unilateral chronic serous otitis media justifies an evaluation for nasopharynx carcinoma.
- Unilateral nasal polyps, nasal obstruction, and/or epistaxis are common presenting complaints of nasal cavity or paranasal sinus neoplasm.
- Trismus—Tonsillar tumors can involve muscles of the temporomandibular joint or the joint itself resulting in difficulty in fully opening the mouth. A quick method of assessing trismus is to ask the patient to open his or her mouth as wide as possible. If less than three fingers can fit in the mouth, trismus is probably present (Buchbinder, Currivan, Kaplan, & Urken, 1993). In latent trismus, a sensation of tightness will be present.
- Cranial nerve involvement—Inflammation and pressure from the tumor can cause cranial nerve impingement. Symptoms depend on the nerve involved and can include diplopia, facial numbness or weakness, dysarthria (stuttering), and difficulty swallowing.
- Unexplained neck mass—Indurated unilateral neck masses are highly suspicious of cancer. Usually 50% of such lumps are malignant (Taylor, 1999). Adenopathy is typically nontender and may not be associated with any other symptoms.

Referrals to other services may be necessary to complete the physical assessment. These may include:

- Dental Evaluation—Chronically diseased teeth should be extracted prior to radiation therapy, since dental work after radiation therapy is extremely difficult. Extractions, root canals, fillings, and crowns should be completed 2 to 3 weeks prior to beginning radiation treatments. If preprosthetic surgery is required, this should also be performed before beginning radiation treatments, since surgical procedures are contraindicated on irradiated bone. Fluoride treatments should be discussed and instituted after completion of treatments to prevent radiation-induced dental caries (Mood, 1997).

■ Speech Therapy Evaluation—Patients are evaluated by a speech therapist for functional impairments in speech or swallowing resulting from both tumor and treatment.

■ Physical Therapy Evaluation—If range of motion in the neck is expected to decrease or shoulder disability may be a potential problem, a physical therapy evaluation is justified. Baseline function should be established prior to treatment.

■ Nutritional Evaluation—Ideally, nutritional assessments should be performed on all head and neck patients. Typically, nutritional support is required and the insertion of a gastrostomy tube is preferred over hyperalimentation (Lutz & Przytulski, 1997).

■ Smoking Cessation Program—Smoking irritates the mucosal membranes and radiation can intensify this reaction. The patient's motivational level to quit, environmental support, and individual risk factors should be assessed. Patients should be encouraged to enroll early in group or individualized sessions that pertain to nonsmoking. Several methods are available: pharmacological therapy, behavorial therapy, hypnosis, acupuncture, or individual aids.

DIAGNOSTIC TESTING

With most head and neck cancers, tumors can be directly visualized. However, diagnostic imaging procedures are necessary for additional evaluation. Studies may include the following:

■ Computerized Tomography Scan (CT) and Magnetic Resonance Imaging (MRI)—assist in defining the extent of the primary tumor and establishing regional lymph node involvement.

■ Radiological Films—plain films can be utilized to evaluate bony involvement of the mandible.

■ PET Scan—used in the staging, posttreatment, and monitoring phases of head and neck cancer management.

■ Cine-esophagography/Barium Swallow—identifies any swallowing difficulties.

If a second primary or distant metastases is suspected, other diagnostic procedures would include:

■ Radiological Films—chest x-ray aids in detecting pulmonary nodules. Lung metastases are the most common metastatic site. Panoramic x-ray of the mandible may be helpful.
■ Bone Scan—to assess for any bone involvement.
■ Liver Scan and/or Liver Function Tests—to ascertain any liver metastases.

Confirmation of pathological type can be obtained by a variety of procedures that can include:

■ Punch Biopsy—most common technique utilized for mucosal biopsies.
■ Curettage—scrapings of tissue are provided for examination.
■ Fine Needle Aspiration (FNA)—widely accepted and typically recommended first, if feasible.
■ Excisional Biopsy—cutting away or taking out the lesion may be preferred.
■ Incisional Biopsy—a procedure that provides diagnosis and may be the treatment necessary to eradicate the tumor.

STAGING

Most cancers of the head and neck are found in the oral cavity and pharynx, nasal cavity and paranasal sinuses, larynx, and salivary glands. Subsites in these areas are listed in Table 10–1. Skin lesions on the face and neck and cervical lymph nodes are also included under head and neck cancers. These cancers however are discussed in other chapters.

Although head and neck cancers are easily detected, many tumors go undiagnosed for long periods of time. Therefore, it is estimated that approximately 60% of newly diagnosed head and neck cancers are in advanced stages (Gale & Charette, 1994). The majority of the head and neck cancers are squamous cell carcinomas. These tumors are pathologically graded and well-differentiated and moderately well-differentiated tumors are generally less aggressive and have a better prognosis than poorly differentiated or anaplastic tumors. The tumors are also staged and pretreatment staging is the

TABLE 10–1   SUBSITES IN HEAD AND NECK AREAS

Oral Cavity	Lips, oral tongue, floor of the mouth, buccal mucosa, upper and lower gingivae, retromolar trigone, and hard palate
Pharynx	Nasopharynx (posterosuperior wall, lateral wall, eustachian tube orifice and adenoids)
	Oropharynx (tonsil, base of tongue, and pharyngeal wall) and soft palate
	Hypopharynx (pyriform sinus, postcricoid area, posterior wall)
Larynx	Supraglottis (ventricular bands (false cords), arytenoids, suprahyoid and infrahyoid epiglottis)
	Glottis (true vocal cords, including anterior and posterior commissures)
	Subglottis
Other locations	Nasal cavity, paranasal sinuses, and salivary glands

most predictive factor of overall survival (Forastiere, Schuller, & Spencer, 1998). Staging criteria for cancers arising in the upper aerodigestive tract, paranasal sinuses, and salivary glands have been developed by the American Joint Committee on Cancer and are site-specific. This system regularly undergoes reevaluation. Staging is based on T (primary tumor size and extent), N (regional nodes evaluation), and M (presence of distant metastasis). Refer to Tables 10–2 and 10–3 for the TNM staging of primary head and neck tumors. The TNM staging can be collected in groups, which is also very important (Table 10–4). Generally, stage I and II tumors are considered early cancers with a more favorable prognosis than those in stage III and IV (more advanced disease).

OUTCOMES MANAGEMENT

After the histologic diagnosis and the extent of involvement have been determined, the treatment depends on a multitude of variables. The objectives of treating head and neck cancer are to eliminate the cancer, preserve function, and offer acceptable cosmetic results. Surgical resection and radiation are the mainstays of curative treatment options for head and neck cancer. In general, for small primary cancers (stage I or II), wide surgical excision alone or curative radiation therapy alone is preferred with the specific recommendations based on a number of factors. Tumor site, patient performance

TABLE 10–2   TNM STAGING OF PRIMARY HEAD AND NECK TUMORS (T)

Lip and Oral Cavity:

T_x	Primary tumor cannot be assessed
T_0	No evidence of primary tumor
T_{is}	Carcinoma in situ
T_1	Tumor < 2 cm in greatest dimension
T_2	Tumor > 2 cm, but ≤ 4 cm in greatest dimension
T_3	Tumor > 4 cm in greatest dimension
T_4(lip)	Tumor invades adjacent structures, i.e., through cortical bone, alveolar nerve, floor of mouth, skin of face
T_4(oral cavity)	Tumor invades adjacent structures, i.e., through cortical bone, deep muscle of tongue, maxillary sinus, skin

Nasopharynx:

T_1	Tumor confined to the nasopharynx
T_2	Tumor extends to soft tissues of oropharynx and/or nasal fossa:
T_{2a}	without parapharyngeal extension
T_{2b}	with parapharyngeal extension
T_3	Tumor invades bony structures and/or paranasal sinuses
T_4	Tumor with intracranial extension and/or involvement of cranial nerves, infratemporal fossa, hypopharynx, or orbit

Oropharynx:

T_1	Tumor < 2 cm in greatest dimension
T_2	Tumor > 2 cm, but ≤ 4 cm in greatest dimension
T_3	Tumor > 4 cm in greatest dimension
T_4	Tumor invades adjacent structures, i.e., pterygoid muscle, mandible, hard palate, deep muscle of tongue, larynx

Hypopharynx:

T_1	Tumor limited to one subsite of hypopharynx and < 2 cm in greatest dimension
T_2	Tumor involves > one subsite of hypopharynx and > 2 cm, but < 4 cm in greatest dimension
T_3	Tumor > 4 cm in greatest dimension or without fixation of hemilarynx
T_4	Tumor invades adjacent structures, i.e., thyroid/cricoid cartilage, carotid artery, soft tissues of neck, prevertebral fascia/muscles, thyroid, and/or esophagus

Supraglottis:

T_1	Tumor limited to one subsite of supraglottis with normal vocal cord mobility
T_2	Tumor invades mucosa of > one adjacent subsite of supraglottis or glottis or region outside the supraglottis without fixation of the larynx

| T_3 | Tumor limited to larynx with vocal cord fixation and/or invades any of the following: postcricoid area, preepiglottic tissues |
| T_4 | Tumor invades through the thyroid cartilage and/or extends into soft tissues of the neck, thyroid, and/or esophagus |

Glottis:

T_1	Tumor limited to the vocal cord(s) with normal mobility:
T_{1a}	limited to one vocal cord
T_{1b}	involves both vocal cords
T_2	Tumor extends to supraglottis and/or subglottis, and/or with impaired vocal cord mobility
T_3	Tumor limited to the larynx with vocal cord fixation
T_4	Tumor invades through the thyroid cartilage and/or to other tissues beyond larynx

Subglottis:

T_1	Tumor limited to the subglottis
T_2	Tumor extends to vocal cord(s) with normal or impaired mobility
T_3	Tumor limited to larynx with vocal cord fixation
T_4	Tumor invades through cricoid or thyroid cartilage and/or extends to other tissues beyond the larynx

Maxillary Sinus:

T_1	Tumor limited to antral mucosa with no erosion or destruction of bone
T_2	Tumor with erosion or destruction of the infrastructure including the hard palate and/or the middle nasal meatus
T_3	Tumor invades any of the following: skin of cheek, posterior wall of the maxillary sinus, floor or medial wall of orbit, anterior ethmoid sinus
T_4	Tumor invades orbital contents and/or any of the following: cribriform plate, posterior ethmoid or sphenoid sinuses, nasopharynx, soft palate, pterygomaxillary or temporal fossae or base of skull

Salivary Glands:

T_1	Tumor ≤ 2 cm in greatest dimension without extraparenchymal extension
T_2	Tumor > 2 cm but ≤ 4 cm in greatest dimension without extraparenchymal extension
T_3	Tumor > 4 cm but ≤ 6 cm in greatest dimension with extraparenchymal extension without 7th nerve involvement
T_4	Tumor > 6 cm in greatest dimension and invades the base of skull, 7th nerve

TABLE 10–3   TNM STAGING OF HEAD AND NECK TUMORS (N)

N_x	Regional lymph nodes cannot be assessed
N_0	No regional lymph node metastasis
N_1	Metastasis in a single ipsilateral lymph node, $\leq$ 3 cm in greatest dimension
N_2	Metastasis in a single ipsilateral lymph node $>$ 3 cm but $\leq$ 6 cm in greatest dimension, or multiple ipsilateral lymph nodes, none $>$ 6 cm in greatest dimension, or bilateral or contralateral lymph nodes, none $>$ 6 cm in greatest dimension
N_{2a}	Metastasis in a single ipsilateral lymph node $>$ 3 cm but $\leq$ 6 cm in greatest diameter
N_{2b}	Metastasis in multiple ipsilateral lymph nodes, none $>$ 6 cm in greatest diameter
N_{2c}	Metastasis in bilateral or contralateral lymph nodes, none $>$ 6 cm in greatest dimension
N_3	Metastasis in a lymph node $>$ 6 cm in greatest dimension

Used with the permission of the American Joint Committee on Cancer (AJCC®), Chicago, Illinois. The original source for this material is the AJCC® Cancer Staging Manual, 5th edition (1997) published by Lippincott-Raven Publishers, Philadelphia, Pennsylvania.

TABLE 10–4   STAGE GROUPING OF HEAD AND NECK TUMORS

Stage 0	T_{is}	N_0	M_0
Stage I	T_1	N_0	M_0
Stage II	T_2	N_0	M_0
Stage III	T_3	N_0	M_0
	T_1	N_1	M_0
	T_2	N_1	M_0
	T_3	N_1	M_0
Stage IV	T_4	N_0	M_0
	T4	N_1	M_0
	Any T	N_2	M_0
	Any T	N_3	M_0
	Any T	Any N	M_1

Used with the permission of the American Joint Committee on Cancer (AJCC®), Chicago, Illinois. The original source for this material is the AJCC® Cancer Staging Manual, 5th edition (1997) published by Lippincott-Raven Publishers, Philadelphia, Pennsylvania.

status, nutritional status, age, concomitant health problems, social and logistic factors, patient preference, morbidity of various treatment options, and the potential for recurrence are all important issues in selecting treatment modality (Clayman, Lippman, Laramore,

& Hong, 1997). In addition, elective treatment of the regional lymph nodes, either surgically or with radiation, may be indicated if the risk of involvement is greater than 20%. Sixty percent of patients with stage III or IV disease require combined-modality treatment (surgery, radiation, and chemotherapy) to improve survival and locoregional control.

The National Comprehensive Cancer Network (NCCN) has developed treatment guidelines and recommendations for squamous cell carcinoma involving six areas within the head and neck region (Forastiere et al., 1998). Selection of radiation dose depends on the size and location of tumor, and the aforementioned patient variables. There are different modes of radiation delivery: external beam, interstitial implantation, and intracavitary. In general, palliation of inoperable tumors requires at least 45 to 50 Gy over 5 to 6 weeks. Early tumors (T_1) require $\geq$ 66 Gy, moderate-size tumors (T_2) require 66 to 70 Gy, and larger tumors (T_3 and T_4) require $\geq$ 70 Gy (Forastiere et al., 1998). When postoperative irradiation is recommended, high doses (60 to 65 Gy) are required for treatment of microscopic disease.

Acute side effects of irradiation may need aggressive management. Patients may experience:

- Laryngitis—Vocal cords may become edematous with treatment, leading to hoarseness. Typically, this is temporary and resolves after completing treatments. Patients can minimize the swelling by avoiding straining their voice, avoiding irritants (alcohol, smoking, spicy or acidic foods), gargling with warm saline solution, and utilizing analgesic medications as needed (Bruner, Bucholtz, Iwamoto, & Strohl, 1998). Occasionally, steroids or alpha-adrenergic agents may become necessary if edema becomes more severe. In rare instances, temporary tracheostomy is necessary because of airway compromise as a result of laryngeal edema.
- Stomatitis—Acute mucosal reaction in the mouth, oropharynx, and hypopharynx with radiation treatment leads to pain, odynophagia, and predisposition to infection. These symptoms are dose dependent and exacerbated by concurrent chemotherapy. Typically, this irritation begins about the third week of treatment and can become quite uncomfortable by the time treatment concludes. The sore mouth/throat generally resolves in 1 to 3 months following treatments, but can require pain medicines during or after treatment. Suggestions for mild pain include nonopioid analgesics or nonsteroidal antiinflammatory drugs (NSAIDs) such as diflunisal

(Dolobid®), etodolac (Lodine®), ketoprofen (Orudis®), ke-
torolac (Toradol ®), or naproxen (Naprosyn®). For moderate
pain Class III or IV narcotics such as hydrocodone bitartrate
and acetaminophen (Lortab®, Lorcet®, Vicodin®) may be appropriate. For severe pain Class II narcotics such as fentanyl
transdermal system (Duragesic®), hydromorphone (Dilau-
did®), oxycodone hydrochloride (Oxycontin®), or morphine
sulfate elixir will be helpful. Topical anesthetics (viscous lidocaine or related medications) can also be useful, especially
prior to eating. Other recommendations include Carafate®
slurries, aloe-containing compounds (Radiocare Oral Rinse®),
and topical mouthwashes. Also, when patients experience
stomatitis they may need to change their eating habits such as
eating small, frequent, high-caloric, high-protein meals; taking
supplemental drinks (Ensure®, Resource®, Sustacal®, Nutri-
Shakes®, Carnation Instant Breakfast®), or inserting a tube for
feeding. Early recognition and treatment of thrush with Diflu-
can® or troches can help improve acute mucosal irritation.

■ Xerostomia and thickened secretions—Acute xerostomia
and chronic xerostomia are among the most common and
clinically significant toxicities that arise from radiotherapy
for head and neck cancer. Xerostomia is characterized as severe dry mouth because of a lack of saliva caused by the salivary glands being exposed in the radiated field. This side effect can greatly affect the quality of life of these patients by
affecting their ability to swallow, eat, taste, speak, and sleep.
Lack of saliva can also lead to major dental problems such
as cavities and tooth decay. Patients may begin to notice
these symptoms at doses as low as 10 Gy. Concurrent
chemotherapy may exacerbate the condition. Treatment options for this condition are limited. An oral mouth rinse regimen includes frequent salt/soda gargles (1 tsp baking soda
and ½ tsp salt in 1 qt water) or diluted hydrogen peroxide
rinses (50/50 mixture, H_2O_2/water). Commercial artificial
saliva products are also available including Salivart®, Xerol-
ube®, Saliva Substitute®, or Moi-Stir®. Patients who have
some functioning salivary tissue may find relief with pilocarpine hydrocholoride (Salagen®). Oral administration of
pilocarpine 5 mg, qid during and 3 months posttreatment
can help increase salivary flow (Guchelaar, Vermes, & Meerwaldt, 1997; Rode et al., 1999; Zimmerman, Mark, Tran, &
Juillard, 1997). However, if the parotid and submandibular

glands are completely irradiated and there is no function left in these glands, these products will not work very effectively (Ward, 1999). Amifostine (Ethyol®) is a recent FDA-approved drug that helps reduce moderate to severe xerostomia in patients undergoing postoperative radiation therapy for head and neck cancers. Amifostine is the first broad-spectrum cytoprotective agent to be approved by the FDA. Laboratory and clinical studies have shown that amifostine protects cells in virtually all organ systems except the central nervous system (Capizzi, 1999a & b). Extensive studies have shown that amifostine selectively protects normal tissues without protecting the tumor. The drug accumulates in epithelial tissues with the highest concentrations in the salivary glands. Amifostine is a pro-drug (WR-2721) converted to the active-free thiol (WR-1065) by alkaline phosphatase. In the cells, amifostine protects DNA by acting as a free radical scavenger and donating hydrogen to repair damaged target molecules (Wagner, Pratt, & Schonekas, 1998). The administration guideline for this indication is amifostine 200 mg/m^2, slow intravenous push, over 3 to 5 minutes, 15 minutes prior to radiation each day. Daily administration of amifostine reduces the severity of acute and late xerostomia in patients undergoing radiotherapy for head and neck cancer without compromising the antitumor.

■ Taste alterations—Taste buds are affected at low doses (10 Gy). These changes can become frustrating to the patient and his or her caregiver. Supportive measures include disguising the taste with marinating sauces, varying food temperatures, and avoiding unpleasant odors with mints, lemons, or other hard candies. Loss of taste is usually a temporary side effect and can last 2 to 6 months after treatments.

■ Radiodermatitis—During the treatment, the skin may develop a red, tender reaction similar to a sunburn that may then be followed by darkening and/or peeling of the skin within the treatment field. This reaction usually resolves within several weeks to months after the treatment, but there may be permanent hair loss and possible skin darkening within the treated areas, which is similar to changes seen with chronic sun exposure.

Support groups are available to assist patients and families with coping after head and neck treatments. Following are some of these resources:

- SPOHNC—Support for People with Oral and Head and Neck Cancer—is a patient-directed support group that maintains a nationwide newsletter (www.spohnc.org)
- Laryngectomy Support Groups

Outcomes Measures

Head and neck cancer patients experience major physical and psychological problems. The physical distress that head/neck patients experience with treatments can be devastating. There are changes in appearance and ongoing symptoms that interfere with their quality of life. Quantitative instruments are being developed to measure the physical changes that impact the cancer patient's quality of life. These instruments include the following:

- FACT-H&N (Functional Assessment of Cancer Therapy for Head and Neck) was developed specifically to evaluate the performance and quality of life in head and neck cancer patients. It is a self-reported instrument consisting of 28 general and 11 head and neck specific items each rated on a 0 to 4 Likert Scale. Questions describe the patient's physical, social, emotional, and functional well-being along with the patient's relationship with the physician and the patient's head and neck symptoms. The FACT-G (Functional Assessment of Cancer Therapy-General) instrument has been validated in numerous studies with cancer patients and proved to be reliable, valid, and responsive to clinical change (Scott, 1998). The validity of the head and neck symptoms items within the FACT-H&N is still under examination (List, Ritter-Sterr, & Lansky, 1990; List et al., 1996).
- Head and Neck Performance Status Scale (PSS)—This is a clinician-rated instrument that rates patients in three subscales from 0 to 100. Patients are rated in several performance areas: ability to eat in public, speech clarity, and normalcy of diet (List et al., 1990). The higher the score, the more normal the function (100 representing normal).
- SOMA Scale for late toxicities (Subjective, Objective, Management, and Analytical evaluation of injury) was developed by the RTOG and EORTC. Grades 1–5 are assigned (1 representing minor symptoms to 5 representing death or loss of the organ) (Pavy et al., 1995). The eight scales are useful for these head/neck sites: eye, ear, mucosa, salivary gland, mandible, teeth, larynx, and thyroid/hypothalamic/pituitary.

- Memorial Symptom Assessment Scale (MSAS)—This is a symptom management tool that measures 32 physical and psychological cancer-related symptoms (Portenoy et al., 1994).

Psychological distress is another major problem confronting a patient who is diagnosed with head and neck cancer. Depression may develop because of the changes in body image, loss of speech, scars or distorted features, poor nutritional status, pain, and the inability to cope. Instruments that can help clinicians identify disfigurement and depression are as follows:

- Dysfunction/Disfigurement Scale—Developed by Dropkin at Memorial Sloan-Kettering Cancer Center it identifies how the patient is coping with the debilitating physical changes (Dropkin, 1989).
- Center for Epidemiologic Studies Depression (CES-D) is a self-reported depression scale (Radloff, 1977).

EXPECTED OUTCOMES

The overall 5-year survival for head and neck cancers is poor, averaging 55% for Whites and 34% for African Americans (Mood, 1997). This low survival is the result of a combination of poor local control of advanced tumors, a moderately high distant metastatic rate, a relatively high rate of second primaries of the upper aerodigestive tract, and a high incidence of comorbid condition in this patient population. Of those patients who recur within 5 years of diagnosis, 30% to 50% will die of the disease and 60% will have distant metastases (Gale and Charette, 1994). As mentioned earlier, survival rates are strongly associated with the stage of disease. Patients who present with early stage (I or II) have an 85% probability of surviving for 5 years as compared with patients in late stages (III or IV) who have a 34% 5-year survival rate (Mood, 1997).

Most of the head/neck quality of life outcome studies focus on the physical effect of radiation on the body, both during and after radiation treatments. The acute treatment toxicities were discussed in the previous section, "Outcomes Management." Certainly, the Phase III randomized trial of amifostine as a radioprotectant in head and neck cancer, which evaluated 315 patients with newly diagnosed and previously untreated head and neck squamous cell carcinoma is a breakthrough for reducing xerostomia. Amifostine significantly reduced the incidence of ≥ grade 2 acute xerostomia from 78% to 51% ($p < 0.0001$). The median dose required to cause this side effect was 50% higher in patients receiving amifostine (60 Gy vs. 42 Gy, $p = 0.0001$). Chronic xerostomia $\geq$ grade 2 was significantly less frequent in the amifostine patients 1 year after the completion of treatment (34% vs. 57%, $p = 0.002$). Antitumor treatment efficacy was preserved (Brizel, 1999).

While most patients report functional and physical measures returning to normal after 12 months, some patients experience residual effects. Delayed effects or functional impairments may include:

- Osteoradionecrosis—Occurs when there is an impairment in the vascularity and cellularity of the bony matrix, causing necrosis of bony structures (Beumer, Curtis, & Harrison, 1979). Usual time frame is 6 months to several years after irradiation. Osteoradionecrosis develops in 5% to 37% of patients following head and neck irradiation with the most common sites being the mandible, temporal bone, and maxilla (Hsu & Phillips, 1998).

- Trismus—Results when the muscles of the jaw become fibrotic making the patient unable to fully open his or her jaw. Severe trismus affects the mechanical process of chewing, inhibits eating, and leads to nutritional problems. Trismus also can affect a patient's speech, oral hygiene, and lifestyle. Monitor the patient for trismus by checking for pain or weakness in masticating muscles in the field of radiation. Instruct the patient to exercise the jaw muscles three times a day by opening and closing the mouth as far as possible without pain and repeating 20 times. Also, exerting gentle pressure against the midline mandible and then opening the mouth will assist in stretching the jaw muscles. These simple exercises may assist in preventing muscle weakness, which could lead to fibrosis. Referrals to physical therapy during and after the radiation is administered may be helpful.

- Decreased Hearing—Occurs when the auditory structures are within the treatment field, resulting in a loss of hearing on the affected side. Also, serous otitis can damage the middle ear bones or inner ear structures, thus causing the hearing loss.

- Permanent Xerostomia—May occur when the salivary glands receive 40 Gy or more. A dry mouth interferes with the patient's comfort, overall nutrition, and activities of daily living. While commercial saliva substitutes are available, they do not offer long-lasting relief. Water bottles may provide temporary relief.

- Dental Caries—With xerostomia comes changes in IgA levels of saliva. These changes increase the risk for developing

dental caries. Typically, this is seen 6 to 12 months after irradiation (Iwamoto, 1997). Topical fluoride treatments and
close dental follow-ups are advised postirradiation.

■ Fibrosis—Some degree of thickening or scarring of the soft
tissues in the treatment field over time may occur. Some
people may develop swelling underneath the chin in the
weeks to months following treatment. This swelling is usually temporary and resolves in several months.

■ Thyroid Dysfunction—The thyroid gland is also generally included in the head/neck radiation treatment field. Because
of this there is a long-term risk of developing decreased
function of the gland that could require replacement of thyroid hormones.

■ Spinal Cord Involvement—When the spinal cord is included
in the treatment field for part of the treatments, there is a
very small risk of permanent damage to the spinal cord from
the treatments. This could result in paralysis or loss of sensation, although the risk is very small. More common is the
development of a temporary Lhermitte's syndrome (shock-
like sensations running down the spinal cord) in the months
following radiation. Typically, this resolves on its own and is
not dangerous.

After treatment, close surveillance is imperative (Shaha &
Strong, 1995). Standard follow-up includes:

■ Physical Examination—Close monitoring is extremely important for this patient population. Follow-up visits should occur
4 to 6 weeks for the first 2 years, then every 2 to 3 months for
the third year, and every 4 months for the fourth and fifth
years. Beginning the sixth year, visits can be scheduled every
6 to 12 months thereafter. Lifelong follow-up is required.

■ Chest X-ray—Initially every 6 months, then annually after 2
to 3 years.

REFERENCES

American Cancer Society. (1999). Cancer facts and figures. New York:
American Cancer Society.
American Joint Committee on Cancer. (1998). AJCC *cancer staging handbook*.
Philadelphia: Lippincott-Raven.
Beumer, J., Curtis, T., & Harrison, R. (1979). Radiation therapy of the oral
cavity: Sequelae and management. *Head and Neck Surgery*, 1, 301–312.

Bockmuhl, U., Wolf, G., Schmidt, S., Schwendel, A., Jahnke, V., Dietel, M., & Petersen, I. (1998). Genomic alterations associated with malignancy in head and neck cancer.*Head and Neck*, 20(2), 145–151.

Brizel, D., Wasserman, T., Stmad, V., Wannemacher, M., Henke, M., Monnier, A., Eschwege, F., Zhang, J., Russell, L., & Sauer, R. (1999). *Final report of a Phase III randomized trial of amifostine as a radioprotectant in head and neck Cancer* [Abstract]. 41st Annual Meeting of The American Society for Therapeutic Radiology and Oncology.

Bruner, D., Bucholtz, J., Iwamoto, R., & Strohl, R. (1998). *Manual for radiation oncology nursing practice and education* (2nd ed.). Pittsburgh, PA: Oncology Nursing Press.

Buchbinder, D., Currivan, R., Kaplan, A, & Urken, M. (1993). Mobilization regimens for the prevention of jaw hypomobility in the radiated patient: A comparison of three techniques. *Oral Maxillofacial Surgery*, 51, 863–867.

Capizzi, R. (1999a). Clinical status and optimal use of amifostine. *Oncology*, 13(1), 47–59.

Capizzi, R. (1999b). The preclinical basis for broad-spectrum selective cytoprotection of normal tissues from cytotoxic therapies by amifostine. *Seminars in Oncology*, 26(2) (Suppl. 7), 3–21.

Clayman, G., Lippman, S., Laramore, G., & Hong, W. (1997). Head and neck cancer. In J. Holland, R. Bast, D. Morton, E. Frei, D. Kufe, & R. Weichselbaum (Eds.), *Cancer medicine*. Baltimore: Williams & Wilkins.

Curran, W. (1998). Radiation-induced toxicities: The role of radioprotectants. *Seminars in Radiation Oncology*, 8(4) (Suppl. 1), 2–4.

DeWys, W., Begg, C, Lavin, P., Band, P., Bennett, J., Bertino, J., Cohen, M., Douglass, H., Engstrom, P., Ezdinli, E., Horton, J., Johnson, G., Moertel, C., Oken, M., Perlia, C., Rosenbaum, C., Silverstein, M., Skeel, R., Sponzo, R., & Tormey, D. (1980). Prognostic effect of weight loss prior to chemotherapy in cancer patients. Eastern Cooperative Oncology Group. *American Journal of Medicine*, 69, 491–497.

Dropkin, M. (1989). Coping with disfigurement and dysfunction after head and neck cancer surgery. *Seminars in Oncology Nursing*, 5, 213–219.

Forastiere, A., Schuller, D., & Spencer, S. (1998). NCCC practice guidelines for head and neck cancer. *Oncology*, 12(7A), 39–145.

Gale, D., & Charette, J. (1994). *Oncology nursing care plans*. El Paso, TX: Skidmore-Roth.

Guchelaar, H., Vermes, A., & Meerwaldt, J. (1997). Radiation-induced xerostomia: Pathophysiology, clinical course and supportive treatment. *Support Care Cancer*, 5(4), 281–288.

Hsu, I., & Phillips, T. (1998). Oral cavity cancer. In S. Leibel & T. Phillips (Eds.), *Textbook of radiation oncology*. Philadelphia: W. B. Saunders.

Iwamoto, R. (1997). Cancers of the head and neck. *Nursing care in radiation oncology*. K. Dow, J. Bucholtz, R. Iwamoto, V. Fieler, & L. Hilderley (Eds.). Philadelphia: W. B. Saunders.

Landis, S., Murray, T., Bolden, S., & Wingo, P. (1998). Cancer statistics, 1999. *CA: A Cancer Journal for Clinicians*, 49(1), 8–31.

List, M., Ritter-Sterr, C., Baker, T., Colangelo, L., Matz, G., & Pauloski, B. (1996). A longitudinal assessment of quality of life in laryngeal cancer patients. *Head and Neck*, 18, 1–10.

List, M., Ritter-Sterr, C., & Lansky, S. (1990). A performance status scale for head and neck cancer patients. *Cancer*, 66, 5649.

Lutz, C., & Przytulski, K. (1997). *Nutrition and diet therapy*. Philadelphia: F. A. Davis.

Mood, D. (1997). "Cancers of the Head and Neck" in A *cancer source book for nurses*. In C. Varricchio, M. Pierce, C. Walker & T. Ades (Eds.). Atlanta, GA: American Cancer Society.

Pavy, J., Denekamp, J., Letschert, J., Littbrand, B., Mornex, F., Bernier, J., Gonzales-Gonzales, D., Horiot, J., Bolla, M., & Bartelink, H. (1995). Late effects toxicity scoring: The SOMA Scale. *International Journal of Radiation Oncology, Biology, Physics*, 31(5), 1043–1091.

Portenoy, R., Thaler, H., Kornblith, A., Lepore, J., Friedlander-Kar, H., Coyle, N., Smart-Curley, T., Kemeny, N., Norton, L. & Hoskins, W. (1994). The Memorial Symptom Assessment Scale: An instrument for the evaluation of symptom prevalence, characteristics and distress. *European Journal of Cancer*, 30A, 1326.

Radloff, L. (1977). The CES-D Scale: A self-report depression scale for research in the general population. *Applied Psychological Measurement*, 1, 385–401.

Rode, M., Smid, L., Budihna, M., Soba, E., Rode, M., & Gaspersic, D. (1999). The effect of pilocarpine and biperiden on salivary secretion during and after radiotherapy in head and neck cancer patients. *International Journal of Radiation Oncology, Biology, Physics*, 45(2), 373–378.

Scott, C. (1998). Issues in quality of life assessment during cancer therapy. *Seminars in Radiation Oncology*, 8(4) (Suppl. 1), 5–9.

Shaha, A., & Strong, E. (1995). Cancer of the head and neck. In G. Murphy, W. Lawrence, & R. Lenhard (Eds.) *American cancer society textbook of clinical oncology*. Atlanta, GA: American Cancer Society.

Sheen, T., Ko, J., Chang, Y. L., Chang, Y. S., Huang, Y., Chang, Y., Tsai, C. & Hsu, M. (1998). Nasopharyngeal swab and PCR for the screening of nasopharyngeal carcinoma in the endemic area: A good supplement to the serologic screening. *Head and Neck*, 20(8), 732–738.

Taylor, S. (1999). Head and neck carcinomas. In J. Foley, J. Vose, & J. Armitage (Eds.), *Current therapy in cancer*. Philadelphia: W. B. Saunders.

Wagner, W. Prott, F., & Schonekas, K. (1998). Amifostine: a radioprotector in locally advanced head and neck tumors. *Oncology Reports*, 5, 1255–1257.

Ward, J. (1999). Oasis in the desert of dry mouth. *Advance*, 10, 10–11.

Zimmerman, R., Mark, R., Tran, L., & Juillard, G. (1997). Concomitant pilocarpine during head and neck irradiation is associated with decreased post-treatment xerostomia. *International Journal of Radiation Oncology, Biology, Physics*, 37(3), 571–575.

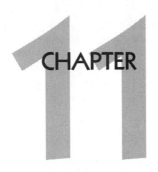

CHAPTER 11

BREAST CANCER

Giselle J. Moore-Higgs, ARNP, MSN
Nancy P. Mendenhall, MD

PROBLEM

- Breast cancer is the most common cancer worldwide among women (Parkin, Pisani, & Ferlay, 1993). It is the most common cancer in women in all developed countries other than Japan (Moss, 1999). Incidence rates of female breast cancer have been highest in North America and northern Europe, intermediate in southern Europe and Central and South America, and lowest in Asia and Africa (Bernstein, 1998). In the United States, the American Cancer Society (ACS) estimates that 184,200 new cases of breast cancer will be diagnosed in 2000 (Greenlee, Murray, Bolden, & Wingo, 2000).

- Breast cancer is the leading cause of death from cancer worldwide (Pisani, 1985). In the United States, the ACS estimates 41,200 deaths from breast cancer in 2000 (Greenlee et al., 2000).

- After increasing about 4% per year in the 1980s, breast cancer incidence rates in women in the United States have leveled off in the 1990s to about 110 cases per 100,000 women (ACS, 1999).

RISK FACTORS

- Age is the most important demographic risk factor for breast cancer (Bernstein, 1998). Risk increases steadily with age from about 100 cases per 100,000 at age 35 to almost 500 cases per 100,000 by age 75 (Offit, 1998).
- Gender—Breast cancer rarely occurs in males. The ACS estimates approximately 1,400 new cases of male breast cancer in 2000, with approximately 400 related deaths (Greenlee et al., 2000). The mean age at diagnosis is 60 to 70 years of age. Predisposing risk factors appear to include radiation exposure, estrogen administration, and diseases associated with hyperestrogenism, such as cirrhosis or Klinefelter's syndrome (Jaiyesimi, Buzdar, Sahin & Ross, 1992; Hultborn, Hanson, Kopf, Verbiene, Warnhammar and Weimarck, 1997). An increased risk of male breast cancer has been reported in families in which the BRCA2 mutation on chromosome 13q has been identified (Thorlacius et al., 1995; Wooster et al., 1995).
- Hormonal Factors—The substantial body of experimental, clinical, and epidemiologic evidence on breast cancer indicates that hormones play a major role in breast cancer (Henderson, Ross, & Bernstein, 1988). A majority of the known nondemographic risk factors for breast cancer can be understood as measures of the cumulative exposure of the breast to estrogen and perhaps to progesterone (Bernstein, 1998).
  - Early age at menarche, late age at menopause, and late age at first pregnancy increase the risk of breast cancer (Bernstein, & Ross, 1993). Nulliparity or age at birth of first child after 30 also has been associated with an increased risk for intraductal breast cancer (Kerlikowske, Barclay, Grady, Sickles, & Ernester, 1997).
  - The role of oral contraceptives as a risk for breast cancer has been controversial. A recent reanalysis of data from 54 studies found that women were at a small increased risk of having breast cancer diagnosed while taking combined oral contraceptives and in the first 10 years after stopping, as compared with a relative risk in current users of 1.24 (95% CI 1015-1.33) (Collaborative Group on Hormonal Factors in Breast Cancer, 1996). Ten or more years after stopping oral contraceptives, there was no evidence

of increased risk. The frequency of oral contraceptive use rather than duration of use was most predictive of breast cancer. The effect of recent use was strongest among those women who first used oral contraceptives before age 20. The greatest increase in breast cancer risk was observed among women who were youngest at the time of their diagnosis. Progestin-only oral contraceptives and the long-acting injectable progestogen contraceptive, depot-medroxyprogesterone acetate (DMPA), do not appear to affect breast cancer risk (Standford & Thomas, 1993).

- The role of hormone replacement therapy on breast cancer risk remains unclear. Most studies that have evaluated long-term users of estrogen replacement therapy indicate a modest increase among women who have used the estrogen with risk increasing approximately 3% per year of use (Pike, Bernstein, & Spicer, 1993). In the United States, breast cancer risk increases about 2.2% per year of use of a standard dose regimen of conjugated equine estrogen (0.625 mg/day) (Bernstein, 1998). This translates into increases in risk of 10% after 5 years, 20% after 10 years, and 40% after 15 years of use. Data are not complete on the evaluation of estrogen and progesterone in combination therapy.
- Diethylstilbestrol (DES) exposure in utero has been found in most studies to be associated with a small increase in the risk of breast cancer (Malone, 1993).

■ Diet—A number of dietary factors have been previously associated with an increased risk for breast cancer including a diet high in fat intake. However, recent data from the Nurses Health Study (Helzlsouer, 1995; Willett, Hunter, & Stampfer, 1992) found no association between varying fat consumption and risk for breast cancer.

- The role of alcohol consumption as a risk factor is not clear (Moss, 1999). Longnecker (1994) in a meta-analysis of 38 studies concluded that a modest, linear, statistically significant dose-response relationship exists. In relation to nondrinkers, the breast cancer risks of women consuming one, two, and three alcoholic drinks daily were increased 11%, 24%, and 38%, respectively.
- High levels of body fat have also been associated with breast cancer risk in postmenopausal women (de Waard,

Cornelis, Aoki, & Yoshida, 1977). The increased risk is probably attributable to the higher levels of circulating endogenous estrogen as a result of the conversion of the androgen precursor androstenedione to estrone in adipose tissue.

■ Genetics—A family history of breast cancer is associated with an increased risk for development of the disease. It is estimated that approximately 5% of all women with breast cancer may have germline mutation(s) in the BRCA1 gene localized to chromosome 17q21. Specific mutations of the BRCA1 gene may be more common in certain ethnic groups (Offit et al., 1996). First-degree relatives of women with breast cancer have a two- to threefold increased risk of the disease as compared with women without a family history. First-degree relatives of premenopausal women with bilateral breast cancer have nearly nine times the risk of women without a family history (Bernstein, 1998). The American Society of Clinical Oncology has developed the following criteria to identify women with a genetic predisposition for breast cancer (ASCO, 1996):

1. Family has more than two breast cancer cases and one or more cases of ovarian cancer diagnosed at any age.
2. Family has more than three breast cancer cases diagnosed before the age of 50.
3. Family has sister pairs with two of the following cancers diagnosed before the age of 50: two breast cancers, two ovarian cancers, or a breast and ovarian cancer.

■ Environmental—exposure to ionizing radiation in moderate to high doses has been found to increase the risk of breast cancer among women under age 40 at the time of exposure. Results from the Late Effects Study Group (Bhatia et al., 1996) indicate that women who received thoracic irradiation in their second or third decade of life have a 35% risk of developing breast cancer by the age of 40. The overall risk associated with prior thoracic irradiation at a young age is 75 times greater than the risk of breast cancer in the general population (NCCN, 1998).

■ Risk Prevention—several studies have identified several factors that may decrease the risk of breast cancer. Thune, Brann, Lund, and Gaard (1997) found that women who exercise at least 4 hours per week have a 40% decrease in breast cancer risk. Lactation has been increasingly reported to protect against breast cancer development, particularly among premenopausal women (Bernstein, 1998). The evidence is not as certain with regard to the risk of postmenopausal breast cancer. A diet high in fiber, fruits, and vegetables has been associated with a decreased risk as has the consumption of phytoestrogens from foods such as soybean products (Bernstein, 1998).

- Estrogen receptor modulators such as tamoxifen may reduce the risk of developing breast cancer. Results of a large chemoprevention trial, NSABP P-1, evaluated 13,366 high-risk premenopausal and postmenopausal women who took tamoxifen or a placebo in a double-blind fashion for 5 years. Women who took tamoxifen for 5 years had a 50% decrease in invasive and noninvasive breast cancer, compared with women who took a placebo (Fisher, Constantino, et al., 1998). The role of raloxifene is currently under evaluation.

ASSESSMENT

- ■ X-ray mammography and physical examination of the breast are the recognized screening tests for breast cancer, together with self-screening by breast self-examination (Moss, 1999). Other imaging studies that have been considered include thermography, ultrasound, and MRI.
  1. Physical Examination
     - No randomized trials of physical exam alone. In measurement of its effectiveness as compared with mammograms, sensitivity of the physical examination alone was estimated to be 66% (UK Trial, 1992).
  2. Mammography
     - Several screening trials have evaluated the sensitivity and specificity of mammography to detect breast cancer. Although studies have shown a sensitivity range of 73% to 85% (Shapiro, Venet, Strax, & Venet, 1988; Tabar, Fagerberg, Day, & Holmberg, 1987; Baines, McFarlane, & Miller, 1988), current imaging technology has improved significantly since these studies were published.
     - High-density mammographic patterns as measured by the proportion of breast area composed of epithelial and stromal tissue have an impact on breast cancer

risk. Byrne et al. (1995) found that mammographic features are associated with known breast cancer risk factors. The high-density pattern effects were independent of family history, age at first birth, alcohol consumption, and benign breast disease. Compared with women with no visible breast density, women who had a breast density of 75% or greater had an almost fivefold increased risk of breast cancer. Of the breast cancers in this study, 28% were attributable to having 50% or greater breast density.

- The U.S. Food and Drug Administration (FDA) recently approved the use of digital, or computerized, images instead of film x-rays to screen breast cancer.
- American College of Radiology Recommendations (Feig et al., 1998):
  Asymptomatic women 40 years old and older should have an annual mammographic screening; monthly breast self-examination and annual clinical breast examination should be performed, although their benefit is scientifically unproven; mammographic screening before the age of 40 years may benefit women who are at high risk for breast cancer. These recommendations apply only to women without signs and symptoms of breast cancer.
- National Comprehensive Cancer Network Breast Cancer Screening Panel Practice Guidelines—Modified (NCCN, 1998):
  Asymptomatic women with a negative clinical examination should be stratified based on risk factors into one of three basic categories for the purpose of screening recommendations:
  1. Women at low to moderate risk:
     a. Age 20 to 39 years—physical breast exam every three years
     b. Age 40 years and older—annual physical breast examination and bilateral screening mammography
  2. Women who have received prior thoracic irradiation:
     a. Physical breast examination every 6 months
     b. Annual bilateral screening mammogram
     c. Initiate screening no later than 10 years after radiation exposure.

   3. Women with a genetic predisposition:
- **a.** Annual bilateral screening mammogram
- **b.** Physical breast examination every 6 months
- **c.** Initiate screening 5 to 10 years before the earliest age of diagnosis of breast or ovarian cancer in a relative

- Breast Imaging Reporting and Data System (ACR, 1993) is the current system for reporting mammography results with recommendations associated with each category.
  1. Negative—negative mammogram
  2. Benign finding—negative mammogram but with an actual finding that a questionable area is benign
  3. Probably benign finding—short interval follow-up suggested
  4. Suspicious abnormality—biopsy should be considered
  5. Highly suggestive of malignancy

   3. Ultrasound is currently used as a diagnostic tool in the evaluation of a positive finding on screening exam. Sonography helps to define solid versus cystic masses as well as defining the borders.

   4. MRI remains under evaluation for its role in screening for breast cancer.

■ Most early-stage breast cancers are found on physical examination or on screening mammogram and are asymptomatic. Patients occasionally may report slight tenderness, feeling of fullness, or discomfort in an area of the breast during certain activities. Symptoms associated with locally advanced breast cancer include pain, nipple discharge, pruritis, shrinkage or enlargement of the breast, inflammation, breast skin changes, skin ulceration, and/or hand or arm swelling, heaviness, and pain.

■ Initial evaluation should include the following:
  1. Complete history and physical examination. History should include breast-related symptoms as well as personal and family history of breast disease.
  2. Karnofsky performance status (KPS)—an individual's performance status should be considered when deciding on the method of evaluation and treatment.
  3. Careful visual inspection for evidence of breast contour and skin changes including skin dimpling, ulceration, rash, erythema, and peau d'orange. Visual inspection of

the chest and arm for evidence of fullness or skin changes in nodal areas.

4. Physical examination of the breast and regional lymphatics (axilla, supraclavicular fossa, parasternal spaces, and infraclavicular area) should be performed. Palpation of the breast should be performed in the upright and supine position. Document the size and position of the mass or abnormality. Detailed drawings or color photographs provide additional documentation that may be useful for comparison later.

5. A biopsy of the suspicious mass or abnormality should be performed. The choice of biopsy procedure depends on whether the mass is palpable and the characteristics (fluid-filled versus solid).

   a. Fine Needle Aspiration—may be performed in the office under local anesthetic. The diagnostic accuracy has been estimated at 80% (Kline & Neal, 1975).

   b. Cutting Needle Biopsy—incises a core of tissue from the breast. Provides more tissue for evaluation thus improving accuracy over fine needle aspiration.

   c. Incisional Biopsy—removes a portion of the mass. Usually indicated in locally advanced breast cancer to provide histologic confirmation of diagnosis prior to initiation of neoadjuvant chemotherapy.

   d. Needle Localization Excision Biopsy—placement of a flexible hooked wire via a localizing needle under the guidance of ultrasonography. The wire provides the surgeon with accurate localization of the abnormal tissue at the time of excision.

   e. Stereotactic Core Biopsy—large core stereotactic breast biopsy is now the technique of choice in many institutions for the biopsy of nonpalpable breast masses and abnormal microcalcifications. It shortens the time from detection at mammography to diagnosis and breast-conserving therapy, permits appropriate discussion of treatment alternatives, reduces the positive margin rate and reexcision rate, and may represent a significant cost savings in the management of nonpalpable breast cancer (Lind et al., 1998).

6. A skin biopsy, either punch or incisional should be performed if there is evidence of skin changes including erythema, peau d'orange, rash, or ulcerative lesion.

7. Nipple discharge should be collected on a glass slide, fixed, and sent for cytologic evaluation.
8. Imaging studies may include:
    a. Bilateral mammogram with ultrasound—evaluate for evidence of synchronous disease (more common in infiltrating lobular cancer)
    b. Chest x-ray
    c. Bone scan if there is evidence of locally advanced disease or clinical suspicion because of symptoms of bone pain
    d. CT scan of the chest, abdomen, and pelvis if there is evidence of locally advanced disease or clinical suspicion of metastatic disease. Useful to evaluate evidence of internal mammary and mediastinal lymph node involvement, liver, and ovaries.
9. Complete blood count with complete chemistry to evaluate renal and liver function.
10. Additional metastatic evaluation studies will depend on clinical stage of disease, reported symptoms, and physical examination findings.
11. Additional studies may be warranted to assess overall medical condition, particularly when considering surgical resection or combined modality therapy.

■ Approximately 85% to 90% of invasive carcinomas are ductal in origin (NCCN, 1997). See Table 11–1 for a list of breast cancer histologic classifications.

■ Inflammatory carcinoma is a clinicopathologic entity characterized by erythema, increased warmth of the skin, peau d'orange, ridging, and diffuse brawny induration of the skin of the breast with an erysipeloid edge. There may not be an underlying palpable mass. Radiologically there is characteristic thickening of the skin of the breast with or without other signs of malignancy in the parenchyma.

■ Important prognostic factors include age, menopausal status, stage of disease, number of involved axillary lymph nodes, pathologic characteristics of the primary tumor including the presence of tumor necrosis, estrogen and progesterone receptor levels, and measures of proliferative capacity. Other factors under investigation include DNA index and oncogene expression, location, age, and KPS.

■ The AJCC staging system is used for breast cancer (Table 11–2).

TABLE 11–1   HISTOPATHOLOGY OF BREAST CANCER

Ductal carcinoma, NOS (not otherwise specified)
    Intraductal (in situ)
        Comedo
        Micropapillary
        Cribriform
    Invasive with predominant intraductal component
    Invasive, NOS
Medullary with lymphocytic infiltrate
Mucinous (colloid)
Papillary
Scirrhous
Tubular
Other
Lobular
    In situ
    Invasive with predominant in situ component
    Invasive
Nipple
    Paget's disease NOS
    Paget's disease with intraductal carcinoma
    Paget's disease with invasive ductal carcinoma
Other
    Undifferentiated carcinoma
    Cystosarcoma phyllodes
    Angiosarcoma
    Primary lymphoma

OUTCOMES MANAGEMENT

- Treatment of breast cancer is influenced by patient age, menopausal status, tumor stage, tumor histopathology, and estrogen- and progesterone-receptor status.
- A multidisciplinary team approach to the treatment of breast cancer is important during the evaluation and treatment phases. The team should include a surgeon, medical oncologist, radiation oncologist, radiologist (specialty of mammography), pathologist, nurse, and social worker. Many institutions conduct a weekly conference to review new cases and make treatment recommendations.

TABLE 11–2 PRIMARY TUMOR (T)

Primary Tumor (T)

T_x — Primary tumor cannot be assessed

T_0 — No evidence of primary tumor

T_{is} — Carcinoma in situ; intraductal carcinoma, lobular carcinoma in situ, or Paget's disease of the nipple with no tumor. Note: Paget's disease associated with a tumor is classified according to the size of the tumor.

T_1 — Tumor 2.0 cm or less in greatest dimension

T_{1mic} — Microinvasion 0.1 cm or less in greatest dimension

T_{1a} — Tumor more than 0.1 but not more than 0.5 cm in greatest dimension

T_{1b} — Tumor more than 0.5 cm but not more than 1.0 cm in greatest dimension

T_{1c} — Tumor more than 1.0 cm but not more than 2.0 cm in greatest dimension

T_2 — Tumor more than 2.0 cm but not more than 5.0 cm in greatest dimension

T_3 — Tumor more than 5.0 cm in greatest dimension

T_4 — Tumor of any size with direct extension to (a) chest wall or (b) skin, only as described below. Note: Chest wall includes ribs, intercostal muscles, and serratus anterior muscle but not pectoral muscle.

T_{4a} — Extension to chest wall

T_{4b} — Edema (including peau d'orange) or ulceration of the skin of the breast or satellite skin nodules confined to the same breast

T_{4c} — Both of the above (T_{4a} and T_{4b})

T_{4d} — Inflammatory carcinoma

Regional Lymph Nodes (N)

N_x — Regional lymph nodes cannot be assessed (e.g., previously removed)

N_0 — No regional lymph node metastasis

N_1 — Metastasis to movable ipsilateral axillary lymph node(s)

N_2 — Metastasis to ipsilateral axillary lymph node(s) fixed to each other or to other structures

N_3 — Metastasis to ipsilateral internal mammary lymph node(s)

Pathologic Classification (pN)

pN_x — Regional lymph nodes cannot be assessed (not removed for pathologic study or previously removed)

pN_0 — No regional lymph node metastasis

pN_1 — Metastasis to movable ipsilateral axillary lymph node(s)

pN_{1a} — Only micrometastasis (none larger than 0.2 cm)

pN_{1b} — Metastasis to lymph node(s), any larger than 0.2 cm

pN_{1bi}	Metastasis in 1 to 3 lymph nodes, any more than 0.2 cm and all less than 2.0 cm in greatest dimension		
pN_{1bii}	Metastasis to 4 or more lymph nodes, any more than 0.2 cm and all less than 2.0 cm in greatest dimension		
pN_{1biii}	Extension of tumor beyond the capsule of a lymph node metastasis less than 2.0 cm in greatest dimension		
pN_{1biv}	Metastasis to a lymph node 2.0 cm or more in greatest dimension		

pN_2 Metastasis to ipsilateral axillary lymph node(s) fixed to each other or to other structures

pN_3 Metastasis to ipsilateral internal mammary lymph node(s)

Distant Metastasis (M)

M_x Presence of distant metastasis cannot be assessed

M_0 No distant metastasis

M_1 Distant metastasis present (includes metastasis to ipsilateral supraclavicular lymph nodes)

AJCC Stage Groupings

Stage 0	T_{is}	N_0	M_0
Stage I	T_1	N_0	M_0
Stage IIA	T_0	N_1	M_0
	T_1*	N_1**	M_0
	T_2	N_0	M_0
Stage IIB	T_2	N_1	M_0
	T_3	N_0	M_0
Stage IIIA	T_0	N_2	M_0
	T_1*	N_2	M_0
	T_2	N_2	M_0
	T_3	N_1	M_0
	T_3	N_2	M_0
Stage IIIB	T_4	Any N	M_0
	Any T	N_3	M_0
Stage IV	Any T	Any N	M_1

---

*T_1 includes T_{1mic}.

**The prognosis of patients with pN_{1a} disease is similar to that of patients with pN_0 disease.

Used with the permission of the American Joint Committee on Cancer (AJCC®), Chicago, Illinois. The original source for this material is the AJCC® Cancer Staging Manual, 5th edition (1997) published by Lippincott-Raven Publishers, Philadelphia, Pennsylvania.

DUCTAL CARCINOMA IN SITU (DCIS)

Surgery

■ Standard surgical treatment options include breast conservation therapy with lumpectomy followed by radiation therapy or mastectomy. The National Surgical Adjuvant Breast and Bowel Project (NSABP) study B-17, randomized patients with localized intraductal carcinoma and negative margins after excision to breast irradiation or no further therapy (Fisher, Dignam, et al., 1998). At 8 years, the cumulative incidence of recurrent DCIS was reduced by the addition of postoperative radiation from 13.4% to 8.2% ($p = 0.007$), and the occurrence of invasive cancer decreased from 13.4% to 3.9% ($p < 0.001$). Pathologic evaluation found that only the absence of clear tumor margins and moderate to marked comedo necrosis were independent predictors of ipsilateral tumor recurrence. Currently, there is no prospective randomized trial data evaluating what constitutes an adequate margin in terms of adjuvant therapy. There are single institution experiences with lumpectomy alone that suggest that appropriately selected patients may do well with conservative surgery alone if margins are adequate (≥ 1 cm). Patients with persistent microscopic involvement of the margins after local excision or evidence of multicentric disease should be treated with mastectomy.

Radiation Therapy

■ Radiation therapy to the breast may be given following complete excision of the area of abnormality with negative margins. The treatment usually consists of 50 Gy to the intact breast followed by a boost to the tumor bed of 10 to 20 Gy depending on the adequacy of the surgical margins. Radiation may be offered after mastectomy if there is evidence of T_3 disease, multicentric disease, or close surgical margins.

Hormone Therapy

■ Tamoxifen may be offered to lower subsequent risk of invasive carcinoma. The NSABP currently has a trial (B-24) to evaluate the role of tamoxifen following treatment for intraductal disease.

LOBULAR CARCINOMA IN SITU (LCIS)

■ Lobular carcinoma in situ is commonly multicentric and frequently bilateral. Careful evaluation of both breasts is necessary. Treatment options include lumpectomy, segmental mastectomy, or mastectomy. The natural history of untreated LCIS suggests that the majority of patients do not develop invasive disease and half of those who do develop it in the contralateral side. In NSABP Trial B-17, 182 patients who underwent excision alone for LCIS were evaluated at 5 years (Fisher et al., 1996). There was a 2.2% incidence of invasive ipsilateral tumor recurrence and a 1.1% incidence of contralateral breast tumor occurrence. Because of this the most frequent management of LCIS is close surveillance only with bilateral prophylactic mastectomy occasionally offered. The options for postexcision management remain controversial.

EARLY-STAGE DISEASE (STAGE I & II)

Surgery

■ Surgery for early-stage breast cancer may include lumpectomy, segmental mastectomy, or modified radical mastectomy with axillary dissection. A number of long-term, prospective, randomized studies have found that survival is equivalent with either breast conservation surgery with postoperative radiation or modified radical mastectomy (Fisher et al., 1995; Blichert-Toft et al., 1992; van Dongen et al., 1992; Sarrazin et al., 1989; Jacobson et al., 1995; Veronesi et al., 1995). In the largest trial—NSABP B-06—there was no difference in survival between the three treatment arms (modified radical mastectomy, lumpectomy plus axillary dissection followed by local breast radiation, or lumpectomy and axillary dissection alone) at a median follow-up of 12.5 years (Fisher et al., 1995). However, for all patients who received lumpectomy followed by irradiation, the rate of local recurrence in the breast was substantially lower than that of patients treated with lumpectomy alone (10% vs. 35%, $p < 0.001$). The rate of local control in the breast varies with surgical technique. Several contraindications exist for breast conservation procedures in early-stage disease:

a. Large tumor size > 4 to 5 cm in small-breasted women
b. Multicentric disease and/or diffuse indeterminate microcalcifications on mammography
c. Positive surgical margins on reexcision
d. Poor cosmetic outcome (breast to tumor ratio requires excision of large volume of breast tissue)

    e. Current first or second trimester pregnancy
    f. Previous history of radiation therapy to the chest or axilla
    g. History of collagen vascular disease

■ Axillary dissection (Level I/II) has been the standard of care in early breast cancer. The rationale for dissection grows from two factors: (1) physical examination is an inadequate method of detecting axillary lymph node involvement, having a false-negative and false-positive rate of 30% in either case (Harris & Hellman, 1996), and (2) lymph node status is the single best predictor of breast cancer prognosis (Osuch, 1999). Unfortunately, axillary dissection is associated with increased morbidity including axillary fibrosis, pain, and decreased range of motion of the shoulder and lymphedema. Recently, sentinel lymph node biopsy has been introduced into the care of early-stage breast cancer. It is based on the rationale that the pathologic status of the sentinel lymph node that drains the tumor site will be reflective of the pathological status of the remainder of the lymph nodes in the axilla. Currently, a number of trials are ongoing to evaluate the accuracy of the procedure and the minimal requirements for pathologic evaluation as well as determining the criteria for selecting patients for the procedure.

RADIATION THERAPY

Intact Breast

■ Radiation therapy to the breast may be given following complete excision of the area of abnormality with negative margins. The treatment usually consists of 50 Gy to the intact breast followed by a boost to the tumor bed of 10 Gy. The boost technique may be altered to include an interstitial radioactive implant if there is evidence of close or positive surgical margins after excision. Radiation should be started as soon as possible after surgery, when the surgical wound has healed. The optimal sequencing of chemotherapy and radiation has not been clearly defined, but delays in radiation of ≥ 4 months have been associated with increased recurrence rates (Dubay, Recht, Come, Shulman, & Harris, 1998).

Postmastectomy Chest Wall and Regional Lymphatics

■ Radiation therapy to the chest wall and regional lymphatics after mastectomy for early-stage breast cancer has been used at many institutions to reduce the risk of local recurrence and distant metastasis and improve survival (Overgaard et al., 1997; Ragaz et al., 1997). The popularity of postoperative chest wall and regional nodal radiation has significantly increased in response to new data published in 1997. In a meta-analysis by the Early Breast Cancer Trialists' Collaborative Group (1995), which analyzed all the randomized trials begun before 1985, a 67% reduction in rates of locoregional relapse ($p < 0.001$) and a 6% reduction in mortality from breast cancer ($p = 0.03$) was found, but no improvement in overall survival. More recent studies have found that postmastectomy radiation therapy in premenopausal women with breast cancer reduces the rate of locoregional and systemic relapses and may improve overall survival (Overgaard et al., 1997; Ragaz et al., 1997). Overgaard (1997) in a randomized trial of radiotherapy after mastectomy in high-risk premenopausal women, all of whom received systemic chemotherapy, found the frequency of locoregional recurrence alone or with distant metastases was 9% among the women who received radiation and chemotherapy as compared to 32% with chemotherapy alone ($p < 0.001$). Overall survival at 10 years was 54% among those given radiotherapy and chemotherapy as compared with 45% among those who received chemotherapy alone ($p < 1.001$). Therefore, postmastectomy radiotherapy is recommended in patients at high risk for local regional failure ($\geq T_2$, any N_1, and any close surgical margin).

■ Fields treated may include chest wall, supraclavicular fossa, axillary, and internal mammary fields. The treatment usually consists of 50 Gy in 1.8 to 2.0 Gy fractions. The mastectomy scar may be boosted with an additional 10 Gy.

Chemotherapy

■ Adjuvant systemic therapy should be considered in patients with tumors greater than 0.5 to 1 cm, positive lymph nodes, and aggressive histology. Prognostic features such as angiolymphatic invasion, high S-phase, high nuclear grade, and high histologic grade should be taken into account. In addition, age, menopausal status, and comorbid disease status should be taken into account. The appropriate adjuvant therapy is also dependent on an assessment efficacy and toxicity data of the treatment regimen. The protocols used include CMF (cyclophosphamide, methotrexate, and 5-fluorouracil), AC (doxorubicin and cyclophosphamide),

CAF (cyclophosphamide, doxorubicin, and 5-fluorouracil), and AT (doxorubicin and taxanes). Currently, high-dose chemotherapy with bone marrow rescue is not standard practice.

Hormone Therapy

■ For women ages 50 years and older with estrogen receptor positive tumors, tamoxifen for 5 years is recommended (NCCN, 1997).

ADVANCED STAGE DISEASE (STAGE III & IV) AND INFLAMMATORY BREAST CANCER

■ Patients with advanced breast cancer should be carefully evaluated for evidence of metastatic disease prior to initiation of treatment. Patients who have locally advanced disease (stage IIIA) should receive systemic treatment, radiation, and surgery with the sequencing tailored to individual cases and institution protocols. Surgery usually consists of a modified radical mastectomy with axillary lymph node dissection. Radiation therapy may be given preoperatively but is usually given after surgery. Chemotherapy may precede or follow surgery. A recent NSABP study comparing preoperative and postoperative chemotherapy showed no survival difference related to time of chemotherapy (Fisher, Bryant et al., 1998) or neoadjuvant chemotherapy followed by surgery and radiation. For patients with T_0, T_1, or T_2 tumors, breast conservation may be an option.

■ Patients with inoperable breast disease usually require neoadjuvant systemic treatment. If the disease responds sufficiently, mastectomy with axillary lymph node dissection precedes radiation therapy. If the tumor remains inoperable after chemotherapy, preoperative radiation may be given, which frequently renders the tumor operable. Further systemic chemotherapy with or without tamoxifen may be considered.

BREAST CANCER AND PREGNANCY

■ Occurs in 1 in 3,000 pregnancies. The natural tenderness and engorgement of the pregnant breast may hinder detection of discrete masses and may delay diagnosis. Diagnostic procedures such as ultrasound and mammography may be used with adequate shielding of the fetus to evaluate dominant masses and occult carcinomas in the presence of other suspicious clinical findings (Barnavon & Wallack, 1990). Staging radiology studies should be limited due to potential risk to the fetus, and should only be used when essential for making a treatment decision. Termination of pregnancy may be considered based on the age of the fetus, if maternal options such as chemotherapy and radiation therapy are significantly limited by the continuation of the pregnancy.

TOXICITY OF TREATMENT

Acute Toxicities

1. Fatigue is a common side effect of radiation therapy. In a study evaluating fatigue related to different treatment methods for breast cancer, women who received combination therapy (chemotherapy and radiation) had the highest fatigue scores; those who received only radiation therapy had the lowest fatigue scores (Woo, Dubble, Piper, Keating & Weiss, 1998). Fatigue significantly increases over the course of treatment, is the highest in the last week of treatment, and returns to pretreatment levels by about 3 months after treatment (Irvine, Vincent, Graydon, & Bubela, 1998). It has been related to symptom distress, psychologic distress, and impairs quality of life (Irvine et al., 1998). Specific management options are found in Chapter 20.

2. Skin reaction occurs frequently in women receiving radiation therapy for breast cancer. The severity of the reaction depends on radiation dose, energy used, and fields treated. The total effect for the dose schedule applied has been found to be the strongest factor for acute and late skin reactions (Turesson, Nyman, Holmberg, & Oden, 1996). In addition to radiation dose, weight, breast size, lymphocele aspiration, smoking, age, history of skin cancer, and tumor stage have been found to be important factors in predicting the severity of an acute radiation skin reaction in women with breast cancer (Porock, Kristjanson, Nikoletti, Cameron & Pedler, et al., 1998). Specific management options may be found in Chapter 21.

   a. Breast conservation—the breast will become gradually erythematous approximately 2 to 3 weeks after initiation of treatment. Patients may experience pruritus particularly in the upper medial area of the breast field associated with folliculitis. Areas of moist desquamation may occur in the inframammary fold and in the axilla.

    b. Chest wall—the chest wall will gradually become erythematous approximately 2 to 3 weeks into treatment. Areas of moist desquamation are common after 40 Gy and may require a treatment break.

3. Breast edema is found commonly in women treated with breast-conservation radiation therapy. The onset of breast swelling is gradual and continues until completion of treatment. It is commonly associated with mild discomfort and breast tenderness. Resolution of the swelling is also gradual. The majority of swelling disappears within the first 6 months in most women. However, in large-breasted women, the swelling may persist for a much longer period of time. In a prospective assessment of late changes in the breast, Moody et al. (1994) found that only 6% of women with small breasts developed moderate or severe late changes as compared with 22% of women with moderate-size breasts and 39% with large breasts ($p < 0.001$). A significant correlation was found between breast size and dose inhomogeneity that may account for the marked changes in breast appearance in the larger breast.

Chronic Toxicities

1. Lymphedema is the buildup of lymph in the tissues, mainly in the fat just under the skin. The incidence of lymphedema of the upper extremity, a disabling complication of treatment, has been reported to range from 2% to 89%, depending on the type of surgery performed (Hardy & Baum 1991; Segerstrom, Bjevle, Graffman, & Nystrom et al., 1992). These data are similar to those occasionally included as part of the analysis of complications associated with therapeutic clinical trials. Lymphedema results from a disturbance of the equilibrium between the transport capacity of the clearing system and the amount of lymph fluid to be cleared (Twycross & Lack, 1990). It is associated with tightness, discomfort, hyperkeratosis, and Stemmer's sign. Since lymphedema cannot be cured, the aim is to achieve maximum improvement and long-term control (Twycross & Lack, 1990). The earlier treatment is initiated, the better the result.

Prevention (Burt & White, 1999)

    1. Avoid breaks in the skin of the affected limb

    2. Treat evidence of cellulitis aggressively with antibiotic therapy

3. Avoid pressure on the involved extremity
4. Avoid constrictive clothing
5. Avoid vigorous activity with the limb
6. Use an electric razor under the affected arm
7. Avoid extremes of heat including sunbathing and hot tubs
8. Keep the skin in good condition
9. Maintain ideal weight
10. Avoid extended use of diuretics
11. Exercise regularly—do not overdo
12. Choose a light prosthesis
13. Eat healthy foods—avoid caffeine, alcohol, and excessive salt intake. Increase water consumption.
14. Plan ahead when you travel. Avoid long airline flights. Take frequent rest breaks and avoid lifting heavy luggage.

Treatment Approaches

1. Manual Lymphatic Massage/Drainage (MLD)—special form of very gentle, rhythmic, pumping massage movements that remove excess fluid and protein from an extremity. Stimulates contraction of the skin lymphatics which improves superficial drainage (Twycross & Lack, 1990).
2. Compression with Bandages or Garments—apply external pressure to swollen limb to support the skin and underlying vessels.
3. Compression with Vasopneumatic Pumps—limb placed in an inflatable sleeve connected to a motor-driven air pump that inflates and deflates cyclically. Multichamber compression stimulates superficial lymph flow, decreases tissue fibrosis, and encourages fluid out of the limb. Compression should be used for a total of 2 hours per day. Pressure of the machine should not exceed 60 mm Hg (Twycross & Lack, 1990).
4. Complete decongestive physiotherapy (CDP) is a combination of manual lymphatic drainage and compression bandaging. It has been found to be superior to pneumatic pumps and surgery in treating lymphedema (Lerner, 1998). Several methods are described in the literature—Lerner School, Vodder School, and Casley Smith method. Boris, Weindorf, and Lasinkski (1997) found that patients who are compliant with treatment showed a significant reduction in lymphedema and maintained that after 36 months.

2. Soft Tissue Fibrosis—mild atrophic and telangiectatic skin changes may occur after radiation to the breast or chest wall. The skin may become tight and some soft tissue fibrosis may occur in the breast, which may affect cosmetic outcome.

    a. Breast—A number of variables have been studied in regard to cosmetic outcome in breast conservation radiation therapy. Kramer and colleagues found on univariate analysis of women receiving an interstitial implant as part of breast-conservation therapy that total excision volume and dose homogeneity index were significantly related to cosmetic outcome (Kramer, Arthur, Ulin, Schmidt-Ullrich, Zwicker, & Wazer, 1999). In multivariate analysis, only the total excision volume remained significant. The mean total excision volume $\pm$ SD (standard deviation) in patients with excellent cosmetic outcome (81.8 cm^3 $\pm$ 84.0) was significantly less than that in patients with less than excellent cosmetic outcome (120 cm^3 $\pm$ 84). The probability of excellent cosmetic outcome linearly increased with an increase in the dose homogeneity index. Vrieling et al. (1999) evaluated the influence of the boost and found that 86% of patients in the no-boost group had an excellent or good global result as compared with 71% of patients in the boost group (16 Gy) ($p = 0.0001$) at 3 years.

    b. Breast Augmentation—Victor et al. (1998) evaluated cosmetic outcome of patients with prosthetically augmented breasts. With a median follow-up of 32 months, good/excellent cosmetic results were found in 100% of women. Bolus application and increasing stage were associated with a worse cosmetic result.

3. Brachial Plexopathy—Secondary to radiation is a rare complication usually related to high total doses of radiation or nonstandard fractionation schemes (Svensson, Westling, & Larsson, 1975). Patients present without pain, but with edema (Thomas & Colby, 1972) and signs of upper trunk (C-5 through C-7) dysfunction (Kori, Foley, & Posner, 1981). When associated with lymphedema, the symptoms of the brachial plexopathy may improve with treatment of the lymphedema (Ganel, Engel, Sela, & Brooks, 1979). Treatment may include nerve blocks, cordotomy, rhizotomy, or oral narcotic management for uncontrolled chronic pain.

4. Rib Fracture—Spontaneous rib fractures occur in approximately 10% of patients who receive radiation to the chest wall following mastectomy (Mendenhall, Fletcher, & Million, 1987).

The fractures may be asymptomatic and only found on chest x-ray or bone scan or they may be quite painful. Typically, the fractures heal spontaneously within 6 to 8 weeks. Overgaard (1988) found that patients treated with a large dose per fraction had a significantly higher incidence of late bone damage (19%) than patients treated with a standard dose per fraction (6%). There was a clear dose-response relationship, especially in the 12-fraction regimen as compared with the 22-fraction regimen.

5. Cardiac Toxicity—Radiation therapy has been associated with an increased risk of cardiac mortality and morbidity in early-stage, left-sided breast cancer. The anterior left ventricle is frequently included in tangential chest wall fields and in en face fields treating the internal mammary nodes (Mendenhall et al., 1987). Cardiac mortality has been found to positively correlate with cardiac dose-volume (Gyenes, Rutquist, Liedberg, & Fornander, 1998). Patients who receive high-dose volumes appear to have an increased mortality of ischemic heart disease, but not of myocardial infarction (Gyenes et al., 1998). However, with modern technology including CT simulation, it is possible to decrease the volume of heart in the irradiation of the left breast.

6. Pulmonary Toxicity—Pulmonary complications following radiation for breast cancer are related to radiation dose, technique, and volume of lung included in the treatment field. Depending on patient anatomy and treatment technique, a variable amount of lung is always irradiated when either the breast, chest wall, or regional lymphatics are treated (Mendenhall et al., 1987). Acute pneumonitis is more likely when larger volumes of lung are irradiated. Acute pneumonitis is characterized by a dry, hacking cough and occasionally febrile episodes and shortness of breath. It may last 2 to 3 weeks or longer, but is usually self-limiting. In severe cases, steroids may be given to manage acute symptoms. Asymptomatic pulmonary fibrosis limited to the treatment volume is usually seen on chest x-ray and CT imaging including the apical region when the supraclavicular/axillary region is irradiated.

7. Shoulder Movement—The range of motion of the shoulder may be limited after treatment. Sugden and colleagues evaluated women at 18 months after surgery and postoperative radiation (Sugden, Rezvani, Harrison & Hughes (1998). Half of the patients reported that the function was reduced when compared with before treatment. Overall, 48% of the patients

had measured limitation of at least one shoulder movement as compared with the other shoulder. Mastectomy patients had more problems than those patients with breast conservation (79% vs. 35%). Patients who had axillary irradiation also had more problems (73% vs. 35%). Patients with dysfunction of the shoulder movement before radiation therapy had a 60% chance of persistent movement problems at 18 months as compared with 24% of patients with normal postoperative function. Similar findings were reported by Hack, Cohen, Katz, Robson, & Goss, 1999. Seventy-two percent of women experienced arm/shoulder pain, weakness or numbness, and impaired range of motion of the impaired arm/shoulder. Pain severity correlated positively with the number of lymph nodes removed and treatment with chemotherapy, but was not significantly related to length of time since surgery or treatment with radiation therapy. Early physical therapy intervention can make a significant contribution to normal function without increasing the incidence of postoperative complications (Wingate, Croghan, Natarajan, Michalek, & Jordan, 1989).

8. Menopausal Symptoms—With the introduction of estrogen suppression therapy as a treatment modality for breast cancer, premenopausal and perimenopausal women are experiencing menopausal symptoms and the consequences of estrogen deprivation much earlier than would naturally occur. The organ systems most commonly affected are the central nervous system, cardiovascular, musculoskeletal, genitourinary, and integumentary. Sequelae include urogenital atrophy, vasomotor instability, osteoporosis, osteopenia, and diminished gender-related cardiovascular protection. Common vulvovaginal and urinary symptoms found in postmenopausal women include irritation, itching, burning, dyspareunia, and urinary difficulties. With these physiologic changes comes change in sexual health, with the dyspareunia due to vaginal dryness being the most common clinical symptom affecting sexual activity (Lamont, 1997).

OUTCOMES MEASURES

■ The NCI Toxicity Criteria (CTC) Version 2, with the Radiation Therapy Oncology Group (RTOG) and European Organization for Research and Treatment of Cancer (EORTC) Acute Effects Criteria Instrument provides a scale for many different organ systems and some symptoms (NCI, 1999). This is a very useful tool for grading severity of acute effects of radiation therapy in all sites.

■ The Radiation Therapy Patient Care Record: A Tool for Documenting Nursing Care (ONS, 1994) provides a tool for weekly assessment and grading of severity of acute effects of radiation therapy in all sites.

■ A follow-up evaluation should be performed every 3 months for a minimum of 3 years, then every 6 to 12 months for the next 2 years, then annually (ASCO, 1999). The evaluation should include:

1. Self-examination of breast monthly
2. History and physical examination
3. Careful visual inspection and physical examination of the breast and regional lymphatic bearing areas
4. Measure the circumference of the midhand, wrist, forearm, and upper arm of both upper extremities for evidence of lymphedema.
5. Mammogram—
   a. Women treated with breast-conserving therapy should have their first posttreatment mammogram 6 months after completion of radiation therapy, then annually or as indicated for surveillance of abnormalities. If stability of mammographic findings is achieved, mammography can be performed yearly thereafter (ASCO, 1999).
      • Radiotherapy causes fat necrosis, fibrosis, skin thickening, and other parenchymal distortion of the breast, making it more difficult to interpret after radiotherapy. In addition, masses, fluid collections, scarring, edema, and calcifications are posttreatment findings that may mimic or mask local tumor recurrence (Krishnamurthy, Whitman, Stelling, & Kushwaha, 1999). Holli and colleagues found that further diagnostic tests prompted by difficulties in interpreting mammograms were performed to the extent of 0.19 per mammography exam in those who had prior breast radiation as compared with 0.15 in those without radiotherapy (approximately 1.3 times more often) (Holli, Saaristo, Isola, Hyoty, & Hakama, 1998). Findings that turned out to be negative at confirmation were two times more common in the radiotherapy group.

   b. All women with a prior diagnosis of breast cancer
should have yearly mammographic evaluation of the
contralateral breast. Of importance is the mammographic changes associated with tamoxifen, specifically
a decrease in breast parenchyma (Son & Oh, 1999).
  6. Radiograph or laboratory studies as clinically indicated.
There is insufficient data to suggest routine use of complete blood counts, automated chemistries, chest radi-
ographs, bone scans, liver ultrasounds, CT scans, CEA,
CA-15-3, or CA-27.29 tumor markers for breast cancer surveillance (ASCO, 1999).
  7. Pelvic examination with appropriate Pap smear annually.
If patient is on tamoxifen, ultrasonography examination
or endometrial biopsy should be performed annually to
evaluate for evidence of endometrial carcinoma.

EXPECTED OUTCOMES

SURVIVAL

■ Relative survival rates for breast cancer increase with age at
diagnosis. Women who develop breast cancer when they are
younger than age 45 have a 5-year relative survival rate of 79%.
This rate increases to 84% for women aged 45 to 64 years, and
87% for women ages 65 and over (Ries, Kosary, Hankey, Miller,
Harras, & Edwards, 1997).

CHILDBEARING AFTER BREAST CANCER

■ Pregnancy does not appear to have adverse effects on the
survival among women diagnosed with stage I and II invasive breast cancer (Velentgas et al., 1999). In a recent evaluation of 53 women who became pregnant after the diagnosis of breast cancer, 5 women died of recurrent disease.
After adjusting for age and stage of disease, the overall relative risk of mortality associated with subsequent pregnancy was 0.8.

QUALITY OF LIFE

■ Four key points can be abstracted from the data that describe breast cancer survivors. The first is that surviving
breast cancer is a process of adjustment that occurs over

time and may be influenced at any point by psychosocial and physical sequelae related to the diagnosis and treatment. Second, depression may be the most common emotional sequela after diagnosis, and may continue or recur in response to treatment-related physical problems in the succeeding years. The third point is that there are insufficient data accurately describing the chronic physical effects of surgery and radiation therapy and their impact on quality of life. Finally, menopausal symptoms related to estrogen suppression after breast cancer may be responsible for a significant effect on a woman's sexual health, and ultimately on quality of life.

- Irvine and colleagues conducted a meta-analysis of the literature investigating psychosocial adjustment in women with breast cancer (Irvine, Brown, Crooks, Roberts, & Browne, 1991). The review suggested that the majority of women with breast cancer did not experience long-term emotional distress, although 20% to 30% experienced a disruption in their quality of life through loss of roles, loss of functional abilities, and problems with social relationships.
- Numerous studies have evaluated specific outcomes related to mastectomy versus breast-conservation therapy. Curran et al. (1998) reported on EORTC Trial 10801 that compared quality of life outcomes of early-stage breast cancer patients treated with radical mastectomy or breast conservation. Significant benefit in body image and satisfaction with treatment was observed in the breast-conservation group. Ratings of cosmetic results decreased in time and in line with clinical observations of long-term side effects of radiotherapy. However, there was no significant difference observed between the two groups in relation to fear of recurrence. This data confirm previous reports of the importance of body image and quality of life in this patient population.
- Only minimal information is available on the incidence of factors that impact physical well-being. Polinsky (1994) found a number of physical sequelae including arm weakness and heaviness, phantom breast syndrome, numbness of the arm and breast, arm swelling, breast changes after irradiation, increased skin sensitivity, pain, and menopausal symptoms from hormonal therapy.
- Data from several studies support the existence of one or more of these themes in long-term breast cancer survivors. A case-control comparison study by Craig, Comstock, and

Geiser (1974) revealed that quality of survival, as defined by physical and psychosocial criteria, was similar among 134 long-term breast cancer survivors ($\geq$ 5 years) and 260 controls. Physical disability was reported by 19% of the women with breast cancer and 16% of the controls. The slight excess of disability among the breast cancer cases was attributed to surgical treatment. There was no evidence of increased psychosocial disability among the women with breast cancer.

- Woods & Earp (1978) explored the quality of survival of 49 women 4 years after mastectomy. They reported a positive association between the number of physical symptoms the women experienced and depressive symptoms. Many of these women continued to experience physical symptoms and depression 4 years after treatment. Although these two studies provided early evidence of chronic psychosocial and physical problems after treatment for breast cancer, they were conducted prior to the availability of many new surgical and radiotherapy techniques used today that alter the extent of surgical resection and physical disability. In addition, Woods' and Earp's study did link the occurrence of physical disability with long-term psychosocial sequelae.

- Vinokur (1989) compared 5-year survivors of breast cancer with a matched control group of asymptomatic women. Women with breast cancer did not differ from the control group on indicators of mental health, social and psychological well-being, or physical functioning. They did report a greater number of diagnosed medical conditions, and took more medications than the control group. Within the breast cancer group, stage and timing of the cancer in relationship to the exam had strong independent adverse effects on several of the indicators of mental health and physical functioning.

- Using a different research method, Carter (1993) analyzed the stories of 25 long-term breast cancer survivors. Each of the women was interviewed during a period of time 5 years or more after diagnosis. Informants described "going through" a survival process that involved movement through several phases. The phases included interpreting the diagnosis, confronting mortality, reprioritizing, coming to terms, moving on, and flashing back. Each of the informants experienced the phases differently; some did not experience all phases and for some two or more phases occurred simultaneously. Four content themes emerged from the stories: the sense of self, the response of others, the meaning of cancer, and changes made as a result of cancer.

- Wyatt, Kurtz, and Liken (1993) found very similar themes in an exploratory study of long-term breast cancer survivorship. Using focus group discussions the following issues were addressed: integration of the disease process into current life, changes in relationships with others, restructuring of one's life perspective, and unresolved issues. In addition, the study found that individuals do not fit their lives into specific domains of QOL. Instead, concerns and issues often cross over into two or more domains.

- In a descriptive phenomenological study, Pelusi (1997) explored women's perspectives of the experience of surviving breast cancer. Eight women participated in open-ended interviews that were transcribed and analyzed using Colaizzi's method. Nine theme categories were identified: a future of uncertainty, abandonment, sanctuaries along the way, self-transcendence, finding resolution to the financial cost of cancer, mediating expectations of others, survivors' lifelines, circle of influences, and the journey. Many of these themes were similar to those previously identified. Pelusi found that the essential structure of the experience of surviving breast cancer is one of facing the unknown and experiencing many losses. At the same time, this journey evolves into one of growth and enlightenment, providing the woman with many unexpected and new opportunities.

- In 1996, Ganz and colleagues reported one of the first prospective studies to specifically address QOL, rehabilitation needs, and psychological distress among breast cancer survivors. Furthermore, this study included repeat evaluations on a regular basis during the period of close surveillance. One hundred and thirty-nine breast cancer survivors were interviewed on four occasions during the first year after primary therapy, and again at 2 or 3 years. They found that at 2 and 3 years after treatment participants did not differ from each other on their prior assessments of quality of life. A significant decline in global quality of life, sexual functioning, and marital functioning occurred between the 1-year and 3-year evaluations. For the 2-year sample, only sexual functioning showed a deterioration. These survivors reported a number of problems associated with physical and recreational activities, body image, sexual interest, and sexual functioning. The authors concluded that breast cancer survivors appear to plateau or reach maximum recovery from the physical and psychological trauma of cancer treatment by 1 year after surgery and decline in some areas in the following 2 years. Many physical, psychosocial, and sexual functioning problems persist or even worsen over time. Physical problems include paresthesia, pain, skin sensitivity, changes in hair, changes in the irradiated breast, and endocrine problems. Psychosocial problems include a reduction in energy, changes in communication and affection with partner, body image, cognitive problems, a decreased interest in sexual activity, and feelings of decreased sexual attractiveness. They suggested that there were many hormone-related reasons why breast cancer patients experience profound menopausal symptomatology including hot flashes, sleep disturbances, vaginal dryness, and emotional lability, which may ultimately impact on sexual health.

- The following are general quality of life instruments that are appropriate:

   1. Functional Assessment of Cancer Therapy - Breast (FACT-B) (Brady et al., 1997)—A measurement system of self-report and 33-item scale of quality of life for people with breast cancer. An 18-item endocrine subscale is currently under evaluation (Fallowfield et al., 1999).

   2. European Organization for Research and Treatment of Cancer (EORTC) QLQ-C30 (Aaronson et al., 1993)—A 36-item questionnaire for assessing the quality-of-life of cancer patients participating in international clinical trials. It has been validated and extensively used in a wide range of cancer clinical trials in Europe and worldwide including breast cancer (McLachlan, Devins, & Goodwin, 1998).

   3. Life Satisfaction Questionnaire (LSQ-32) (Carlsson & Hamrin, 1996)—A tool for measuring quality of life in

women with breast cancer. The instrument was designed for use within conventional cancer therapy as well as in complementary care.

REFERENCES

Aaronson, N. K., Ahmedzai, S., Bergman, B., Bullinger, M., Cull, A., Duez, N. J., Filiberti, A., Flechtner, H., Fleishman, S. B., de Haes, J. C. J. M., Kaasa, S., Klee, M., Osoba, D., Razavi, D., Rofe, P. B., Schraub, S., Sneeuw, K., Sullivan, M., & Takeda, F. (1993). The European Organization for Research and Treatment of Cancer QLQ-C30: A quality-of-life instrument for use in international clinical trials in oncology. *Journal of the National Cancer Institute*, 85(5), 365–376.

American Cancer Society. (1999). *Cancer facts and figures*. Atlanta, GA: American Cancer Society.

American College of Radiology. (1993). *Breast imaging reporting and data system* (BIRADS). Reston, VA: American College of Radiology.

American Society of Clinical Oncology. (1996). ASCO statement on genetic testing for cancer susceptibility. *Journal of Clinical Oncology*, 14(5), 1730–1736.

American Society of Clinical Oncology. (1999). Recommended breast cancer surveillance guidelines. *Journal of Clinical Oncology*, 17(3), 1080–1082.

Baines, C. J., McFarlane, D. V., & Miller, A. B. (1988). Sensitivity and specificity of the first screen mammography in 15 NBSS centers. *Journal of Canadian Radiology Association*, 39(4), 273–276.

Barnavon, Y., & Wallack, M. K. (1990). Management of the pregnant patient with carcinoma of the breast. *Surgical Gynecology and Obstetrics*, 171(4), 347–352.

Bernstein, L. (1998). The epidemiology of breast cancer. *Women and Cancer*, 1(Suppl. 1), 7–13.

Bernstein, L., & Ross, R. (1993). Endogenous hormones and breast cancer risk. *Epidemiologic Reviews*, 15(1), 48–65.

Bhatia, S., Robison, L. L., Oberlin, O., Greenberg, M., Bunin, G., Fossati-Bellani, F., & Meadows, A. T. (1996). Breast cancer and other second neoplasms after childhood Hodgkin's disease. *New England Journal of Medicine*, 334(12), 745–751.

Blichert-Toft, M., Rose, C., Andersen, J. A., Overgaard, M., Axelsson, C. K., Anderson, K. W., & Mouridsen, H. T. (1992). Danish randomized trial comparing breast conservation therapy with mastectomy: Six years of life-table analysis. *Journal of the National Cancer Institute Monographs*, 11, 15–18.

Boris, M., Weindorf, S., & Lasinkski, S. (1997). Persistence of lymphedema reduction after noninvasive complex lymphedema therapy. *Oncology Huntington*, 11(1), 99–109.

Brady, M. J., Cella, D. F., Mo, F., Bonomi, A. E., Tulsky, D. S., Lloyd, S. R., Deasy, S., Cobleigh, M, & Shiomoto, G. (1997). Reliability and validity of the Functional Assessment of Cancer Therapy—Breast quality-of-life instrument. *Journal of Clinical Oncology*, 15(3), 974–986.

Burt, J., & White, G. (1999). *Lymphedema: A breast cancer patient's guide to prevention and healing*. Alameda, CA: Hunter House Publications.

Byrne, C., Schairer, C., Wolfe, J., Parekh, N., Salane, M., Brinton, L. A., Hoover, R., & Haile, R. (1995). Mammographic features and breast cancer risk: Effects with time, age, and menopause status. *Journal of the National Cancer Institute*, 87(21), 1622–1629.

Carlsson, M., & Hamrin, E. (1996). Measurement of quality of life in women with breast cancer. Development of a Life Satisfaction Questionnaire (LSQ-32) and a comparison with the EORTC QLQ-C30. *Quality of Life Research*, 5(2), 265–274.

Carter, B. J. (1993). Long-term survivors of breast cancer. A qualitative descriptive study. *Cancer Nursing*, 16(5), 354–362.

Collaborative Group on Hormonal Factors in Breast Cancer. (1996). Breast cancer and hormonal contraceptives: Collaborative reanalysis of individual data on 53,297 women with breast cancer and 100,239 women without breast cancer from 54 epidemiologic studies. *Lancet*, 347(9017), 1713–1727.

Craig, T. J., Comstock, G. W., & Geiser, P. B. (1974). The quality of survival in breast cancer: A case-control comparison. *Cancer*, 33(5), 1451–1457.

Curran, D., van Dongen, J. P., Aaronson, N. K., Kiebert, G., Fentiman, I. S., Mignolet, F., & Bartelink, H. (1998). Quality of life of early-stage breast cancer patients treated with radical mastectomy or breast-conserving procedures: Results of EORTC Trial 10801. The European Organization for Research and Treatment of Cancer (EORTC), Breast Cancer Cooperative Group (BCCG). *European Journal of Cancer*, 24(3), 307–314.

de Waard, F., Cornelis, J. P., Aoki, K., & Yoshida, M. (1977). Breast cancer incidence according to weight and height in two cities of the Netherlands and in Aichi prefecture, Japan. *Cancer*, 40(3), 1269–1275.

Dubay, A. K., Recht, A., Come, S., Shulman, L., & Harris, J. (1998). Why and how to combine chemotherapy and radiation therapy in breast cancer patients. *Recent Results in Cancer Research*, 152, 247–254.

Early Breast Cancer Trialists' Collaborative Group. (1995). Effects of radiotherapy and surgery in early breast cancer. An overview of the randomized trials. *New England Journal of Medicine*, 333(22), 1444–1455.

Fallowfield, L. J., Leaity, S. K., Howell, A., Benson, S., & Cella, D. (1999). Assessment of quality of life in women undergoing hormonal therapy for breast cancer: Validation of an endocrine symptom subscale for FACT-B. *Breast Cancer Research and Treatment*, 55(2), 189–199.

Feig, S. A., D'Orsi, C. J., Hendrick, R. E., Jackson, V. P., Kopans, D. B., Monsees, B., Sickles, E. A., Stelling, C. B., Zinninger, M., & Wilcox-Buchalla, P. (1998). American College of Radiology guidelines for breast cancer screening. *American Journal of Roentgenology*, 171(1), 29–33.

Fisher, B., Anderson, S., Redmond, C. K., Wolmark, N., Wickerham, D. L., & Cronin, W. M. (1995). Reanalysis and results after 12 years of follow-up in a randomized clinical trial comparing total mastectomy with lumpectomy with or without irradiation in the treatment of breast cancer. *New England Journal of Medicine*, 333(22), 1456–1461.

Fisher, B., Bryant, J., Wolmark, N., Mamounas, E., Brown, A., Fisher, E. R., Wickerham, D. L., Begovic, M., DeCillis, A., Robidoux, A., Margolese, R. G., Cruz, A. B. Jr., Hoehn, J. L., Lees, A. W., Dimitrov, N. V., & Bear, H. D. (1998). Effect of preoperative chemotherapy on the outcome of women with operable breast cancer. *Journal of Clinical Oncology*, 16(8), 2672–2685.

Fisher, B., Constantino, J. P., Wickerham, D. L., Redmond, C. K., Kavanah, M., Cronin, W. M., Vogel, V., Robidoux, A., Dimitrov, N., Atkins, J., Daly, M., Wieand, S., Tan-Chiu, E., Ford, L., & Wolmark, N. (1998). Tamoxifen for prevention of breast cancer: Report of the National Surgical Adjuvant Breast and Bowel Project P-1 study. *Journal of the National Cancer Institute*, 90(18), 1371–1388.

Fisher, B., Dignam, J., Wolmark, N., Mamounas, E., Costantino, J., Poller, W., Fisher, E. R., Wickerham, D. L., Deutsch, M., Margolese, R., Dimitrov, N., & Kaanah, M. (1998). Lumpectomy and radiation therapy for the treatment of intraductal breast cancer: Findings from the National Surgical Adjuvant Breast and Bowel Project B017. *Journal of Clinical Oncology*, 16(2), 441–452.

Fisher, E. R., Costantino, J., Fisher, B., Palekar, A. S., Paik, S. M., Suarez, C. M., & Wolmark, N. (1996). Pathologic findings from the National Surgical Adjuvant Breast and Bowel Project (NSABP) Protocol B-17. *Cancer*, 78(7), 1403–1416.

Ganel, A., Engel, J., Sela, M., & Brooks, M. (1979). Nerve entrapments associated with postmastectomy lymphedema. *Cancer*, 44(6), 2254–2259.

Ganz, P. A., Coscarelli, A., Fred, C., Kahn, B., Polinsky, M. L, & Petersen, L. (1996). Breast cancer survivors: Psychosocial concerns and quality of life. *Breast Cancer Research and Treatment*, 38(2), 183–199.

Greenlee, R. T., Murray, T., Bolden, S., & Wingo, P. A. (2000). Cancer statistics, 2000. *CA: A Cancer Journal for Clinicians*, 50(1), 7–33.

Gyenes, G., Rutqvist, L. E., Liedberg, A., & Fornander, T. (1998). Long-term cardiac morbidity and mortality in a randomized trial of pre- and postoperative radiation therapy versus surgery alone in primary breast cancer. *Radiotherapy and Oncology*, 48(2), 185–190.

Hack, T. F., Cohen, L., Katz, J., Robson, L. S., & Goss, P. (1999). Physical and psychological morbidity after axillary lymph node dissection for breast cancer. *Journal of Clinical Oncology*, 17(1), 143–149.

Hardy, J. R., & Baum, M. (1991). Lymphoedema—prevention rather than cure. *Annals of Oncology*, 2(8), 532–533.

Harris, J. R., & Hellman, S. (1996). Natural history of breast cancer. In J. R. Harris, M. E. Lippman, M. Morrow, & S. Hellman (Eds.), *Disease of the breast*, (pp. 375–391). Philadelphia: Lippincott-Raven.

Helzlsouer, K. (1995). Epidemiology, prevention, and early detection of breast cancer. *Current Opinion in Oncology*, 7(6), 489–494.

Henderson, B. E., Ross, R. K., & Berstein, L. (1988). Estrogens as a cause of human cancer. The Richard and Hinda Rosenthal Foundation Award Lecture. *Cancer Research*, 48(2), 246–253.

Holli, K., Saaristo, R., Isola, J., Hyoty, M., & Hakama, M. (1998). Effect of radiotherapy on the interpretation of routine follow-up mammography after conservative breast surgery: A randomized study. *British Journal of Cancer*, 78(4), 542–545.

Hultborn, R., Hanson, C., Kopf, I., Verbiene, I., Warnhammar, E., & Weimarck, A. (1997). Prevalence of Klinefelter's syndrome in male breast cancer patients. *Anticancer Research*, 17(6D), 4293–4298.

Irvine, D. M., Vincent, L., Graydon, J. E., & Bubela, N. (1998). Fatigue in women with breast cancer receiving radiation therapy. *Cancer Nursing*, 21(2), 127–135.

Irvine, D., Brown, B., Crooks, D., Roberts, J., & Browne, G. (1991). Psychosocial adjustment in women with breast cancer. *Cancer*, 67(4), 1097–1117.

Jacobson, J. A., Danforth, D. N., Cowan, K. H., d'Angelo, T., Steinberg, S. M., Pierce, L., Lippman, M. E., Lichter, A. S., Glatstein, E., & Okunieff, P. (1995). Ten year results of a comparison of conservation with mastectomy in the treatment of stage I and II breast cancer. *New England Journal of Medicine*, 332(14), 907–911.

Jaiyesimi, I. A., Buzdar, A. U., & Sahin, A. A., Ross, M. A. (1992). Carcinoma of the male breast. *Annals of Internal Medicine*, 117(9), 771–777.

Kerlikowske, K., Barclay, J., Grady, D., Sickles, E. A., & Ernster, V. (1997). Comparison of risk factors for ductal carcinoma in situ and invasive breast cancer. *Journal of the National Cancer Institute*, 89(1), 76–82.

Kline, T. S., & Neal, H. S. (1975). Role of needle aspiration biopsy in diagnosis of carcinoma of the breast. *Obstetrics and Gynecology*, 46(1), 89–92.

Kori, S. H., Foley, K. M., & Posner, L. R. (1981). Brachial plexus lesions in patients with cancer: 100 cases. *Neurology*, 31(1), 45–50.

Kramer, B. A., Arthur, D. W., Ulin, K., Schmidt-Ullrich, R. K., Zwicker, R. D., & Wazer, D. E. (1999). Cosmetic outcome in patients receiving interstitial implant as part of breast-conservation therapy. *Radiology*, 213(1), 61–66.

Krishnamurthy, R., Whitman, G. J., Stelling, C. B., & Kushwaha, A. C. (1999). Mammographic findings after breast conservation therapy. *Radiographics*, 19, 53–62.

Lamont, J. A. (1997). Sexuality. In S. E. Stewart & G. E. Robinson (Eds.). A *clinician's guide to menopause* (pp. 63–76). London: Health Press International.

Lerner, R. (1998). Complete decongestive physiotherapy and the Lerner Lymphedema Services Academy of Lymphatic Studies. *Cancer*, 83, 2861–2863.

Lind, D. S., Minter, R., Steinbach, B., Abbitt, P., Lanier, L., Haigh, L., Vauthey, J. N., Russin, M., Hackett, R., & Copeland, E. M. (1998). Stereotactic core biopsy reduces the re-excision rate and the cost of mammographically detected cancer. *Journal of Surgical Research*, 78(1), 23–26.

Longnecker, M. P. (1994). Alcoholic beverage consumption in relation to risk of breast cancer: Meta-analysis and review. *Cancer Causes Control*, 5(1), 73–82.

Malone, K. E. (1993). Diethylstilbestrol (DES) and breast cancer. *Epidemiologic Reviews*, 15(1), 108–109.

McLachlan, S. A., Devins, G. M., & Goodwin, P. J. (1998). Validation of the European Organization for Research and Treatment Quality of Life Questionnaire (QLQ-C30) as a measure of psychosocial function in breast cancer patients. *European Journal of Cancer*, 34(4), 510–517.

Mendenhall, N. P., Fletcher, G. H., & Million, R. R. (1987). Adjuvant radiation therapy following modified radical or radical mastectomy. In K. I. Bland & E. M. Copeland (Eds.), *The breast: comprehensive management of benign and malignant diseases* (pp. 770–780). Philadelphia: W. B. Saunders.

Moody, A. M., Mayles, W. P., Bliss, J. M., A'Hern, R. P., Owen, J. R., Regan, J., Broad, B., & Yarnold, J. R. (1994). The influence of breast size on late radiation effects and association with radiotherapy dose inhomogeneity. *Radiotherapy and Oncology*, 33(2), 106–112.

Moss, S. M. (1999). Breast cancer. In B. Kramer, J. K. Gohagen, & P. C. Prorok (Eds.), *Cancer screening: theory and practice*. New York: Marcel Dekker.

National Cancer Institute. (1999). *NCI Common Toxicity Criteria (CTC) Version 2 with the Radiation Therapy Oncology Group (RTOG) and European Organization for Research and Treatment of Cancer (EORTC) Acute Effects Criteria*. Bethesda, MD. National Cancer Institute.

National Comprehensive Cancer Network. (1997). Update of the NCCN Guidelines for Treatment of Breast Cancer. *Oncology Huntington*, 11(11A), 199–220.

National Comprehensive Cancer Network. (1998). NCCN Practice Guidelines: Screening for and evaluation of suspicious breast lesions. *Oncology Huntington*, 12(11), 89–138.

Offit, K. (1998). *Clinical cancer genetics*. New York: Wiley-Liss.

Offit, K., Gilewski, T., McGuire, P., Schluger, A., Hampel, H., Brown, K., Swensen, J., Neuhausen, S., Skolnick, M., Norton, L., & Goldgar, D. (1996). Germline BRCA1 185delAG mutations in Jewish women with breast cancer. *Lancet*, 347(9016), 1643–1645.

Oncology Nursing Society—Radiation Therapy Special Interest Group Documentation Project Core Committee. (1994). *Radiation therapy patient care record: A tool for documenting nursing care*. Pittsburgh, PA: Oncology Nursing Society.

Osuch, J. R. (1999). Surgical approaches to breast cancer. *LOWAC Journal*, 1(Suppl. 1), 22–28.

Overgaard, M., Hansen, P. S., Overgaard, J., Rose, C., Andersson, M., Bach, F., Kjaer, M., Gadeberg, C. C., Mouridsen, H. T., Jensen, M. B., & Zedeler, K. (1997). Postoperative radiotherapy in high-risk premenopausal women with breast cancer who receive adjuvant chemotherapy. *New England Journal of Medicine*, 337(14), 949–955.

Overgaard, M. (1988). Spontaneous radiation-induced rib fractures in breast cancer patients treated with postmastectomy irradiation. A clinical radiobiological analysis of the influence of fraction size and dose-response relationships on late bone damage. *Acta Oncologica*, 27(2), 117–122.

Parkin, D. M., Pisani, P., & Ferlay, J. (1993). Estimates of the worldwide incidence of eighteen major cancers in 1985. Implications for prevention and projections of future burden. *International Journal of Cancer*, 55(6), 891–903.

Pelusi, J. (1997). The lived experience of surviving breast cancer. *Oncology Nursing Forum*, 24(8), 1343–1353.

Pike, M. C., Bernstein, L., & Spicer, D. V. (1993). The relationship of exogenous hormones to breast cancer risk. In J. E. Niederhuber (Ed.), *Current therapy in oncology* (pp. 292–303). St. Louis: Mosby-Year Book.

Pisani, P., Parkin, D. M., & Ferlay, J. (1993). Estimates of the worldwide mortality of 18 major cancers in 1985. *International Journal of Cancer*, 54(4), 594–606.

Polinsky, M. L. (1994). Functional status of long-term breast cancer survivors: Demonstrating chronicity. *Health and Social Work*, 19(3), 165–173.

Porock, D., Kristjanson, L., Nikoletti, S., Cameron, F., & Pedler, P. (1998). Predicting the severity of radiation skin reactions in women with breast cancer. *Oncology Nursing Forum*, 35(6), 1019–1029.

Ragaz, J., Jackson, S. M., Le, N., Plenderleith, I. H., Spinelli, J., Basco, V. E., Wilson, K. S., Knowling, M. A., Coppin, C. M., Paradis, M., Coldman, A. J., & Olivotto, I. A. (1997). Adjuvant radiotherapy and chemotherapy in node-positive premenopausal women with breast cancer. *New England Journal of Medicine*, 337(14), 956–962.

Ries, L. A. G., Kosary, C. L., Hankey, B. F., Miller, B. A., Harras, A., & Edwards, B. K. (1997). SEER *cancer statistics review, 1973-1994: Tables and graphs* (NIH Publication No. 97-2789). Bethesda, MD: National Cancer Institute.

Sarrazin, D., Le, M. G., Arriagada, R., Contesso, G., Fontaine, F., Spielmann, M., Rochard, F., Le-Chevalier, T., & Lacour, J. (1989). Ten-year results of a randomized trial comparing a conservative treatment to mastectomy in early breast cancer. *Radiotherapy and Oncology*, 14(3), 177–184.

Segerstrom, K., Bjerle, P., Graffman, S., & Nystrom, A. (1992). Factors that influence the incidence of brachial oedema after treatment of breast cancer. *Scandinavian Journal of Reconstructive Hand Surgery*, 26(2), 223–227.

Shapiro, S., Venet, W., Strax, P., & Venet, L. (1988). Periodic screening for breast cancer. In *The health insurance plan project and its sequelae*, 1963–1986. Baltimore: Johns Hopkins University Press.

Son, H. J., & Oh, K. K. (1999). Significance of follow-up mammography in estimating the effect of tamoxifen in breast cancer patients who have undergone surgery. *American Journal of Roentgenology*, 173(4), 905–909.

Standford, J. L., & Thomas, D. B. (1993). Exogenous progestins and breast cancer. *Epidemiologic Review*, 15, 98–107.

Sugden, E. M., Rezvani, M., Harrison, J. M., & Hughes, L. K. (1998). Shoulder movement after the treatment of early stage breast cancer. *Clinical Oncology*, 10(3), 173–181.

Svensson, H., Westling, P., & Larsson, L. G. (1975). Radiation-induced lesions of the brachial plexus correlated to the time-dose-fraction schedule. *Acta Radiologica Therapy, Physics, Biology*, 14(3), 228–238.

Tabar, L., Fagerberg, G., Day, N. E., & Holmberg L. (1987). What is the optimum interval between mammographic screening examinations? An analysis based on the results of the Swedish two-county breast cancer screening trial. *British Journal of Cancer*, 55(5), 547–551.

Thomas, J. E., & Colby, M. Y. (1972). Radiation-induced or metastatic brachial plexopathy? A diagnostic dilemma. JAMA, 222(11), 1392–1395.

Thorlacius, S., Tryggvadottir, L., Olafsdottir, G. H., Thorlacius, S., Jonasson, J. G., Ogmundsdottir, H. M., Tulinius, H., & Eyfjord, J. E. (1995). Linkage to BRCA2 region in hereditary male breast cancer. Lancet, 346(9874), 544–545.

Thune, I., Brenn, T., Lund, E., & Gaard, M. (1997). Physical activity and the risk of breast cancer. New England Journal of Medicine, 336(18), 1269–1275.

Turesson, I., Nyman, J., Holmberg, E., & Oden, A. (1996). Prognostic factors for acute and late skin reactions in radiotherapy patients. International Journal of Radiation Oncology, Biology, Physics, 36(5), 1065–1067.

Twycross, R. G., & Lack, S. A. (1990). Therapeutics in terminal cancer (2nd ed.). Edinburgh: Churchill Livingstone.

United Kingdom Trial of Early Detection of Breast Cancer Group. (1992). Specificity of screening in United Kingdom trial of early detection of breast cancer. British Medical Journal, 304(6823), 346–349.

van Dongen, J. A., Bartelink, H.,Fentiman, I. S., Lerut, T., Mignolet, F., Olthuis, G., van-der-Schueren, E., Sylvester, R., Winter, I., & van-Zijl, K. (1992). Randomized clinical trial to assess the value of breast-conserving therapy in stage I and II breast cancer, EORTC 10801 trial. Journal of the National Cancer Institute Monograph, 11, 15–18.

Velentgas, P., Daling, J. R., Maline, K. E., Weiss, N. S., Williams, M. A., Self, S. G., & Mueller, B. (1999). Pregnancy after breast carcinoma: Outcomes and influence on mortality. Cancer, 85(11), 2424–2432.

Veronesi, U., Salvadori, B., Luini, A., Greco, M., Saccozzi, R., del-Vecchio, M., Mariani, L., Zurrida, S., & Rilke, F. (1995). Breast conservation is a safe method in patients with small cancer of the breast: Long term results of three randomized trials on 1,973 patients. European Journal of Cancer, 31A(10), 1574–1579.

Victor, S. J., Brown, D. M., Horwitz, E. M., Martinez, A. A., Kini, V. R., Pettinga, J. E., Shaheen, K. W., Benitez, P., Chen, P. Y. & Vicini, F. A. (1998). Treatment outcome with radiation therapy after breast augmentation or reconstruction in patients with primary breast carcinoma. Cancer, 82(7), 1303–1309.

Vinokur, A. (1989). Physical and psychosocial functioning and adjustment to breast cancer. Long term follow-up of a screening population. Cancer, 63(2), 394–405.

Vrieling, C., Collette, L., Fourquet, A., Hoogenraad, W. J., Horiot, J. C., Jager, J. J., Pierart, M., Poortmans, P. M., Struikmans, H., Van-der-Hulst, M., Van-der-Schueren, E., & Bartelink, H. (1999). The influence of the boost in breast-conserving therapy on cosmetic outcome in the EORTC "boost versus no boost" trial. EORTC Radiotherapy and Breast Cancer Cooperative Groups. European Organization for Research and Treatment of Cancer. International Journal of Radiation Oncology, Biology, Physics, 45(3), 677–685.

Willett, W. C., Hunter, D. J., Stampfer, M. J. (1992). Dietary fat and fiber in relation to risk of breast cancer: An 8 year follow-up. JAMA, 268(15), 2037–2044.

Wingate, L., Croghan, I., Natarajan, N., Michalek, A. M., & Jordan, C. (1989). Rehabilitation of the mastectomy patient: A randomized, blind, prospective study. *Archives of Physical Medicine and Rehabilitation*, 70(1), 21–24.

Woo, B., Dibble, S. L., Piper, B. F., Keating, S. B., & Weiss, M. C. (1998). Differences in fatigue by treatment methods in women with breast cancer. *Oncology Nursing Forum*, 25(5), 915–920.

Woods, N., & Earp, J. L. (1978). Women with cured breast cancer: A study of mastectomy patients in North Carolina. *Nursing Research*, 27(5), 279–285.

Wooster, R., Bignell, G., Lancaster, J., Swift, S., Seal, S., Mangion, J., Collins, N., Gregory, S., Gumbs, C., & Micklem, G. (1995). Identification of the breast cancer susceptibility gene BRCA2. *Nature*, 378(6559), 789–792.

Wyatt, G., Kurtz, M. E., & Liken, M. (1993). Breast cancer survivors: An exploration of quality of life issues. *Cancer Nursing*, 16(6), 440–448.

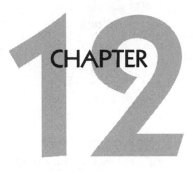

CHAPTER 12

LUNG CANCER

Giselle J. Moore-Higgs, ARNP, MSN
Roberta A. Strohl, RN, MN, AOCN
Mohan Suntharalingam, MD

PROBLEM

- The American Cancer Society (ACS) estimates that there will be 164,100 new cases of lung cancer diagnosed in the United States in 2000—89,500 in men and 74,600 in women (Greenlee, Murray, Bolden, & Wingo, 2000).
- Lung cancer is the leading cause of cancer deaths in the United States, with 156,900 estimated deaths in 2000 (Greenlee et al., 2000).
- Since 1988, lung cancer has become the number one cause of cancer death in American women. From 1991 to 1995 deaths from lung cancer in men declined (−1.6% per year) while rates for women continued to rise (Wingo et al., 1999). However, the rate of increase has begun to slow recently (Khuri, Keller, & Wagner, 1999).
- The highest incidence of lung cancer is found in Scotland and Wales. In the United States, the highest incidence is found in northern urban areas and along the southern coast from Texas to Florida (Khuri et al., 1999).
- In the United States, the highest incidence of lung cancer is found in Hawaiians and African Americans (Khuri et al., 1999).

■ The global incidence of lung cancer is increasing at a rate of 0.5% per year.

■ The median age at diagnosis is ~60 years (Khuri et al., 1999).

RISK FACTORS

■ Cigarette smoking is the leading risk factor for lung cancer. Of the 164,100 new cases of lung cancer estimated each year, 80% will be related to cigarette smoking. Smoking is the cause of all four types of lung cancer: squamous cell, adenocarcinoma, large cell, and small cell cancer. The incidence of lung cancer is related to the duration of smoking and the daily dose of smoke. The relative risk of lung cancer in smokers is 10 to 15 times that of nonsmokers. Nonsmokers exposed to smoke have a 1 to 2 times greater relative risk of developing lung cancer than the nonexposed individual (Schottenfeld, 1996).

■ Polynuclear aromatic hydrocarbons and nitrosamines have been strongly implicated as the causative agents of lung cancer in cigarette smoke. They are also found in aluminum production, coal gasification, coke production, and exposure to soot (Schottenfeld, 1996).

■ Radon gas exposure has been shown to increase lung cancer risk among underground miners (Schottenfeld, 1996). This is particularly true in uranium miners who have been exposed to radioactive dust and radon gas (Khuri et al., 1999). There is some controversy about the risk posed by exposure to residential radon gas.

■ Exposure to metals such as arsenic, nickel, and cadmium has been linked to increased risk of lung cancer.

■ Exposure to asbestos is a major risk factor in the development of mesothelioma. Smoking and asbestos exposure result in a strong additive effect. The highest risk is found among miners, millers, and textile employees as well as insulation and cement workers (Schottenfeld, 1996).

■ Air pollution has been cited as a cause of lung cancer because urban air contains a number of known or suspected lung carcinogens. These include nickel, arsenic, asbestos, uranium, cadmium, and chromium. It is difficult to separate air quality from smoking as a risk factor, and air quality alone may not confer a significant risk (Schottenfeld, 1996).

■ In a preliminary study, Neugut and colleagues found that the risk of developing lung cancer increased in women smokers treated with radiation therapy for breast cancer before 1980 (Neugut, Weinberg, Ahsan and Rescigno, 1999).

ASSESSMENT

■ The treatment of lung cancer has been hampered by the lack of a sensitive and cost-effective early detection test. Screening trials have failed to demonstrate a survival advantage for individuals screened by sputum cytology or annual chest x-rays. Currently, routine screening is not recommended. However, patients at risk (including present and former smokers) who present with symptoms consistent with lung cancer should receive an appropriate evaluation.

■ Recent advances in the understanding of the biology of lung cancer hold promise in early detection. The process of the development of lung cancer takes many years. The following techniques are under investigation:

1. Sputum cytology can be combined with an analysis of cancer specific antigens. Studies are looking prospectively at high-risk individuals to determine if periodic sputum analysis can identify developing neoplasms (Shaw & Mulshine, 1996).

2. Oncogense—The dominant ras oncogene Ki-ras has been found in one-third of patients with adenocarcinoma. If the presence of oncogenes proves to be specific enough serum studies might be possible to predict the development of cancer.

3. Tumor suppressor genes have also been implicated in lung cancer (retinoblastoma gene). Abnormalities of Rb protein are seen in 90% of small cell lung cancers but only 15% of non-small-cell tumors. Abnormalities in p53 occur in 50% of both small cell and non-small-cell lung cancers. Immunohistochemical analysis affords a potential for screening (Shaw & Mulshine, 1996).

4. Low-dose CT screening is currently under evaluation in the Early Lung Cancer Action Program (ELCAP). In a

recent update of the study, the authors reported that of 1,000 persons screened, CT scanning had detected non-calcified nodules in 233 patients and conventional chest x-rays had found nodules in 68 patients. Twenty-seven cancers were detected by CT, only seven of which were detected by chest x-ray. Of these 27, 23 were diagnosed as stage I lung cancers (Henschke et al., 1999).

5. Xillix LIFE-Lung—A fluorescence imaging system used during bronchoscopy that uses blue rather than white light to take advantage of natural differences in fluorescence between normal and cancerous or precancerous tissues. This assists the physician in identifying sites for biopsy during bronchoscopy. The device received FDA approval in August 1996.

■ The clinical manifestations of lung cancer depend on the location and extent of the tumor. In patients who have localized disease, the most common symptoms are related to obstruction of major airways, infiltration of lung parenchyma, and invasion of surrounding structures including the chest wall, major blood vessels, and viscera (Khuri et al., 1999). Patients with advanced disease present with symptoms of systemic disease including pain, anorexia, and weight loss. The following is a list of common signs and symptoms:

1. Cough is a common manifestation of lung cancer. Patients with chronic coughs related to smoking or other respiratory illness should be asked about a change in the cough such as an increase in frequency, severity, or production of sputum.

2. Dyspnea is a more common symptom of later-stage lung cancer as a result of obstruction of an airway.

3. Hemoptysis—Result of tumor eroding into surrounding tissue & blood vessels.

4. Chest pain is a result of invasion of the chest wall.

5. Pneumonia—Postobstructive pneumonia occurs as a result of a partial or complete obstruction of the bronchus by the tumor.

6. Shoulder and arm pain—Apical tumors (also known as Pancoast tumors) that infiltrate surrounding structures produce shoulder and arm pain as a result of brachial plexus compression.

7. Horner's syndrome—Apical tumors may invade the sympathetic ganglia resulting in ptosis, myosis, and ipsilateral anhydrosis.

8. Hoarseness—Compression of the recurrent laryngeal nerve by central tumors or mediastinal lymphadenopathy may result in vocal cord paresis or paralysis. This is most common in left-sided tumors.

9. Other symptoms may be related to advanced disease including superior vena cava syndrome, systemic paraneoplastic syndrome, or Lambert-Eaton syndrome.

■ Initial evaluation should include the following:

1. Complete history and physical examination. The history should include lung-related symptoms as well as history of exposure to tobacco and other environmental agents listed under risk factors.

2. Karnofsky performance status (KPS)—An individual's performance status should be considered when deciding on the method of evaluation and treatment.

3. Careful physical examination of the peripheral lymphatics (neck, supraclavicular fossa, and axilla). Visual inspection and physical examination of the chest wall for evidence of chest wall involvement and/or skin involvement.

4. Physical examination that includes evaluation of neurologic status and musculoskeletal status to identify potential sites of metastasis.

5. Imaging studies are important in the evaluation process. Lung cancer may appear as peripheral or central chest tumors. Small cell lung cancer often presents with large bulky chest disease. Peripheral tumors may present with cavitation especially in squamous cell tumors. Central tumors often present with obstruction or atelectasis from tumor occlusion of the bronchus. Collapse of the lung is seen most often in squamous cell tumors (Shaw & Mulshine, 1996). Imaging studies may include the following:

   a. Chest x-ray (CXR) should be performed in all high-risk individuals who present with new respiratory symptoms. PA and lateral films will reveal evidence of a pulmonary mass(s), widened mediastinum, pleural effusion, synchronous pulmonary nodules, and/or evidence of osseous metastases (Khuri et al., 1999). Having prior CXRs is useful for comparison, especially if there is a history of abnormal findings (including benign lesions).

   b. CT scan of the chest (including the liver and adrenal glands) is performed to evaluate the primary tumor and to identify lymphatic or parenchymal metastases (Khuri et al., 1999).

    c. MRI may be performed to evaluate the extent of tumor invasion into or destruction of peripheral structures including the brachial plexus, vertebral body, and spinal canal.

6. Histologic or cytologic diagnosis is necessary to confirm a malignancy and identify the specific type of tumor prior to initiation of treatment. Obtaining a tissue diagnosis can be done via several of the following methods:

    a. Sputum cytologies—Sputum is collected for 3 consecutive days to provide cytologic diagnosis in the presence of central tumors. Not a very effective method in peripheral tumors.

    b. Bronchoscopy—Used in centrally located tumors to establish both cytologic and histologic diagnosis. Also provides staging information (involvement of distal trachea or carina) (Khuri et al., 1999).

    c. Mediastinoscopy provides a histologic diagnosis as well as staging information by obtaining biopsies from lymph nodes at several levels to determine extent of disease.

    d. CT-guided needle aspirate is useful in peripheral lesions. There is a significant risk of pneumothorax and therefore it is primarily used in patients unable to undergo surgical procedures or those with extensive metastatic disease.

    e. Thoracentesis and thoracoscopy—Thoracentesis may be used in patients with pleural effusions to obtain cytologic diagnosis. Thoracoscopy allows direct visualization of the pleural surface and direct biopsy of a pleural nodule(s).

7. Complete blood count with complete chemistry to evaluate renal and liver function. Additional studies may be ordered depending on the patient's status at the time of evaluation.

8. Additional metastatic evaluation studies will depend on the clinical stage of the disease, reported symptoms, and physical examination findings. Common studies in lung cancer include:

    a. Bone Scan—The presence of skeletal metastasis would alter the treatment plan and is an essential part of the evaluation of a patient thought to be a surgical or combined modality therapy candidate.

b. CT Scan—Lung cancer commonly spreads to the liver, brain, adrenals, kidney, or other lung. A CT scan or MRI may be performed to evaluate for brain metastasis. A CT scan of the abdomen will evaluate for liver, kidney, or adrenal metastases.

9. Additional studies may be warranted to assess overall medical conditions, particularly when considering surgical resection or combined modality therapy.

10. Pulmonary function studies are performed before surgery to determine the volume of lung that can be removed without compromising the patient's respiratory ability.

■ There are two major subdivisions of lung cancer: small cell carcinoma (SCLC) and non-small-cell carcinoma (NSCLC). SCLC accounts for approximately 20% of all lung cancers while NSCLC accounts for approximately 80% (Table 12–1). The three major types of NSCLC are adenocarcinoma, squamous cell carcinoma, and large-cell carcinoma (Khuri et al., 1999).

■ Histologic cell type and anatomic extent of disease are the primary prognostic factors in lung cancer. In addition, performance status, age, and severity of symptoms are considered.

TABLE 12–1 HISTOPATHOLOGIC TYPES OF LUNG CANCER

Squamous Cell Carcinoma (Epidermoid)
Spindle cell variant

Small Cell Carcinoma
Oat cell carcinoma
Intermediate cell type
Combined oat cell carcinoma

Adenocarcinoma
Acinar adenocarcinoma
Papillary adenocarcinoma
Bronchiolo-alveolar carcinoma
Solid carcinoma with mucus formation

Large Cell Carcinoma
Giant cell carcinoma variant
Clear cell carcinoma variant

Table 12–2 AJCC Staging of Lung Cancer

Primary Tumor (T)

T_x Primary tumor cannot be assessed, or tumor proven by presence of malignant cells in sputum or bronchial washings but not visualized by imaging or bronchoscopy

T_0 No evidence of primary tumor

T_{is} Carcinoma in situ

T_1 Tumor 3 cm or less in greatest dimension, surrounded by lung or visceral pleura without bronchoscopic evidence of invasion more proximal than the lobar bronchus* (i.e., not in main bronchus)

T_2 Tumor with any of the following features of size or extent:

    More than 3 cm in greatest dimension

    Involves main bronchus, 2 cm or more distal to the carina

    Invades the visceral pleura

    Associated with atelectasis or obstructive pneumonitis that extends to the hilar region but does not involve the entire lung

T_3 Tumor of any size that directly invades any of the following: chest wall (including superior sulcus tumors), diaphragm, mediastinal pleura, parietal pericardium; or tumor in the main bronchus less than 2 cm distal to the carina but without involvement of the carina; or associated atelectasis of obstructive pneumonitis of the entire lung

T_4 Tumor of any size that invades any of the following: mediastinum, heart, great vessels, trachea, esophagus, vertebral body, carina; separate tumor nodule(s) in the same lobe; or tumor with a malignant pleural effusion

Regional Lymph Nodes (N)

N_x Regional lymph nodes cannot be assessed

N_0 No regional lymph node metastasis

N_1 Metastasis to ipsilateral peribronchial and/or ipsilateral hilar lymph nodes and intrapulmonary nodes involved by direct extension of the primary tumor

N_2 Metastasis to ipsilateral, mediastinal, and/or subcarinal, lymph node(s)

N_3 Metastasis in contralateral mediastinal, contralateral hilar, ipsilateral or contralateral scalene, or supraclavicular lymph node(s)

Distant Metastasis (M)

M_x Distant metastasis cannot be assessed

M_0 No distant metastasis

M_1 Distant metastasis present (includes synchronous separate nodule(s) in a different lobe)

Stage Grouping

Stage grouping of the TNM subsets has been revised as follows:

Occult carcinoma	T_x	N_0	M_0
Stage 0	T_{is}	N_0	M_0
Stage IA	T_1	N_0	M_0
Stage IB	T_2	N_0	M_0
Stage IIA	T_1	N_1	M_0
Stage IIB	T_2	N_1	M_0
	T_3	N_0	M_0
Stage IIIA	T_1	N_2	M_0
	T_2	N_2	M_0
	T_3	N_1	M_0
	T_3	N_2	M_0
Stage IIIB	Any T	N_3	M_0
	T_4	Any N	M_0
Stage IV	Any T	Any N	M_1

Used with the permission of the American Joint Committee on Cancer (AJCC®), Chicago, Illinois. The original source for this material is the AJCC® Cancer Staging Manual, 5th edition (1997) published by Lippincott-Raven Publishers, Philadelphia, Pennsylvania.
*The uncommon superficial tumor of any size with its invasive component united to the bronchial wall, which may extend proximal to the main bronchus.

■ Clinical staging of NSCLC is based on the assessment of the anatomic extent of disease before definitive therapy is instituted. This includes a medical history, physical examination, various imaging procedures, and the results of selected studies (including bronchoscopy, esophagoscopy, mediastinoscopy, mediastinotomy, thoracentesis, and thoracoscopy) and other tests designed to demonstrate extrathoracic metastasis and regional extension. Pathologic staging is based on information obtained from clinical staging, from thoracotomy, and from examination of the resected specimen including lymph nodes (Fleming et al., 1998). See Table 12–2 for complete AJCC staging.

■ The TNM staging classification is generally not utilized in SCLC, since it does not predict well for survival. Rather, SCLC is usually described as either limited (M) or extensive (M_1). For surgical staging, the TNM system is usually used (Khuri et al., 1999).

OUTCOMES MANAGEMENT

- While resectable early stage NSCLC may be treated with surgery alone, most patients with lung cancer are treated with a combined modality approach. SCLC is considered primarily a nonsurgical disease.
- Since the overall prognosis of lung cancer has not changed significantly despite many advances in treatment, all patients with lung cancer are potential candidates for clinical trials to evaluate new forms of treatment.

NON-SMALL-CELL LUNG CANCER (NSCLC)

Surgery

- For more than 60 years pulmonary resection has been the accepted treatment for early stage NSCLC (stage I & II). As surgical techniques improved, less extensive methods of pulmonary resections were developed in an attempt to reduce morbidity and mortality.
- Although surgery is the treatment of choice for localized resectable NSCLC tumors, less than one-third of patients are considered resectable at initial diagnosis (Morice, 1998).
- A comprehensive preoperative evaluation is essential in identifying patients who are at risk for serious intraoperative and postoperative complications. In addition to patient age, KPS, and overall health, the evaluation should include the following:
  1. Pulmonary function studies
  2. Cardiovascular function studies (Morice, 1998)
- Adequate resection for lung cancer includes removal of the primary tumor plus the draining local-regional lymph nodes. For early-stage lung cancer a lobectomy is usually performed. The surgery involves resection of the lobe of the lung containing the tumor. With thoracoscopic-assisted surgery limited resection may be possible in small tumors. In small peripheral lung tumors lobectomy may not be indicated and segmentectomy can be an alternative procedure (Luketich & Ginsberg, 1996). Wedge resection may be performed in patients with pulmonary compromise, although there is little data to support wide spread use. There is a four-fold higher local recurrence rate found in wedge resections as compared to lobectomy (Luketich & Ginsberg, 1996).

■ For more advanced lesions sleeve pneumonectomy may be indicated. This procedure is used when carinal involvement occurs with large central tumors. Anastomotic complications are frequent.

■ In stages IA, IB, IIA, and IIB lung cancer, surgery provides the best chance for cure. The extent of resection depends on the size of the tumor and the functional ability of the patient to tolerate surgery (Ettinger et al., 1996).

Radiation Therapy

■ External-beam therapy is one of the primary modalities in the management of lung cancer. It has been used extensively in the definitive and postoperative setting and more recently in trials evaluating preoperative treatment.

■ Complex anatomy of the lung with the proximity of the spinal cord makes treatment difficult. Three-dimensional (3-D) conformal radiotherapy provides a means for increasing tumor dose while limiting dose to the critical structures such as the spinal cord (Emani & Graham, 1998).

Preoperative Radiation Therapy

• Preoperative radiation therapy with or without chemotherapy may be used for patients with stage III disease. Advantages of preoperative therapy include delivery of therapy to better oxygenated tumors and better vascularized tissue. Research from the Cleveland Clinic shows promising results in terms of tumor response, disease control, survival, and toxicity after short-course induction chemoradiotherapy and surgical resection in patients with stage III non-small-cell lung carcinoma (NSCLC). Patients received 12-day induction therapy of a 96-hour continuous infusion of cisplatin (20 mg/m^2 per day), 24-hour infusion of paclitaxel (175 mg/m^2), and concurrent accelerated fractionation radiation therapy (1.5 Gy twice daily) to a dose of 30 Gy, followed by surgical resection 4 weeks later and a second postoperative identical course of chemotherapy and concurrent radiation therapy (30 to 33 Gy). This regime resulted in good tumor response and downstaging with 71% of those who underwent thoracotomy able to be resected for cure and 31% of patients being downstaged to mediastinal node negative (stage 0, I, or II). The median survival was modestly improved compared with historical controls.

Induction toxicity resulted in hospitalization of 18 (40%) patients for neutropenic fever (Rice et al., 1998).

Postoperative Radiation Therapy

- The role of radiation therapy in stage I and II disease has been primarily as postoperative adjuvant therapy in patients with close or positive margins, or N_1 or N_2 disease. However, the appropriate role of postoperative radiation therapy remains ill-defined despite a number of randomized trials. The trials have been hindered by a lack of uniformity of patient selection and the use of non-CT–guided treatment planning approaches. In a meta-analysis of nine randomized trials assessing postoperative radiation therapy in NSCLC, there was no significant improvement in disease-free or overall survival and a 21% increase in mortality (PORT MTG, 1998).

Primary Radiation Therapy

- Medically inoperable patients with early-stage disease (stage I and II) should be offered radiation therapy with or without chemotherapy. Although the results are not as good as those for patients selected for surgery, definitive radiation offers patients a chance of cure (50 to 65 Gy).
- Radiation therapy was considered the standard therapy for patients with stage IIIA or IIIB NSCLC until recently. Recent randomized trials have compared standard daily radiation therapy (60 Gy) with twice-daily treatment of a higher dose (69.6 Gy) and with an accelerated regimen that delivered 54 Gy over 2.5 weeks. Both altered fractionation schedules resulted in improved survival (Khuri et al., 1999).
- Recent randomized trials have introduced combined chemotherapy and radiation as a method to improve outcomes in stage III disease. Current approaches include induction chemotherapy for several cycles followed by radiation therapy or concurrent chemoradiation. Cisplatin, vinblastine, carboplatin, and paclitaxel have all been used in these trials. Radiation therapy is usually given to a dose of 50 to 60 Gy.
- A recent analysis of five RTOG trials studying chemoradiotherapy for NSCLC (88-04, 88-08 (chemo-RT arm), 90-15, 91-06, 92-04) was undertaken to determine if patients with non-small-cell lung carcinoma (NSCLC) and positive supra-

clavicular nodes (SN⁺) have a similar outcome to other patients with stage IIIB NSCLC (SN⁻) when treated with modern chemoradiotherapy. In this series, the outcome for patients with supraclavicular metastases treated with modern chemoradiotherapy appeared to be similar to that of other stage IIIB patients. This supports the rationale for continuing to enroll SN⁺ patients in aggressive chemoradiotherapy clinical trials for locally advanced NSCLC (Machtay, Seuferheld, Komaki, Cox, Sause, & Byhardt, 1999).

- In advanced disease (stage IV), patient care is individualized and usually palliative. The goal of treatment is to relieve symptoms including shortness of breath, airway obstruction, pain, or neurologic symptoms. The primary site is treated with radiation therapy consisting of ~30 Gy. Bone, brain, and adrenal metastasis may also be treated with short courses of palliative radiation therapy (8 to 30 Gy).

- Endobronchial occlusion is a common and potentially life-threatening complication. Endobronchial irradiation has also been used to palliate symptoms arising from partial airway obstruction (Khuri et al., 1999). In palliative care, 50% to 100% of patients have reported symptomatic relief. Studies also report that from two-thirds to three-fourths of the remainder of the patient's life is symptom improved or symptom-free (Mehta, 1996).

Chemotherapy

■ There is no evidence that adjuvant chemotherapy significantly increases survival in patients with stage I or II disease. Chemotherapy is primarily used in stage III and IV disease in combination with radiation therapy. However it may also be used in patients with recurrent or widely metastatic disease in a palliative approach. Agents that have been used include cisplatin, etoposide, paclitaxel, docetaxel, vinorelbine, gemcitabine, and irinotecan.

SMALL CELL LUNG CANCER (SCLC)

■ SCLC is one of the most sensitive solid tumors to cytotoxic chemotherapy. In spite of this, the median survival for extensive stage SCLC is 8 to 10 months and almost all patients die within 2 years.

■ The NCCN guidelines (Demetri et al., 1996) for SCLC stress the importance of the pretreatment evaluation. In addition to the evaluation described earlier in the chapter, a baseline EKG, pulmonary function studies, and a MUGA scan should be performed before the start of treatment.

■ Treatment of the primary site with local therapy (radiation therapy or surgery) is usually not adequate due to the propensity for distant metastasis. Therefore, the major focus of treatment regimens is systemic therapy.

LIMITED STAGE DISEASE

Surgery

■ Surgery is not usually indicated in SCLC. However, if a patient presents with a small solitary nodule, surgery may be indicated. This is usually followed by chemotherapy with or without chest radiation therapy.

Chemotherapy

■ In limited stage disease, the results of prospective randomized trials suggest that combined modality therapy produces a modest but significant improvement in survival compared with chemotherapy alone. Two meta-analyses showed an improvement in 3-year survival rates of about 5% for those receiving chemotherapy and radiation therapy compared to those receiving chemotherapy alone (Pignon et al., 1992; Warde & Payne, 1992). The current standard therapy is etoposide and cisplatin with or without vincristine. The radiation component is 45 Gy to the primary site. In patients with poor pulmonary function studies or poor KPS, current standard therapy is combined chemotherapy alone.

Radiation Therapy

■ In addition to radiation therapy to the chest, prophylactic cranial irradiation (PCI) may be considered. The physician and patient should discuss the role of PCI as part of the treatment protocol. Recommendations have been made limiting its use to those who have a complete response or at least an "extremely good partial response" (Demetri et al., 1996). PCI has been shown to improve both overall survival and disease-free survival among patients with small cell lung cancer in complete remission. A recent meta-analysis indicated that the relative risk of death in the group treated with prophylactic cranial irradiation as compared with the control group was 0.84 (95% confidence interval, 0.73 to 0.97; $p = 0.01$), which corresponds to a 5.4% increase in the rate of survival at 3 years. Prophylactic cranial irradiation also increased the rate of disease-free survival and decreased the cumulative incidence of brain metastasis. Although higher doses of radiation led to greater decreases in the risk of brain metastasis, according to an analysis of four total doses (8 Gy, 24 to 25 Gy, 30 Gy, and 36 to 40 Gy), the effect on survival did not differ significantly according to the dose. Earlier administration of cranial irradiation after the initiation of induction chemotherapy is associated with a decreased risk of brain metastasis (Auperin et al., 1999).

Extensive Stage Disease

Chemotherapy

■ Combination chemotherapy is the standard of care for patients with extensive stage small cell lung cancer. The following regimens are current standard therapy and produce similar survival outcomes:

1. Cyclophosphamide, doxorubicin, and vincristine
2. Cyclophosphamide, doxorubicin, and etoposide
3. Etoposide, cisplatin or carboplatin
4. Ifosfamide, carboplatin, and etoposide

■ Oral etoposide alone is often used in patients with poor performance status. A recent Southwest Oncology Group (SWOG) clinical trial of an all-oral regimen of etoposide-cyclophosphamide given days 1 to 14 every 28 days has demonstrated a 7-month median survival in poor-prognosis extensive disease small cell lung cancer patients. Granulocytopenia and alopecia were the most common toxicities seen. A trough etoposide level should be obtained within 24 hours after the start of therapy to predict severe granulocytopenia (Grunberg et al., 1999).

■ A number of studies are ongoing in the evaluation of new chemotherapy agents for small cell lung cancer. This includes new drug combinations, dose intensity, alternative drug schedules, and high-dose protocols. However, currently there are no clinical trials that have shown significant improvement in disease response or survival using higher doses of the current standard chemotherapy protocols.

Radiation

■ Radiation therapy is primarily used in a palliative setting to sites of metastatic disease including skeletal and brain metastases.

TOXICITY OF TREATMENT

Acute Toxicities

Respiratory Symptoms

1. Cough may increase during treatment and become more productive as radiation opens obstructed airways. Eventually the respiratory mucosa becomes dry and the cough becomes nonproductive. Patients may be concerned that the increase in cough means that the therapy is not working when indeed the opposite may be true. If coughing disrupts ability to eat, rest, or sleep, an over-the-counter cough suppressant can be used at bedtime (Knopp, 1997). Some patients may require a narcotic cough suppressant to manage the symptoms. Other measures that may help include:
   a. Decreased activity—short walks and resting between activities (bathing, work, etc.)
   b. Use of oxygen supplementation as needed
   c. Avoid irritants such as smoke, paint, etc.
   d. Maintain an adequate food and fluid intake
2. Dyspnea or breathlessness is a problem commonly encountered in patients with advanced cancer. It can also be caused by general disability, cancer treatment, and other conditions such as obesity or chronic lung disease. It is an unpleasant sensation that can be frightening and can increase a patient's fatigue. It can symbolize a threat to life itself. In a study to evaluate the effectiveness of nursing intervention for breathlessness in patients with lung cancer, a 6-hospital multicenter controlled trial was conducted. Most of the 119 patients who completed the study had a poor prognosis and breathlessness was typically a symptom of their deteriorating condition (Bredin et al., 1999). All patients had completed first-line treatment for their disease and had reported breathlessness and were randomized to either attend a nursing clinic offering intervention for their breathlessness or receive

best supportive care. The nursing intervention consisted of a range of strategies combining breathing control, activity pacing, relaxation techniques, and psychosocial support. Best supportive care involved receiving the standard management and treatment available for breathlessness and breathing assessments. Participants completed a range of self-assessment questionnaires at baseline, 4 and 8 weeks. The intervention group improved significantly at 8 weeks in 5 of the 11 items assessed including breathlessness at best, WHO performance status, levels of depression, and two Rotterdam symptom checklist measures (physical symptom distress and breathlessness), and showed slight improvement in 3 of the remaining 6 items as compared with control patients.

Treatment options should be directed toward relieving the problem that has resulted in the dyspnea. This may include primary treatment of the cancer or secondary treatment of the symptoms. Some of these options include the following:

  a. Pharmaceutical steroids may alleviate the symptoms: antibiotics for pneumonia, bronchodilators for chronic lung disease such as asthma, and recombinant human erythropoietin (r-HuEPO) for anemia

  b. Oxygen therapy

  c. Breathing exercises and positioning techniques

  d. Relaxation and coping strategies

3. Pharyngitis/esophagitis occurs as a result of mucositis of the esophagus and pharynx during radiation therapy and chemotherapy and usually begins in the third week of therapy. Patients report a sensation that they cannot swallow and feel as though food is "stuck." Treatment options are discussed in Chapter 21.

4. Fatigue is a multifactoral problem commonly associated with lung cancer. Patients with advanced disease usually present with weight loss, anorexia, pain, and dyspnea, which can all contribute to fatigue. Radiation therapy and chemotherapy can compound fatigue making it more severe. Treatment options can be found in Chapter 20.

5. Anorexia and weight loss—Most patients with advanced lung cancer present with anorexia and weight loss. Treatment-related symptoms such as nausea, vomiting, and esophagitis also impact nutritional intake. Patients should have a nutrition consultation with a dietician and follow an individualized plan to maintain and if possible gain weight. Included in the plan should be the use of nutritional supplements. McCarthy & Weihofen (1999) found that patients who ingested nutritional supplements between meals significantly increased their total caloric and protein intake above that of controls and did not reduce their food-derived caloric or protein intake compared with controls.

6. Skin changes—Patients who receive radiation therapy will develop an acute skin reaction depending on the dose and the type of skin within the treatment field. In most patients who receive radiation therapy to the chest, the skin reaction will become a dry desquamation with erythema and rarely become moist. Patients who receive palliative radiation therapy for a large lung mass, bone metastasis, or brain metastasis usually develop only a mild case of dry desquamation. For symptom management options please see Chapter 21.

7. Pain—Pain related to lung cancer may be due to tumor compression of an organ structure, direct nerve compression, bone erosion, or brain metastasis (headaches). Patients may also experience pain caused by treatment-induced tissue reactions (esophagitis, dry desquamation, mucositis). For symptom management options see Chapter 20.

8. Radiation pneumonitis—The incidence and severity of this response is related to the volume of lung irradiated, total dose and fractionation, and concomitant chemotherapy. Patients present with a dry persistent cough, low-grade fevers, and dyspnea approximately 8 to 12 weeks after completion of radiation therapy. Pneumonitis is often transient and does not require aggressive management. However, some patients may develop severe dyspnea requiring hospitalization and steroid therapy.

9. Hoarseness occurs in patients who experience pharyngitis or in patients who present with compression of the recurrent laryngeal nerve by central tumors or mediastinal lymphadenopathy (vocal cord paresis or paralysis). Symptom management should be focused on resting the voice as much as possible and treatment of the pharyngitis. Alternative methods of communication (such as note writing) should be encouraged.

CHRONIC TOXICITIES

1. Radiation fibrosis of the lung—Fibrosis is a permanent response to the lung tissue reaction that occurs during radiation therapy. Most patients do not experience clinical symptoms related to the fibrosis. However, some patients may experience chronic dyspnea, cough, and increased sensitivity to pollutants and irritants. A specific treatment for fibrosis is not available, and the focus should be on individual symptom management.
2. Esophageal stenosis—Esophageal stenosis, ulceration, and fistula formation are rare. Management is individualized depending on degree of injury and symptoms.
3. Hoarseness may be a permanent result of nerve injury.
4. Skin changes/alopecia—Patients who receive > 50 Gy to the chest may experience hyperpigmentation and alopecia of the skin within the treatment field(s). Mild fibrosis of the skin may also occur.

OUTCOMES MEASURES

- The NCI Toxicity Criteria (CTC) Version 2, with the Radiation Therapy Oncology Group (RTOG) and European Organization for Research and Treatment of Cancer (EORTC) Acute Effects Criteria Instrument provides a scale for many different organ systems and some symptoms (NCI, 1999). This is a very useful tool for grading severity of acute effects of radiation therapy in all sites.
- The Radiation Therapy Patient Care Record: A Tool for Documenting Nursing Care (ONS, 1994) provides a tool for weekly assessment and grading of severity of acute effects of radiation therapy in all sites.

FOLLOW-UP

- Surveillance of patients after initial treatment depends on the response to treatment. For patients who have a partial response or progressive disease, surveillance should be individualized to evaluate for alternative treatment protocols or symptom management. Patients with an initial complete response require close surveillance with appropriate diagnostic evaluation for relapse.

■ A follow-up evaluation should be performed every 3 months for a minimum of 3 years, then every 6 to 12 months for the next 2 years, then annually. The evaluation should include:
  1. Complete history and physical examination
  2. Careful visual inspection and physical examination of the chest and regional lymphatic-bearing areas
  3. Chest x-ray
  4. Laboratory studies: CBC, electrolytes, BUN, creatinine and liver function studies (Demetri et al., 1996)
  5. Additional studies would depend on presenting symptoms or abnormal physical or radiographic findings

EXPECTED OUTCOMES

SURVIVAL

■ The 1-year relative survival rates for lung cancer have increased from 34% in 1975 to 41% in 1995, largely as a result of improvements in surgical techniques. The 5-year relative survival rate for all stages combined is only 14%. The survival rate is 49% for cases detected when the disease is still localized, but only 15% of lung cancers are discovered that early (American Cancer Society, 2000).

QUALITY OF LIFE

■ Because lung cancer is often diagnosed late in the disease process and survival rates are poor, quality of life is an important focus of care. In a review of the literature on quality of life in patients with lung cancer (1970–1995), Montazeri, Gillis, and McEwen (1998) found 155 English citations and over 50 different instruments used to measure quality of life. The review identified several problems in the evaluation of quality of life in lung cancer. The first is the inconsistent use of instruments resulting in the inability to compare and contrast results in different treatment settings. The second is the inconsistent method of obtaining serial evaluations because of the overall poor prognosis and short life span of most lung cancer patients.

■ Most of the studies that report quality of life data in lung cancer are studies comparing single versus combination chemotherapy agents, single versus combined modality therapies, and comparing oral versus combination intravenous chemotherapy agents. In addition, a few studies have been conducted to evaluate the palliation response to different therapy options. However, most of the studies have used instruments to measure symptoms and their impact on quality of life and have avoided the evaluation of the psychosocial and spiritual aspects of quality of life.

■ Several examples of studies that are reflective of the data available on quality of life in lung cancer are as follows:

  • The relationship between quality of life and survival was examined in a group of 206 patients with advanced non-small-cell lung cancer on CALGB 8931. The European Organization for Research and Treatment of Cancer (EORTC) Quality of Life Scale and the Duke-UNC Social Support Scale were used. The study did not confirm the prognostic importance of overall quality of life. After adjustment for significant clinical factors a patient-provided pain report had the greatest prognostic importance for survival (Herndon, Fleishman, Kornblith, Kosty, Green, & Holland, 1999).

  • In a study evaluating quality of life after surgery for lung cancer, Fielder, Neef, and Rosendahl (1999) found that 6 months after pneumonectomy patients reported a persistent increase in dyspnea, lack of sleep and pain, and a decrease in the global quality of life.

■ Quality of life was assessed in 57 patients with limited small cell lung carcinoma using scales that measured mood, functional status, and cognitive impairment. All patients received chemotherapy and some received radiation. Patients who received combined therapy and CNS had improved survival but a decrease in quality of life because of increased toxicity (Ahles et al., 1994).

■ Sarna and Brecht (1997) evaluated the structure of symptom distress in women with advanced lung cancer. They found that fatigue, disruptions in outlook, frequent pain, and difficulties sleeping were rated the most distressing and were the most prevalent serious disruptions. Symptoms were significantly related to KPS.

■ There are several general quality of life instruments that are applicable to lung cancer. In addition, there are a number of symptom-specific instruments used in the terminal setting that are appropriate.

1. Functional Assessment of Cancer Therapy-Lung (FACT-L) (Cella et al., 1995)—A measurement system of self-report (33-item) scale of quality of life for people with cancer with an additional 9-question lung cancer subscale.

2. European Organization for Research and Treatment of Cancer (EORTC) QLQ-LC13 (Bergman, Sullivan, & Sorenson, 1992)—A 36-item questionnaire for assessing the quality of life of cancer patients participating in international clinical trials. The lung module has 13 questions to assess dyspnea, coughing, sore mouth, dysphagia, peripheral neuropathy, alopecia, and hemoptysis. It has been validated and used extensively in a wide range of cancer clinical trials in Europe and throughout the world.

3. Lung Cancer Symptom Scale—A patient-rated quality of life measure that evaluates symptom distress, activity, and overall quality of life (Hollen et al, 1994).

4. Hospice Quality of Life Index (HQLI) (McMillan & Weitzner, 1998)—A 28-item self-report instrument that includes three subscales: psychophysiological well-being, functional well-being, and social/spiritual well-being. Allows patients the opportunity to express beliefs about quality-of-life issues and to maintain direction over a critical aspect of their care.

5. Missoula-VITAS Quality of Life Index (MVQOLI) (Byock & Merriman, 1998)—Instrument developed to provide a measure of quality of life of terminally ill patients.

6. McGill Quality of Life Questionnaire (MQOL) (Cohen, Mount, & Strobel, 1995)—Instrument designed to measure overall quality of life in people with a life-threatening illness and to indicate the areas in which the patient is doing well or poorly. Correlates with the Spitzer Quality of Life and SIS instruments. Internal consistency reliability rating of 0.89.

7. The McMaster Quality of Life Scale (MQLS) (Sterkenburg & Woodward, 1996)—Instrument developed to measure quality of life in a palliative patient population including cancer patients. Has been correlated with the Spitzer Quality of Life instrument and has a good internal consistency (0.62 to 0.79) and inter-rater reliability (0.83 to 0.95).

8. The Symptom Distress Scale (McCorkle & Young, 1978)—Instrument developed for patients with a life-threatening disease, either cancer or heart disease. It concentrates mainly on the symptoms and mood in relation to quality of life. Has been correlated with global quality of life measures and has an internal consistency of 0.78 to 0.89. It has been found to be sensitive to changes in treatment over time.

REFERENCES

Ahles, T., Silberfarb, P., Rundle, A., et al. (1994). Quality of life in patients with limited small-cell carcinoma of the lung receiving chemotherapy with or without radiation therapy, for cancer and leukemia groups. *Psychotherapy and Psychosomatics, 62*(3–4), 193–199.

American Cancer Society. (2000). 2000 facts and figures. http://www.cancer.org/statistics. Accessed May 7, 2000.

Auperin, A., Arriagada, R., Pignon, J. P., Le-Pechoux, C., Gregor, A., Stephens, R. J., Kristjansen, P. E., Johnson, B. E., Ueoka, H., Wagner, H., & Aisner, J. (1999). Prophylactic cranial irradiation for patients with small-cell lung cancer in complete remission. Prophylactic Cranial Irradiation Overview Collaborative Group. *New England Journal of Medicine, 341*(7), 476–484.

Bergman, B., Sullivan, M., & Sorenson, S. (1992). Quality of life during chemotherapy for small cell lung cancer. II. A longitudinal study of the EORTC core quality of life questionnaire and comparison with the Sickness Impact profile. *Acta Oncologica, 31*(1), 19–28.

Bredin, M., Corner, J., Krishnasamy, M., et al. (1999). Multicenter randomized controlled trial of nursing intervention for breathlessness in patients with lung cancer. *BMJ, 318*(7188), 901–904.

Byock, I. R., & Merriman, M. P. (1998). Measuring quality of life for patients with terminal illness: The Missoula-VITAS quality of life index. *Palliative Medicine, 12*(4), 231–244.

Cella, D. F., Bonomi, A. E., Lloyd, S. R., Tulsky, D. S., Kaplan, E., Bonomi, P. (1995). Reliability and validity of the functional assessment of cancer therapy-lung (FACT-L) quality of life instrument. *Lung Cancer, 12*(3), 199–220.

Cohen, S. R., Mount, B. M., & Strobel, M. G. (1995). The McGill Quality of Life Questionnaire: A measure of quality of life appropriate for people with advanced disease. A preliminary study of validity and acceptability. *Palliative Medicine, 9*(3), 207–219.

Demetri, G., Elias, A., Gershenson, D., Fossella, F., Grecula, J., Mittal, B., Raschko, J., & Robertson, J. (1996). NCCN small-cell lung cancer practice guidelines. The National Comprehensive Cancer Network. *Oncology Huntington, 10* (Suppl. 11), 179–194.

Emami, B., & Graham, M. (1998). Three-dimensional conformal radiotherapy in bronchogenic carcinoma. In J. Roth, J. Cox, & W. Hong (Eds.), *Lung cancer*, (2nd ed., pp. 181–195). Malden, MA: Blackwell Science.

Ettinger, D. S. Cox, J. D., Ginsberg, R. J., Komaki, R., Kris. M. G., Livingston, R. B., & Sugarbaker, D. J. (1996). NCCN non-small-cell lung cancer practice guidelines. The National Comprehensive Cancer Network. *Oncology Huntington,* 10 (Suppl. 11): 81–111.

Fiedler, R., Neef, H., & Rosendahl, W. (1999). Functional outcome and quality of life at least 6 months after pneumonectomy effect of operation, adjuvant therapy, tumor stage, sex, type of pneumonia and recurrence. *Pneumonologie,* 53(1), 45–49.

Fleming, I. D., Cooper, J. S., Henson, E. D., Hutter, R. V. P., Kennedy, B. J., Murphy, G. P., O'Sullivan, B., Sobin, L. H., & Yarbro, J. W. (1998). *AJCC cancer staging handbook.* (5th ed., pp. 117–129). Philadelphia: Lippincott-Raven.

Greenlee, R. T., Murray, T., Bolden, S., & Wingo, P. A. (2000). Cancer statistics, 2000. *CA: A Cancer Journal for Clinicians,* 50(1), 7–33.

Grunberg, S. M., Crowley, J., Hande, K. R., Girous, D., Munshi, N. C., Lau, D. H. M., Schroder, L. E., Zangmeister, M. H., Balcerzak, S. P., Hynes, H. E., & Gandara, D. R. (1999). Treatment of poor-prognosis extensive disease small-cell lung cancer with an all-oral regimen of etoposide and cyclophosphamide: A Southwest Oncology Group clinical and pharmacokinetic study. *Cancer Chemotherapy and Pharmacology* 44(6), 461–468.

Henschke, C. I., McCauley, D. I., Yankelevitz, D. F., Naidich, D. P., McGuinness, G., Miettinen, O. S., Libby, D. M., Pasmantier, M. W., Koizumi, J., Altorki, N. K., & Smith, J. P. (1999). Early Lung Cancer Action Project: Overall design and findings from baseline screening. *Lancet,* 354(9173), 99–105.

Herndon, J. E., Fleishman, S., Kornblith, A. B., Kosty., M., Green, M. R. & Holland, J. (1999) Is quality of life predictive of the survival of patients with advanced non-small cell lung cancer. *Cancer,* 85(27), 333–340.

Hollen, P. J., Gralla, R. J., Kris, M. G., & Cox, C. (1994). Quality of life during clinical trials: Conceptual model for the Lung Cancer Symptom Scale (LCSS). *Supportive Care Cancer,* 2(4), 213–222.

Khuri, F. R., Keller, S. M., & Wagner, H., Jr. (1999). Non-small-cell lung cancer and mesothelioma. In R. Pazdur & W. J. Hoskins (Eds.), *Cancer management: A multidisciplinary approach* (3rd ed.). Melville, NY: Research and Representation.

Knopp, J. (1997). Lung cancer. In K. Dow, J. Bucholtz, R. Iwamoto, V. Fieler, & L. Hilderley (Eds.), *Nursing care in radiation oncology* (2nd ed. pp. 293–316). Philadelphia: W.B. Saunders.

Luketich, J., & Ginsberg, R. (1996) Limited resection versus lobectomy for Stage I non-small-cell lung cancer. In H. Pass, J. Mitchell, D. Johnson, & A. Turrisi (Eds.), *Lung cancer: Principles and practice* (pp. 561–567). New York: Lippincott-Raven.

Machtay M., Seiferheld, W., Komaki. R., Cox, J. D., Sause, W. T., & Byhardt, R. W. (1999). Is prolonged survival possible for patients with supraclavicular node metastases in non-small-cell lung cancer treated with chemoradiotherapy?: Analysis of the Radiation Therapy Oncology Group experience. *International Journal of Radiation Oncology, Biology, Physics,* 44(4), 847–853).

McCarthy, D., & Weihofen, D. (1999). The effect of nutritional supplements on food intake in patients undergoing radiotherapy. *Oncology Nursing Forum,* 26(5), 897–900.

McCorkle, R., & Young, R. (1978). Development of a symptom distress scale. *Cancer Nursing,* 1(5), 373–378.

McMillan, S. C., & Weitzner, M. (1998). Quality of life in cancer patients: Use of a revised hospice index. *Cancer Practices,* 6(5), 282–288.

Mehta, M. (1996). Endobronchial radiotherapy for lung cancer. In H. Pass, J. Mitchell, A. Johnson, & A. Turrisi (Eds.), *Lung cancer: Principles and practice,* (pp. 741–751). Philadelphia: Lippincott-Raven.

Montazeri, A., Gillis, C. R., & McEwen, J. (1998). Quality of life inpatients with lung cancer. A review of the literature from 1970–1995. *Chest,* 113(2), 467–481.

Morice, R. (1998). Preoperative evaluation of the patient with lung cancer. In J. Roth, J. Cox, & W. Hong, (Eds.), *Lung cancer,* (2nd cd., pp. 73–87). Malden, MA: Blackwell Science.

National Cancer Institute. (1999). NCI *Common Toxicity Criteria (CTC) Version 2 with the Radiation Therapy Oncology Group (RTOG) and European Organization for Research and Treatment of Cancer (EORTC) Acute Effects Criteria.* Bethesda, MD: National Cancer Institute.

Neugut, A. I., Weinberg, M. D., Ahsan, H., & Rescigno, J. (1999). Carcinogenic effects of radiotherapy for breast cancer. *Oncology Huntington,* 13(9), 1245–1265.

Oncology Nursing Society—Radiation Therapy Special Interest Group Documentation Project Core Committee. (1994). *Radiation Therapy Patient Care Record: A tool for documenting nursing care.* Pittsburgh, PA: Oncology Nursing Society.

Pignon, J. P., Arriagada, R., Ihde, D. C., Johnson, D. H., Perry, M. C., Souhami, R. L., Brodin, O., Joss, R. A., Kies, M. S., & Lebeau, B. (1992). A meta-analysis of thoracic radiotherapy for small-cell lung cancer. *New England Journal of Medicine,* 327(23), 1618–1624.

PORT Meta-analysis Trialists' Group. (1998). Postoperative radiotherapy in non-small-cell lung cancer: Systematic review and meta-analysis of individual patient data from nine randomized controlled trials. *Lancet,* 352(9124), 257–263.

Rice, T. W., Adelstein, D. J., Ciezki, J. P., Becker, M. E., Rybicki, L. A., Farver, C. F., Larto, M. A., & Blackstone, E. H. (1998). Short-course induction chemoradiotherapy with paclitaxel for stageIII non-small-cell lung cancer. *Annals of Thoracic Surgery,* 66(6), 1909–1914.

Sarna, L. & Brecht, M. (1997). Dimensions of symptom distress in women with advanced lung cancer: A factor analysis. *Heart Lung Journal of Acute Critical Care,* 26(1), 23–30.

Schottenfield, D. (1996). Epidemiology of lung cancer. In H. Pass, J. Mitchell, D. Johnson, & A. Turrisi, (eds.). *Lung cancer: Principles and practice* (pp. 305–323). New York: Lippincott-Raven.

Shaw, G., & Mulshine, J. (1996). General strategies for early detection: New ideas and future directions. In H. Pass, J. Mitchell, D. Johnson, & A. Turrisi (Eds.), *Lung cancer: Principles and practice* (pp. 329–341). New York: Lippincott-Raven.

Sterkenburg, C. A. & Woodward, C. A. (1996). A reliability and validity study of the McMaster Quality of Life Scale (MQLS) for a palliative population. *Journal of Palliative Care*, 12(1), 18–25.

Warde, P., & Payne, D. (1992). Does thoracic irradiation improve survival and local control in limited-stage small-cell carcinoma of the lung? A meta-analysis. *Journal of Clinical Oncology*, 10(6), 890–895.

Wingo, P. A., Ries, L. A., Giovino, G. A., Miller, D. S., Rosenberg, H. M., Shopland, D. R., Thun, M. J., & Edwards, B. K. (1999). Annual report to the nation on the status of cancer, 1973–1996, with a special section on lung cancer and tobacco smoking. *Journal of the National Cancer Institute*, 91(8), 675–690.

CHAPTER 13

GASTROINTESTINAL MALIGNANCIES

Giselle J. Moore-Higgs, ARNP, MSN
William M. Mendenhall, MD

PROBLEM

Cancers of the gastrointestinal tract account for approximately 24% of all cancer deaths that occur in the United States annually (Greenlee, Murray, Bolden, & Wingo, 2000). The American Cancer Society (ACS) estimates 226,600 new cases of cancer of the gastrointestinal tract with 129,800 deaths in 2000 (Greenlee et al., 2000). This includes cancers of the esophagus, stomach, pancreas, hepatobiliary system, small bowel, colon, rectum, and anus.

ESOPHAGUS AND GASTROESOPHAGEAL JUNCTION CANCER

- Cancer of the esophagus is the ninth most common malignant disease worldwide, and it is endemic in many developing nations (Day & Varghese, 1994). In the United States, it constitutes 1.5% of all cancers and 7% of all gastrointestinal cancers, with approximately 12,300 new cases and 12,100 deaths estimated in 2000 (Harras, 1996; Greenlee et al., 2000). The highest incidence occurs in Linhsien county of northern China, in the Caspian region of Iran, and in the former Soviet Union.
- The incidence varies by age, sex, and race. In Western countries, esophageal cancer is far more common in men than women. However, in high-risk countries such as China the incidence is almost equally distributed in men and women.

■ In the United States, squamous cell carcinoma is more common in the African American population, while adenocarcinoma is more common in the Caucasian population.

GASTRIC CANCER

■ Some estimates place gastric cancer as the second most common malignant disorder in the world. However, its incidence has been declining globally since World War II (NCCN, 1998). It is one of the least-common cancers in the United States, with more than 21,500 new cases and 13,000 deaths estimated in 2000 (Greenlee et al., 2000). Countries in eastern Asia, Central and South America, Eastern Europe, and the former Soviet Union have the highest incidences of gastric cancer.

■ Gastric cancer is primarily a disease of older people with peak incidence in the seventh or eighth decade of life.

■ Incidence for men is about twice that for women in both high- and low-risk countries (Parkin & Pisani, 1999).

CANCER OF THE PANCREAS

■ An estimated 28,300 new cases of pancreatic cancer will be diagnosed in the United States in 2000 with approximately 28,200 deaths (Greenlee et al., 2000). Over the past 20 years, rates of pancreatic cancer have declined in men and remained approximately constant among women. During the same period of time, there has been a significant slight decrease in mortality rates among men (about 1.0% per year) while rates have increased slightly among women (Greenlee, 2000).

HEPATOBILIARY CANCER

■ Hepatocellular cancer is one of the 10 most common cancers in the world (Curley, 1998). It is a relatively uncommon cancer in Western countries mostly occurring in sub-Saharan Africa, the southeastern coastline of China, Southeast Asia, Taiwan, Singapore, and Hong Kong (Curley, 1998). In the United States, the ACS estimates 15,300 new cases of liver cancer with 13,800 deaths in 2000 (Greenlee et al., 2000).

■ Adenocarcinoma of the gallbladder is the fifth most common gastrointestinal malignancy. It accounts for fewer than 10% of all cases of hepatobiliary cancer worldwide (Curley,

1998). However in the United States and countries of Western Europe with a low incidence of hepatocellular cancer, gallbladder cancer is relatively more prevalent. It is estimated that there will be 6,900 new cases of gallbladder cancer in 2000 with 3,400 deaths (Greenlee et al., 2000).

■ Cholangiocarcinoma arises from the intrahepatic or extrahepatic bile ducts and comprises less than 10% of primary cancers of the liver.

COLORECTAL CANCER

■ The ACS estimates 93,800 new cases of colon cancer in 2000 with 47,700 deaths. It is the fourth most common form of cancer worldwide (Greenlee et al., 2000). The disease is most common in economically developed countries, in particular North America, Australia, New Zealand, and parts of Europe (Boyle, 1998). The ACS estimates 36,400 new cases of rectal cancer in 2000 with 8,600 deaths (Greenlee et al., 2000). In the United States, the incidence is higher for men than for women (53.8 vs. 37.2 per 100,000) and higher for Black men than for White men (59.4 vs. 53.8 per 100,000)(NCI, 1998).

ANAL CANCER

■ Anal cancer incidence in the United States has increased significantly during the past 30 years and is now higher for women than for men, for Blacks than for Whites, and for residents of metropolitan rather than for residents of rural areas (Melbye, Rabkin, Frisch, & Biggar, 1994). It is more common for homosexual and bisexual men than cervical cancer is for women (Palefsky et al., 1998). The ACS estimates 3,400 new cases of anal cancer with 500 deaths in 2000 (Greenlee et al., 2000).

ASSESSMENT

RISK FACTORS

Esophagus and Gastroesophageal Junction

■ Tobacco and alcohol consumption constitute the principal risk factors for esophagus cancer. In addition, nutritional factors including vitamin deficiencies and nitrosamines in food increase the likelihood of developing this malignancy.

■ Medical conditions that may contribute include hiatal hernia, reflux esophagitis, and diverticula. Barrett's esophagus, which develops as a sequela of chronic esophageal reflux, is considered a precursor to esophageal cancer, in particular adenocarcinoma (Hesketh, Clapp, Doos, & Spechler, 1989). Gastric Helicobacter pylori (H-pylori) infection may also have a role in gastroesophageal reflux disease (GERD) resulting in esophageal dysplasia.

■ Untreated achalasia is associated with a seven- to eightfold greater risk of developing esophageal cancer.

■ Patients with head and neck cancer are at increased risk of developing esophageal cancer. Goldstein and Zornoza (1978) evaluated approximately 10,000 patients treated for squamous cell cancer of the head and neck who were over the age of 40. They found that 89 patients developed esophageal cancers: 16 synchronous and 73 metachronous lesions (latency period of 2 months to 16 years, average 46 months).

■ Approximately 95% of persons with tylosis palmaris et plantaris, a rare inherited syndrome characterized by hyperkeratosis of the palms or soles and papillomata of the esophagus, will develop esophageal cancer by the age of 65 (Helm, 1979).

Gastric Cancer

■ The pathologic changes that are assumed to precede cancer development are chronic atrophic gastritis, metaplasia, and dysplasia. The risk factors for gastric cancer act at different stages of this process by modifying progression or regression of precancerous lesions (Parkin & Pisani, 1999).

■ Infection with Helicobacter pylori as well as a high intake of irritants such as salt and nitrates causes chronic inflammation and superficial gastritis that can develop into atrophic gastritis (Correa, 1992). Dietary risk factors include ingestion of pickled vegetables, salted fish, excessive dietary salt, and smoked meats.

■ Other factors that have been reported include age over 40, low socioeconomic status, family history, pernicious anemia, hypochlorhydria, achlorhydria, diffuse adenomatous gastric polyps, prior low-dose radiation therapy (peptic ulcer disease), prior gastrectomy for benign disease, and peptic ulcer disease. In addition, individuals who work in coal mines, nickel refineries, or the rubber and timber industry are at increased risk because of environmental exposure to harmful by-products.

■ Gastric cancer is a feature of familial adenomatous polyposis as well as hereditary nonpolyposis colorectal cancer (Keller et al., 1996).

Cancer of the Pancreas

■ Blot, Fraumeni, and Stone (1978) found a correlation in the geographic pattern in the United States for lung cancer and pancreatic cancer, suggesting that tobacco may be a contributing factor. The use of two or more packs of cigarettes per day substantially increases the risk (Hiatt, Klatsky, & Armstrong, 1988).

■ In the United States, the known risk factors are older age, male gender, African American race, Jewish ancestry, low socioeconomic status, high-fat/low-fiber diet, and occupational exposure to certain chemicals (Gold, 1995).

■ Medical diseases associated with development of pancreatic cancer include peptic ulcer disease, diabetes mellitus, and chronic pancreatitis.

■ Clinical syndromes associated with increased risk of pancreatic cancer include hereditary breast-ovarian cancer, dyskeratosis congenita, Li-Fraumeni syndrome, MEN1, von Hippel-Lindau syndrome, Peutz-Jeghers, familial atypical multiple mole melanoma (FAMMM), ataxia telangiectasia, familial pancreatitis, site-specific pancreatic cancer, and hereditary nonpolyposis colorectal cancer (HNPCC) (Hruban, Yeo, & Kern, 1999; Offit, 1998).

Hepatobiliary Cancer

■ Factors that have been associated with increased risk of developing hepatocellular carcinoma include the following (Curley, 1998):
  - Hepatitis B and C viral infections causing liver damage and cirrhosis
  - Aflaxin B_1 (mycotoxin) ingestion
  - Alcohol-induced, nutritional, or posthepatic cirrhosis
  - Primary biliary cirrhosis
  - Hemochromatosis
  - α_1 - Antitrypsin deficiency
  - Glycogen storage diseases
  - Hypercitrullinemia
  - Porphyria

- Hereditary tyrosinemia
- Wilson's disease
- Hepatotoxin exposure
■ In a series from Japan, the cumulative risk of developing hepatocellular cancer at 3 years was 12.5% among patients with cirrhosis and almost 4% among patients with clinical histories of hepatitis. In the presence of hepatitis C antibody, the risk ratio was 4 as compared with 7 in patients positive for hepatitis B surface antigen (Tsukuma et al., 1993).
■ There is a significant association between gallstones and gallbladder cancer, with gallstones present in 74% to 92% of patients (Nagorney & McPherson, 1988). The risk of developing gallbladder cancer increases directly with increasing gallstone size (Diehl, 1983). The mechanism associated is a chronic inflammation of the gallbladder mucosa that may induce a series of premalignant changes. Left untreated they may progress to invasive disease.
■ The peak incidence of gallbladder cancer occurs during the sixth and seventh decades of life. It has a higher incidence in women than in men, with a ratio of 3:1 (Piehler & Crichlow, 1978). It also develops more commonly in Hispanic populations than in Black or Caucasian populations (Strom et al., 1995).
■ Gallbladder cancer is most prevalent in the Southwest American Indian populations, with its incidence being six times higher than that in non-Indian populations (Curley, 1998).
■ In cholangiocarcinoma the following have been proposed as possible risk factors: flukes, ulcerative colitis, Crohn's disease, congenital abnormalities, biliary atresia, Caroli's disease, multiple biliary papillomatosis, and ingestion of nitrosamines (Schoenthaler, 1998).

Colorectal Cancer
■ Most colorectal cancers (between 67% and 90%) arise from benign, adenomatous polyps lining the wall of the bowel. Those that grow to a large size and have a villous appearance or contain dysplastic cells are most likely to progress to cancer (Peipens & Sandler, 1994). Adenomatous polyps (villous or tubular) are outcroppings caused by tissue overgrowth that account for 50% of polyps less than 5 mm in size and 95% of polyps larger than 1 cm (Offit, 1998). The time to pro-

gression from adenoma to cancer is approximately 5 years. Forty percent of villous adenomas progress to malignancy compared with only 5% of tubular adenomas.

■ Approximately 2% to 5% of colon cancer is associated with highly penetrant dominant susceptibility syndromes (Mecklin, 1987). The most common is hereditary nonpolyposis colon cancer (HNPCC) (Offit, 1998). Members of HNPCC families have a 70% to 75% risk of developing colon cancer by age 65 (Offit, 1998).

■ Familial adenomatous polyposis (FAP) is a rare syndrome characterized by a presentation with hundreds of colonic polyps in the late teens or early twenties. In the absence of prophylactic colectomy, death occurs in virtually all FAP cases by age 50 with 37% affected by colon cancer by age 37 (Offit, 1998).

■ Other possible risk factors include physical inactivity, high-fat and/or low-fiber diet. There is some contradiction in the literature about the role of hormone replacement therapy (HRT) in women and colorectal cancer (Boyle, 1998). In a meta-analysis of the literature between January 1974 and December 1993, MacLennan and Ryan (1995) found that the overall relative risk of estrogen replacement therapy use and colorectal cancer was 0.92 (95% confidence interval, 0.74–1.15), which was not significantly different from unity ($p > 0.05$). The separate overall relative risks of estrogen replacement therapy use for colon or rectal cancer were also not significantly different from unity. They concluded that when the results of all studies published to date are combined there is no association between estrogen replacement therapy and the incidence of colorectal cancer.

Anal Cancer

■ Risk factors for anal cancer include tobacco smoking and human papilloma viral infection. Frisch and colleagues (1999a) in an evaluation of smoking found that premenopausal women who smoked had a higher risk of anal cancer than did postmenopausal women. In another study, Frisch et al. (1999b) evaluated the role of high-risk types of human papilloma virus (hrHPV) and found that homosexual men and women were more often hrHPV positive ($p < 0.01$) than heterosexual men. It was also associated with higher lesions in the anal canal. It is assumed that anal intercourse is the likely means of transmission of hrHPV into the anal canal. Women with primary invasive cervical cancer have also been found to have a relative risk of 4.6 for subsequent invasive anal cancer (Rabkin, Beggar, Melbye, & Curtis, 1992).

SCREENING AND DIAGNOSTIC TESTS

Esophagus and Gastroesophageal Junction

■ Currently, there are no routine recommended screening practices for this disease in the United States. Brush or balloon cytologies have been employed in high-risk areas such as parts of China and Iran. Endoscopic surveillance of patients with Barrett's esophagus is recommended to detect dysplasia and early cancer, however, controversy exists regarding how frequent this surveillance should be.

■ Symptoms of cancer of the esophagus include dysphagia, weight loss, pain, anorexia, and vomiting. Additional symptoms may include retrosternal or epigastric pain, dyspnea, cough, hoarseness, aspiration pneumonia, hematemesis, or a neck mass (Mendenhall & Million, 1990). The location of the tumor can influence the nature of the symptoms.

■ Most lesions occur at the esophageal gastric junction (47.9%), followed by the upper thoracic region of the esophagus (26.2%), the lower thoracic (17.8%), and cervical section (8.1%). In the upper third most cancers are squamous cell and in the lower third they are adenocarcinoma (Reed, 1995).

■ Esophageal cancer lesions spread locally through direct extension into surrounding tissue. Tracheoesophageal or bronchoesophageal fistulas occur in approximately 15% of patients. The incidence of lymph node involvement by lymph node location relates to the site of the primary tumor in the esophagus. Lymph node sites at risk include the mediastinum, supraclavicular, and sites in the upper abdomen. The most common sites of hematogenous metastasis are lung, liver, pleura, bone, kidney, and adrenal gland (Phillips, Minsky, & Dicker, 1998).

■ Initial evaluation should include the following:
   1. Complete history and physical examination.
   2. Karnofsky performance status (KPS): An individual's performance status should be considered when deciding on the method of evaluation and the treatment approach.

3. Initial diagnosis is usually made on flexible endoscopy, which allows visualization of the esophageal wall and biopsy of abnormal tissue.
4. Imaging studies may include the following:
    a. Barium esophagram—allows delineation of the upper and lower margins and detects fistulas
    b. CT scan—identifies evidence of metastatic disease in the regional lymphatics and lung
    c. Endoscopic ultrasound—measures the depth of penetration of the lesion through the esophageal wall
5. Bronchoscopy may be performed for tumors near the level of the carina to look for evidence of tracheoesophageal fistula.
6. Complete blood count and complete chemistry with electrolyte analysis.
7. Laparoscopic staging of the peritoneal cavity is an option for lesions of the gastroesophageal junction.
8. Metastatic evaluation may include a CT scan of the abdomen to evaluate liver and celiac nodes. Additional studies will depend on clinical stage of disease, reported symptoms, and physical examination findings.
9. Additional studies may be warranted to assess overall medical condition, particularly when considering surgical resection or combined modality therapy.

■ Although squamous cell carcinoma is the most common cell type in the endemic regions of the world, adenocarcinoma is most common in the world's nonendemic areas such as North America and many western European countries (NCCN, 1998).

■ Factors that improve overall prognosis include lesions in the upper one-third of the esophagus, lesions < 5 cm in length, female gender, age < 65 years, and KPS > 80. In addition, lesions that have a deep ulceration, sinus tract formation, or fistulae have a poor prognosis.

■ Staging can be either clinical or pathologic. The 1997 AJCC staging system (Table 13–1) is a pathologic staging system. For clinical preoperative or nonoperative staging, T stage can be assessed by CT scans and endoscopic ultrasound, but N stage is poorly assessed clinically. An alternative to the 1997 AJCC system for nonoperative patients is the 1983 AJCC staging system that is clinically based on endoscopic findings including length and obstruction rather than depth of penetration.

TABLE 13–1 AJCC STAGING SYSTEM FOR CANCER OF THE ESOPHAGUS

Primary Tumor (T)

T_x	Primary tumor cannot be assessed
T_0	No evidence of primary tumor
T_{is}	Carcinoma in situ
T_1	Tumor invades lamina propria or submucosa
T_2	Tumor invades muscularis propria
T_3	Tumor invades adventitia
T_4	Tumor invades adjacent structures

Regional Lymph Nodes (N)

N_x	Regional lymph nodes cannot be assessed
N_0	No regional lymph node metastasis
N_1	Regional lymph node metastasis

Distant Metastasis (M)

M_x	Distant metastasis cannot be assessed
M_0	No distant metastasis
M_1	Distant metastasis
	Tumors of the lower thoracic esophagus:
M_{1a}	Metastasis in celiac lymph nodes
M_{1b}	Other distant metastasis
	Tumors of the midthoracic esophagus:
M_{1a}	Not applicable
M_{1b}	Nonregional lymph nodes and/or other distant metastasis
	Tumors of the upper thoracic esophagus:
M_{1a}	Metastasis in cervical nodes
M_{1b}	Other distant metastasis

Stage Grouping

Stage 0	T_{is}	N_0	M_0
Stage I	T_1	N_0	M_0
Stage IIA	T_2	N_0	M_0
	T_3	N_0	M_0
Stage IIB	T_1	N_1	M_0
	T_2	N_1	M_0
Stage III	T_3	N_1	M_0
	T_4	N_1	M_0
Stage IV	Any T	Any N	M_1
Stage IVA	Any T	Any N	M_{1a}
Stage IVB	Any T	Any N	M_{1b}

Gastric Cancer

- Several screening tests have been suggested for gastric cancer and some are currently in use in Japan (Parkin & Pisani, 1999). However, these tests have not been included in any randomized controlled trials to determine the efficacy of such screening. They include:
    1. Fetal sulfaglycoprotein antigen (FSA) tumor marker
    2. Photofluorography, which involves the use of double-contrast radiology to outline small lesions of the gastric mucosa with detection by radiography, either directly or under an image intensifier.
    3. Serologic tests to determine serum pepsinogen or antibody to *Helicobacter pylori*
- The most common presenting symptoms are loss of appetite, weight loss, upper abdominal pain, nausea, vomiting, dyspepsia, anemia, and tarry stools.
- Gastric cancer spreads by direct extension into the abdomen including the omentum, pancreas, diaphragm, transverse colon, and duodenum. Lymphatic drainage follows the arterial supply. Nodal sites at risk include the celiac axis, splenic hilum, suprapancreatic nodes, porta hepatis, and gastroduodenal areas (Chao, Perez, & Brady, 1999).
- Initial evaluation should include the following:
    1. Complete history and physical examination.
    2. Karnofsky performance status (KPS): An individual's performance status should be considered when deciding on the method of evaluation and the treatment approach.
    3. Initial diagnosis is usually made on esophagogastroduodenoscopy, which allows visualization of the gastric wall, cytology, brushings, and biopsy of abnormal tissue. In the West, the most frequent site of gastric cancer is in the proximal half of the stomach (Blot, Devesa, Kreller, Fraumeni 1991).
    4. Imaging studies may include the following:
        a. Double-contrast upper gastrointestinal series x-ray—reveals small lesions limited to the inner layers of the gastric wall
        b. CT scan of the abdomen—identifies evidence of metastatic disease in the regional lymphatics and liver
        c. Endoscopic ultrasound (EUS) to assess depth of penetration and size of lesion

5. Complete blood count and complete chemistry with electrolyte analysis.
6. Metastatic evaluation may include a CT scan of the chest.
   Additional studies will depend on clinical stage of disease, reported symptoms, and physical examination findings.
7. Laparoscopy may be performed to evaluate the peritoneal cavity and liver.
8. Additional studies may be warranted to assess overall
   medical condition, particularly when considering surgical
   resection or combined modality therapy.

■ Adenocarcinoma accounts for 90% to 95% of all gastric malignancies followed by lymphoma (Chao et al., 1999).
■ At diagnosis, approximately 50% of patients have gastric
  cancer that extends beyond the local-regional confines
  (Landis et al., 1998). Important prognostic factors include
  the extent of the tumor and the number and location of any
  involved lymph nodes.
■ Staging can be done using the TNM system (Table 13–2) or
  the Astler-Coller rectal system.

Pancreatic Cancer

■ Currently, there are no specific methods available to screen
  for pancreatic cancer. Radiographic techniques including octreotide scanning and echo-planar MRI have shown promise
  in imaging the pancreas, but their usefulness in screening and
  detecting small pancreatic cancers is limited. In addition, the
  sensitivity and specificity of currently available serum markers
  for pancreatic cancer including CA19-9, carcinoembryonic
  antigen (CEA), CA 125, DU-PAN-2, and pancreatic oncofetal
  antigen are unacceptably low (Hruban et al., 1999).
■ Brentnall and colleagues (1999) recently published data on
  a series of tests performed on 14 members of high-risk families. Two imaging tests, endoscopic ultrasound (EUS) and
  endoscopic retrograde cholangiopancreatography (ERCP),
  paired together were found to identify dysplasia in the pancreas. Ten of fourteen patients had abnormal findings on
  EUS. Of these ten, seven also had abnormal ERCP studies
  and underwent pancreatectomy that revealed dysplasia on
  pathology, confirming the radiographic findings. These studies are small and further studies need to be performed to determine appropriate use of these procedures in screening
  high-risk individuals.

TABLE 13–2 AJCC STAGING OF GASTRIC CANCER

Primary Tumor (T)

T_x	Primary tumor cannot be assessed
T_0	No evidence of primary tumor
T_{is}	Carcinoma in situ; intraepithelial tumor without invasion of the lamina propria
T_1	Tumor invades lamina propria or submucosa
T_2	Tumor invades muscularis propria or subserosa*
T_3	Tumor penetrates serosa (visceral peritoneum) without invasion of adjacent structures **
T_4	Tumor invades adjacent structures***

Regional Lymph Nodes (N)

N_x	Regional lymph nodes cannot be assessed
N_0	No regional lymph node metastasis
N_1	Metastasis in 1 to 6 regional lymph nodes
N_2	Metastasis in 7 to 15 regional lymph nodes
N_3	Metastasis in more than 15 regional lymph nodes

Distant Metastasis (M)

M_x	Distant metastasis cannot be assessed
M_0	No distant metastasis
M_1	Distant metastasis

Stage Grouping

Stage 0	T_{is}	N_0	M_0
Stage IA	T_1	N_0	M_0
Stage IB	T_1	N_1	M_0
	T_2	N_0	M_0
Stage II	T_1	N_2	M_0
	T_2	N_1	M_0
	T_3	N_0	M_0
Stage IIIA	T_2	N_2	M_0
	T_3	N_1	M_0
	T_4	N_0	M_0
Stage IIIB	T_3	N_2	M_0
Stage IV	T_4	N_1	M_0
	T_1	N_3	M_0
	T_2	N_3	M_0
	T_3	N_3	M_0
	T_4	N_2	M_0
	T_4	N_3	M_0
	Any T	Any N	M_1

*Note: A tumor may penetrate the muscularis propria with extension into the gastrocolic or gastrohepatic ligaments, or into the greater or lesser omentum without perforation of the visceral peritoneum covering these structures. In this case, the tumor is classified T_2. If there is perforation of the visceral peritoneum covering the gastric ligaments or the omentum, the tumor should be classified T_3.

** Note: The adjacent structures of the stomach include the spleen, transverse colon, liver, diaphragm, pancreas, abdominal wall, adrenal gland, kidney, small intestine, and retroperitoneum.

*** Note: Intramural extension to the duodenum or esophagus is classified by the depth of greatest invasion in any of these sites including stomach.

Used with the permission of the American Joint Committee on Cancer (AJCC®), Chicago, IL. The original source for this material is the AJCC® Cancer Staging Manual, 5th ed. (1997). Philadelphia: Lippincott-Raven. **289**

■ Presenting symptoms include jaundice, abdominal pain, abdominal distention, anorexia, depression, and weight loss. Tumors of the head of the pancreas commonly invade or compress the common bile duct, causing jaundice and dilation of the bile ducts and gallbladder (Chao et al., 1999). Other less-common symptoms include diabetes mellitus, acute pancreatitis, migratory thrombophlebitis, or palpable gallbladder.

■ The most common sites of metastasis are liver, peritoneum, and lung. Other sites include ovary, spleen, and bone.

■ Initial evaluation should include the following:
1. Complete history and physical examination.
2. Karnofsky performance status (KPS): An individual's performance status should be considered when deciding on the method of evaluation and the treatment approach.
3. Imaging studies may include:
   a. Ultrasonography—may distinguish between obstructive and nonobstructive jaundice
   b. CT scan of the abdomen—detects dilation of pancreatic and bile ducts, extent of the tumor and status of surrounding structures, and evidence of liver metastasis
4. Endoscopic retrograde cholangiopancreatography (ERCP) to define the level of biliary obstruction and obtain biopsy of tumor.
5. Complete blood count, serum chemistry with liver function tests, lipase and amylase tests, CEA and CA 19-9 tests.
6. Percutaneous ultrasonography-guided or CT-guided biopsy of the tumor to obtain pathologic diagnosis.
7. Metastatic evaluation may include a CT scan of the chest. Additional studies will depend on clinical stage of disease, reported symptoms, and physical examination findings.
8. Additional studies may be warranted to assess overall medical condition, particularly when considering surgical resection or combined modality therapy.

■ The most common type of pancreatic cancer is of ductal origin, constituting 75% to 90% of cases (Cubilla & Fitzgerald, 1985). The remaining are cancers of endocrine origin. Important prognostic factors include degree of local extension and number of involved lymph nodes.

■ The staging for pancreatic cancer is by the AJCC staging system (Table 13–3).

TABLE 13-3   AJCC STAGING FOR CANCER OF THE PANCREAS

Primary Tumor (T)

T_x	Primary tumor cannot be assessed
T_0	No evidence of primary tumor
T_{is}	Carcinoma in situ
T_1	Tumor limited to the pancreas 2 cm or less in greatest dimension
T_2	Tumor limited to the pancreas of more than 2 cm in greatest dimension
T_3	Tumor extends directly into any of the following: duodenum, bile duct, peripancreatic tissues
T_4	Tumor extends directly into any of the following: stomach, spleen, colon, adjacent large vessels

Regional Lymph Nodes (N)

N_x	Regional lymph nodes cannot be assessed
N_0	No regional lymph node metastasis
N_1	Regional lymph node metastasis
pN_{1a}	Metastasis is a single regional lymph node
pN_{1b}	Metastasis in multiple regional lymph nodes

Distant Metastasis (M)

M_x	Distant metastasis cannot be assessed
M_0	No distant metastasis
M_1	Distant metastasis

Stage Grouping

Stage 0	T_{is}	N_0	M_0
Stage I	T_1	N_0	M_0
	T_2	N_0	M_0
Stage II	T_3	N_0	M_0
Stage IIB	T_1	N_1	M_0
	T_2	N_1	M_0
	T_3	N_1	M_0
Stage IVA	T_4	Any N	M_0
Stage IVB	Any T	Any N	M_1

Hepatobiliary Cancer

■ Two screening tests are available for hepatocellular cancer. The first is alpha fetoprotein (AFP). It is not a very sensitive test for small preclinical tumors, but high levels are very specific. Serum levels are elevated in 70% to 90% of persons with hepatocellular carcinoma (Tremolda et al., 1989). The second test is ultrasound of the liver, which is an easy, noninvasive, portable, inexpensive test that produces no ionizing radiation. The sensitivity and specificity of ultrasound is low with the overall false-negative rate estimated at 50% (Ferrucci, 1990). A number of factors affect the ability to obtain an adequate exam including obesity, fatty infiltrates of the liver, lesions in the dome of the liver, and operator skill.

■ The National Institutes of Health's (NIH) consensus conference recommended screening for hepatocellular carcinoma in patients with chronic HBV infection (McMahon & London, 1991). Patients at high risk (particularly those with cirrhosis, men, non-Whites, and those with perinatal-acquired infection) are recommended to have AFP screening every 3 to 4 months and ultrasound of the liver every 4 to 6 months. Those at moderate risk, those without cirrhosis, adult-onset HBV infection, Caucasian, or female, should have AFP screening every 3 to 4 months and ultrasound every 12 months.

■ Currently, there are no screening programs for primary gallbladder disease or cholangiocarcinoma. However, patients with symptomatic gallstones should be advised of the risk of malignancy and offered appropriate therapy.

■ The most common symptom of hepatocellular carcinoma and cholangiocarcinoma is right upper quadrant abdominal pain that is not severe but rather dull and aching. The pain may radiate to the right scapula. As the disease progresses, weakness, fatigue, fullness in the epigastrium, constipation, diarrhea, and anorexia occur. Jaundice is present in many cases.

■ Right upper quadrant pain, which may or may not be exacerbated by eating a fatty meal, is the predominant presenting complaint in primary gallbladder cancer (75–97%) (Nagorney & McPherson, 1988). Nausea, vomiting, anorexia, and weight loss may also be present. Jaundice is present in 45% (Curley, 1998).

■ Hepatocellular cancer spreads via direct extension into the other lobes of the liver and surrounding tissue. As the disease grows, complications can occur such as ascites, portal hypertension, and hematemesis secondary to esophageal varices or tumor invasion into the stomach. Common sites of distant metastasis include regional lymph nodes, lung, bone, adrenal glands, and brain.

■ Gallbladder cancer spreads via direct extension into the liver, biliary ductal system, colon, pancreas, and omentum. Common sites of distant metastasis are regional lymph nodes (cystic duct, pericholedochal, gastrohepatic, peripancreatic, periduodenal, periportal, celiac, and superior mesenteric areas), lung, and bone.

■ Cholangiocarcinoma spreads via direct extension into the liver, peritoneum, and regional lymphatics. Distant metastatic sites include lung and bone.

■ Initial evaluation should include the following:
1. Complete history and physical examination.
2. Karnofsky performance status (KPS): An individual's performance status should be considered when deciding on the method of evaluation and the treatment approach.
3. Imaging studies may include the following:
   a. Plain films of the abdomen may reveal hepatomegaly
   b. CT scan with contrast of the abdomen to evaluate for lesions, vascular rearrangements, and metastatic disease
   c. CT during arterial portography (CTAP): more sensitive hepatic imaging and is useful in delineating vascular anatomy
   d. Ultrasonography of the liver and gallbladder to detect lesion and extent of invasion
   e. MRI: more sensitive for hepatic lesions than other noninvasive modalities including CT
   f. Gallium-67 scan: may also be used in hepatocellular disease as 90% will accumulate ^{67}Ga
4. Complete blood count, serum chemistry with liver function tests, PT/PTT, Hepatitis panel, and AFP. Serum alpha-L-fucosidase is a new serum marker under investigation for hepatocellular carcinoma. CEA levels may also be obtained to evaluate for metastatic disease versus primary hepatocellular cancer. Serum alkaline phosphatase levels are elevated in two-thirds of patients with gallbladder cancer (Curley, 1998). Serum levels of CA19-9 are elevated in more than 90% of patients with gallbladder cancer (Curley 1998).
5. Pathologic evaluation—Percutaneous ultrasonography-guided or CT-guided biopsy of the tumor may be used to obtain pathologic diagnosis of lesions in the liver. ERCP is performed to obtain a biopsy of a lesion of the biliary tract. Tumors of the gallbladder may be biopsied during

an ERCP procedure or may not be biopsied prior to laparotomy.

6. Metastatic evaluation may include a CT scan of the chest. Additional studies will depend on clinical stage of disease, reported symptoms, and physical examination findings.

7. Additional studies may be warranted to assess overall medical condition, particularly when considering surgical resection or combined modality therapy.

■ Most primary tumors of the liver are adenocarcinomas of two cell types: approximately 90% are hepatocellular carcinomas arising from liver cells and approximately 7% are cholangiocarcinomas arising from the bile duct cells. A small proportion are hepatoblastomas, angiosarcomas, or sarcomas (Ahlgren, Wanebo, & Hill, 1992).

■ Adenocarcinoma accounts for 90% of all gallbladder cancers with the remaining lesions being adenosquamous carcinomas, anaplastic carcinomas, carcinoid tumors, or sarcomas (Nagorney & McPherson, 1988).

■ Over 90% of cholangiocarcinomas are adenocarcinomas (papillary, nodular, or sclerosing) (Schoenthaler, 1998).

■ Prognostic factors for these disease sites include extent of local involvement including adjacent organs and nodal status.

■ The staging systems for hepatocellular and cholangiocarcinoma are based on the TNM system (Table 13–4).

■ The staging systems used for gallbladder cancer are based on the pathologic characteristics of local invasion by the tumor and lymph node metastasis (Table 13–5).

Colorectal Cancer

■ Screening tests for colorectal cancer include digital rectal examination (DRE), guaiac-based occult blood tests, sigmoidoscopy, barium enema, and colonoscopy. A brief description of each test follows:

• DRE: Sensitivity of this test is severely limited by the short region that can be investigated and the skill of the examiner.

• *Guaiac-based fecal occult blood tests*: Low-cost test aimed at the detection of early asymptomatic cancer. These tests are based on the assumption that such cancer will bleed and small quantities of blood will be lost in the stool, which may be detected chemically or immunologically (Boyle, 1998). The sensitivity of this test to detect a malignancy is

TABLE 13–4 AJCC STAGING OF THE LIVER (INCLUDING INTRAHEPATIC BILE DUCTS)

Primary Tumor (T)

T_x — Primary tumor cannot be assessed

T_0 — No evidence of primary tumor

T_1 — Solitary tumor 2 cm or less in greatest dimension without vascular invasion

T_2 — Solitary tumor 2 cm or less in greatest dimension with vascular invasion or multiple tumors limited to one lobe, none more than 2 cm in greatest dimension without vascular invasion, or a solitary tumor more than 2 cm in greatest dimension without vascular invasion.

T_3 — Solitary tumor more than 2 cm in greatest dimension with vascular invasion, or multiple tumors limited to one lobe, none more than 2 cm in greatest dimension with vascular invasion, or multiple tumors limited to one lobe, any more than 2 cm in greatest dimension with or without vascular invasion.

T_4 — Multiple tumors in more than one lobe or tumor(s) involve(s) a major branch of the portal or hepatic vein(s) or invasion of adjacent organs other than the gallbladder or perforation of the visceral peritoneum.

Regional Lymph Nodes (N)

N_x — Regional lymph nodes cannot be assessed

N_0 — No regional lymph node metastasis

N_1 — Regional lymph node metastasis

Distant Metastasis (M)

M_x — Distant metastasis cannot be assessed

M_0 — No distant metastasis

M_1 — Distant metastasis

Stage Grouping

Stage I	T_1	N_0	M_0
Stage II	T_2	N_0	M_0
Stage IIIA	T_3	N_0	M_0
Stage IIIB	T_1	N_1	M_0
	T_2	N_1	M_0
	T_3	N_1	M_0
Stage IVA	T_4	Any N	M_0
Stage IVB	Any T	Any N	M_1

Table 13–5   AJCC Staging System for Cancer of the Gallbladder

Primary Tumor (T)

T_x	Primary tumor cannot be assessed
T_0	No evidence of primary tumor
T_{is}	Carcinoma in situ
T_1	Tumor invades lamina propria or muscle layer
T_{1a}	Tumor invades laminae propria
T_{1b}	Tumor invades muscle layer
T_2	Tumor invades perimuscular connective tissue; no extension beyond serosa or into liver
T_3	Tumor perforates the serosa (visceral peritoneum) or directly invades an adjacent organ, or both (extension 2 cm or less into liver)
T_4	Tumor extends more than 2 cm into liver, and/or into two or more adjacent organs (stomach, duodenum, colon, pancreas, omentum, extrahepatic bile ducts, any involvement of liver)

Regional Lymph Nodes (N)

N_x	Regional lymph nodes cannot be assessed
N_0	No regional lymph node metastasis
N_1	Metastasis in cystic duct, pericholedochal, and/or hilar lymph nodes
N_2	Metastasis in peripancreatic (head only), periduodenal, periportal, celiac, and/or superior mesenteric lymph nodes

Distant Metastasis (M)

M_x	Distant metastasis cannot be assessed
M_0	No distant metastasis
M_1	Distant metastasis

Stage Grouping

Stage 0	T_{is}	N_0	M_0
Stage I	T_1	N_0	M_0
Stage II	T_2	N_0	M_0
Stage III	T_1	N_1	M_0
	T_2	N_1	M_0
	T_3	N_0	M_0
	T_3	N_1	M_0
Stage IVA	T_4	N_0	M_0
	T_4	N_1	M_0
Stage IVB	Any T	N_2	M_0
	Any T	Any N	M_1

Used with the permission of the American Joint Committee on Cancer (AJCC®), Chicago, IL. The original source for this material is the AJCC® *Cancer Staging Manual*, 5th ed. (1997). Philadelphia: Lippincott-Raven.

approximately 40% to 70% (Cuzick, 1999). A number of foods can produce false-positive results including certain fresh fruits and vegetables that contain peroxides, oral iron preparations, and aspirin. High-dose vitamin C supplementation may lead to a false-negative result (Cuzick, 1999).

- *Sigmoidoscopy*: Currently, two large randomized trials are evaluating the efficacy of screening by flexible sigmoidoscopy.
- *Barium enema and colonoscopy*: Currently cannot be proven to reduce mortality rates from colorectal cancer.

■ Current screening recommendations (endorsed by the American Cancer Society) for medium-risk individuals (both men and women) aged 50 years include one of the following (Smith, Mettlin, Johnston-Davis, & Eyre, 2000):

1. Annual fecal occult blood testing plus flexible sigmoidoscopy every 5 years,* or
2. Colonoscopy every 10 years,* or
3. Double-contrast barium enema every 5 to 10 years.*
4. Colonoscopy every 10 years.

■ For individuals at high risk, screening should start at age 40 if a first-degree blood relative had cancer before the age of 55 years. If a strong family history of cancer is present, screening exam of the entire colon should start between ages 20 and 30. Individuals with large or multiple adenomatous polyps should be advised to have a repeat exam of the colon after 3 years.

■ About 70% of HNPCC families have mutations in one of the four known genes: HMSH2, *h*MLH1, *h*PS1 and *h*PMS2 (Offit, 1998). Of these, mutations of *h*MSH2 and *h*MLH1 are far more frequent than the others, accounting for about 30% of each of the HNPCC families. These genetic mutations provide the basis for genetic testing in HNPCC families and should be offered to high-risk patients with appropriate counseling.

■ Colon and rectal cancer spreads via direct extension, peritoneal seeding, and lymphatic and hematogenous spread.

■ Hematochezia is the most common presenting symptom in rectal and lower sigmoid cancers. Abdominal pain, changes in bowel habits, nausea, vomiting, anemia, or abdominal mass may also be present.

*A digital rectal examination (DRE) should be performed at the time of each screening sigmoidoscopy, colonoscopy, or barium enema examination.

■ Initial evaluation should include the following:
   1. Complete history and physical examination with DRE and pelvic exam in women.
   2. Karnofsky performance status (KPS): An individual's performance status should be considered when deciding on the method of evaluation and the treatment approach.
   3. Imaging studies may include the following:
      a. Barium enema
      b. CT scan with contrast of the abdomen and pelvis to evaluate for extent of disease and metastasis
      c. Proctosigmoidoscopy or colonoscopy to visualize the lesion and obtain biopsy for pathologic confirmation and to exclude the presence of other large bowel lesions
      d. Endorectal ultrasound to define extent and depth of penetration of rectal lesion
   4. Complete blood count with serum chemistry and electrolytes and liver function studies and CEA test.
   5. Chest x-ray to evaluate for metastasis.
   6. Metastatic evaluation may include a CT scan of the chest. Additional studies will depend on clinical stage of disease, reported symptoms, and physical examination findings.
   7. Additional studies may be warranted to assess overall medical condition, particularly when considering surgical resection or combined modality therapy.
■ Most tumors of the colon are adenocarcinomas.
■ Discontinuous spread of colon and rectal cancer occurs by peritoneal seeding, lymphatic spread, hematogenous spread, and surgical implantation (Chao et al., 1999).
■ The depth of tumor penetration and nodal status are the most important prognostic factors.
■ The AJCC system based on TNM evaluation can be used as a clinical or postoperative pathologic staging system. The Duke's system is based on extent of disease penetration through the bowel wall and presence or absence of nodal metastasis (Table 13–6).

Anal Cancer
■ Routine screening of the anal canal has not been advocated until recently. Anal canal cancer may be preceded by anal squamous intraepithelial lesions (ASIL), but the natural history of ASIL is poorly understood. Palefsky and colleagues (1997) conducted an assessment of anal cytology as a

TABLE 13-6 AJCC STAGING FOR COLON AND RECTAL CANCER

Primary Tumor (T)

T_x	Primary tumor cannot be assessed
T_0	No evidence of primary tumor
T_{is}	Carcinoma in situ; intraepithelial or invasion of lamina propria*
T_1	Tumor invades submucosa
T_2	Tumor invades muscularis propria
T_3	Tumor invades through the muscularis propria into the subserosa, or into nonperitonealized pericolic or perirectal tissues
T_4	Tumor directly invades other organs or structures, and/or perforates visceral peritoneum**

Regional Lymph Nodes (N)

N_x	Regional lymph nodes cannot be assessed
N_0	No regional lymph node metastasis
N_1	Metastasis in 1 to 3 regional lymph node
N_2	Metastasis in 4 or more regional lymph nodes

Distant Metastasis (M)

M_x	Distant metastasis cannot be assessed
M_0	No distant metastasis
M_1	Distant metastasis

Stage Grouping

AJCC/UICC				DUKES*
Stage 0	T_{is}	N_0	M_0	
Stage I	T_1	N_0	M_0	A
	T_2	N_0	M_0	
Stage II	T_3	N_0	M_0	B
	T_4	N_0	M_0	
Stage III	Any T	N_1	M_0	C
	Any T	N_2	M_0	
Stage IV	Any T	Any N	M_1	

* Note: T_{is} includes cancer cells confined within the glandular basement membrane (intraepithelial) or lamina propria (intramucosal) with no extension through the muscularis mucosae into the submucosa.
** Note: Direct invasion in T_4 includes invasion of other segments of the colorectum by way of the serosa.
Used with the permission of the American Joint Committee on Cancer (AJCC®), Chicago, IL. The original source for this material is the AJCC® *Cancer Staging Manual*, 5th ed. (1997). Philadelphia: Lippincott-Raven.

screening tool for anal disease. Defining abnormal cytology as including atypical squamous cells of undetermined significance and ASIL, the sensitivity of anal cytology for detection of biopsy-proven ASIL was 69% in HIV-positive men and 47% in HIV-negative men during their first visit and 81% and 50%, respectively, for all subsequent visits combined. In a further analysis of the data, Palefsky et al. Holly, Hogeboom, Berry, Jay & Darragh, (1998) found that among HIV-positive men, those with lower baseline CD_4 counts and persistent infection with one or more human papilloma virus types, were more likely to develop high-grade ASIL lesions. They concluded that anal cytology and HPV studies are a useful screening method for high-grade intraepithelial lesions and anal canal cancer, particularly in HIV-positive individuals.

■ Squamous cell cancers of the anal canal spread most commonly by direct extension and lymphatic pathways. Lymph nodes that may be involved include superior hemorrhoidal, external iliac, obturator, hypogastric nodes, and inguinal nodes.

■ Presenting symptoms include bleeding, anal discomfort, pruritus, anal discharge, anal fullness or mass, and occasionally pain or fecal incontinence.

■ Initial evaluation should include the following:

1. Complete history and physical examination with DRE and pelvic exam in women and careful visual inspection of perianal and perineal skin.
2. Karnofsky performance status (KPS): An individual's performance status should be considered when deciding on the method of evaluation and the treatment approach.
3. Imaging studies may include the following:
    a. Transanorectal ultrasound to determine depth of tumor penetration
    b. CT scan with contrast of the abdomen and pelvis to evaluate for extent of disease and metastasis
    c. Biopsy for pathologic confirmation
4. Complete blood count with serum chemistry and electrolytes and liver function studies, and HIV serum studies if not already documented.
5. Chest x-ray to evaluate for metastasis.
6. Metastatic evaluation may include a CT scan of the chest. Additional studies will depend on clinical stage of disease, reported symptoms, and physical examination findings.

7. Additional studies may be warranted to assess overall medical condition, particularly when considering surgical resection or combined modality therapy.

■ Squamous cell cancer represents approximately 80% of all malignant tumors of the anal canal and is subdivided into large-cell keratinizing, large-cell nonkeratinizing, and basaloid (Chao et al., 1999).

■ Prognostic factors include size of the lesion, extent of invasion into adjacent tissue, nodal status, and HIV status.

■ UICC and AJCC staging systems are used to stage anal cancers (Table 13–7).

OUTCOMES MANAGEMENT

Esophagus and Gastroesophageal Junction

Surgery

• Patients with cancer of the proximal esophagus are sometimes not optimal surgical candidates. Surgery should be considered strongly in patients with early-stage disease of the lower third of the thoracic esophagus and gastroesophageal junction. A wide resection of the primary tumor should be performed including > 5 cm resection margins plus regional lymphadenectomy. Procedures currently in use include the Ivor-Lewis technique, the McKeown approach, the transhiatal approach, and a left throracoabdominal approach with a high anastomosis (NCCN, 1998).

Radiation Therapy

• Radiation therapy alone is used primarily for palliation of symptoms rather than with curative intent. The dose most often selected is 30 Gy in 10 fractions over 2 weeks.

   • Preoperative radiation to reduce marginal tumors to resectable size has been compared with surgery alone in a number of studies with mixed results. The patients are given 45 to 50 Gy at 180 to 200 cGy per fraction. In general, it has not been shown to improve survival.

   • Postoperative radiation therapy may be beneficial to sterilize residual microscopic disease and to control bulky local regional disease. It is usually necessary to use a higher total dose of 50 to 60 Gy. However, there has not been any clear impact on overall survival.

TABLE 13-7   AJCC STAGING SYSTEM FOR ANAL CANCER

Primary Tumor (T)

T_x	Primary tumor cannot be assessed
T_0	No evidence of primary tumor
T_{is}	Carcinoma in situ
T_1	Tumor 2 cm or less in greatest dimension
T_2	Tumor more than 2 cm but not more than 5 cm in greatest dimension
T_3	Tumor more than 5 cm in greatest dimension
T_4	Tumor of any site invades adjacent organ(s), e.g., vagina, urethra, bladder (involvement of the sphincter muscles(s) alone is not classified as T_4)

Regional Lymph Nodes (N)

N_x	Regional lymph nodes cannot be assessed
N_0	No regional lymph node metastasis
N_1	Metastasis in perirectal lymph node(s)
N_2	Metastasis in unilateral internal iliac and/or inguinal lymph node(s)
N_3	Metastasis in perirectal and inguinal lymph nodes and/or bilateral internal iliac and/or inguinal lymph nodes

Distant Metastasis (M)

M_x	Distant metastasis cannot be assessed
M_0	No distant metastasis
M_1	Distant metastasis

Stage Grouping

Stage 0	T_{is}	N_0	M_0
Stage I	T_1	N_0	M_0
Stage II	T_2	N_0	M_0
	T_3	N_0	M_0
Stage IIIA	T_1	N_1	M_0
	T_2	N_1	M_0
	T_3	N_1	M_0
	T_4	N_0	M_0
Stage IIIB	T_4	N_1	M_0
	Any T	N_2	M_0
	Any T	N_3	M_0
Stage IV	Any T	Any N	M_1

Used with the permission of the American Joint Committee on Cancer (AJCC®), Chicago, IL. The original source for this material is the AJCC® *Cancer Staging Manual*, 5th ed. (1997). Philadelphia: Lippincott-Raven.

- The role of intracavitary brachytherapy remains under investigation.

Chemoradiotherapy

- The National Cancer Data Base reported an increased use of combined chemotherapy and radiation therapy reflecting the results of recent randomized trials demonstrating improved response and outcome for combined modality therapy as compared with radiation therapy alone (Daly, Karnell & Menck, 1996). The RTOG randomly assigned patients to receive either radiotherapy alone (64 Gy) or fluorouracil (5-FU) plus cisplatin and concurrent radiotherapy (50 Gy). The randomization was terminated after an interim analysis demonstrated a median survival advantage for patients receiving combined-modality therapy (Herskovic et al., 1992). Al-Sarraf et al. (1997) updated this data and concluded that cisplatin and 5-FU infusion given with radiation therapy (50 Gy) was statistically superior to standard radiation therapy (64 Gy) alone. With a minimum follow-up time of 5 years for all patients the median survival duration was 14.1 months and the 5-year survival rate was 27% in the combined treatment group, while the median survival duration was 9.3 months with no patients alive at 5 years in the radiation therapy alone group ($p <$ 0.0001). Other randomized trials have had similar findings. Based on these results, chemoradiotherapy for local-regional carcinoma of the esophagus, particularly with squamous cell histology, is now an established alternative to surgical therapy (NCCN, 1998).

  Chemoradiation may also be given before planned resection. Several randomized trials have been performed that have yielded mixed results.

Chemotherapy

- Chemotherapy is not effective as a single modality. It may provide some short-term palliation for some patients with advanced local-regional disease.

Gastric Cancer

Surgery

- Surgery is the treatment of choice for patients with apparent local-regional carcinoma (stages I to III). The goal of surgery is to accomplish a curative resection with negative margins and > 5 cm proximal and distal margins. A D_2 lymphadenectomy is preferred (NCCN, 1998). For cancers located in the distal stomach (body and antrum), a subtotal gastrectomy is preferred. For cancers located proximally (in the cardia), a total or proximal gastrectomy is preferred (NCCN, 1998). If there is evidence of peritoneal involvement or encasement of major blood vessels, the disease should be considered unresectable.

Radiation Therapy

- Adjuvant therapy including radiation to 45 Gy with concurrent 5-FU may be given if there is evidence of positive margins or local gross residual disease (NCCN, 1998). The gastric tumor bed, anastomosis and stump, and regional lymphatics should be included in the treatment fields (Chao et al., 1999).
  - Patients with advanced disease who are considered inoperable may be offered radiation to 45 Gy with concurrent 5-FU, palliative chemotherapy, or participation in a clinical trial (NCCN, 1998).

Pancreatic Cancer

Surgery

- Surgery is the standard treatment for pancreatic cancer using an operation called a pancreaticoduodenectomy, or Whipple procedure. This procedure consists of resecting the distal stomach, the duodenum, the first portion of the jejunum, and the head and a portion of the body of the pancreas. The bile duct is anastomosed to the jejunal remnant as is the pancreatic remnant. A gastrojejunostomy is then performed along with a vagotomy to prevent upper gastrointestinal hemorrhage (Lillis-Hearne & Castro, 1998). In a recent national patterns of care study (Janes et al., 1996), survey results showed that for a highly selective category of patients cancer-directed surgery offered a chance for cure with excellent operative mortality rates and acceptable complication rates, especially when performed in institutions that treat at least 20 cases per year.
  - Most patients present with advanced disease and are not candidates for resection. In this setting, stents may be placed endoscopically to relieve obstructive jaundice, and palliative therapy is offered.

Radiation Therapy

- Radiation therapy is the most common treatment for patients with unresectable disease. The unresected or residual tumor and nodal areas at risk are included in the treatment field and receive a total dose of 45 to 50 Gy. Concurrent 5-FU infusion given with the radiation improves median survival but not overall survival (GITSG, 1987).

Chemotherapy

- Chemotherapy is not effective as a single modality. It may provide some short-term palliation for some patients with advanced local-regional disease. Burris et al. (1997) evaluated the effectiveness of gemcitabine in patients with newly diagnosed advanced pancreas cancer. Patients were randomized to gemcitabine or 5-FU. The primary efficacy measure was clinical benefit response, which was a composite of measurements of pain, KPS, and weight. Other measures included response rate, time to progressive disease, and survival. The study demonstrated that gemcitabine was more effective than 5-FU in alleviation of some disease-related symptoms in patients with advanced disease and also conferred a modest survival advantage.

Hepatocellular Cancer

Surgery

- Surgical resection is the primary treatment for primary hepatocellular cancer. Unfortunately, in the high-incidence regions of the world only 10% to 15% of newly diagnosed patients are candidates for resection, whereas in lower-incidence Western countries 15% to 30% of patients present with potentially resectable lesions (Liver Cancer Study Group of Japan, 1990; Nagorney, van Heerden, Ilstrup, & Adson, 1989). All patients should be evaluated for functional hepatic reserve before undergoing a surgical procedure. Findings that may contraindicate hepatic resection include direct tumor invasion into segmental or main portal or hepatic vein branches, multicentric tumor, satellite nodules, tumor proximity to major vascular structures, and severe liver cirrhosis (Curley, 1998). The size and location of the lesion will mandate the type of surgery that is needed to achieve negative resection margins.

Cryosurgery

- Hepatic cryosurgery is based on the principle that the rapid freezing of tumor tissue using an intratumoral circulating liquid nitrogen probe causes tumor cell death by a combination of mechanisms. In a series of 107 patients with hepatocellular carcinoma treated with cryosurgery, the 5- and 10-year survival rates were 22% and 8%, respectively (Zhou et al., 1993). The size of the lesion has a significant impact on outcome, with tumors < 5 cm having a better outcome than those > 5 cm.

Liver Transplantation

- With a limited number of available organs, transplantation for hepatocellular cancer remains highly controversial.

Radiation Therapy

- Single-modality therapies such as radiotherapy fail to provide long-term survival benefit for most patients (Curley, 1998). One of the factors restricting the use of radiotherapy is the inability of a substantial part of the liver to tolerate a dose of more than 25 to 30 Gy in 3 to 4 weeks (Chao et al., 1999). Therefore, radiation has primarily provided palliation for painful lesions in the liver. However, new technology may provide opportunities for higher doses to small areas of the liver with minimal surrounding liver damage.

Chemotherapy

- To date, there is no evidence that any systemically administered agent or regimen has reproducible response rates in excess of 20% in selected patients, and systemic therapy has no effect on survival rates (Jones, 1998).

Gallbladder Cancer

Surgery

- Surgical evaluation via laparotomy is recommended for patients with clinically early-stage disease. If there is no evidence of peritoneal carcinomatosis or noncontiguous liver disease, patients may be eligible for en-bloc extended cholecystectomy and regional lymphadenectomy.

Palliation

- Most patients with gallbladder cancer are diagnosed at an advanced stage. Palliation of symptoms due to gastroduodenal obstruction may include a bypass procedure or placement of a decompressing gastrostomy tube and feeding jejunostomy tube (Curley, 1998). Radiation therapy to a total dose of 20 to 45 Gy may provide some temporary reduction in tumor and relief of obstructive symptoms. External-beam or intraoperative radiation therapy has been used in this setting. Currently, there are no chemotherapy agents with a proven role in this patient population.

Cholangiocarcinoma

Surgery

- Surgery is the primary treatment for early-stage disease, namely a Whipple procedure. However, similar to gallbladder cancer, most patients present with advanced unresectable disease.

Palliation

- Palliation may include surgical bypass procedures and placement of biliary stents to relieve obstructive symptoms. Radiation therapy has shown some improvement in disease-free intervals for patients with minimal residual disease after resection. However, there has not been a significant benefit from aggressive treatment overall.

Colon Cancer

Surgery

- Radical surgery is the only potentially curative treatment for colon cancer, despite recent advances in multidisciplinary treatment (Morton & Fielding, 1998). The surgical procedure of choice for resectable colon cancer is an en-bloc resection of the involved colon, or hemicolectomy (NCCN, 1996). The principles of radical surgical resection for colon cancer are ligation of the major vascular pedicle, resection of primary cancer with tumor-free margins, resection of any contiguous organs involved by tumor, and resection of the mesenteric nodes (Morton & Fielding, 1998). If the patient's tumor is unresectable, a diverting colostomy or palliative resection may be considered.
- The role of laparoscopy in the surgical treatment of colon cancer remains controversial. Concern about the risk of dissemination and partial seeding has been raised. Currently,

the procedure is used for left colectomy in a select group of patients with early-stage disease. Further research is necessary to improve technique. However, two recent studies evaluated outcomes in terms of symptoms and length of stay. The first study evaluated the symptoms of pain and fatigue associated with laparoscopy versus conventional colon resection (Schwenk, Bohm, & Muller, 1998b). The PCA dose of morphine given immediately after surgery until postoperative day 4 was higher in the conventional group (median, 1.37 mg/kg; 5–95 percentile, 0.71–2.46 mg/kg) than in the laparoscopic group (0.78 mg/kg; 0.24–2.38 mg/kg, $p < 0.01$). Postoperative fatigue was higher after conventional than after laparoscopic surgery from the second to the seventh day ($p < 0.05$). In the second study, postoperative ileus and earlier oral alimentation was evaluated (Schwenk et al., 1998a). Peristalsis was first noticed 26 ± 9 h after laparoscopic and 38 ± 17 h after conventional colorectal resection ($p < 0.01$). First flatus occurred 50 ± 19 h after laparoscopic and 79 ± 21 h after conventional surgery ($p < 0.01$). The incidence of postoperative vomiting was similar in both groups. The first bowel movement occurred 70 ± 32 h after laparoscopic and 91 ± 22 h after conventional resection ($p < 0.01$). Oral feeding without additional parenteral alimentation was tolerated 3.3 ± 0.7 days after laparoscopic and 5.0 ± 1.5 days after conventional surgery ($p < 0.01$).

Radiation Therapy

- The role of adjuvant radiation therapy in colon cancer is not well defined. In all stages combined, the most common site of failure is the abdomen rather than local failure. Patients who are at increased risk of developing local or regional failure as a result of stage, site, close or positive margins, perforation, or abcess may benefit from postoperative radiotherapy. In a study by Willett et al. (1993), three groups of patients appeared to benefit from postoperative radiation therapy. First, there was a significant improvement in local control and disease-free survival rates for patients with stage $T_4N_0M_0$ or $T_4N_{1-2}M_0$ disease. Second, among patients with stage $T_4N_0M_0$ disease with a perforation or fistula, local control and disease-free survival rates were improved. Third, radiation therapy salvaged some patients with residual disease after subtotal resection (37% 5-year, disease-free survival). There was no benefit in local control or disease-free survival for patients with $T_3N_0M_0$ or $T_3N_{1-2}M_0$ disease.

Chemotherapy

- The standard adjuvant therapy for node-positive or high-risk resectable colon cancer is postoperative 5-fluorouracil (5-FU) and leucovorin for 1 year. This protocol has been shown to confer a small disease-free survival advantage and borderline prolongation in overall survival when compared with treatment with 5-FU and levamisole (Wolmark et al., 1999). It is a regimen with a well-characterized toxicity profile. Several new agents are under investigation. One of the most promising is irinotecan. The role for intraperitoneal chemotherapy continues to be investigated.

Rectal Cancer

■ The National Cancer Data Base (1996) report on patterns of care for adenocarcinoma of the rectum (1985–1995) observed several treatment trends: 1) There was an increase in the frequency with which local excision was used as all or part of the primary treatment for Stage I disease; 2) Stage for stage, there was an increase in the frequency with which anterior/posterior resections were used and a corresponding decline in the use of abdominoperineal resections; and 3) Multimodal treatment regimens were being used with greater frequency, particularly in patients with Stage II and III disease (Jessup, Stewart & Menck, 1998).

Surgery

- Patients with early-stage disease (T_1–T_2) lesions may be treated with a low anterior resection, or in very favorable cases a transanal or posterior local resection. However, abdominoperineal resection is the standard approach for lesions that are low in the rectum and for which a sphincter-sparing procedure is not possible.

Radiation Therapy

- In a very select group of patients with well-differentiated, nonulcerated lesions, endocavitary radiotherapy may be used. Preoperative radiation therapy may be used for patients with resectable disease with the goal of sphincter

preservation (45 to 54 Gy). In addition, patients with locally advanced or unresectable radiation may be treated
with combined modality therapy including radiation and
chemotherapy with a 5-FU–based regimen. Radiation
therapy and chemotherapy are standard in the postoperative management of transmural and node-positive (stage
II and III) resectable lesions.

Anal Canal Cancer

■ The National Cancer Data Base report on carcinoma of the
anus found a trend in patterns of care favoring nonsurgical
management with radiochemotherapy for epidermoid carcinomas of the anus (Myerson, Karnell, & Menck, 1997). For
adenocarcinomas, there was a trend toward increasing use
of multimodality therapy with surgery and adjuvant radiochemotherapy.

Surgery

• Surgery was once the treatment of choice for patients with
anal cancer. It is now reserved primarily for patients who
develop locally recurrent disease after radiation therapy.

Radiation Therapy

• Most patients with anal cancer are treated with radiation
therapy concurrent with chemotherapy. The drugs of
choice are 5-fluorouracil and mitomycin C. It may be possible to substitute cisplatin for mitomycin C with equivalent long-term results. The UKCCCR Anal Cancer Working
Trial (1996) compared radiation therapy alone to radiation
therapy with chemotherapy for patients with anal cancer.
They found a 46% reduction in the risk of local failure for
the patients receiving chemotherapy. In locally advanced
($T_{3-4}N_{0-3}$ or $T_{1-2}N_{1-3}$) disease, Bartelink et al. (1997) evaluated concomitant radiotherapy and chemotherapy com-
pared with radiotherapy alone. They found that adding
chemotherapy to radiotherapy resulted in a significant increase in the complete remission rate (from 54% for radiotherapy alone to 80% for chemoradiation). The local-
regional control rate improved by 18% at 5 years. The
colostomy-free rate at that time increased by 32% with the
addition of chemotherapy to radiation. Patients with T_1
well-to moderately differentiated squamous cell carcinomas (and those with medical problems that contraindicate chemotherapy) are treated with radiotherapy alone.

TOXICITY OF TREATMENT: ESOPHAGUS

Acute Toxicities

- Esophagitis can cause substantial morbidity. Patients will complain of chest pain, dysphagia, odynophagia, and/or heartburn. Candidiasis infection is common and may significantly increase symptoms. For treatment options see Chapter 21.

- Acute skin reaction usually occurs with erythema and dry desquamation. Patients rarely experience moist desquamation. For treatment options see Chapter 21.

- Fatigue is very common, particularly for patients who have experienced significant weight loss due to dysphagia. For treatment options see Chapter 20.

- Weight loss is a common presenting symptom, and will continue during treatment due to esophagitis, dysphagia, and nausea. Patients should be considered for alternate nutritional methods. For treatment options see Chapter 22.

- Pneumonitis may occur if large volumes of lung are included in the treatment field. Use of CT-planning may help in the design of fields to reduce this risk. Symptoms usually begin 6 to 8 weeks after completion of treatment and may include shortness of breath, dry cough, malaise, and low-grade fevers. Symptom management is usually sufficient, however, a small number of patients may require a short course of corticosteroids.

- Fistulae formation between the esophagus and trachea is a rare but often fatal complication of tumors close to the carina. An increased risk of fistulae has been observed with the aggressive combination of brachytherapy, external-beam radiation, and chemotherapy. Patients may complain of substernal chest pain, fever, and tachycardia. An esophagogram should be obtained and treatment stopped if there is documented evidence of fistulae. An esophageal stent may be used to occlude the fistula.

Latent Toxicities

- Esophageal stenosis, strictures, or ulceration may occur 4 to 6 months or more after radiation in about 5% of patients treated to 63 Gy (Coia, 1998). When doses exceed 70 Gy, as many as 50% of patients may experience this complication. Patients may need dilation to reduce associated discomfort and dysphagia.

■ Other rare complications include esophageal perforation and mediastinitis, myelitis, and pericarditis (Coia, 1998).

TOXICITIES OF TREATMENT: UPPER ABDOMEN

Acute Toxicities

■ Anorexia and weight loss are common symptoms in patients receiving radiation therapy to the upper abdomen. It is commonly associated with heartburn, nausea, and vomiting. Uncontrolled symptoms can result in rapid weight loss and dehydration, often compromising the course of radiation. Prophylactic use of antiemetics and H_2 blockers can prevent these symptoms or at least reduce their impact. For treatment options, see Chapter 22.

■ Fatigue is a common symptom that is often a result of significant weight loss and anorexia, in addition to the effects of radiation. See Chapter 20 for management options.

■ Skin reactions are usually mild with erythema and dry desquamation occurring. However, patients may have biliary drains that enter through the skin and excoriation may occur. Careful evaluation of the drain sites should be performed each day for evidence of leakage and infection. Clean, dry dressing should be applied twice a day. See Chapter 21 for further management of radiation-induced skin reactions.

Latent Toxicities

■ The major late toxicity is small bowel obstruction. This is relatively uncommon and is managed conservatively, if possible. It is more common in patients with prior surgery or pelvic infection and in patients treated with fields that include a large amount of small bowel. Surgical management may be required and entails bypass of the affected bowel.

■ Gastritis and gastric ulcers may occur 2 or more months after radiation therapy that includes the gastric mucosa (> 50 Gy) (Coia, 1998). Treatment requires antacids or H_2-blocker medications to allow healing.

■ Another rare toxicity is nephritis, which may occur if two-thirds of one kidney is not excluded from the treatment field (Coia, 1998).

■ Radiation hepatitis may occur occasionally (< 5%) with radiation doses of 25 Gy to the whole liver. The risk increases to 50% at 40 Gy (Coia, 1998). Symptoms associated with acute radiation hepatitis include hepatomegaly, ascites, and elevated liver enzymes 2 to 6 weeks after irradiation. Chronic radiation hepatitis occurs 4 to 6 months or more after irradiation and is treated like chronic nonradiation hepatitis (Coia, 1998).

TOXICITIES OF TREATMENT: LOWER ABDOMEN AND PELVIS

Acute Toxicities

■ Diarrhea due to enteritis is a common side effect of radiation to the lower abdomen and pelvis. It usually occurs after approximately 8 Gy and continues until completion of treatment. Uncontrolled diarrhea can lead to anorexia, weight loss, and dehydration, ultimately impacting quality of life and compromising treatment. See Chapter 23 for treatment options.

■ In women, vaginal mucositis may occur. See Chapter 21 for treatment options.

■ Cystitis (due to bladder irritation) may occur and consists of urinary frequency and dysuria. Urinary tract infection should be excluded before initation of symptom management. See Chapter 23 for treatment options.

■ Skin reactions including erythema and moist desquamation occur when the perineum is included in the treatment field. These reactions can be very painful and difficult to manage. See Chapter 21 for treatment options.

■ In patients with HIV disease, particularly if the pretreatment CD_4 count is $\leq$ 200, acute toxicity may require treatment break. In particular, these patients experience intractable diarrhea and moist desquamation (Hoffman, Welton, & Klencke, 1999).

Latent Toxicities

■ The major latent complication is small bowel obstruction, which may occur in a small subset of patients.

■ Radiation proctitis, ulceration, and bleeding are rarely seen with doses under 55 to 60 Gy (Coia, 1998). Onset is usually 6 to 12 months after radiation. See Chapter 23 for treatment recommendations.

■ Loss of vaginal elasticity and vaginal stenosis occur in women treated to the pelvis, which may have a significant impact on sexual function and quality of life. See Chapter 26 for treatment recommendations.

Outcomes Measures

- The NCI Common Toxicity Criteria (CTC) Version 2 with the Radiation Therapy Oncology Group (RTOG) and European Organization for Research and Treatment of Cancer (EORTC) Acute Effects Criteria instrument provides a scale for many different organ systems and some symptoms (NCI, 1999). It is a very useful tool for grading severity of acute effects of radiation therapy in all sites.
- The Radiation Therapy Patient Care Record: A Tool for Documenting Nursing Care (ONS, 1994) provides a tool for weekly assessment and grading of severity of acute effects of radiation therapy in all sites.

Follow-Up

Esophagus and Gastroesophageal Junction Cancer

- A follow-up evaluation should be performed every 3 months for a minimum of 2 years. The evaluation should include the following:
  1. History and physical examination.
  2. Complete blood count with chemistry and electrolyte analysis.
  3. Chest x-ray every 6 months.
  4. Radiographic or endoscopic exams as clinically indicated.
- Patients who develop an anastomotic or chemoradiation-induced stricture may require dilation as needed.

Gastric Cancer

- Follow-up evaluation should be conducted every 3 months for the first 2 years and every 6 months for the following 3 years. The following procedures should be included:
  1. Complete history and physical examination.
  2. Complete blood count with chemistry and electrolyte evaluation.
  3. Chest x-ray every 6 to 12 months.

4. Endoscopy as clinically indicated.
5. Long-term vitamin B_{12} supplementation for patients who have proximal or total gastrectomy.

PANCREAS AND HEPATOBILIARY CANCER

■ Cancers of the pancreas, liver, biliary tract, and gallbladder in general have a poor prognosis. Most patients have advanced disease at diagnosis and treatment is usually palliative. Only a small percentage of patients benefit from radical surgery; however, there is a high incidence of local-regional recurrence. Therefore, follow-up should be individualized to the patient and to the treatment provided. Symptom management of progressive disease may include the following:
1. Pain: pain may be difficult to control because of intolerance of oral medications. Percutaneous neurolysis of the celiac ganglion may provide relief of severe abdominal pain associated with tumor progression.
2. Maintenance of biliary drainage tubes can relieve jaundice and associated pruritus and skin irritation. Marcy, Chevallier, and Granon (1999) evaluated the costs and benefits of percutaneous interventional radiological procedures in terminal cancer patients. Procedures included placement of endovenous or urinary stents, percutaneous gastrostomy tubes, celiac plexus block, tumor embolization, and others. A retrospective analysis of the consequences of each procedure in terms of survival, quality of life, and cost ratios was conducted, and findings justified the use of interventional radiology in palliative oncology.

COLORECTAL CANCER

■ Follow-up evaluation should be conducted every 3 months for the first 2 years and every 6 months for the following 3 years. The following procedures should be included:
1. Complete history and physical examination.
2. A CEA should be done if the CEA was elevated at diagnosis and had decreased after resection (NCCN, 1996). If resection of liver metastasis would be clinically indicated, it is recommended that postoperative serum CEA testing should be performed every 2 to 3 months for patients with

stage II or III disease for ≥ 2 years after diagnosis (ASCO, 1999). Regular monitoring of liver function studies is not recommended.

3. Chest x-ray every 6 to 12 months.
4. Sigmoidoscopy should be performed 1 year after completion of treatment and repeated annually. Colonoscopy should be performed every 3 years.
5. Fecal Occult Blood Test—ASCO (1999) does not recommend periodic fecal occult blood test in surveillance for colorectal cancer recurrence.
6. Routine CT scan of the abdomen and pelvis and other pelvic imaging is not recommended (ASCO, 1999).

■ There is much controversy about the cost-effectiveness of follow-up of patients diagnosed with colorectal cancer. Audisio and colleagues (1996) conducted a study evaluating cost. Five hundred five patients who survived curative surgery for stage I-III colorectal adenocarcinoma had close follow-up for at least 4 years. One hundred forty-one patients (28%) had recurrence. Of these, 32 underwent one or more surgical procedures for cure, whereas 109 could only benefit from palliation. Eighteen were cured. The mean survival of all recurrent cases was 44.4 months. Of those operated on with curative intent, the mean survival was 69.3 months compared with 37.1 months in those who had surgery with palliative intent. Of those 18 patients who were cured by reoperative surgery, the average survival was 81.4 months. The overall follow-up cost was $1,914,900 (U.S.) for the 505 patients; $13,580 (U.S.) for each recurrence; $59,841 (U.S.) for each case treated for cure; and $136,779 (U.S.) for those effectively cured. Careful postoperative monitoring is expensive yet effective when one considers that one-quarter of the detected recurrences were suitable for potentially curative second surgery, however, only 3.6% of the original group were effectively cured. To reduce costs, follow-up programs should be tailored according to the stage and site of the primary lesion.

ANAL CANCER

■ Follow-up evaluation should be conducted every 3 months for the first 2 years and every 6 months for the following 3 years. The following procedures should be included:

1. Complete history and physical examination.
2. Complete blood count with chemistry and electrolyte evaluation. A CEA should be done if the CEA was elevated at diagnosis and decreased after resection (NCCN, 1996).
3. Chest x-ray every 6 to 12 months.

■ Patients with recurrent disease may be eligible for salvage therapy if the disease is found early. Pocard, Tiret, and Nugent (1998) evaluated the role of salvage abdominoperineal resection for anal cancer after radiation therapy failure. The overall survival rate at 3 years after salvage resection was 58%. The overall survival rate for patients with residual disease after radiation was 72% at 3 years and 60% at 5 years.

EXPECTED OUTCOMES

ESOPHAGUS AND GASTROESOPHAGEAL JUNCTION CANCER

Survival
■ Despite improvement in the diagnostic modalities, surgical technique, chemotherapy, and radiotherapy, mortality and morbidity as a result of esophagus cancer remain dismal. The five-year survival rate for all stages is 12%, with 24% for early-stage disease, and only 2% for stage IV disease (NCI, 1998).

Quality of Life
■ In a critical review of the literature, Micallef, Macquart-Moulin, Auquier, Seitz & Moatti (1998) found only five studies that used validated quality-of-life measures in the evaluation of surgical treatment for esophageal carcinoma. There are currently no studies evaluating the role of radiotherapy or chemoradiation in this population. However, the European Organization for Research and Treatment of Cancer (EORTC) has recently developed a module to be used to assess quality of life in this particular patient population—the QLQ-OES 24 (Blazeby et al., 1996).
■ The following instruments are also appropriate for evaluation of overall quality of life in this patient population:
  1. Functional Assessment of Cancer Therapy (FACT-G) (Cella, Tulsky, & Gray, 1993)—A measurement system of

self-report (33-item) scale of quality of life for people with cancer. The general version has been validated in English and has been used extensively in the United States.

2. European Organization for Research and Treatment of Cancer (EORTC) QLQ-C30 (Aaronson et al., 1993)—A 36-item questionnaire for assessing the quality of life of cancer patients participating in international clinical trials. It has been validated and used extensively in a wide range of cancer clinical trials in Europe and worldwide.

■ With most patients with cancer of the esophagus presenting with advanced disease, palliative therapy is commonly used. Quality of life must still be evaluated in this patient population. The following are instruments that may be used:

1. Hospice Quality of Life Index (HQLI) (McMillan & Weitzner, 1998)—A 28-item self-report instrument that includes three subscales: psychophysiological well-being, functional well-being, and social/spiritual well-being. Allows patients the opportunity to express beliefs about quality-of-life issues and to maintain direction over a critical aspect of their care.

2. Missoula-VITAS Quality of Life Index (MVQOLI) (Byock & Merriman, 1998)—Developed to provide a measure of quality of life of terminally ill patients.

3. McGill Quality of Life Questionnaire (MQOL) (Cohen, Mount, & Strobel, 1995)—Designed to measure overall quality of life in people with a life-threatening illness and to indicate the areas in which the patient is doing well or poorly. Correlates with the Spitzer Quality of Life and SIS instruments. Internal consistency reliability rating of 0.89.

4. The McMaster Quality of Life Scale (MQLS) (Sterkenburg & Woodward, 1996)—Instrument developed to measure quality of life in a palliative patient population including cancer patients. Has been correlated with the Spitzer Quality of Life instrument and has a good internal consistency (0.62 to 0.79) and inter-rater reliability (0.83 to 0.95).

5. The Symptom Distress Scale (McCorkle & Young, 1978)—Developed for patients with a life-threatening disease, either cancer or heart disease. It concentrates mainly on the symptoms and mood in relation to quality of life. Has been correlated with global quality-of-life measures and has an internal consistency of 0.78 to 0.89. It has been found to be sensitive to changes in treatment over time.

GASTRIC CANCER

Survival

■ Overall survival for gastric cancer is poor, with 5-year survival rates of 21% for all stages. Survival rates at 5 years for early-stage local disease are 60%, but quickly drop to 2% for stage IV disease (NCI, 1998).

Quality of Life

■ The impact of gastric cancer on health-related quality of life has been limited in terms of quality and quantity. The effect of different treatments including surgical procedures, pharmacological and nonpharmacological therapies, and procedures for symptom management have dominated this area of research (Schmier, Elixhauser, & Halpern, 1999). Variables that do appear to influence health-related quality in this patient population related to tolerance of food, ability to eat, weight loss, and depression (Wu et al., 1997; Andreyeve, Norman, Oates, & Cunningham, 1998; Jentschura, Weakler, Strohmeier, Rumstadt & Hagmuller, 1997; and Davies et al., 1998).

■ The following instruments are appropriate for evaluation of overall quality of life evaluation in this patient population:
  1. Functional Assessment of Cancer Therapy (FACT-G) (Cella et al., 1993)
  2. European Organization for Research and Treatment of Cancer (EORTC) QLQ-C30 (Aaronson et al., 1993)

■ In late-stage disease, the following measures are appropriate:
  1. Hospice Quality of Life Index (HQLI) (McMillan & Weitzner, 1998)
  2. Missoula-VITAS Quality of Life Index (MVQOLI) (Byock & Merriman, 1998)
  3. McGill Quality of Life Questionnaire (MQOL) (Cohen et al., 1995)
  4. The McMaster Quality of Life Scale (MQLS) (Sterkenburg & Woodward, 1996)
  5. The Symptom Distress Scale (McCorkle & Young, 1978)

PANCREATIC CANCER

Survival

■ Survival in pancreatic cancer is very dismal. Five-year survival for all stages is 4%, with only a 17% survival in stage I disease (NCI, 1998).

Quality of Life

- There is a paucity of studies conducted to evaluate the quality of life of patients with pancreatic cancer. The available data focus on surgical outcomes. One example is a study by McLeod (1999) who evaluated the QOL of 25 patients after a Whipple procedure. The patients appeared to have few gastrointestinal symptoms, were not clinically malnourished, and had excellent quality of life. The suggestion that median survival and performance status are improved for patients having a resection may be biased by the disease being more favorable to allow a resection rather than the treatment being beneficial.

- However, most available studies focus on specific problems related to advanced disease. Ballinger and colleagues (1994) evaluated symptom relief and quality of life after stent placement for malignant bile duct obstruction. They found that the stent insertion not only helped to relieve the symptoms of jaundice and pruritis, but also improved anorexia and indigestion. Patients reported an improvement in appetite. Mood, physical health, and level of activity were unchanged. These findings were confirmed in another study conducted by Luman, Cull, and Palmer (1997). They reported significant improvement in emotional, cognitive, and global health scores in addition to improvement in diarrhea and sleep patterns.

- Appropriate quality-of-life instruments for this patient population include those related to end-of-life issues. Examples include:
  1. Hospice Quality of Life Index (HQLI) (McMillan & Weitzner, 1998)
  2. Missoula-VITAS Quality of Life Index (MVQOLI) (Byock & Merriman, 1998)
  3. McGill Quality of Life Questionnaire (MQOL) (Cohen et al., 1995)
  4. The McMaster Quality of Life Scale (MQLS) (Sterkenburg & Woodward, 1996)
  5. The Symptom Distress Scale (McCorkle & Young, 1978)

HEPATOBILIARY CANCER

Survival

- The reported long-term survival rates after curative resection of hepatocellular cancer are widely variable. In Western countries, 2- and 3-year survival rates range from 23.5% to 51.0%, and studies with longer follow-up periods report 5-year survival rates ranging from 27% to 49% (Nagorney & McPherson, 1989; Paquet, Koussouris, Mercado, Kalk, Muting & Raubach, 1991; Franco et al., 1990; Ringe, Pichlmayr, Wittekind, & Tusch, 1991). However, in the United States, the 5-year survival for all stages is 5%, with only 15% survival for stage I disease (NCI, 1998).

■ Local recurrence is the site of first failure in 45% to 70% of patients. Most patients develop hepatic recurrences within the first 2 years.

Quality of Life

■ Unresectable hepatocellular carcinoma is virtually (by definition) incurable (Jones, 1998). With this prognosis, focus on quality of life should be in the palliative setting. No studies in the current literature evaluate this patient population. The following instruments would be appropriate to use in this population:
  1. Hospice Quality of Life Index (HQLI) (McMillan & Weitzner, 1998)
  2. Missoula-VITAS Quality of Life Index (MVQOLI) (Byock & Merriman, 1998)
  3. McGill Quality of Life Questionnaire (MQOL) (Cohen et al., 1995)
  4. The McMaster Quality of Life Scale (MQLS) (Sterkenburg & Woodward, 1996)
  5. The Symptom Distress Scale (McCorkle & Young, 1978)

COLORECTAL AND ANAL CANCER

Survival

■ Early diagnosis and treatment of colorectal cancer results in higher 5-year survival rates—91% for local disease (NCI, 1998). Even in patients with regional lymph node metastasis, survival rates at 5 years are 66%. However, individuals with stage IV disease at the time of diagnosis still have a poor outcome with survival of 9% at 5 years.

Quality of Life

■ Most studies evaluating quality of life in patients with colorectal and anal canal cancer have focused on patient adjustment to surgical or chemotherapy outcomes including colostomy. Few studies have evaluated quality of life in patients receiving radiation therapy. Ahmad and Nagle (1996) evaluated the long-term functional outcome of patients treated with chemoradiation for cancer of the anal canal. They found that the impact of concerns about sphincter function on patients' quality of life was minimal in 53%, moderate in 24%, and significant in 24%. Qualitative assessment of sphincter function demonstrated that 41% of patients experienced transient incontinence of solid stool following completion of treatment, and this effect appeared more pronounced in patients receiving > 45 Gy. However with long-term follow-up, most recover continence of solid stool, and impairment of anal sphincter function did not significantly compromise quality of life for most patients. Several instruments have recently been published that focus on this particular disease. They include:

1. EORTC QLQ-CR38 (Spangers, te Velde, & Aaronson, 1999)—Consists of 38 items covering symptoms and side effects related to different treatment modalities, body image, sexuality, and future perspective. The instrument has been found to be clinically valid as a supplementary questionnaire for assessing specific quality of life issues relevant to patients with colorectal cancer.

2. FACT-C (Ward, Hahn, Mo, Hernandez, Tulsky, & Cella, 1999)—A self-report instrument that combines specific concerns related to colorectal cancer with concerns that are common to all cancer patients as assessed with the FACT-General (FACT-G). The instrument has been found to be reliable and valid in both English and Spanish.

■ One interesting study that crosses both treatment modalities focused on the role of exercise and QOL. Courneya & Friedenreich (1997) evaluated the relationship between exercise patterns and current quality of life in colorectal cancer survivors. Colorectal cancer survivors exhibited four main exercise patterns across the cancer experience that were labeled maintainers (active at all three time points), temporary relapsers (active prediagnosis, inactive during treatment, active posttreatment), permanent relapsers (active prediagnosis, inactive during treatment, inactive posttreatment), and nonexercisers (inactive at all three time points). Statistical analyses showed that functional QOL was the least possessed but most important QOL dimension underlying overall SWL, exercise levels decreased from prediagnosis to active treatment and then increased from active treatment to posttreatment but not back to prediagnosis levels, and permanent relapsers reported the lowest QOL of the four main exercise patterns. It was concluded that cancer treatment has a negative impact on exercise levels and that those previously active individuals who fail to reinitiate exercise after cancer treatment experience the lowest QOL 1 to 4 years later.

REFERENCES

Aaronson, N. K., Ahmedzai, S., Bergman, B., Bullinger, M., Cull, A., Duez, N. J., Filiberti, A., Flechtner, H., Fleishman, S. B., de Haes, J. C. J. M., Kaasa, S., Klee, M., Osoba, D., Razavi, D., Rofe, P. B., Schraub, S., Sneeuw, K., Sullivan, M., & Takeda, F. (1993). The European Organization for Research and Treatment of Cancer QLQ-C30: A quality-of-life instrument for use in international clinical trials in oncology. *Journal of the National Cancer Institute*, 85(5), 365–376.

Ahlgren, J. D., Wanebo, H. J., & Hill, M. C. (1992). Hepatocellular carcinoma. In J. D. Ahlgren & J. S. McDonald (Eds.), *Gastrointestinal oncology* (pp. 417–436). Philadelphia: Lippincott.

Ahmad, N. R., & Nagle, D. (1996). Long-term functional outcome of patients treated with chemoradiation therapy for carcinoma of the anal canal [Abstract No. 1055]. Proceedings of the 38th Annual ASTRO Meeting. *International Journal of Radiation Oncology, Biology, Physics*, 36 (Suppl. 1), 271.

Al-Sarraf, M., Martz, K., Herskovic, A., Leichman, L., Brindle, J. S., Vaitkevicius, V. K., Cooper, J., Byhardt, R., Davis, L., & Emami, B. (1997). Progress report of combined chemoradiotherapy versus radiotherapy alone in patients with esophageal cancer: An intergroup study. *Journal of Clinical Oncology*, 15(1), 277–284.

Andreyev, H. J., Norman, A. R., Oates, J., & Cunningham, D. (1998). Why do patients with weight loss have a worse outcome when undergoing chemotherapy for gastrointestinal malignancies? *European Journal of Cancer*, 24(4), 503–509.

American Society of Clinical Oncology. (1999). Recommended colorectal cancer surveillance guidelines by the American Society of Clinical Oncology. *Journal of Clinical Oncology*, 17(4), 1312–1321.

Audisio, R. A., Setti-Carraro, P., Segala, M., Capko, D., Andreoni, B., & Tiberio, G. (1996). Follow-up in colorectal cancer patients: A cost-benefit analysis. *Annals of Surgical Oncology*, 3(4), 349–357.

Ballinger, A. B., McHugh, M., Catnach, S. M., Alstead, E. M., & Clark, M. L. (1994). Symptom relief and quality of life after stenting for malignant bile duct obstruction. *Gut*, 35(4), 467–470.

Bartelink, H., Roelofsen, F., Eschwege, F., Rougier, P., Bosset, J. F., Gonzalez, D. G., Peiffert, D., van-Glabbeke, M., Pierart, M. (1997). Concomitant radiotherapy is superior to radiotherapy alone in the treatment of locally advanced anal cancer: Results of a phase III randomized trial of the European Organization for Research and Treatment of Cancer Radiotherapy and Gastrointestinal Cooperative Groups. *Journal of Clinical Oncology*, 15(5), 2040–2049.

Blazeby, J. M., Alderson, D., Winstone, K., Steyn, R., Hammerlid, E., Arraras, J., & Farndon, J. R. (1996). Development of an EORTC questionnaire module to be used in quality of life assessment for patients with esophageal cancer. The EORTC Quality of Life Study Group. *European Journal of Cancer*, 32A(11), 1912–1917.

Blot, W. J., Fraumeni, J. F. Jr, & Stone, B. J. (1978). Geographic correlates of pancreas cancer in the United States. *Cancer*, 42(1), 373–380.

Blot, W. J., Devesa, S. S., Kneller, R. W., & Fraumeni, J. F. Jr. (1991). Rising incidence of adenocarcinoma of the esophagus and gastric cardia. JAMA, 265(10), 1287–1289.

Boyle, P. (1998). Relative value of incidence and mortality data in cancer research. *Recent Results in Cancer Research*, 114, 41–63.

Brentnall, T. A., Bronner, M. P., Byrd, D. R., Haggitt, R. C., & Kimmey, M. B. (1999). Early diagnosis and treatment of pancreatic dysplasia in patients with a family history of pancreatic cancer. *Annals of International Medicine*, 131(4), 247–255.

Burris, H. A., III, Moore, M. J., Anderson, J., Green, M. R., Rothenberg, M. L., Modiano, M. R., Cripps, M. C., Portenoy, R. K., Storniolo, A. M., Tarassoff, P., Nelson, R., Dorr, F. A., Stephens, C. D., & Von-Hoff, D. D. (1997). Improvements in survival and clinical benefit with gemcitabine as first-line therapy for patients with advanced pancreas cancer: A randomized trial. *Journal of Clinical Oncology*, 15(6), 2403–2413.

Byock, I. R., & Merriman, M. P. (1998). Measuring quality of life for patients with terminal illness: The Missoula-VITAS Quality of Life Index. *Palliative Medicine*, 12(4), 231–244.

Cella, D. F., Tulsky, D. S., & Gray, G. (1993). The Functional Assessment of Cancer Therapy Scale: Development and validation of the general measure. *Journal of Clinical Oncology*, 11(3), 570–579.

Chao, K. S. C., Perez, C. A., & Brady, L. W. (1999). *Radiation oncology: Management decisions*. Philadelphia: Lippincott-Raven.

Choi, T. K., Edward, C. S., Fan, S. T., Francis, P. T., & Wong, J. (1990). Results of surgical resection for hepatocellular carcinoma. *Hepatogastroenterology*, 37(2), 172–175.

Cohen, S. R., Mount, B. M., & Strobel, M. G. (1995). The McGill Quality of Life Questionnaire: A measure of quality of life appropriate for people with advanced disease. A preliminary study of validity and acceptability. *Palliative Medicine*, 9(3), 207–219.

Coia, L. R. (1998). Gastrointestinal Cancers. In L. R. Coia & D. J. Moylan, (Eds.), *Introduction to clinical radiation oncology* (pp. 243–283). Madison, WI: Medical Physics Publishing.

Correa, P. (1992). Human gastric carcinogenesis: A multistep and multifactorial process. First American Cancer Society Award lecture on cancer epidemiology and prevention. *Cancer Research*, 52(24), 6735–6740.

Courneya, K. S., & Friedenreich, C. M. (1997). Relationship between exercise pattern across the cancer experience and current quality of life in colorectal cancer survivors. *Journal of Alternative and Complementary Medicine*, 3(3), 215–226.

Cubilla, A. L., & Fitzgerald, P. J. (1985). Cancer of the exocrine pancreas: The pathologic aspects. CA: *Cancer Journal for Clinicians*, 35(1), 2–18.

Curley, S. A. (1998). Diagnosis and treatment of primary gallbladder cancer. In S. A. Curley (Ed.), *Liver cancer*. New York: Springer-Verlag.

Cuzick, J. (1999). Colorectal cancer. In B. S. Kramer, J. K. Gohagan & P. C. Prorok (Eds.), *Cancer screening* (pp. 219–265). New York: Marcel Dekker.

Daly, J. M., Karnell, L. H., & Menck, H. R. (1996). National Cancer Data Base report on esophageal carcinoma. *Cancer*, 78(8), 1820–1828.

Davies, J., Johnston, D., Sue-Ling, H., Young, S., May, J., Griffith, J., Miller, G., & Martin, I. (1998). Total or subtotal gastrectomy for gastric carcinoma? A study of quality of life. *World Journal of Surgery*, 22(10), 1048–1055.

Day, N. E., & Varghese, C. (1994). Esophageal cancer. *Cancer Surveys*, 19/20, 43–54.

Diehl, A. K. (1983). Gallstone size and the risk of gallbladder cancer. *JAMA*, 250(17), 2323–2326.

Ferrucci, J. T. (1990). Liver tumor imaging: Current concepts. AJR. *American Journal of Roentgenology*, 155(3), 473–484.

Franco, D., Capussotti, L., Smadja, C., Bouzari, H., Meakins, J., Kemeny, F., Grange, D., & Dellepiane, M. (1990). Resection of hepatocellular carcinoma: Results in 72 European patients with cirrhosis. *Gastroenterology*, 98(3), 733–738.

Frisch, M., Glimelius, B., Wohlfahrt, J., Adami, H. O., & Melbye, M. (1999). Tobacco smoking as a risk factor in anal carcinoma: An antiestrogenic mechanism? *Journal of the National Cancer Institute*, 91(8), 708–715.

Frisch, M., Fenger, C., van-den-Brule, A. J., Sorensen, P., Meijer, C. J., Walboomers, J. M., Adami, H. O., Melbye, M., & Glimelius, B. (1999). Variants of squamous cell carcinoma of the anal canal and perianal skin and their relation to human papilloma viruses. *Cancer Research*, 59(3), 753–757.

Gastrointestinal Tumor Study Group. (1987). Further evidence of effective adjuvant combined radiation and chemotherapy following curative resection of pancreatic cancer. *Cancer*, 59(12), 2006–2010.

Gold, E. B., (1995). Epidemiology of and risk factors for pancreatic cancer. *Surgical Clinics of North America*, 75(5), 819–843.

Goldstein, H. M., & Zornoza, J. (1978). Association of squamous cell carcinoma of the head and neck with cancer of the esophagus. *American Journal of Roentgenology*, 131(5), 791–794.

Greenlee, R. T., Murray, T., Bolden, S., & Wingo, P. A. (2000). Cancer statistics, 2000. CA: A *Cancer Journal for Clinicians*, 50(1): 7–33.

Harras, A. (Ed.). (1996). *Cancer: Rates and risks* (4th ed.). (NIH Publication No. 96-691). Bethesda, MD: National Institutes of Health, National Cancer Institute.

Helm, F. (1979). *Cancer dermatology* (pp. 48–49). Philadelphia: Lea and Feibiger.

Herskovic, A., Martz, K., al-Sarraf, M., Leichman, L., Brindle, J., Vaitkevicius, V., Cooper, J., Byhardt, R., Davis, L., & Emami, B. (1992). Combined chemotherapy and radiotherapy compared with radiotherapy alone in patients with cancer of the esophagus. *New England Journal of Medicine, 326*(24), 1593–1598.

Hesketh, P. J., Clapp, R. W., Doos, W. G. & Spechler, S. J. (1989). The increasing frequency of adenocarcinoma of the esophagus. *Cancer, 64*(2), 526–530.

Hiatt, R. A., Klatsky, A. L., & Armstrong, M. A. (1988). Pancreatic cancer, blood glucose and beverage consumption. *International Journal of Cancer, 41*(6), 794–797.

Hoffman, R., Welton, M. L., & Klencke, B. (1999). The significance of pretreatment CD4 count on the outcome and treatment tolerance of HIV-positive patients with anal cancer. *International Journal of Radiation Oncology, Biology, Physics, 44*(1), 127–131.

Hruban, R. H., Yeo, C. J., & Kern, S. E. (1999). Pancreatic cancer. In B. S. Kramer, J. K. Gohagan & P. C. Prorok (Eds.) *Cancer screening* (pp. 441–459). New York: Marcel Dekker.

Janes, R. H., Jr, Niederhuber, J. E., Chmiel, J. S., Winchester, D. P., Ocwieja, K. C., Karnell, J. H., Clive, R. E., & Menck, H. R. (1996). National patterns of care for pancreatic cancer. Results of a survey by the Commission on Cancer. *Annals of Surgery, 223*(3), 261–272.

Jentschura, D., Winkler, M., Strohmeier, N., Rumstadt, B., & Hagmuller, E. (1997). Quality-of-life after curative surgery for gastric cancer: A comparison between total gastrectomy and subtotal gastric resection. *Hepatogastroenterology, 44*(16), 1137–1142.

Jessup, J. M., Stewart, A. K., & Menck, H. R. (1998). The National Cancer Data Base report on patterns of care for adenocarcinoma of the rectum, 1985–1995. *Cancer, 83*(11), 2408–2418.

Jones, D. V. (1998). Chemotherapy for hepatocellular carcinoma. In S. A. Curley (Ed.), *Liver cancer* (pp. 53–68). New York: Springer-Verlag.

Keller, G., Grimm, V, Vogelsang, H., Bischoff, P., Mueller, J., Siewert, J. R., & Hofler, H. (1996). Analysis of microsatellite instability and mutations of the DNA mismatch repair gene hMLH1 in familial gastric cancer. *International Journal of Cancer, 68*(5), 571–576.

Landis, S. H., Murray, T., Bolden, S., & Wingo, P. A. (1998). Cancer statistics. *CA: Cancer Journal for Clinicians, 48*(1), 6–29.

Lillis-Hearne, P., & Castro, J. R. (1998). Pancreatic cancer. In S. A. Leibel & T. L. Phillips (Eds.), *Textbook of radiation oncology* (pp. 641–658). Philadelphia: W. B. Saunders.

Liver Cancer Study Group of Japan. (1990). Primary liver cancer in Japan: Clinicopathologic features and results of surgical treatment. *Annals of Surgery, 211*(3), 277–287.

Luman, W., Cull, A., & Palmer, K. R. (1997). Quality of life in patients stented for malignant biliary obstructions. *European Journal of Gastroenterology Hepatology, 9*(5), 481–484.

Marcy, P. Y., Chevallier, P., & Granon, C. (1999). Cost-benefit analysis of percutaneous interventional radiological procedures in cancer patients, *Supportive Care in Cancer, 7*(5), 635–637.

MacLennan, S. C. & Ryan, A. H. (1995). Colorectal cancer and oestrogen replacement therapy: A meta-analysis of epidemiologic studies. *Medical Journal of Australia, 162*(9), 491–493.

McCorkle, R., & Young, R. (1978). Development of a symptom distress scale. *Cancer Nursing, 1*(5), 373–378.

McLeod, R. S. (1999). Quality of life, nutritional status and gastrointestinal hormone profile following the Whipple procedure. *Annals of Oncology,* 10(Suppl. 4), 281–284.

McMillan, S. C., & Weitzner, M. (1998). Quality of life in cancer patients: Use of a revised hospice index. *Cancer Practice, 6*(5), 282–288.

McMahon, B. J., & London, T. (1991). Workshop on screening for hepatocellular carcinoma. *Journal of the National Cancer Institute, 83*(13), 916–919.

Mecklin, J. P. (1987). Frequency of hereditary nonpolyposis colorectal carcinoma. *Gastroenterology, 93*(5), 1021–1025.

Melbye, M., Rabkin, C., Frisch, M., & Biggar, R. J. (1994). Changing patterns of anal cancer incidence in the United States, 1940–1989. *American Journal of Epidemiology, 139*(8), 772–780.

Mendenhall, W. M., & Million, R. R. (1990). Esophageal cancer. In R. R. Dobelbower, Jr. (Ed.), *Gastrointestinal cancer radiation therapy* (pp. 73–97). Berlin: Springer-Verlag.

Micallef, J., Macquart-Moulin, G., Auquier, P., Seitz, J. F., & Moatti, J. P. (1998). Assessment of the quality of the life in the surgery of cancer of the esophagus: Critical review of the literature. *Bulletin du Cancer, 85*(7), 644–650.

Morton, D. G., & Fielding, J. W. (1998). Surgery for colonic cancer. In H. Bleiberg, P. Rougier, & H. J. Wilke (Eds.), *Management of colorectal cancer,* (pp. 79–92). St. Louis: Mosby.

Myerson, R. J., Karnell, L. H., & Menck, H. R. (1997). The National Cancer Data Base report on carcinoma of the anus. *Cancer, 80*(4), 805–815.

Nagorney, D. M., van Heerden, J. A., Ilstrup, D. M. & Adson, M. A. (1989). Primary hepatic malignancy: Surgical management and determinants of survival. *Surgery, 106*(4), 740–748.

Nagorney, D. M., & McPherson, G. A. D. (1988). Carcinoma of the gallbladder and extrahepatic bile ducts. *Seminars in Oncology, 15*(2), 106–115.

National Cancer Institute. (1999). *NCI Common Toxicity Criteria (CTC) Version 2 with the Radiation Therapy Oncology Group (RTOG) and European Organization for Research and Treatment of Cancer (EORTC) Acute Effects Criteria.* Bethesda, MD: National Cancer Institute.

National Cancer Institute. (1998). *Surveillance, epidemiology, and end results program, 1998.* Bethesda, MD: National Cancer Institute.

National Comprehensive Cancer Network. (1996). NCCN *practice guidelines for colorectal cancer. Oncology,* 10(Suppl. 11), 140–175.

National Comprehensive Cancer Network. (1998). NCCN *practice guidelines for upper gastrointestinal carcinomas. Oncology,* 12(11A), 179–223.

Offit, K. (1998). *Clinical cancer genetics* (pp. 210). New York: Wiley-Liss.

Oncology Nursing Society—Radiation Therapy Special Interest Group Documentation Project Core Committee. (1994). *Radiation Therapy Patient Care Record: A tool for documenting nursing care.* Pittsburgh, PA: Oncology Nursing Society.

Palefsky, J. M., Holly, E. A., Hogeboom, C. J., Berry, J. M., Jay, N., & Darragh, T. M. (1997). Anal cytology as a screening tool for anal squamous intraepithelial lesions. *Journal of Acquired Immune Deficiency Syndromes and Human Retrovirology,* 14(5), 415–422.

Palefsky, J. M., Holly, E. A., Ralston, M. L., Jay, N., Berry, J. M., & Darragh, T. M. (1998). High incidence of anal high-grade squamous intraepithelial lesions among HIV-positive and HIV-negative homosexual and bisexual men. *AIDS,* 12(5), 495–503.

Paquet, K. J., Koussouris, P., Mercado, M. A., Kalk, J. F., Muting, D., & Rambach, W. (1991). Limited hepatic resection for selected cirrhotic patients with hepatocellular or cholangiocellular carcinoma: A prospective study. *British Journal of Surgery,* 78(4), 459–462.

Parkin, D. M., & Pisani, P. (1999). Gastric cancer. In B. S. Kramer, J. K. Gohagan & P. C. Prorok (Eds.), *Cancer screening* (pp. 515–529). New York: Marcel Dekker.

Peipens, L. A., & Sandler, R. S. (1994). Epidemiology of colorectal adenomas. *Epidemiology Review,* 16(2), 273–297.

Phillips, T. L., Minsky, B. D., & Dicker, A. P. (1998). Cancer of the esophagus. In S. A. Leibel & T. L. Phillips (Eds.), *Textbook of radiation oncology* (pp. 601–623). Philadelphia: W. B. Saunders.

Piehler, J. M., & Crichlow, R. W. (1978). Primary carcinoma of the gallbladder. *Surgical Gynecology and Obstetrics,* 147(6), 929–942.

Pocard, M., Tiret, E., & Nugent, K. (1998). Results of salvage abdominoperineal resection for anal cancer after radiotherapy. *Diseases of the Colon and Rectum,* 41(12), 1488–1493.

Rabkin, C. S., Biggar, R. J., Melbye, M., & Curtis, R. E. (1992). Second primary cancers following anal and cervical carcinoma: Evidence of shared etiologic factors. *American Journal of Epidemiology,* 136(1), 54–58.

Reed, C. E. (1995). Cancer of the esophagus: Clinical presentation and stricture management. In J. A. Roth, J. C. Ruckdeschel, & T. H. Weisenburder (Eds.), *Thoracic oncology* 2nd ed., (pp. 356–367). Philadelphia: W. B. Saunders.

Ringe, B. Pichlmayr, R., Wittekind, C. & Tusch, G. (1991). Surgical treatment of hepatocellular carcinoma: Experience with liver resection and transplantation in 198 patients. *World Journal of Surgery,* 15(2), 270–285.

Schmier, J., Elixhauser, A., & Halpern, M. T. (1999). Health-related quality of life evaluations of gastric and pancreatic cancer. *Hepatogastroenterology,* 46(27), 1998–2004.

Schoenthaler, R. (1998). Hepatobiliary carcinomas. In S. A. Leibel & T. L. Phillips (Eds.), *Textbook of radiation oncology* (pp. 659–675). Philadelphia: W. B. Saunders.

Schwenk, W., Bohm, B., Haase, O., Junghans, T., & Muller, M. (1998). Laparoscopic versus conventional colorectal resection: A prospective randomized study of postoperative ileus and early postoperative feeding. *Langenbecks Archives of Surgery*, 383(1), 49–55.

Schwenk, W., Bohm, B., & Muller, J. M. (1998b). Postoperative pain and fatigue after laparoscopic or conventional colorectal resections. A prospective randomized trial. *Surgical Endoscopy*, 12(9), 1131–1136.

Smith, R. A., Mettlin, C. J., Johnston-Davis, K., & Eyre, H. (2000). American Cancer Society guidelines for early detection of cancer. CA: *Cancer Journal for Clinicians*, 50(1), 34–49.

Spangers, M. A., te Velde, A., & Aaronson, N. K. (1999). The construction and testing of the EORTC colorectal cancer-specific quality of life questionnaire module (QLQ-CR38). European Organization for Research and Treatment of Cancer Study Group on Quality of Life. *European Journal of Cancer*, 35(2), 238–247.

Sterkenburg, C. A. & Woodward, C. A. (1996). A reliability and validity study of the McMaster Quality of Life Scale (MQLS) for a palliative population. *Journal of Palliative Care*, 12(1), 18–25.

Strom, B. L., Soloway, R. D., Rios-Dalenz, J. L., Rodriguez-Martinez, H. A., West, S. L., Kinman, J. L., Polansky, M., & Berlin, I. A. (1995). Risk factors for gallbladder cancer. An international collaborative case-control study. *Cancer*, 76(10), 1747–1756.

Tremolda, F., Benevegnu, L., Drago, C., Casarin, C., Cechetto, A., Realdi, G., & Ruol, A. (1989). Early detection of hepatocellular carcinoma inpatients with cirrhosis by alphaprotein, ultrasound and fine-needle biopsy. *Hepatogastroenterology*, 36(6), 519–521.

Tsukuma, H., Hiyama, T., Tanaka, S., Nakao, M., Yabuuchi, T., Kitamura, T., Nakanishi, K., Fujimoto, I., Inoue, A., & Yamazaki, H., (1993). Risk factors for hepatocellular carcinoma among patients with chronic liver disease. *New England Journal of Medicine*, 328(25), 1797–1801.

UK Coordinating Committee on Cancer Research. (1996). Epidermoid anal cancer: Results from the UKCCCR randomized trial of radiotherapy alone versus radiotherapy, 5-fluorouracil, and mitomycin. UKCCCR Anal Cancer Trial Working Party. *Lancet*, 349(9046), 205–206.

Ward, W. L., Hahn, E. A., Mo, F., Hernandez, L., Tulsky, D. S., & Cella, D. (1999). Reliability and validity of the Functional Assessment of Cancer Therapy—Colorectal (FACT-C) quality of life instrument. *Quality of Life Research*, 8(3), 181–195.

Willett, C. G., Fung, C. Y., & Kaufman, D. S., Efird, J., & Shellito, P. C. (1993). Postoperative radiation for high-risk colon cancer. *Journal of Clinical Oncology*, 11(6), 1112–1117.

Wolmark, N., Rockette, H., Mamounas, E., Jones, J., Wieand, S., Wickerham, D. L., Bear, H. D., Atkins, J. N., Dimitrov, N. V., Glass, A. G., Fisher, E. R., Fisher, B. (1999). Clinical trial to assess the relative efficacy of fluorouracil and leucovorin, fluorouracil and levamisole, and fluorouracil, leucovorin, and levamisole in patients with Dukes' B and C carcinoma of the colon: Results from National Surgical Adjuvant Breast and Bowel Project C-04. *Journal of Clinical Oncology*, 17(11), 3553–3559.

Wu, C. W., Hsieh, M. C., Lo, S. S., Lui, W. Y. & P'eng, F. K. (1997). Quality of life of patients with gastric adenocarcinoma after curative gastrectomy. *World Journal of Surgery*, 21(7), 777–782.

Zhou, X. D., Tang, Z. Y., Yu, Y. Q., Weng, J. M., Ma., Z. C., Zhang, B. H., & Zheng, Y. X. (1993). The role of cryosurgery in the treatment of hepatic cancer: A report of 113 cases. *Journal of Cancer Research and Clinical Oncology*, 120(1–2), 100–102.

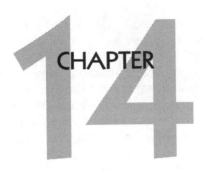

CHAPTER 14

BLADDER CANCER

Deborah Watkins Bruner
Mark Hurwitz

PROBLEM

Bladder cancer is the most common urinary tract malignancy with 53,200 new cases and 12,200 deaths predicted in 2000 (Greenlee, Murray, Bolden, & Wingo, 2000). Superficial bladder tumors (T_{is}, T_a, and T_1 lesions) account for approximately 70% to 80% of cases, with muscle-invading tumors accounting for the remainder. Bladder cancer constitutes almost 5% of all new cancer cases and approximately 2.2% of all cancer deaths. More than half of new cases occur in patients 70 years and older (Smart, 1990).

ASSESSMENT

PATHOLOGIC CLASSIFICATION

- ■ Approximately 92% of bladder cancers are transitional cell carcinomas, 6% are squamous cell carcinomas, and the remaining 2% include adenocarcinomas, sarcomas, lymphomas, and other rare variants.

RISK FACTORS/EPIDEMIOLOGY

- ■ Bladder cancer rarely occurs below the age of 40. The median age at diagnosis is 65 years (Scher et al., 1998).

- There is a men to women ratio of 4:1 (American Cancer Society, 1999). This difference is not accounted for in full by tobacco use or occupational exposure. Risk of death from bladder cancer may be significantly greater for women. It has been suggested that this may be due to the difference in the higher stage at diagnosis of women (Micheli, Mariotto, Rossi, Gatta, & Muti, 1998; van der Poel, Mungan, & Witjes, 1999).
- Race provides mixed outcomes. Although African Americans have a lower risk of developing bladder cancer, overall survival is worse compared with American Whites. Poorer survival has been attributed to the higher incidence of advanced disease at diagnosis (only 50% of Blacks have localized disease at diagnosis as compared with 72% for Whites) and poor follow-up (Smart, 1990). As with American Whites, African American women have poorer outcomes after bladder cancer than African American men (Hoke, Stone, Klein, & Williams, 1999).
- As with most cancers today, the relationship of genetic predisposition and bladder cancer is being studied most intensely. While several chromosomal abberations have been linked to bladder cancer, loss of all or part of chromosome 9 is the most common chromosomal abnormality noted (Knowles et al., 1994). A tumor suppressor locus involved in bladder cancer has been mapped to human chromosome 9q32–q33 and designated DBC1 (Nishiyama, Hornigold, Davies, & Knowles, 1999). The level of risk this confers is yet to be determined.
- The finding of high rates of transition cell carcinoma in various ethnic groups in association with other disease processes, such as with Balkan nephropathy, suggests a genetic link to the development of bladder cancer (Radovanovic, 1989).
- Smoking is the most important known risk factor for bladder cancer in both men and women, accounting for 47% and 37% of bladder cancer deaths, respectively (American Cancer Society, 1999). In one study, smoking of cigarettes was associated with an elevated relative risk (RR) of RR = 2.80 in males and RR = 5.33 in females as compared with nonsmokers. Factors like daily amount of smoked cigarettes, duration of smoking, age at beginning of cigarette smoking, and time since smoking cessation showed a clear dose- and time-response relationship in males but not in females (Pohlabeln, Jockel, & Bolm-Audorff, 1999).

■ It was estimated that the percentage of bladder cancers attributed to occupational exposure in the United States is 11% in women, compared with 21% in men (Micheli et al., 1998; van der Poel et al., 1999). Associations have been found among multiple occupations that involve a risk of chemical exposure to aromatic amines and dyes. However, numerous other occupational exposures have now been identified including the exposure to rubber workers, among others (Carel, Levitas-Langman, Kordysh, Goldsmith, & Friger, 1999; Carpenter & Roman, 1999). It has been suggested that risk estimates in major occupational groups have been distorted by approximately 10% when not adjusting for smoking. A statistically significant excess risk for bladder cancer has been found in 13 specific occupations and industries (Mannetje et al., 1999).

■ Dietary habits may also be an element in the development of bladder cancer. Diets high in cholesterol and fat have been associated with increased risk while vitamin A and carotene may be associated with decreased risk (Claude et al., 1986; Steineck, Hagman, Gerhardsson, & Norell, 1990). Epidemiologic studies of fruit and vegetable intake that may decrease bladder cancer risk have yielded inconsistent results, with regard to both types and amounts of fruits and vegetables required (Michaud et al., 1999). Phenacetin has been linked with increased risk of bladder cancer (Fokkens, 1979). Other analgesics including acetaminophen are not associated with increased risk (Piper, Tonascia, & Matanoski, 1985). Phenacetin is no longer available in the United States.

■ Squamous cell carcinoma of the bladder is associated with chronic irritation of the bladder mucosa. Chronic urinary tract infections including most notably *Shistosoma haematobium* (El-Bolkainy, Mokhtar, Ghoneim, & Hussein, 1981; Kantor et al., 1984) as well as chronic cystitis as a result of indwelling catheters and calculi all increase the risk of squamous cell carcinoma (Broecker, Klein, & Hackler, 1981).

SCREENING/DIAGNOSTIC TESTS AND STAGING

Presenting symptoms (in order of frequency) include:

■ Gross hematuria (70–80%)
■ Dysuria, frequency and/or urgency (30–50%)
■ Asymptomatic with microscopic hematuria (20%) (Epstein, 1991)

There are currently no standard recommendations for bladder cancer screening because of the low specificity and positive predictive value, which clinically manifests as a high false-positive rate, of current urinary tumor markers. However, several tests are under investigation including two urinary tumor markers, NMP22 and bladder tumor antigen (BTA), both used for the screening of transitional-cell carcinoma of the bladder as well as standard voided urine cytology.

- Several authors have reported that exclusion of the conditions that result in false-positive findings, such as benign inflammatory or infectious conditions, or renal or bladder calculi can increase the specificity and enhance the clinical usefulness of NMP22 and BTA stat tests (Sharma, Zippe, Pandrangi, Nelson, & Agarwal, 1999).
- Although still under investigation, one report suggests that the BTA test may be useful in the detection of recurrence in patients with bladder cancer who have been treated with definitive irradiation for bladder preservation (Crane, Clark, Bissonette, & Theodorescu, 1999).
- Other biomarkers for bladder cancer have been studied including p53, p27, p21, Ki-67, microvascular counts (factor VIII-related antigen), and DNA content/ploidy. A recent study by the National Cancer Institute Bladder Tumor Marker Network of 109 patients with primary transitional-cell cancer (stages T_2–T_3, grade 2 or higher) found no correlation with p53, Ki-67, microvascular counts, or DNA content/ploidy, with the finding of lymph node metastases at cystectomy in patients with muscle invasive, grade $\geq$ 2 bladder cancer (Lianes et al., 1998). Others have noted a positive correlation with survival for patients with T_2 tumors that were p53 negative who underwent bladder preservation (Herr & Donat, 1999).

Diagnostic tests include:

- History and physical including pelvic/rectal examination
- Laboratory studies including CBC, chemistries, liver function tests, urinalysis, and urine cytology
- Radiographic studies include intravenous pyelography, retrograde pyelogram as indicated, CT of the abdomen and pelvis, chest x-ray, and bone scan as indicated
- Cystoscopy and biopsy with bimanual exam performed under anesthesia and transurethral resection performed as indicated
- The AJCC staging system is presented in Table 14–1

TABLE 14-1   TNM STAGING OF URINARY BLADDER

Primary Tumor (T)

T_x	Primary tumor cannot be assessed
T_0	No evidence of primary tumor
T_a	Noninvasive papillary carcinoma
T_{is}	Carcinoma in situ "flat tumor"
T_1	Tumor invades subepithelial connective tissue
T_2	Tumor invades muscle
T_{2a}	Tumor invades superfisial muscle (inner half)
T_{2b}	Tumor invades deep muscle (outer half)
T_3	Tumor invades perivesical tissue
T_{3a}	microscopically
T_{3b}	macroscopically (extravesical mass)
T_4	Tumor invades any of the following: prostate, uterus, vagina, pelvic wall, abdominal wall
T_{4a}	Tumor invades prostate, uterus, vagina
T_{4b}	Tumor invades pelvic wall, abdominal wall

Stage Grouping

Stage 0	T_a	N_0	M_0
Stage 0_{is}	T_{is}	N_0	M_0
Stage I	T_1	N_0	M_0
Stage II	T_{2a}	N_0	M_0
	T_{2b}	N_{2b}	M_0
Stage III	T_{3a}	N_0	M_0
	T_{3b}	N_0	M_0
	T_{4c}	N_0	M_0
Stage IV	T_{4b}	N_0	M_0
	Any T	N_1	M_0
	Any T	N_2	M_0
	Any T	N_3	M_0
	Any T	Any N	M_1

From the AJCC *Cancer Staging Manual* (5th ed.). Copyright 1997 by Lippincott-Raven. Adapted with permission of the publisher.

OUTCOMES MANAGEMENT

SUPERFICIAL BLADDER CANCER

Superficial bladder cancer is a heterogeneous group of preinvasive or minimally invasive tumors including T_a, T_{is}, and T_1 tumors. Five-year survival ranges from greater than 95% for low-grade papillary tumors to 50% for high-grade T_1 lesions. Likewise, recurrence rates after local therapy also vary widely and as such patients with superficial bladder cancers require rigorous follow-up. For patients with multiply recurrent superficial disease, radical cystectomy may be indicated. Radiation therapy has virtually no role in treatment of preinvasive disease except the rare instance in which palliation is required in nonsurgical candidates following failure of standard treatment modalities.

■ For superficial, low-grade lesions transurethral resection is usually the treatment of choice in combination with intravesical chemotherapy or immunotherapy. The low systemic availability of most intravesical agents is consistent with the low frequency of acute and delayed systemic adverse effects, except in the case of thiotepa in which local toxicity is transient and tolerable (Highley, Van Oosterom, Maes, & De Bruijn, 1999).

■ The effectiveness of intravesical therapy with bacillus Calmette-Guerin (BCG) for the treatment of carcinoma in situ of the bladder and for prophylaxis of tumor recurrence in superficial bladder cancer has been well established (Alexandroff, Jackson, O'Donnell, & James, 1999). To enhance the efficacy of BCG, several cytokines have been investigated including interferon, interleukin-2, and keyhole limpet hemocyanin, but there is of yet no firmly standardized role for use of these agents (Schnitz-Drager & Muller, 1998).

■ Other intravesical drug agents used in the treatment of superficial bladder cancer are mitomycin C, thiotepa, anthracyclines such as doxorubicin, and, more recently, taxol (Gan, Wientjes, Badalament, & Au, 1996).

■ Photodynamic therapy has also been used.

INVASIVE DISEASE

Radical cystectomy is the most proven local treatment for muscle-invading bladder cancer, but it is associated with significant morbidity. In men this procedure includes the removal of the prostate, seminal vesicles, proximal vas deferens, and at least the proximal portion of the urethra. In women, the uterus, fallopian tubes, ovaries, anterior vaginal wall, and urethra are excised. Lymphadenectomy is usually performed also.

■ Innovations in surgical techniques now allow for continent diversions in a majority of patients. Continent diversions may include stomal reservoirs such as the Kock pouch (Kock, Nilson, Nilsson, Norlen, & Philipson, 1982) requiring periodic catheterization or anastomosis of the reservoir directly to the male urethra employing the external sphincter to achieve continence. Voiding is accomplished by abdominal straining (Kock, Ghoneim, Lycke, & Mahran, 1989). With this technique daytime continence of greater than 90% and nighttime continence of about 75% can be achieved (Ghoneim, Shaaban, Mahran, & Kock, 1992; Skinner, Boyd, Lieskovsky, Bennett, & Hopwood, 1991). Differences in tumor extent, patient age, performance status, renal and mental function, and acceptance make different diversion techniques necessary (Turner & Studer, 1997).

The propensity for distant spread despite local treatment combined with the potential complications of surgery and the impact on quality of life, all foster debate about the indications for cystectomy (Turner & Studer, 1997). Organ preservation with aggressive combined radiochemotherapy has been used in an attempt to improve clinical and quality-of-life outcomes.

Organ preservation with a combination of transurethral resection of bladder tumor (TURBT), radiation, and chemotherapy can be achieved in selected patients with overall survival comparable to similarly staged patients undergoing radical prostatectomy. A discussion of studies concerning the importance of bladder preservation follows:

■ In a key study establishing the efficacy of bladder preservation, 53 consecutive patients with muscle-invading bladder cancer (stages T_2 through T_4, N_xM_0) were treated with transurethral surgery followed by two cycles of MCV (methotrexate, cisplatin, and vinblastine), and then radiation (40 Gy) with concurrent cisplatin administration. Patients who had complete responses received additional chemotherapy and radiotherapy (64.8 Gy). With median follow-up of 48 months, 45% were alive and free of detectable tumor. In 58% the bladder was free of invasive tumor and functioning well. Of the 28 patients who had complete responses after initial treatment, 89% had functioning tumor-free bladders (Kaufman et al., 1993).

■ A recently reported phase III study of bladder preservation with or without neoadjuvant TURBT has revealed no advantage to the use of MCV before radiation with concurrent cisplatin. Overall survival was comparable to historical surgical series. The decreased toxicity resulting from exclusion of MCV may lead to bladder preservation in a greater number of patients (Shipley et al., 1998).

■ A National Cancer Institute of Canada (NCIC) study as well as a European study has confirmed the importance of cisplatin in combination with radiation therapy in both the preoperative and definitve settings. Concurrent cisplatin administration was associated with increased complete response and decreased risk of local recurrence. While the Ehrlangen study demonstrated improved survival with concurrent cisplatin, the NCIC study revealed no impact on distant metastases or overall survival (Coppin et al., 1996; Sauer et al., 1998).

■ Evidence of hydronephrosis is a contraindication to bladder preservation (Kaufman et al., 1993). In addition, patients undergoing bladder preservation should have a complete response on second-look cystoscopy following moderate dose radiation (approximately 40 Gy) and chemotherapy, otherwise cystectomy should be considered.

■ Close follow-up of patients undergoing bladder preservation is required as 20% to 30% will develop superficial recurrences amenable to transurethral resection of bladder tumor TURBT with or without intravesical therapy. A smaller number of patients may experience an invasive recurrence (Kachnic et al., 1997).

■ Radiation therapy as single modality therapy is indicated for patients medically unsuitable for cystectomy and chemotherapy. Local control rates of 25% to 45% have been obtained with total dose of approximately 65 Gy (Duncon & Quilty, 1986; Gospodarowicz et al., 1989; Mameghan, Fisher, Mameghan, & Brook, 1995; Moonen et al., 1998). Hyperfractionation may result in increased complete response and enhanced survival with acceptable toxicity (Naslund, Nilsson, & Littbrand, 1994). Interstitial brachytherapy has also been used in Europe with encouraging results (Rozan et al., 1992; Wijnmaalen et al., 1997).

■ Guidelines for the appropriate type and timing of bladder cancer therapies for initial and salvage treatments are further delineated in the NCCN oncology practice guidelines (Scher et al., 1998).

SIDE EFFECTS

Several recent studies have evaluated the acute toxicity of simultaneous radiochemotherapy for bladder cancer.

■ Patients treated with transurethral resection followed by cisplatin with or without 5-FU plus radiation therapy to the pelvis have reported dysuria and gastrointestinal symptoms including diarrhea and rectal tenesmus.

■ Hematological toxicity following chemotherapy has commonly included leukopenia and thrombocytopenia.

■ In most cases the acute side effects of radiochemotherapy are tolerable and can be managed by supportive care (Birkenhake, Leykamm, Martus, & Sauer, 1999; Saracino et al., 1998).

■ Acute cystitis including pain with urination, urinary frequency, and urgency have been reported in 23% to 80% of patients receiving pelvic radiation (Marks, Carroll, Dugan, & Anscher, 1995). Acute symptoms after radiation therapy usually subside about 2 weeks after therapy.

■ Chronic cystitis, continuing 6 months after therapy, is dose dependent. Bladder contraction or hemorrhagic cystitis may occur in less than 5% of patients treated to 50 Gy, 15% of patients treated to 70 Gy, and in over 50% of patients treated above 70 Gy (Epstein, 1991).

■ Bladder preservation results in good long-term organ function for a majority of patients. A series from Ehrlangen indicated that only 3 of 192 (1.6%) required cystectomy for bladder shrinkage (Sauer et al., 1998). At Massachusetts General Hospital a total of 106 patients received chemoradiotherapy. Seventy-one patients had preserved bladders with median follow-up of 59 months with no cystectomies required (Kachnic et al., 1997). Another review of patients treated with definitive radiation therapy ($\geq$ 50 Gy) for bladder cancer and surviving 10 years found 68% to have well-functioning bladders and 10% with contracted bladders, 4% of which required cystectomy (Goodman, Hislop, Elwood, & Balfour, 1981).

■ Salvage cystectomy is more difficult than primary cystectomy but can be performed with acceptable complications. In one report, the records of 69 patients who had undergone postradiation salvage cystectomy for bladder cancer were reviewed, looking specifically at surgical complications. There were three postoperative deaths (5%), three pulmonary emboli, and three fistulae—with some overlap of complications. Five patients who underwent cystectomy for intractable symptoms in the apparent absence of recurrent tumor were found to have residual cancer in the excised specimens (Lynch, Jenkins, Fowler, Hope-Stone, & Blandy, 1992).

To improve the management and outcomes of bladder cancer a combination of medical and behavioral interventions are required (Bruner, Bucholtz, Iwamoto, & Strohl, 1998). Cystitis can be treated medically with an oral analgesic phenazopyridine hydrochloride (100–200 mg tid), which causes the patient's urine to turn red/orange in color. Oxybutynin chloride (5 mg tid) and flavoxate hydrochloride (100–200 mg tid-qid) are antispasmodics that are useful in relieving urinary urgency and frequency (Marks et al., 1995).

- The risk of developing chronic cystitis can be diminished if the administration of radiation can be held until 4 to 6 weeks following transurethral resection. Catheterization should be avoided or minimized when possible (Epstein, 1991).
- Behavior modification with increased fluid intake of 3 liters per day of water or cranberry juice, and decreased intake of caffeine may help minimize the risk of cystitis or minimize symptoms when it does occur (Bruner et al., 1998).

OUTCOMES MEASURES

Urinary outcomes should include assessment of frequency, urgency, dysuria, nocturia, obstructive symptoms, and urge or stress incontinence (Bruner et al., 1998). Urinalysis and urine cultures should be done for fever, pain, hematuria, or cloudy urine. Instruments that measure the impact these symptoms have on quality of life include:

- Functional Alterations due to Changes in Elimination (FACE) is an experimental instrument being piloted in two National Cancer Clinical Trial Groups: the Radiation Therapy Oncology Group (RTOG), and the Gynecologic Oncology Group (GOG). FACE is an expansion of CUF (Changes in Urinary Function) developed by Bruner et al. (1994). CUF was developed specifically to assess symptoms related to prostate and bladder cancer therapies and their impact on quality of life. FACE is a 15-item, Likert-type, self-rating scale divided into two subscales, one assessing urinary function and one assessing bowel function. The questionnaire was designed to measure the construct of intrusion on daily functioning caused by changes in elimination as measured by these two subscales. Dimensions of intrusion include control, fear, anxiety, sexual activity/body image, and incontinence.

■ American Urologic Association (AUA) Symptom Problem Index (SPI)/Benign Prostatic Hyperplasia Impact Index (BPHII). The SPI is a 7-item, Likert-type scale designed to assess the difficulty patients experience with their urinary symptoms. The BPHII is a 4-item scale that measures how much their urinary symptoms affect various domains of health including discomfort, worry, distress, and daily activities. Both indices have demonstrated acceptable reliability and validity in patients with prostate cancer and may be useful in assessing the QOL impact of bladder cancer therapies (Barry et al., 1995).

■ Several authors have developed self-administered questionnaires for assessing quality of life after treatment for bladder cancer. Caffo and colleagues developed a questionnaire for patients who were treated either with a conservative approach based on radiotherapy with or without chemotherapy, or with cystectomy followed by urostomy. The questionnaire demonstrated acceptable psychometric properties. The items were grouped into seven subscales reflecting different QOL domains (Caffo, Fellin, Graffer, & Luciani, 1996). In addition, Biermann and colleagues developed a QOL questionnaire for bladder cancer surgery (Biermann, Schmidt, & Kuchler, 1995).

■ Measures of sexual function are discussed in Chapter 16, "Prostate Cancer," and include The Sexual Adjustment Questionnaire (SAQ).

■ Additional outcomes that impact QOL after bladder cancer therapy such as fatigue or anxiety can be measured with symptom checklists or with measures that incorporate the multidimensional outcomes of interest. One such example is the Functional Assessment Cancer Therapy-Bladder (FACT-Bl).

  • FACT-Bl developed by Cella et al. (1993) is an instrument designed to assess the multidimensional aspects of QOL including physical well-being, social/family well-being, emotional well-being, functional well-being, treatment satisfaction, and specific concerns of bladder cancer. The 27 core items of the questionnaire were tested for validity and reliability and the total score correlated highly with other measures of aspects of quality of life. FACT-Bl includes 13 "Additional Concerns" developed to address specific symptoms of bladder cancer that may impact quality of life.

EXPECTED OUTCOMES

■ An analysis of published data from three institutions and two prospective trials conducted by the RTOG of combined modality therapy for patients with muscle-invading bladder cancer using selective bladder preservation or cystectomy was recently reported (Shipley, Kaufman, Heney, Althausen, & Zietman, 1999). The analysis indicated that the overall 5-year survival rates were comparable to other series of immediate cystectomy. Of patients treated with the bladder-preserving approach of transurethral resection, radiation therapy, and concurrent chemotherapy followed by either bladder conservation with surveillance for complete responders, or prompt cystectomy in those whose tumors persisted after induction therapy, 20% to 30% cured of muscle invading cancer were found to have subsequently developed a new superficial tumor. Intravesical drug therapy has demonstrated efficacy in the treatment of these superficial tumors, however, radiochemotherapy has the potential for acute morbidity. The authors suggested that based on this data the ideal candidate for bladder preservation has primary clinical stage T_2 tumor, no associated ureteral obstruction, visibly complete transurethral resection, and complete response after induction radiochemotherapy based on endoscopic evaluation including rebiopsy and cytology (Shipley et al., 1999).

■ In another recent study on postradiochemotherapy, restaging transurethral resection of the bladder resulted in 88% complete remissions, and 8% were nonresponders. After a median follow-up of 38 months, 80% of patients were alive (Birkenhake et al., 1999).

Five-year actuarial survival after treatment for bladder cancer:

■ For T_2 and T_3 bladder cancer treated with combination radiochemotherapy the results at 5 years in the RTOG 89-03 series was 49% regardless of whether neoadjuvant MCV was used or not (Shipley et al., 1998). These results are similar to other series (Kachnic et al., 1997; Sauer et al., 1998).

■ Overall survival has improved by more than 45% since the 1950s within each stage. The relative 5-year survival rates for American Whites versus African Americans are overall, 81% versus 58%; for localized disease, 88% versus 74%; for regional disease, 44% versus 30%; for distant disease, 9% versus 8%; and for unknown stage, 61% versus 35% (Smart, 1990).

QUALITY OF LIFE

Quality-of-life outcome studies after treatment for bladder cancer have focused mainly on acute and chronic cystitis, although other symptoms are recognized to impact QOL including sexual dysfunction, diarrhea, proctitis, and fatigue.

■ In a study comparing the quality of life of patients receiving preoperative radiation therapy (40 Gy) and cystectomy with radical radiation therapy (60 Gy) and salvage cystectomy, there were no consistent differences between the two treatment groups. At 6 months after treatment, patients treated with radical radiation therapy and salvage cystectomy expressed a slightly more pessimistic outlook than patients treated with preoperative irradiation and cystectomy. There was no such difference at 12 to 18 months, but the latter group reported the largest reduction of social (sports, hobbies, etc.) and sexual activities (Mommsen, Jakobsen, & Sell, 1989).

■ The quality of life in 72 patients with bladder cancer who had shown a complete response to radiation therapy, using a modified bladder symptom score and the Nottingham health profile, was compared with the quality of life in a similar control group matched for age and sex. There was no significant difference in either group in the domains assessed (Lynch et al., 1992).

■ One study compared the adjustments reported by male patients with ileal conduits and the problems related to management and body image with the more recent neobladder replacements developed in an effort to return the body to its more natural structure and function. The analysis indicated no statistically significant differences in sickness impact

scores between the ileal conduit (12 patients) and neobladder (11 patients) groups who responded to a questionnaire.
Few patients with ileal conduits reported problems with the
device as compared with all of the patients with neobladders
who reported some continued incontinence primarily at
night. This was in contrast to previous reports by Kock et al.
(1989) and Skinner et al. (1991). However, the patients with
ileal conduits reported impact on their social activities more
frequently. All of the patients, regardless of the type of urinary diversion, reported erectile dysfunction (Raleigh, Berry,
& Montie, 1995).

■ In contrast, another study assessing the quality of life in patients with continent urinary diversions after cystectomy
found an acceptable rate of complications, with stone formation and urinary tract infection as the most common
morbidities. Continence was rated as good in most patients,
with no patient reporting complete incontinence. Urinary
symptoms were reported by less than 20% of the patients.
Although there was a significant effect on sex life, the overall quality of life appeared to be very good because 70% of
the patients had no limitations to their activities (Sullivan,
Chow, Ko, Wright, & McLoughlin, 1998).

■ In a retrospective study conducted by mail of patients with
invasive bladder cancer treated either with a conservative
radiation therapy approach (with or without chemotherapy),
or with cystectomy followed by urostomy, group differences
were reported in QOL adjustment. QOL after cystectomy,
marked by stoma presence, was reduced by a lack of sexual
activity and a worsened physical condition, but social and
recreational life was little affected. Conversely, a low incidence of urinary symptoms and acceptable physical, psychologic, social, and sexual adjustments were found in the
radiation therapy group. QOL in the radiation therapy group
was consistently better than in the cystectomy group (Caffo
et al., 1996).

Impotence, although a recognized outcome of combined radiochemotherapy for bladder cancer, has not been well studied.

■ In a rare study to assess sexual function in men before and
after radiation therapy for bladder cancer, patients were
queried using an anonymous questionnaire regarding libido, frequency of sexual function, erectile capacity, orgasm,

and ejaculation in the 6 months prior to radiation therapy and following treatment. Serum testosterone was measured in 10 patients. Seventy-one percent felt their sex life was worse following radiation therapy, but only 56% were concerned about the deterioration. Testosterone levels were normal in all but one patient (Little & Howard, 1998).

■ In comparison, a similar study was carried out to compare the postoperative sexual adjustment problems in men after cystectomy and using the urethral Kock reservoir or the ileocecal reservoir. Of the 76 men who completed the questionnaire, 82% reported they were able to achieve an erection preoperatively, whereas only 9% of all patients could achieve an erection at least every second time postoperatively. Thirty-eight percent of all patients were able to achieve orgasm and 26% were coitally active to some degree. Reasons for decrease or cessation of coitus were loss of potency among 77% of those with bladder substitution, and 96% among those with an ileal conduit diversion, respectively. Other reasons reported for sexual inactivity included decreased libido (29%), partner refusal (13%), and feeling less sexually attractive (20%). No differences between groups were shown. The type of operation did not influence sexual outcomes, however age above 68 years influenced orgasmic ability and coital activity (Bjerre, Johansen, & Steven, 1998).

REFERENCES

Alexandroff, A. B., Jackson, A. M., O'Donnell, M. A., & James, K. (1999). BCG immunotherapy of bladder cancer:20 years on. *Lancet*, 353(9165), 1689–1694.

American Cancer Society. (1999). *Cancer facts and figures*. New York: American Cancer Society.

Barry, M., Fowler, F., O'Leary, M., Bruskewitz, R., Holtgrewe, H., Mebust, W., & American Urologic Association. (1995). Measuring disease-specific health status in men with benign prostatic hyperplasia. *Medical Care*, 33 (Suppl. 4), AS145–AS155.

Biermann, C. W., Schmidt, C., & Kuchler, T. (1995). Development of a life quality questionnaire in bladder cancer surgery. *British Journal of Urology*, 76(3), 412–413.

Birkenhake, S., Leykamm, S., Martus, P., & Sauer, R. (1999). Concomitant radiochemotherapy with 5-FU and cisplatin for invasive bladder cancer. Acute toxicity and first results. *Strahlentherapie und Onkologie*, 175(3), 97–101.

Bjerre, B. D., Johansen, C., & Steven, K. (1998). Sexological problems after cystectomy: Bladder substitution compared with ileal conduit diversion. A questionnaire study of male patients. *Scandinavian Journal of Urology and Nephrology, 32*(3), 187–193.

Broecker, B. H., Klein, F. A., & Hackler, R. H. (1981). Cancer of the bladder in spinal cord injury patients. *Journal of Urology, 125*(2), 196–197.

Bruner, D. W., Bucholtz, J., Iwamoto, R., & Strohl, R. (1998). *Manual for radiation oncology nursing practice and education* (2nd ed.). Pittsburgh, PA: Oncology Nursing Press.

Bruner, D. W., Scott, C., Byhardt, R., Coughlin, C., Friedland, J., & DelRowe, J. (1994). *Changes in Urinary Function (CUF): Pilot data on the development and validation of a measure of the intrusion of quality of life caused by changes in urinary function after cancer therapy.* Paper presented at the Drug Information Association 2nd Symposium on Quality of Life Evaluation, Charleston, SC.

Caffo, O., Fellin, G., Graffer, U., & Luciani, L. (1996). Assessment of quality of life after cystectomy or conservative therapy for patients with infiltrating bladder carcinoma. A survey by a self-administered questionnaire. *Cancer, 78*(5), 1089–1097.

Carel, R., Levitas-Langman, A., Kordysh, E., Goldsmith, J., & Friger, M. (1999). Case-referent study on occupational risk factors for bladder cancer in southern Israel. *International Archives of Occupational and Environmental Health, 72*(5), 304–308.

Carpenter, L., & Roman, E. (1999). Cancer and occupation in women: Identifying associations using routinely collected national data. *Environmental Health Perspectives, 107*(Suppl. 2), 299–303.

Cella, D. F., Tulsky, D., Gray, G., Sarafian, B., Linn, E., Bonomi, A., Silberman, M., Yellen, S., Winicour, P., Brannon, J., Eckberg, K., Lloyd, S., Purl, S., Blendowski, L., Goodman, M., Barnicle, M., Stewart, I., McHall, M., Bonomi, P., Kaplan, E., Taylor, S., IV, Thomas, C., Jr., & Harris, J. (1993). The Functional Assessment Cancer Therapy Scale: Development and validation of the general measure. *Clinical Oncology, 11,* 570–579.

Claude, J., Kunze, E., Frentzel-Beyme, R., Paczkowski, K., Schneider, J., & Schubert, H. (1986). Life-style and occupational risk factors in cancer of the lower urinary tract. *American Journal of Epidemiology, 124*(4), 578–589.

Coppin, C. M., Gospodarowicz, M. K., James, K., Tannock, I. F., Zee, B., Carson, J., Pater, J., & Sullivan, L. D. (1996). Improved local control of invasive bladder cancer by concurrent cisplatin and preoperative or definitive radiation. The National Cancer Institute of Canada Clinical Trials Group. *Journal of Clinical Oncology, 14*(11), 2901–2907.

Crane, C. H., Clark, M. M., Bissonette, E. A., & Theodorescu, D. (1999). Prospective evaluation of the effect of ionizing radiation on the bladder tumor-associated (BTA) urine test. *International Journal of Radiation Oncology, Biology, Physics, 43*(1), 73–77.

Duncon, W., & Quilty, P. M. (1986). The results of a series of 963 patients with transitional cell carcinoma of the urinary bladder primarily treated by radical megavoltage x-ray therapy. *Radiotherapy Oncology*, 7(4), 299–310.

El-Bolkainy, M. N., Mokhtar, N. M., Ghoneim, M. A., & Hussein, M. H. (1981). The impact of schistosomiasis on the pathology of bladder carcinoma. *Cancer*, 48(12), 2643–2648.

Epstein, B. (1991). Genitourinary cancer. In L. Coia & D. Moylan (Eds.), *Introduction to clinical radiation oncology* (pp. 299–332). Madison, WI: Medical Physics Publishing.

Fokkens, W. (1979). Phenacetin abuse related to bladder cancer. *Environmental Research*, 20(1), 192–198.

Gan, Y., Wientjes, M. G., Badalament, R. A., & Au, J. L. (1996). Pharmacodynamics of doxorubicin in human bladder tumors. *Clinical Cancer Research*, 2(8), 1275–1283.

Ghoneim, M. A., Shaaban, A. A., Mahran, M. R., & Kock, N. G. (1992). Further experience with the urethral Kock pouch. *Journal of Urology*, 147(2), 361–365.

Goodman, G. B., Hislop, T. G., Elwood, J. M., & Balfour, J. (1981). Conservation of bladder function in patients with invasive bladder cancer treated by definitive irradiation and selective cystectomy. *International Journal of Radiation Oncology, Biology, and Physics*, 7, 569–573.

Gospodarowicz, M. K., Hawkins, N. B., Rawlings, G. A., Connolly, J. G., Jewett, M. A., Thomas, G. M., Herman, J. G., Garrett, P. G., Chua, T., & Juncan, W. (1989). Radical radiotherapy for muscle invasive transitional cell carcinoma of the bladder: Failure analysis. *Journal of Urology*, 142(6), 1448–1453.

Greenlee, T. R., Murray, T., Bolden, S., & Wingo, A. P. (2000). Cancer Statistics, 2000. *Journal of the American Cancer Society*, 50(1), 7–33.

Herr, H. W., & Donat, S. M. (1999). Prostatic tumor relapse in patients with superficial bladder tumors: 15-year outcome. *Journal of Urology*, 161(6), 1854–1857.

Highley, M. S., Van Oosterom, A. T., Maes, R. A., & De Bruijn, E. A. (1999). Intravesical drug delivery. Pharmacokinetic and clinical considerations. *Clinical Pharmacokinetics*, 37(1), 59–73.

Hoke, G. P., Stone, B. A., Klein, L., & Williams, L. (1999). The influence of gender on incidence and outcome of patients with bladder cancer in Harlem. *Journal of the National Medical Association*, 91(3), 144–148.

Kachnic, L. A., Kaufman, D. S., Heney, N. M., Althausen, A. F., Griffin, P. P., Zietman, A. L., & Shipley, W. U. (1997). Bladder preservation by combined modality therapy for invasive bladder cancer. *Journal of Clinical Oncology*, 15(3), 1022–1029.

Kantor, A. F., Hartge, P., Hoover, R. N., Narayana, A. S., Sullivan, J. W., & Fraumeni, J. F., Jr. (1984). Urinary tract infection and risk of bladder cancer. *American Journal of Epidemiology*, 119(4), 510–515.

Kaufman, D. S., Shipley, W. U., Griffin, P. P., Heney, N. M., Althausen, A. F., & Efird, J. T. (1993). Selective bladder preservation by combination treatment of invasive bladder cancer. *New England Journal of Medicine,* 329(19), 1377–1382.

Knowles, M. A., Elder, P. A., Williamson, M., Cairns, J. P., Shaw, M. E., & Law, M. G. (1994). Allelotype of human bladder cancer. *Cancer Research,* 54(2), 531–538.

Kock, N. G., Ghoneim, M. A., Lycke, K. G., & Mahran, M. R. (1989). Replacement of the bladder by the urethral Kock pouch: Functional results, urodynamics and radiological features. *Journal of Urology,* 141(5), 1111–1116.

Kock, N. G., Nilson, A. E., Nilsson, L. O., Norlen, L. J., & Philipson, B. M. (1982). Urinary diversion via a continent ileal reservoir: Clinical results in 12 patients. *Journal of Urology,* 1128(3), 469–475.

Lianes, P., Charytonowicz, E., Cordon-Cardo, C., Fradet, Y., Grossman, H. B., Hemstreet, G. P., Waldman, F. M., Chew, K., Wheeless, L. L., & Faraggi, D. (1998). Biomarker study of primary nonmetastatic versus metastatic invasive bladder cancer. National Cancer Institute Bladder Tumor Marker Network. *Clinical Cancer Research,* 4(5), 1267–1271.

Little, F. A., & Howard, G. C. (1998). Sexual function following radical radiotherapy for bladder cancer. *Radiotherapy and Oncology,* 49(2), 157–161

Lynch, W. J., Jenkins, B. J., Fowler, C. G., Hope-Stone, H. F., & Blandy, J. P. (1992). The quality of life after radical radiotherapy for bladder cancer. *British Journal of Urology,* 70(5), 519–521.

Mameghan, H., Fisher, R., Mameghan, J., & Brook, S. (1995). Analysis of failure following definitive radiotherapy for invasive transitional cell carcinoma of the bladder. *International Journal of Radiation Oncology, Biology, Physics,* 31(2), 247–254.

Mannetje, A., Kogevinas, M., Chang-Claude, J., Cordier, S., Gonzalez, C. A., Hours, M., Jockel, K. H., Bolm-Audorff, U., Lynge, E., Porru, S., Donato, F., Ranft, U., Serra, C., Tzonou, A., Vineis, P., Wahrendorf, J., & Boffetta, P. (1999). Smoking as a confounder in case-control studies of occupational bladder cancer in women. *American Journal of Industrial Medicine,* 36(1), 75–82.

Marks, L. B., Carroll, P. R., Dugan, T. C., & Anscher, M. S. (1995). The response of the urinary bladder, urethra, and ureter to radiation and chemotherapy. *International Journal of Radiation Oncology, Biology, Physics,* 31(5), 1257–1280.

Michaud, D. S., Speigelman, D., Clinton, S. K., Rimm, E. B., Willett, W. C., & Giovannucci, E. L. (1999). Fruit and vegetable intake and incidence of bladder cancer in a male prospective cohort. *Journal of the National Cancer Institute,* 91(7), 605–613.

Micheli, A., Mariotto, A., Rossi, A. G., Gatta, G., & Muti, P. (1998). The prognostic role of gender in survival of adult cancer patients. EUROCARE Working Group. *European Journal of Cancer,* 34(14), (Spec No. 14) 2271–278.

Mommsen, S., Jakobsen, A., & Sell, A. (1989). Quality of life in patients with advanced bladder cancer. A randomized study comparing cystectomy and irradiation—the Danish Bladder Cancer Study Group (DAVECA protocol 8201). *Scandinavian Journal of Urology and Nephrology Supplement*, 125, 115–120.

Moonen, L., v d Voet, H., de Nijs, R., Hart, A. A., Horenblas, S., & Bartelink, H. (1998). Muscle-invasive bladder cancer treated with external beam radiotherapy: Pretreatment prognostic factors and the predictive value of cystoscopic reevaluation during treatment. *Radiotherapy Oncology*, 49(2), 149–155.

Naslund, I., Nilsson, B., & Littbrand, B. (1994). Hyperfractionated radiotherapy of bladder cancer. A ten-year follow-up of a randomized clinical trial. *ACTA Oncologica*, 33(4), 397–402.

Nishiyama, H., Hornigold, N., Davies, A. M., & Knowles, M. A. (1999). A sequence-ready 840-kb PAC contig spanning the candidate tumor suppressor locus DBC1 on human chromosome 9q32–q33. *Genomics*, 59(3), 335–338.

Piper, J. M., Tonascia, J., & Matanoski, G. M. (1985). Heavy phenacetin use and bladder cancer in women aged 20–49 years. *New England Journal of Medicine*, 313(5), 292–295.

Pohlabeln, H., Jockel, K. H., & Bolm-Audorff, U. (1999). Non-occupational risk factors for cancer of the lower urinary tract in Germany. *European Journal of Epidemiology*, 15(5), 411–419.

Radovanovic, Z. (1989). Aetiology of Balkan nephropathy: A reapprasisal after 30 years. *European Journal of Epidemiology*, 5(3), 372–377.

Raleigh, E. D., Berry, M., & Montie, J. E. (1995). A comparison of adjustments to urinary diversions: A pilot study. *Journal of Wound Ostomy Continence Nursing*, 22(1), 58–63.

Rozan, R., Albuisson, E., Donnarieix, D., Giraud, B., Mazeron, J. J., Gerard, J. P., Pernot, M., Gerbaulet, A., Baillet, F., & Douchez, J. (1992). Interstitial iridium-192 for bladder cancer (a multicentric survey: 205 patients). *International Journal of Radiation Oncology, Biology, Physics*, 24(3), 469–477.

Saracino, B., Arcangeli, G., Mecozzi, A., Tirindelli Danesi, D., Cruciani, E., Altavista, P., & Giannarelli, D. (1998). Combined hyperfractionated radiotherapy and protracted infusion chemotherapy in bladder cancer for organ preservation. *Clinical Therapeutics*, 49(3), 183–189.

Sauer, R., Birkenhake, S., Kuhn, R., Witekind, C., Schrott, K. M., & Martus, P. (1998). Efficacy of radiochemotherapy with latin derivatives compared to radiotherapy alone in organ-sparing treatment of bladder cancer. *International Journal of Radiation Oncology, Biology, Physics*, 40(1), 121–127.

Scher, H., Bahnson, R., Cohen, S., Eisenberger, M., Herr, H., Kozlowski, J., Lange, P., Montie, J., Pollack, A., Raghaven, D., Richie, J., & Shipley, W. (1998). NCCN urothelial cancer practice guidelines. National Comprehensive Cancer Network. *Oncology*, 12(7A), 255–271.

Schnitz-Drager, B. J., & Muller, M. (1998). Intravesical treatment of bladder cancer: Current problems and needs. *Urologia Internationalis*, 61(4), 199–205.

Sharma, S., Zippe, C. D., Pandrangi, L., Nelson, D., & Agarwal, A. (1999). Exclusion criteria enhance the specificity and positive predictive value of NMP22 and BTA stat. *Journal of Urology*, 62(1), 53–57.

Shipley, W. U., Kaufman, D. S., Heney, N. M., Althausen, A. F., & Zietman, A. L. (1999). An update of combined modality therapy for patients with muscle invading bladder cancer using selective bladder perservation or cystectomy. *Journal of Urology*, 162(2), 445–450.

Shipley, W. U., Winter, K. A., Kaufman, D. S., Lee, W. R., Heney, N. M., Tester, W. R., Donnelly, B. J., Venner, P. M., Perez, A. A., Murray, K. J., Doggett, R. S., & True, L. D. (1998). Phase III trial of neoadjuvant chemotherapy in patients with invasive bladder cancer treated with selective bladder preservation by combined radiation therapy and chemotherapy: Initial results of Radiation Therapy Oncology Group 89-03. *Journal of Clinical Oncology*, 16(11), 3576–3583.

Skinner, D. G., Boyd, S. D., Lieskovsky, G., Bennett, C., & Hopwood, B. (1991). Lower urinary tract reconstruction following cystectomy: Experience and results in 1226 patients using the Kock ileal reservoir with bilateral ureteroileal urethrostomy. *Journal of Urology*, 146(3), 756–760.

Smart, C. R. (1990). Bladder cancer survival statistics. *Journal of Occupational Medicine*, 32(9), 926–928.

Steineck, G., Hagman, U., Gerhardsson, M., & Norell, S. E. (1990). Vitamin A supplements, fried foods, fat, and urothclial cancer. A case-referent study in Stockholm in 1985–87. *International Journal of Cancer*, 45(6), 1006–1011.

Sullivan, L. D., Chow, V. D., Ko, D. S., Wright, J. E., & McLoughlin, M. G. (1998). An evaluation of quality of life in patients with continent urinary diversions after cystectomy. *British Journal of Urology*, 81(5), 699–704.

Turner, W. H., & Studer, U. E. (1997). Cystectomy and urinary diversion. *Seminars in Surgical Oncology*, 13(5), 350–358.

van der Poel, H. G., Mungan, N. A., & Witjes, J. A. (1999). Bladder cancer in women. *International Urogynecologic Journal of Pelvic Floor Dysfunction*, 10(3), 207–212.

Wijnmaalen, A., Helle, P. A., Koper, P. C., Jansen, P. P., Hanssens, P. E., Boiken Kruger, C. G., & van Putten, W. L. (1997). Muscle invasive bladder cancer treated by transurethral resection, followed by external beam radiation and interstitial iridium-192. *International Journal of Radiation Oncology, Biology, Physicis*, 39(5), 1043–1052.

CHAPTER 15

GYNECOLOGIC MALIGNANCIES

Giselle J. Moore-Higgs, ARNP, MSN
Susan M. Chafe, MD

PROBLEM

■ Gynecologic malignancies are a major problem throughout the world. In the United States, the American Cancer Society (ACS) estimates 77,500 new cases of female genital cancer in 2000 with 26,500 associated deaths (Greenlee, Murray, Bolden, & Wingo, 2000).

CANCER OF THE VULVA

■ Cancer of the vulva is relatively rare, accounting for approximately 3% to 5% of all female malignancies (Shepherd et al., 1998). However, some reports indicate an even higher incidence of 8% (Keys, 1993). In the United States, the ACS estimates 3,400 new cases of cancer of the vulva in 2000 with 800 deaths (Greenlee et al., 2000).
■ Two epidemiologic factors should be considered regarding an increase in the incidence of this cancer. The first factor is the rapid growth of the population of women in their seventh and eighth decades of life. The second factor is the increasing number of women under age 65 who have human papilloma viral (HPV) infections and intraepithelial neoplasia of the vulva (VIN).

Cancer of the Vagina

■ Cancer of the vagina accounts for 1% to 2% of all female genital malignancies. In the United States, the ACS estimates 2,100 new cases of cancer of the vagina in 2000 with 600 associated deaths (Greenlee et al., 2000).

Cancer of the Cervix

■ Cancer of the cervix is the second most common cancer in women worldwide, accounting for approximately 437,000 new cases each year (Parkin, Pisani, & Ferday, 1993). In most countries in North America and western Europe, the incidence has been decreasing due to the availability of screening examinations. In the United States, the American Cancer Society estimates 12,800 new cases of cancer of the cervix in 2000 with 4,600 associated deaths (Greenlee et al., 2000). In many developing countries, cervical cancer is the most common cancer among women, with no change in the incidence rate.

■ In the United States, the highest age-adjusted incidence rate occurs among Vietnamese women, followed by Alaskan Native, Korean, and Hispanic women (NCI, 1999a).

■ The African American death rate (6.7 per 100,000 women) continues to be more than twice that of Whites (2.5 per 100,000 women). The higher African American death rate is a result of the high number of cervical cancer deaths among older Black women (NCI, 1999a).

Cancer of the Endometrium

■ Cancer of the endometrium is the most common gynecological malignancy and is the fourth most common malignancy in women in the United States (Walker & Nuñez, 1999). The American Cancer Society predicts 36,100 new cases of endometrial cancer in 2000 with 6,500 associated deaths (Greenlee et al., 2000).

Cancer of the Ovary and Fallopian Tube

■ Cancer of the ovary is the fifth leading cause of cancer death in women in the United States and the most common cause of death from gynecologic malignancy (Seltzer, 1999). The ACS predicts 23,100 new cases of ovarian cancer in the

United States in 2000 with 14,000 deaths, accounting for 4% of all cancer malignancies among American women (Greenlee et al., 2000).

■ Primary fallopian tube cancer is one of the rarest gynecologic malignancies, accounting for 0.1% to 0.8% of all female reproductive cancers (Nordin, 1994).

RISK FACTORS

CANCER OF THE VULVA

■ Historically, cancer of the vulva is associated with medical disorders such as obesity, hypertension, cardiovascular disease, diabetes, and syphilis. However, recent studies did not confirm these as significant factors (Parazzini et al., 1993).

■ Other risk factors identified include a history of HPV infection, a history of cervical cancer, immunosuppression, and tobacco abuse. Human papilloma virus-DNA (HPV 6, 16, and 18) has been detected in many cancers of the vulva, particularly in patients younger than 60 years (Monk, Burger, Lin, Parham, Vasilev & Wilczynski, 1995).

■ Nonneoplastic disorders of the skin of the vulva that have been associated with cancer of the vulva include lichen scleroses and chronic pruritus.

■ The median age at time of diagnosis is 60 to 65 years, however the average age is falling and the disease is now seen more frequently in women in their 20s and 30s (Sturgeon, Brinton, Devesa, & Kurman, 1992).

CANCER OF THE VAGINA

■ The exact etiology of vaginal cancer remains unknown. The proximity of the vagina to the cervix and the similarity of epithelium make it logical to assume that risk factors may be similar. The predominance of lesions in the upper third and on the posterior wall has led to speculation that an accumulation of irritating or macerating substances that pool in the posterior fornix produce a chronic irritation leading to malignant degeneration.

■ Additional predisposing factors that have been postulated, but not validated, include use of a vaginal pessary, prolapse of the vaginal wall, leukorrhea, and leukoplakia. As with cancer of the cervix and vulva, HPV infection may be a significant etiologic factor.

■ Intrauterine exposure to diethylstilbestrol (DES) has been associated with clear cell adenocarcinomas of the vagina.

CANCER OF THE CERVIX

■ Cervical cancer is thought to be the result of a sexually transmitted agent, and it is generally believed that the oncogenic types of HPV are the relevant agents (IARC, 1995). Large studies have found HPV (primarily 16, 18, 31, and 45) in virtually all cases of cervical cancer (> 93%)(NCI, 1999). Therefore, behaviors that increase risk of exposure to HPV place a woman at increased risk for the development of this disease. These behaviors include early age at first intercourse, multiple sexual partners, monogamous women whose husbands had multiple sexual partners, multiparous women, and those with a history of sexually transmitted diseases.

■ Cancer of the cervix has also been associated with lower-socioeconomic status and tobacco use. Nicotine and cotinine have been shown to exert mutagenic activity in the cervical mucus of smokers. Tobacco use may also produce a local immunosuppression in cervical epithelium, which may increase the likelihood of development of HPV-induced neoplastic transformation (Barton et al., 1988).

■ Women who are infected with human immunodeficiency virus (HIV) have an increased risk of cervical dysplasia as well as an increased risk of progression to higher-grade lesions (Holcomb, Maiman, Dimaio, & Gates, 1998).

■ Women who have never had a Pap smear are also at high risk of developing invasive cervical cancer.

■ In the United States, cervix cancer is approximately twice as frequent in Blacks as in Whites, although these rates are slowly declining (Kosary, Reis, Miller, Hankey, Harras, & Edwards, 1995).

■ Rates of cervical carcinoma in situ (CIS) reach a peak in both Black and White women between the ages of 20 and 30 years. After the age of 25, the number of cases of invasive cervical cancer increases with age in White women and Black women, however it increases more notably with age in Black women (NCI, 1999).

CANCER OF THE ENDOMETRIUM

■ Endometrial cancer can occur during both the reproductive and postmenopausal years of a woman's life, but it is more common in postmenopausal women with a median age of 63 years (Walker & Nuñez, 1999). It is widely accepted that prolonged endometrial exposure to estrogen increases the risk for hyperplastic endometrial disorders including cancer and is the basis for many of the identified risk factors.

■ Unopposed estrogen replacement therapy in a woman with a uterus significantly increases the risk of endometrial cancer (relative risk of 2.3) (Grady, Gebutsadik, Kerlikowske, Ernster, & Petitti, 1995).

■ Obese women have increased endogenous estrogen stimulation of the endometrium secondary to the peripheral conversion of ovarian and adrenal androgens to estrone by aromatase in adipose cells. Relative risk is positively associated with the number of pounds over ideal body weight or the body mass index (Walker & Nuñez, 1999).

■ Other risk factors include nulliparity, early menarche, longer days of menstrual flow, late menopause, diabetes mellitus, hyperthyroidism, and hypertension.

■ Women on long-term tamoxifen have a 2 to 7.5 relative risk of endometrial cancer. The increased risk is thought to be due to local estrogenic effects of tamoxifen on the endometrium (Walker & Nuñez, 1999).

■ The low-grade endometrial cancer rate in Whites is five times that of African American women who have a higher incidence of high-grade tumors. This impacts survival, making the prognosis appear better in White women (Walker & Nuñez, 1999).

■ At least two distinct types of endometrial cancer have been recognized: an estrogen-dependent type, which has a better prognosis, and an estrogen-independent type (Walker & Nuñez, 1999). The latter has been associated with genetic predisposition syndromes. Hereditary associations such as the Lynch II syndrome and hereditary nonpolyposis colorectal cancer (HNPCC) include a predisposition for endometrial cancer in which the lifetime risk is estimated to be 20% (Walker & Nuñez, 1999).

CANCER OF THE OVARY AND FALLOPIAN TUBE

- A number of risk factors have been associated with ovarian cancer. They include advancing age, northern European descent, nulliparity, personal history of breast, colon, or endometrial cancer, and family history of ovarian cancer.
- Women in the United States have a 1 in 70 lifetime risk of developing ovarian cancer that increases to 1 in 20 if the woman has a first-degree relative with ovarian cancer and to 7% if she has two first-degree relatives with ovarian cancer (Seltzer, 1999).
- Hereditary associations such as the Lynch II syndrome and hereditary nonpolyposis colorectal cancer (HNPCC) include a predisposition for ovarian cancer. Claus, Schildkraut, Thompson & Risch, (1996) have indicated that 10% of women with ovarian cancer carry a breast/ovarian cancer gene mutation. There are at least three different classes of genes that confer increased risk for ovarian cancer: BRCA1, BRCA2, and P53.
- Factors have also been identified that may decrease ovarian cancer risk. They include reduction in incessant ovulation, use of oral contraceptives, and tubal ligation.

ASSESSMENT

CANCER OF THE VULVA

- Currently, there are no recommended screening guidelines for cancer of the vulva. However, the age-appropriate guidelines for annual physical examination with pelvic exam and Pap smear should be applied. During these examinations, careful visual inspection of the vulva should be performed and suspicious lesions or areas of abnormal pigmentation should be photographed and biopsied.
- Presenting symptoms of cancer of the vulva include a lump or mass, vulvar pruritus, bleeding, discharge, dysuria, dyspareunia, a lesion that will not heal, incontinence, or vulvar pain.
- Approximately two-thirds of patients present with a lesion involving the labia majora. The clitoris, labia minora, posterior fourchette, or perineum constitute the presenting sites

for the other one-third of patients (Blake, Lambert, & Crawford, 1998). The disease spreads via direct extension into the vagina, urethra, and anus. Superficial inguinofemoral lymph nodes are the first regional lymph nodes to be involved, followed by deep inguinofemoral nodes and pelvic nodes. The overall incidence of lymph node involvement in cancer of the vulva is 30% (Figge, Tamimi, & Greer, 1985). Lung, liver, and bone are common sites of distant hematogenous metastasis.

■ Initial evaluation should include the following:
1. Complete history and physical examination.
2. Karnofsky performance status (KPS): An individual's performance status should be considered when deciding on the method of evaluation and treatment.
3. Careful visual inspection of the vulva and vagina, colposcopy, and full-thickness biopsy of any suspicious lesions.
4. A pap smear of the cervix and vagina should also be obtained to evaluate for evidence of disease that may constitute a primary site other than the vulva.
5. Imaging studies such as:
   a. CT scan of abdomen and pelvis to look for evidence of pelvic extension of disease and adenopathy
   b. Chest x-ray to look for evidence of lung metastasis
6. Complete blood count with complete chemistry to evaluate renal and liver function.
7. If clinical evidence of urethral involvement, cystoscopy may be appropriate to document extent of disease.
8. If clinical evidence of anal involvement, proctosigmoidoscopy may be indicated.
9. Additional metastatic evaluation studies will depend on clinical stage of disease, reported symptoms, and physical examination findings.
10. Additional studies may be warranted to assess overall medical condition, particularly when considering surgical resection or combined modality therapy.

■ Most cancers of the vulva are squamous cell. Melanoma accounts for < 5%, with Bartholin's gland adenocarcinoma, basal cell, verrucous carcinoma, and sarcoma comprising the rest.

■ Important prognostic factors include FIGO stage and presence of clinically involved lymph nodes. Additional factors include tumor size and location, age, and KPS. Midline tumors tend to do worse than lateral lesions.

■ The FIGO staging system is used in cancer of the vulva, and is a surgical staging system based on pathologic assessment of the tumor and lymph node specimens. Clinical staging (TNM) may be used in instances when the patient may not be a surgical candidate (Table 15–1).

CANCER OF THE VAGINA

■ Currently, there are no recommended screening guidelines for cancer of the vagina. However, the age-appropriate guidelines for annual physical examination with pelvic exam

TABLE 15–1   FIGO STAGING SYSTEM FOR CANCER OF THE VULVA (1988)

FIGO	TNM			Clinical/Pathologic Findings
Stage 0	T_{is}			Carcinoma in situ, intraepithelial carcinoma
Stage I	T_1	N_0	M_0	Tumor confined to the vulva or perineum, $<$ 2 cm in greatest dimension, nodes are negative
IA				Invasion not $>$ 1 mm
IB				Invasion $>$ 1 mm*
Stage II	T_2	N_0	M_0	Tumor confined to the vulva and/or perineum, $>$ 2 cm in greatest dimension, nodes are negative
Stage III	T_3	N_0	M_0	Tumor of any size with:
	T_3	N_1	M_0	Adjacent spread to the lower urethra and/or the vagina and/or anus
	T_1	N_1	M_0	Unilateral regional lymph node metastasis
	T_2	N_1	M_0	
Stage IVA	T_1	N_2	M_0	Tumor invades any of the following: upper urethra, bladder mucosa, rectal mucosa, pelvic bone, and/or bilateral regional nodes
	T_2	N_2	M_0	
	T_3	N_2	M_0	
	T_4	N_{0-2}	M_0	
Stage IVB	T_{1-4}	N_{0-2}	M_1	Any distant metastases including pelvic lymph nodes

*Note: The depth of invasion is defined as the measurement of the tumor from the epithelial-stromal junction of the adjacent most superficial dermal papilla to the deepest point of invasion.
Used with the permission of the American Joint Committee on Cancer (AJCC®), Chicago, Illinois. The original source for this material is the AJCC® Cancer Staging Manual, 5th edition (1997) published by Lippincott-Raven Publishers, Philadelphia, Pennsylvania.

and Pap smear should be applied. During these examinations, careful visual inspection of the vaginal walls should be performed and suspicious lesions or areas of abnormal pigmentation should be photographed and biopsied.

■ The most common symptoms of cancer of the vagina are intermenstrual or postmenopausal bleeding and/or vaginal discharge as well as urinary symptoms including dysuria or hematuria and pelvic pain.

■ Cancer of the vagina spreads by local invasion to the rest of the vagina, vulva, paravaginal tissues, and parametria. Lymphatic spread occurs in accordance with the site of the primary tumor in the vagina. The lymph nodes in the pelvis drain the upper two-thirds of the vagina and the inguinal nodes drain the lower one-third. Hematogenous spread is rare and occurs late in the disease process.

■ Initial evaluation should include the following:

1. Complete history and physical examination.
2. Karnofsky performance status (KPS): An individual's performance status should be considered when deciding on the method of evaluation and treatment.
3. Careful visual inspection of the vagina, vulva, and cervix with colposcopy and biopsy of any suspicious lesions.
4. A Pap smear of the cervix should also be obtained to evaluate for evidence of disease that may constitute a primary site other than the vagina. Any suspicious lesions on the vulva should also be biopsied.
5. Imaging studies such as:
   a. CT scan or MRI of abdomen and pelvis to look for evidence of pelvic extension of disease and adenopathy
   b. Chest x-ray to look for evidence of lung metastasis
   c. Transrectal or transvaginal ultrasound may help define the size and extent of the disease
6. Complete blood count with complete chemistry to evaluate renal and liver function.
7. Exam under anesthesia allows cystoscopy, proctocsigmoidoscopy, and extensive clinical examination of the vagina.
8. Additional metastatic evaluation studies will depend on clinical stage of disease, reported symptoms, and physical examination findings.
9. Additional studies may be warranted to assess overall medical condition, particularly when considering surgical resection or combined modality therapy.

- Most cancers of the vagina are squamous cell (90%). Melanoma, adenocarcinoma, and sarcoma comprise the rest.
- FIGO stage is the most important prognostic factor. Other prognostic factors include grade of tumor, depth of penetration, and presence of involved lymph nodes.
- The FIGO staging system, which is based on clinical finding, is used in cancer of the vagina (Table 15–2).

CANCER OF THE CERVIX

- Cytological screening using the Pap smear with pelvic examination is the established method of screening for cancer of the cervix. The ACS, American College of Obstetrics and Gynecology (ACOG), and the National Cancer Institute (NCI) recommend initial Pap smear screening in women who have been sexually active or who have reached 18 years of age. After a woman has had three or more consecutive satisfactory annual exams, the Pap test may be performed less frequently at the discretion of the physician (ACOG, 1997; ACS, 1998; NCI, 1998).

TABLE 15–2 FIGO STAGING SYSTEM FOR CANCER OF THE VAGINA

FIGO	TNM			Clinical/Pathologic Findings
Stage 0	T_{is}	N_0	M_0	Carcinoma in situ, intraepithelial carcinoma
Stage I	T_1	N_0	M_0	Tumor confined to the vaginal wall
Stage II	T_2	N_0	M_0	Tumor invades paravaginal tissues, but not to the pelvic wall
Stage III	T_1	N_1	M_0	Tumor extends to the pelvic wall
	T_2	N_1	M_0	
	T_3	N_0	M_0	
	T_3	N_1	M_0	
Stage IVA	T_4	N_{0-2}	M_0	Tumor invades mucosa of the bladder or rectum and/or extends beyond the true pelvis (Bullous edema is not sufficient evidence to classify a tumor as T_4)
Stage IVB	T_{1-4}	N_{0-2}	M_1	Distant metastases

Used with the permission of the American Joint Committee on Cancer (AJCC®), Chicago, Illinois. The original source for this material is the AJCC® Cancer Staging Manual, 5th edition (1997) published by Lippincott-Raven Publishers, Philadelphia, Pennsylvania.

■ Additional screening tools include colposcopy, cervicography, self-administered cervical cancer screening, automated cytology, and ThinPrep. These tools are not currently approved for routine screening.

■ The most common symptoms of cervix cancer are abnormal vaginal bleeding (postcoital, intermenstrual, or postmenopausal) and malodorous discharge. Urinary symptoms including dysuria or hematuria, and pelvic or back pain are usually associated with advanced disease. Anemia secondary to vaginal bleeding may be present.

■ Cancer of the cervix spreads directly to the vaginal mucosa, endometrial cavity, parametrial tissues and ligaments, pelvic side wall, bladder, and rectum. Regional lymphatics that are at risk for metastases include the paracervical, internal iliac, obturator, external iliac, presacral, common iliac, and para-aortic lymph nodes. Hematogenous spread is usually late and may be to lungs, bone, or liver.

■ Initial evaluation should include the following:
   1. Complete history and physical examination.
   2. Karnofsky performance status (KPS): An individual's performance status should be considered when deciding on the method of evaluation and treatment.
   3. Initial cervical abnormality is usually discoverd by Pap smear. However, obvious cervical lesions may proceed directly to biopsy. Careful visual inspection of the cervix and vagina with colposcopy and biopsy of any suspicious lesions follows abnormal cytology results.
   4. Imaging studies may include the following:
      a. CT scan or MRI of abdomen and pelvis for evidence of pelvic extension of disease and adenopathy
      b. Chest x-ray to look for evidence of lung metastasis
      c. Transvaginal ultrasound may help define the size and extent of the disease
   5. Tumor markers including CA125, CA19-9, CEA, and squamous cell carcinoma antigen (SCC) have been shown to be elevated in cervical cancer. However, these are not specific markers for cervical cancer and therefore are not routinely used in clinical practice.
   6. Complete blood count with complete chemistry to evaluate renal and liver function.
   7. Exam under anesthesia allows extensive clinical examination of the cervix, cystoscopy, and proctosigmoidoscopy.

8. Additional metastatic evaluation studies will depend on clinical stage of disease, reported symptoms, and physical examination findings.

9. Additional studies may be warranted to assess overall medical condition, particularly when considering surgical resection or combined modality therapy.

■ Over 90% of tumors of the cervix are squamous cell carcinoma, approximately 7% to 10% are classified as adenocarcinoma, and 1% to 2% are clear cell mesonephric type (Chao, Perez, & Brady, 1999).

■ Important prognostic factors in cervix cancer include stage of disease, tumor volume, lymph node involvement, histologic type of lesion, and vascular or lymphatic invasion. Host factors, such as anemia, also affect the prognosis (Chao et al., 1999).

■ FIGO staging, which is based on clinical evaluation (preferably under anesthesia), is commonly used. The evaluation may also include chest x-ray, intravenous pyelography, cystoscopy, proctoscopy, and pathology results from biopsy (Table 15–3).

CANCER OF THE ENDOMETRIUM

■ Screening for endometrial cancer remains difficult. The ACOG recommendations state that screening techniques to detect endometrial cancer, including ultrasonography and endometrial sampling, have not demonstrated sufficient accuracy and cost-effectiveness and therefore are not acceptable for general use (ACOG, 1996). Cervical cytology alone is not reliable. Therefore, endometrial biopsy should only be used as a diagnostic test for women with unexpected breakthrough bleeding during the perimenopausal period or while on estrogen replacement therapy, and in women with postmenopausal bleeding.

■ The American College of Physicians (ACP) recommends that women on unopposed estrogen should have endometrial evaluation once a year or sooner if bleeding occurs (ACP, 1992).

■ The ACS (1997) recommended the following guidelines: women 40 and older should have an annual pelvic examination by a health care professional. Women at high risk for endometrial cancer should receive counseling to reduce

TABLE 15–3   FIGO STAGING SYSTEM FOR CANCER OF THE CERVIX

FIGO	TNM			Clinical/Pathologic Findings
Stage 0	T_{is}	N_0	M_0	Carcinoma in situ
Stage I	T_1	N_0	M_0	Cervical carcinoma confined to uterus
IA	T_{1a}	N_0	M_0	Invasive carcinoma diagnosed only by microscopy. All macroscopically visible lesions—even with superficial invasion—are T_{1b}/IB. Stromal invasion with a maximal depth of 5.0 mm measured from the base of the epithelium and a horizontal spread of 7.0 mm or less. Vascular space involvement, either venous or lymphatic, does not affect classification
IA$_1$	T_{1a_1}	N_0	M_0	Measured stromal invasion 3.0 mm or less in depth and 7.0 mm or less in horizontal spread
IA$_2$	T_{1a_2}	N_0	M_0	Measured stromal invasion more than 3.0 mm and not more than 5.0 mm with a horizontal spread 7.0 mm or less
IB	T_{1b}	N_0	M_0	Clinically visible lesion confined to the cervix or microscopic lesion greater than T_{1a}/IA$_2$
IB$_1$	T_{1b_1}	N_0	M_0	Clinically visible lesion 1.0 cm or less in greatest dimension
IB$_2$	T_{1b_2}	N_0	M_0	Clinically visible lesion more than 4.0 cm in greatest dimension
Stage II				Cervical carcinoma invades beyond uterus but not to pelvic wall or to the lower third of vagina
IIA	T_{2a}	N_0	M_0	Tumor without parametrial invasion
IIB	T_{2b}	N_0	M_0	Tumor with parametrial invasion
Stage III				Tumor extends to the pelvic wall, and/or involves the lower third of the vagina, and/or causes hydronephrosis or nonfunctioning kidney
IIIA	T_{3a}	N_0	M_0	Tumor involves lower third of the vagina, no extension to pelvic wall
IIIB	T_1	N_1	M_0	Tumor extends to the pelvic wall and/or causes hydronephrosis or nonfunctioning kidney
	T_2	N_1	M_0	
	T_{3a}	N_1	M_0	
	T_{3b}	Any N	M_0	
Stage IVA	T_4	Any N	M_0	Tumor invades mucosa of the bladder or rectum, and/or extends beyond the true pelvis (bullous edema is not sufficient to classify a tumor as T_4)
Stage IVB	T_4	Any N	M_1	Distant metastasis

Used with the permission of the American Joint Committee on Cancer (AJCC®), Chicago, Illinois. The original source for this material is the AJCC® Cancer Staging Manual, 5th edition (1997) published by Lippincott-Raven Publishers, Philadelphia, Pennsylvania.

risk, annual pelvic examinations, and immediate intervention for postmenopausal or irregular vaginal bleeding.

■ The most common presenting symptom is intermenstrual or postmenopausal vaginal bleeding. Additional symptoms in advanced disease include pelvic pain, back pain, and urinary symptoms (dysuria and frequency) secondary to uterine enlargement.

■ Endometrial cancer can spread via direct extension into surrounding organs (cervix, vagina, bladder, rectum, or parametria). Lymphatic spread and hematogenous spread can also occur. Lymph nodes at risk for metastasis include the pelvic and para-aortic nodes. Peritoneal seeding is common with endometrial cancer because an endometrial lesion may penetrate the uterine wall or seed transtubally (Chao et al., 1999).

■ Initial evaluation should include the following:

1. Complete history and physical examination.
2. Karnofsky performance status (KPS): An individual's performance status should be considered when deciding on the method of evaluation and treatment.
3. Endometrial biopsy, aspiration curettage, or fractional dilation and curettage (D&C), by which the initial diagnosis is usually made.
4. Imaging studies may include:
   a. CT scan or MRI of abdomen and pelvis for evidence of pelvic extension of disease and adenopathy
   b. Chest x-ray to look for evidence of lung metastasis
5. Complete blood count with complete chemistry to evaluate renal and liver function.
6. Exam under anesthesia allows extensive clinical examination of the pelvis, with cystoscopy and proctosigmoidoscopy indicated in advanced disease.
7. Additional metastatic evaluation studies will depend on clinical stage of disease, reported symptoms, and physical examination findings.
8. Additional studies may be warranted to assess overall medical condition, particularly when considering surgical resection or combined modality therapy.

■ The most common cancer of the endometrium is endometroid adenocarcinoma (Chao et al., 1999). This is further divided into four subtypes: papillary, secretory, ciliated cells, and adenocarcinoma with squamous differentiation.

Other histologic types of tumors of the endometrium are rare and include papillary serous carcinoma, clear cell carcinoma, and sarcoma.

■ Important prognostic factors include clinical or pathologic stage, histologic grade of the tumor, depth of myometrial invasion, presence of lymphovascular involvement, lymph node involvement, and age.

■ FIGO staging (based on surgical evaluation) is most commonly used. (Table 15–4). For patients unable to undergo a surgical procedure, a FIGO (1971) clinical staging is used. (Table 15–5).

CANCER OF THE OVARY AND FALLOPIAN TUBE

■ Screening for cancer of the ovary and fallopian tube remains controversial. The CA-125 radioimmunoassay is a serum tumor marker that is elevated in 80% of women with epithelial ovarian cancer. However, it is less likely to be elevated in mucinous tumors. Unfortunately, many other medical conditions may result in an elevated CA-125 including endometriosis, pelvic inflammatory disease, benign ovarian neoplasms, fibroids, liver disease, congestive heart failure, and a variety of other benign problems (Seltzer, 1999). CA-125 appears to be more accurate for detecting ovarian cancer in postmenopausal women.

■ Transvaginal and transabdominal ultrasound have been studied as possible noninvasive screening tools. Color flow doppler imaging is also being used in some centers as an investigational adjunct to endovaginal sonograms to measure flow patterns within ovarian vessels. The 1994 NIH Consensus Statement of Ovarian Cancer concluded that, at that time, there was no evidence available that the current screening modalities of CA-125 and transvaginal ultrasound could be used effectively for large population screening to reduce the morality rate from ovarian cancer (NIH, 1995).

■ The NIH Consensus Statement (1994) advised that women with two first-degree relatives should have an annual physical examination with bimanual rectovaginal examination, CA-125 serum levels, and transvaginal ultrasound. At the conclusion of childbearing or at least by age 35 years, prophylactic bilateral oophorectomy may be appropriate (NIH, 1995).

TABLE 15–4 FIGO SURGICAL STAGING OF CANCER
OF THE ENDOMETRIUM

FIGO	Grade	TNM		Clinical/Pathologic Findings
Stage 0	G1,2,3	T_{is}	N_0 M_0	Carcinoma in situ
Stage I				Tumor confined to the corpus uteri
IA	G1,2,3	T_{1a}	M_0 M_0	Tumor limited to endometrium
IB	G1,2,3	T_{1b}	N_0 M_0	Tumor invades up to or less than one-half of the myometrium
IC	G1,2,3	T_{1c}	N_0 M_0	Tumor invades to more than one-half of the myometrium
Stage II				Tumor invades cervix but does not extend beyond uterus
IIA	G1,2,3	T_{2a}	N_0 M_0	Endocervical glandular involvement only
IIB	G1,2,3	T_{2b}	N_0 M_0	Cervical stromal invasion
Stage III				Local and/or regional spread as specified in T3a, b, and/or N_1, and FIGO IIIA, B, and C
IIIA	G1,2,3	T3a	N_0 M_0	Tumor involves serosa and/or adnexa (direct extension or metastasis) and/or cancer cells in ascites or peritoneal washings
IIIB	G1,2,3	T_{3b}	N_0 M_0	Vaginal involvement (direct extension or metastasis)
IIIC	G1,2,3	T_1	N_1 M_0	Metastasis to the pelvic and/or para-aortic lymph nodes
		T_2	N_1 M_0	
		T_{3a}	N_1 M_0	
		T_{3b}	N_1 M_0	
Stage IVA	G1,2,3	T_4	Any N M_0	Tumor invades bladder mucosa and/or bowel mucosa (bullous edema is not sufficient to classify a tumor as T_4)
Stage IVB		Any T	Any N M_1	Distant metastasis

TABLE 15–5 CLINICAL STAGING OF CANCER OF THE ENDOMETRIUM (1971)
(NO LONGER ADOPTED FOR FIGO CLASSIFICATION)

Stage 0	Carcinoma in situ
Stage I	Cancer confined to corpus
IA	Uterine cavity sounds to 8 cm or less
IB	Uterine cavity sounds to over 8 cm
G_1	Highly differentiated adenocarcinoma
G_2	Differentiated adenocarcinoma with partially solid areas
G_3	Predominantly solid or entirely undifferentiated carcinoma
Stage II	Carcinoma involves corpus and cervix
Stage III	Carcinoma extends outside corpus, but not true pelvis (it may not involve bladder or rectum)
Stage IV	Carcinoma involves bladder or rectum or extends outside true pelvis

■ Symptoms associated with ovarian cancer usually do not occur until the disease is advanced. The symptoms include early satiety, abdominal distension, abdominal pain, nausea, and vomiting.

■ Epithelial ovarian cancer arises from the ovarian surface epithelium and spreads through the peritoneal cavity. Lymphatic or hematogenous spread can also occur.

■ Initial evaluation should include the following:

1. Complete history and physical examination.

2. Karnofsky performance status (KPS): An individual's performance status should be considered when deciding on the method of evaluation and treatment.

3. Imaging studies may include the following:
   a. CT scan of the abdomen and pelvis
   b. Chest x-ray to look for evidence of pleural effusion or lung mass

4. Complete blood count with complete chemistry to evaluate renal and liver function and serum CA-125 level.

5. Laparotomy with biopsy will confirm diagnosis and is recommended for staging.

6. Additional metastatic evaluation studies depend on clinical stage of disease, reported symptoms, and physical examination findings.

7. Additional studies may be warranted to assess overall medical condition, particularly when considering surgical resection or combined modality therapy.

■ Epithelial ovarian tumors account for the majority of ovarian tumors. They arise from the germinal epithelium or mesothelium on the surface of the ovary. Almost all Fallopian tube tumors are adenocarcinomas.

■ Staging of ovarian and fallopian tube cancers are based on surgical evaluation and cytoreduction (see Table 15–6 & 15–7).

OUTCOMES MANAGEMENT

Cancer of the Vulva

A better understanding of tumor biology and the consideration of different clinicopathologic factors that bear prognostic significance in therapeutic modalities have allowed individualization of treatment for cancer of the vulva (Maker & Trope, 1992). Although the treatment of choice for cancer of the vulva is surgery, the new modalities have less surgical morbidity and fewer functional and psychosexual impairments without impairing survival.

Surgery

• For patients with early-stage squamous cell cancer of the vulva, a conservative "radical" wide local excision may be performed. This is appropriate in stage I or II lesions and has been associated with decreased complications and 5-year overall survival and recurrence rate similar to those of radical vulvar surgery (Magrina et al., 1998). The procedure may include ipsilateral or bilateral inguinal and femoral lymphadenectomy if there is no clinical suspicion of nodal involvement. Radical vulvectomy and bilateral inguinofemoral lymphadenectomy is usually performed in advanced stage disease (stage III or IV).

• Sentinel lymph node evaluation has recently been reported in several studies. De Hullu et al. (1998) (greater than 6) in a small study of 10 patients, found that identification of the sentinel inguinal femoral lymph node in squamous cell cancer of the vulva was feasible with preoperatively administered technetium-99m-labeled nanocolloid. Similar findings were reported by Terada, Coel, Ko, and Wong (1998) in

TABLE 15–6 FIGO STAGING SYSTEM FOR CANCER OF THE OVARY

FIGO	TNM			Clinical/Pathologic Findings
Stage I				Tumor limited to ovaries (one or both)
IA	T_{1a}	N_0	M_0	Tumor limited to one ovary; capsule intact, no tumor on ovarian surface. No malignant cells in ascites or peritoneal washings*
IB	T_{1b}	N_0	M_0	Tumor limited to both ovaries; capsule is intact, no tumor on ovarian surface. No malignant cells in ascites or peritoneal washings*
IC	T_{1c}	N_0	M_0	Tumor limited to one or both ovaries with any of the following: capsule ruptured, tumor on ovarian surface, malignant cells in ascites or peritoneal washings
Stage II	T_2			Tumor involves one or both ovaries with pelvic extension
IIA	T_{2a}	N_0	M_0	Extension and/or implants on uterus and/or tube(s). No malignant cells in ascites or peritoneal washings
IIB	T_{2b}	N_0	M_0	Extension to other pelvic tissues. No malignant cells in ascites or peritoneal washings
IIC	T_{2c}	N_0	M_0	Pelvic extension (2a or 2b) with malignant cells in ascites or peritoneal washings
Stage III	T_3			Tumor involves one or both ovaries with microscopically confirmed peritoneal metastasis outside the pelvis and/or regional lymph node metastasis
IIIA	T_{3a}	N_0	M_0	Microscopic peritoneal metastasis beyond the pelvis
IIIB	T_{3b}	N_0	M_0	Macroscopic peritoneal metastasis beyond pelvis 2 cm or less in greatest dimension
IIIC	T_{3c}	N_0	M_0	Peritoneal metastasis beyond the pelvis more than 2 cm in greatest dimension and/or regional
	Any T	N_1	M_0	lymph node metastasis
Stage IV	Any T	Any N	M_1	Distant metastasis

*Note: The presence of nonmalignant ascites is not classified. The presence of ascites does not affect staging unless malignant cells are present.

TABLE 15–7 FIGO Staging System for Cancer of the Fallopian Tube

FIGO	TNM			Clinical/Pathologic Findings
Stage I				Tumor limited to the fallopian tube(s)
IA	T_{1a}	N_0	M_0	Tumor limited to one tube without penetrating the serosal surface; no ascites
IB	T_{1b}	N_0	M_0	Tumor limited to both tubes without penetrating the serosal surface; no ascites
IC	T_{1c}	N_0	M_0	Tumor limited to one or both tubes with extension onto or through the tubal serosa, or with malignant cells in ascites or peritoneal washings
Stage II	T_2			Tumor involves one or both fallopian tubes with pelvic extension
IIA	T_{2a}	N_0	M_0	Extension and/or implants on uterus and/or ovaries
IIB	T_{2b}	N_0	M_0	Extension to other pelvic structures
IIC	T_{2c}	N_0	M_0	Pelvic extension with malignant cells in ascites or peritoneal washings
Stage III	T_3			Tumor involves one or both fallopian tubes with peritoneal implants outside the pelvis and/or regional lymph node metastasis
IIIA	T_{3a}	N_0	M_0	Microscopic peritoneal metastasis beyond the pelvis
IIIB	T_{3b}	N_0	M_0	Macroscopic peritoneal metastasis beyond pelvis 2 cm or less in greatest dimension
IIIC	T_{3c}	N_0	M_0	Peritoneal metastasis beyond the pelvis more than 2 cm in greatest dimension and/or regional
	Any T	N_1	M_0	lymph node metastasis
Stage IV	Any T	Any N	M_1	Distant metastasis

Used with the permission of the American Joint Committee on Cancer (AJCC®), Chicago, Illinois. The original source for this material is the AJCC® Cancer Staging Manual, 5th edition (1997) published by Lippincott-Raven Publishers, Philadelphia, Pennsylvania.

five patients. There was minimal morbidity associated with the procedure in both studies. Although further studies are necessary, lymphatic mapping could significantly reduce the amount of surgical resection necessary, and reduce the postoperative complications of wound dehiscence and lymphedema.

Radiation Therapy

- Preoperative therapy may be used alone or adjuvantly with chemotherapy to reduce large-volume disease in preparation for surgical resection. Postoperative radiation therapy can be given to the pelvic and inguinal areas for nodal metastasis (Homesley, 1986). It also has a role in the prevention of local recurrence in the vulva when there is a close or positive surgical margin. Radiation therapy can also be given alone or combined with chemotherapy for medically inoperable patients, or used to palliate symptoms in advanced disease.

Chemotherapy
- Chemotherapy use has been limited for cancer of the vulva, but can be given in the neoadjuvant setting for advanced disease either alone or in combination with radiation therapy.

Cancer of the Vagina

Surgery
- Surgery is used primarily for very early stage I lesions when an adequate margin of tissue can be removed with the tumor. Radical hysterectomy with pelvic lymphadenectomy can be used for stage I lesions of the uppermost part of the vagina.

Radiation Therapy
- Radiation therapy is the preferred method of treatment for most vaginal cancers. It can be given as a combination of external-beam radiation with brachytherapy or brachytherapy alone.

Cancer of the Cervix

Surgery
- Surgery is the primary therapy for very early stage disease (CIS and stage IA). The procedure is individualized to the patient. The patient's desire to maintain fertility may include a therapeutic conization or simple hysterectomy with or without a bilateral salpingo-oophorectomy. However, these patients must have very close follow-up with colposcopy to assure early recognition of recurrent disease. Modified radical hysterectomy with or without bilateral salpingo-oophorectomy is the surgery of choice for stage IB and stage IIA cancers of the cervix (for patients who are surgical candidates). This procedure includes removal of the uterus, the upper one-third of the vagina, the broad ligament, the parametria, and biopsy of the pelvic

lymph nodes. Surgery is not offered to patients who are elderly or obese because of the increased risk of surgical complications. Patients who receive preoperative radiation therapy for a "barrel-shaped or bulky" stage IB lesion may have an extrafascial hysterectomy after completion of radiotherapy. In advanced stage disease, surgical resection is not an option. These patients are treated with radiotherapy alone. Surgery may be considered for patients who have a central recurrence after radiation therapy. In this setting, pelvic exenteration may be offered for a chance of cure in patients with limited disease.

Radiation Therapy

- Radiation therapy may be used in all stages of cervical cancer, but is most often used in stages IB_2 to IV. The procedure is usually a combination of external-beam radiation followed with an intracavitary implant. Occasionally, interstitial needle implants are used after external-beam radiation therapy.

Combined Therapy

- Combined therapy (chemotherapy and radiation therapy) for advanced-stage cervix cancer may offer both long-term disease control and overall survival advantages. Recently the management of advanced cervical cancer has changed. A number of recent studies revealed that the addition of concurrent chemotherapy to radiation improved the outcome in patients with stage IIB, III, IVA, bulky disease, or positive pelvic lymph nodes (Keys et al., 1999; Rose et al., 1999; Morris et al., 1999; Whitney et al., 1999). Keys et al. (1999) found that adding weekly infusions of cisplatin to pelvic radiotherapy followed by hysterectomy significantly reduced the risk of disease recurrence and death in women with bulky stage IB cancers. The rates of both progression-free survival ($p < 0.001$) and overall survival ($p = 0.008$) were significantly higher in the combined-therapy group at 4 years. Toxicities were higher in the combined group, particularly gastrointestinal effects and transient grade 3 and grade 4 hematologic effects. Morris et al. (1999) reported on the effect of radiotherapy to the pelvis with concurrent 5-fluorouracil (5-FU) and cisplatin in women with advanced cancer (stages IIB to IVA, or stage IB or IIA with biopsy-proven pelvic lymph nodes or tumor size of at least 5 cm) versus radiotherapy alone to the pelvis and periaortic nodes. Estimated cumulative rates of survival at 5 years were 73% among patients treated with radiotherapy and chemotherapy and 58% among patients treated with radiotherapy alone ($p = 0.004$). Cumulative rates of disease-free survival at 5 years were 67% in the combined-therapy group and 40% among patients in the radiotherapy group ($p < 0.001$). The rates of both distant metastasis and local-regional recurrence were significantly higher among patients treated with radiotherapy alone. The side effects were similar in both groups, with a higher rate of reversible hematologic effect in the combined-therapy group.

Chemotherapy

- Chemotherapy has primarily been used in the palliative setting in cervix cancer. Agents such as cisplatin, carboplatin, and 5-FU have been used. Newer agents such as paclitaxel remain under study. Brader, Morns, Levenback, Levy, Lucas & Gershenson (1998) identified characteristics that predict response to chemotherapy in patients with advanced or recurrent squamous cell cancer of the cervix. Patients who were older were more likely to respond to therapy. The response rate for patients in whom disease recurred outside the irradiated field was 25.2%, compared with a 5.3% response rate for patients with recurrent disease limited to a previously irradiated field.

Cancer of the Endometrium

Surgery

- Surgery is usually performed for patients with stage I to III disease. The surgery includes a total abdominal hysterectomy with bilateral salpingo-oophorectomy, pelvic and para-aortic lymph node sampling, and peritoneal washings. Based on pathologic findings, patients may be referred for postoperative radiation.

Radiation Therapy

- Radiation therapy is given postoperatively to patients with pathologic findings that place them at risk for local-regional recurrence. This includes stage I patients with grade 1 tumors with greater than two-thirds myometrial invasion, grade 2 tumors with greater than one-third invasion, all grade 3 tumors with invasion (Lanciano & Corn, 1998), and all stage II to IVA patients. Radiation therapy may also be used alone for patients who are not surgical candidates. In certain pathological types of endometrial cancer and in advanced stage disease, whole-abdomen radiotherapy may be considered.

Chemotherapy and Hormonal Therapy

- Systemic therapy with chemotherapy or hormones has been used for patients with metastatic disease (in a palliative approach).

Cancer of the Ovary and Fallopian Tube

Surgery

- The primary treatment approaches for ovarian and fallopian tube cancer are surgery and (when indicated) systemic chemotherapy. Laparotomy and surgical exploration are essential and should include the following, when possible (Lanciano & Corn, 1998):
  1. Peritoneal cytologic examination.
  2. Inspection of pelvis, peritoneal surfaces, diaphragm, omentum, and pelvic/para-aortic lymph nodes. Biopsy of any suspicious areas.
  3. Removal of all tumor possible; this includes a total abdominal hysterectomy and bilateral salpingo-oophorectomy, pelvic and para-aortic lymph node sampling, and partial omentectomy.

Radiation Therapy

- Whole-abdomen radiation or intraperitoneal P-32 have been used adjuvantly in an effort to improve survival after surgical resection and systemic chemotherapy. Currently, this is not standard practice and can be used on an individual basis or as part of a clinical trial.

Chemotherapy

- After a patient has surgical resection, a course of systemic chemotherapy is recommended based on stage and pathologic findings. Currently, platinum-based agents with paclitaxel are the standard first line of agents offered. The extent of treatment varies with the stage of disease. For patients with advanced-stage disease, 6 cycles of chemotherapy are recommended and for early-stage disease, 3 to 6 cycles are recommended (Ozols, 1997). Other chemotherapeutic agents can be offered in clinical trials or in the setting of recurrent disease. Chemotherapy can be given for recurrent disease with or without repeat laparotomy and debulking.

Toxicity of Treatment

Toxicity associated with radiation therapy for gynecologic malignancies depends on the site of treatment. In patients treated with abdomino-pelvic radiation, acute complications include nausea, vomiting, diarrhea, frequency of urination, leukopenia, thrombocytopenia, transient hepatic enzyme elevation, and (on occasion) symptomatic basal pneumonitis (Fyles, Dembo, & Bush, 1992). Late toxicities may include bowel obstruction, enteritis, proctitis, and hemorrhagic cystitis. Patients treated to the pelvis may experience acute toxicities such as cystitis, diarrhea, proctitis, vaginal mucositis, nausea, and moist desquamation within skin folds. Late toxicities may include bowel obstruction, hemorrhagic cystitis, vaginal stenosis, vesicovaginal fistula, rectovaginal fistula, enteritis, proctitis, pelvic nerve damage, and lower extremity edema. If the perineum is included in the treatment field, acute brisk erythema and moist desquamation will occur in the majority of patients. Infertility and menopause will be permanent in women treated with radiotherapy that involves the pelvis.

Acute Toxicities

1. Skin reactions are usually confined to areas with skin folds and the perineum. Treatment to the whole abdomen does not generally result in a skin reaction. Treatment to the pelvis may result in mild hyperpigmentation within the treatment fields, and moist desquamation in folds of abdominal skin, in the groin, and between the buttocks. Treatment to the perineum usually results in brisk erythema 10 to 14 days after treatment is initiated, with moist desquamation shortly thereafter. The presence of numerous skin folds and exposure to urine and fecal material increase the risk of skin breakdown. Wound dehiscence and soft tissue necrosis particularly along suture lines are uncommon, but may occur in patients after recent radical vulvectomy. See chapter 21 for skin care options.

2. Cystitis usually becomes symptomatic after 10 to 14 days of treatment, and results in dysuria, frequency, and urgency. The symptoms usually resolve within 1 month of completing treatment. See chapter 23 for treatment.

3. Diarrhea (radiation-induced) results from a variety of different pathophysiological mechanisms including malabsorption of bile salts and lactose, imbalances in local bacterial flora, and changes in the intestinal patterns of motility. Wang et al. (1998) found that patients with increased acute toxicity and diarrhea during radiation therapy for cervix cancer had

significantly increased risk of late rectal injury, suggesting that early excessive damage of the acute-responding component of the rectal wall can play an important role in the initiation of rectal injury. A number of treatment approaches with antidiarrheal and diet interventions have been used with little research to evaluate efficacy. Henriksson, Franzen, and Littbrand (1992) reported on the use of sucralfate in preventing radiation-induced diarrhea and bowel discomfort. In a double-blind and placebo-controlled study of patients treated to the pelvis with radiation, frequency of defecation and stool consistency were significantly improved by sucralfate. One year later, the patients in the sucralfate group displayed significantly less problems with frequency of defecation, mucus, and blood in the stools compared with the placebo group. Other treatment options may be found in chapter 23.

4. Nausea and vomiting may occur in patients receiving treatment to the whole abdomen. Prophylactic antiemetics before radiotherapy often eliminate this problem. Occasionally patients receiving treatment only to the pelvis report mild nausea. See chapter 22 for treatment options. If persistent nausea with vomiting occurs, evaluation for bowel obstruction may be warranted.

5. Vaginal mucositis usually occurs within the first 14 to 21 days of treatment. Patients will report symptoms of discomfort and dyspareunia. If a foul-smelling or thin, watery discharge begins, cultures should be obtained for infectious agents such as *Candida albicans*, bacterial vaginosis, and chlamydia. Otherwise, patients may be treated symptomatically. See chapter 26 for treatment options.

6. Bone marrow suppression may occur in patients treated with whole-abdomen radiotherapy. In addition, patients with active vaginal bleeding may develop anemia. See chapter 21 for treatment options.

7. Fatigue is also common in patients treated with pelvic or whole-abdomen radiotherapy. See chapter 20 for management options.

Latent Toxicities

1. Enteritis/proctitis—Radiation-induced intestinal injury can result in local ischemia and fibrosis with the development of ulcers, strictures, and rectal bleeding. Montana & Fowler (1989) identified a correlation between rectal dose and proctitis in patients receiving radiation therapy to the pelvis. The

risk of proctitis increased as a function of rectal dose ranging from 2% for patients receiving 50 Gy or less to the rectum to 18% for patients receiving at least 80 Gy to the rectum. Symptoms may include rectal bleeding, painful bowel movements, and chronic or intermittent diarrhea. Occasionally, the rectal bleeding can be severe enough to result in anemia and transfusion dependency. Bleeding typically develops from 6 months to 1 year after completion of radiation therapy and is caused by friable mucosal angioectasias (Swaroop & Gostout, 1998). A number of treatment options are available for rectal bleeding:

a. The utility of formalin rectal instillation for treatment of bleeding was evaluated in a prospective study by Counter, Froese, and Hart (1999). In a single treatment, 4% formalin was instilled into the rectum in four separate 20 cc aliquots with total mucosal contact time of approximately 15 minutes. Patients were evaluated at 7 to 10 days and at 1 month. In a follow-up of 3 to 64 months, 100% had initial success with cessation of bleeding. Twenty-seven percent had recurrent bleeding with only one patient requiring retreatment.

b. Short-term topical sucralfate suspension was evaluated by Kochhar, Sriram, and Sharma (1999). All patients were treated with 20 ml of 10% rectal sucralfate suspension enemas twice a day until bleeding per rectum ceased or until failure of therapy was acknowledged. A good response (severity of bleeding improved by a change of two grades) was found in 77% of patients at 4 weeks, 85% at 8 weeks, and 92% at 16 weeks. Over a median follow-up of 45.5 months (range of 5 to 73 months), 22.2% had recurrence, all of which responded to reinstitution of sucralfate therapy.

c. Endoscopic laser obliteration.

d. Short-chain fatty acids are the main energy source of coloncytes and they may be impaired in chronic radiation proctitis. Pinto et al. (1999) evaluated the use of short-chain fatty acid enemas containing 60 mM sodium acetate, 30 mM sodium propionate, and 40 mM of sodium butyrate. The treatment period lasted 5 weeks and patients had follow-up for 6 months. After 5 weeks, the patients treated with short-chain fatty acid showed a significant decrease in the number of days of rectal bleeding and an improvement of endocospic score. Hemoglobin values were also significantly higher for those patients.

    e. Nutritional intervention including total parenteral nutrition or elemental diets can be useful as adjunctive therapy to maintain hydration and nutritional status.

    f. Surgery should be reserved for severe refractory bleeding, fistulas, or obstruction.

2. Hemorrhagic cystitis occurs in 1% to 2% of patients after pelvic radiation (Mathews, Rajan, & Josefson, 1999). Montana and Fowler (1989) found that the risk of cystitis increased as a function of bladder dose, ranging from 3% for patients receiving 50 Gy or less to 12% in patients receiving at least 80 Gy to the bladder. Management includes endoscopy with obliteration, instillation of sodium pentosanpolysulfate (Parsons, 1986), formalin instillation (Magrina, 1993), and hyperbaric oxygen therapy (Mathews et al., 1999).

3. Vaginal stenosis—High-dose radiation to the pelvis causes varying degrees of sexual dysfunction because of the effects on the ovaries and vagina. Ovarian failure resulting in estrogen deprivation and vaginal stenosis are common sequelae. Bruner, Larciano, Keegan, Corn, Martin & Hanks (1993) evaluated the incidence and degree of vaginal stenosis, sexual activity, and satisfaction in women treated with intracavitary radiation therapy for cervical or endometrial cancer. They found that radiation at standard doses with or without hysterectomy can cause a decrease in vaginal length as compared to the normal vaginal length of 8 to 9 cm documented by Masters and Johnson. Women treated with intracavitary implants remained as sexually active postimplant as preimplant. However, coital frequency and sexual satisfaction decreased and dyspareunia increased.

    Vaginal dilators and sexual intercourse have been the standard recommendations to reduce the risk of vaginal stenosis. However, patient compliance has been a problem, motivating health care providers to look for alternatives. Decruze, Guthrie, and Magnani (1999) designed a vaginal stent to replace the commonly used vaginal dilator. In a retrospective study of the incidence of vaginal stenosis, 57% of the patients who were advised to have regular sexual intercourse developed stenosis, whereas only 11% of patients taught to use the stent had evidence of stenosis. The 11% who developed stenosis were found to be using the stent improperly.

    The success of vaginal dilation depends on patient compliance. Robinson, Faris, and Scott (1999) found a significant improvement in compliance (44.4% vs. 5.6%) with recommendations for dilation when women participated in a group psychoeducational program based on the "information-motivation-behavioral skills" model of behavior change as compared with standard written information with brief counseling. This was particularly true for younger women. Regardless of age, women who received the intervention reported less fear about sex after cancer treatment.

Topical estrogen products, which promote proliferation of the epithelium, can be prescribed to reduce vaginal dryness and dyspareunia. However, this may not be appropriate for patients with estrogen-sensitive tumors. For specific treatment recommendations, see chapter 26.

4. Obliterative endarteritis secondary to ionizing radiation may lead to tissue hypoxia, poor healing, and ultimately to fistulae formation. In women who had radiotherapy to the pelvis for a gynecologic malignancy, fistulae may form between the bladder and vagina, vagina and rectum, bowel and vagina, or bowel and bladder. Patients may present with fecal material draining from the vagina, fecal material in the urine, or urine draining from the vagina. If the small bowel is involved, significant damage can occur to tissue exposed to the small bowel contents. Fistulae require a multidisciplinary team of surgeons, wound care providers, and nutritional experts to design a program to divert the fecal matter or urine and promote healing. Surgery may be necessary to create a diversion around the fistulae. Total parenteral nutrition may be necessary to reduce bowel content and provide adequate calories and protein for healing. Hyperbaric oxygen therapy has been demonstrated to improve angiogenesis and promote healing in radiation-injured tissue. Williams, Clarke, Dennis, Dennis & Smith (1992) evaluated fourteen patients who underwent hyperbaric oxygen therapy for radiation-induced soft tissue necrosis 3 months after the wounds failed to heal with conservative therapy. All patients had a complete resolution of the necrosis and fistula, with only one patient experiencing a recurrent problem.

5. Chronic lymphedema of the lower extremities may occur in response to surgical resection of or radiation to the groin and/or pelvic lymph nodes. Early recognition is necessary to reduce the risk of permanent lymphedema, which can become painful and place the patient at risk for recurrent episodes of lymphangitis and cellulitis. See Chapter 11 for lymphedema management options.

6. A rare complication of radiation therapy to the pelvis (particularly when the groin area is included in the field) is necrosis and fracture of the femoral head/neck. Grigsby, Roberts, and Perez (1995) reported a 5% actuarial 5-year incidence of fractures in patients receiving doses of 50 Gy or greater.
7. Reproductive function is affected by radiation therapy to the pelvis. Women who develop cancer during their childbearing years should receive counseling regarding this loss, and should be referred to a reproductive endocrinologist for fertility options.

OUTCOMES MEASURES

■ The NCI Toxicity Criteria (CTC) Version 2, with the Radiation Therapy Oncology Group (RTOG) and European Organization for Research and Treatment of Cancer (EORTC) Acute Effects Criteria Instrument provides a scale for many different organ systems and some symptoms (NCI, 1999b). This is a very useful tool for grading severity of acute effects of radiation therapy in all sites.
■ The Radiation Therapy Patient Care Record: A Tool for Documenting Nursing Care (ONS, 1994) provides a tool for weekly assessment and grading of severity of acute effects of radiation therapy in all sites.

CANCER OF THE VULVA

■ A follow-up evaluation should be performed every 3 months for a minimum of 2 years. The evaluation should include the following:
  1. History and physical examination.
  2. Careful visual inspection of the vulva and perineum. Colposcopy and biopsy should be performed if there are any suspicious lesions.
  3. Pelvic exam with Pap smear of the cervix every 12 months.
  4. Radiograph or laboratory studies as clinically indicated.
■ In addition to evaluating for recurrence during follow-up visits, patients should be considered at risk for the development of a second primary cancer after vulva cancer. Sturgeon, Curtis, Johnson, Ries, & Brinton (1996) found an increased risk of all second cancers combined among women with cancer of the vulva (observed/expected in situ = 1.5; observed/

expected invasive = 1.3). Most of the excess second cancers were smoking-related (including lung, head and neck sites, and esophagus), or related to infection with human papilloma virus (cervix, vagina, or anus).

CANCER OF THE VAGINA

■ A follow-up evaluation should be performed every 3 months for a minimum of 2 years. The evaluation should include the following:
1. History and physical examination.
2. Careful visual inspection of the vagina with colposcopy and biopsy of any suspicious lesions.
3. Pelvic exam with Pap smear of the cervix and vagina every 3 to 6 months.
4. Radiograph or laboratory studies as clinically indicated.

■ Patients with a history of vaginal squamous cell cancer are also at risk for the development of a second primary tumor in the same manner as patients with a history of vulvar cancer.

CANCER OF THE CERVIX

■ A follow-up evaluation should be performed every 3 months for a minimum of 2 years. The evaluation should include the following:
1. History and physical examination.
2. Pelvic exam with Pap smear of the cervix every 6 to 12 months. Careful examination of the anus and anal canal should be performed. Women with primary invasive cervical cancer have been found to have a relative risk of 4.6 for subsequent invasive anal cancer (Rabkin, Biggar, Melbye, & Curtis, 1992).
3. Radiograph or laboratory studies as clinically indicated.

CANCER OF THE ENDOMETRIUM

■ A follow-up evaluation should be performed every 3 to 6 months for a minimum of 2 years. The evaluation should include the following:
1. History and physical examination.
2. Pelvic exam with Pap smear of the vaginal cuff every 12 months.
3. Radiograph or laboratory studies as clinically indicated.

CANCER OF THE OVARY OR FALLOPIAN TUBE

■ A follow-up evaluation should be performed every 3 months for a minimum of 2 years. The evaluation should include the following:
1. History and physical examination including pelvic exam.
2. CA-125 assay if level was elevated before initial cytore-duction surgery. Median time for clinical relapse after a rising CA-125 is 2 to 6 months (Ozols, 1997).
3. Radiograph or laboratory studies as clinically indicated. No role has been established for routine CT scans of the abdomen or pelvis (Ozols, 1997).

EXPECTED OUTCOMES

SURVIVAL

Cancer of the Vulva
■ The 5-year survival rate for patients with no lymph node spread is about 90% and is only marginally lower for patients with microscopic involvement of one node, providing there is no extracapsular tumor. Patients with two or three in-volved nodes have a survival rate of 66% and those with more than three positive groin nodes have only a 30% sur-vival rate (Burger, Hollema, Emanuels, Krans, Pras, & Bouma, 1995; Origoni, Sideri, Garsia, Carinella, & Ferrari, 1992).

Cancer of the Vagina
■ Kučera and Vavra (1991) reported the outcome of 434 pa-tients with vaginal cancer. Five-year survival for patients with stage I disease was 77%, stage II disease was 45%, stage III disease was 31%, and stage IV was 18%.

Cancer of the Endometrium
■ Five-year survival estimate for all stages is 84%. Patients with disease confined to the uterus have a 96% chance of five-year survival. However, once the disease has extended beyond the uterus or involves regional lymphatics, survival decreases to 66%. Patients with distant metastasis have a five-year survival estimate of 27% (NCI, 1998).

Cancer of the Ovary and Fallopian Tube

■ Despite advances in surgical technology and chemotherapy agents, the prognosis for ovarian and fallopian tube cancer remains poor. The five-year survival rate for all stages is only 50%. Survival of disease confined to the ovary is 95%, but it decreases to 79% for patients with local-regional disease and to 28% for patients with stage III or stage IV disease (NCI, 1998).

QUALITY OF LIFE

■ The measurement of quality-of-life outcomes in women with gynecologic malignancies is sparse in the literature. In addition, there are only a few studies conducted on women receiving radiation therapy. Most studies on quality-of-life outcomes have focused on the physical domain, such as the development of a specific morbidity (such as fistulae development), and have not evaluated psychological, spiritual, or social domains. Of the few quality-of-life studies available, the majority focused on psychological adjustment to the diagnosis, on the treatment, and on the immediate sequelae— usually impact on sexuality. Unfortunately, evaluation of these studies is difficult because of the small populations included, the variety of diagnoses and treatment approaches, and because of differences in design, outcome variability, and end results.

Survivors of gynecologic malignancies face a number of issues in addition to those common in all cancer survivors. These issues include sexual and fertility issues, body image issues, and the impact of treatment-induced early menopause. Only one longitudinal prospective study has been conducted on the incidence and cause of major life difficulties for gynecologic cancer survivors (Andersen, Anderson, & de Prosse, 1989). Women with early-stage cancer were assessed after their diagnosis but prior to treatment and then reassessed at 4, 8, and 12 months posttreatment. Two matched comparison groups (women diagnosed and treated for benign disease and healthy women) were also assessed. The emotional response to the life-threatening diagnosis and anticipation of treatment was characterized by depressed, anxious, and confused moods, whereas the response for women with benign disease was anxious mood only. In both cases, these responses were transitory and resolved posttreatment. There was no evidence for a higher incidence of relationship dissolution or impaired marital adjustment. However, 30% of women treated for disease reported that their sexual partners had some difficulty in reaching orgasm. There was no evidence for impaired social adjustment. Women treated for cancer retained their employment and their occupations. However, their involvement (hours worked per week) was significantly reduced during recovery. The authors suggested that "islands" of significant life disruption after cancer do occur. However, these difficulties do not appear to portend global adjustment vulnerability.

■ Sexual dysfunction has received more attention than any other aspect of quality-of-life research in this patient population. As might be expected because of the organs involved, a high degree of sexual dysfunction is reported among gynecologic cancer survivors, with estimates ranging from 20% to 100% (Anderson & Lutgendorf, 1997). The degree and nature of sexual dysfunction vary according to the type, length, and intensity of treatment. Two surgical procedures, vulvectomy and exenteration result in the most dramatic anatomical changes. Radiation therapy also has a significant impact on vaginal function, with stenosis and loss of elasticity. Induction of early menopause from oophorectomy or ovarian ablation, aggravates other anatomic changes.

Andersen, Anderson, and de Prosse (1989a) found that global sexual behavior changes in women did not occur, but frequency of intercourse declined for women with early-stage gynecologic cancer and those with benign disease. Of the women who had no sexual dysfunction before the diagnosis and treatment of cancer, approximately 50% eventually were diagnosed with at least one dysfunction during the year after treatment. Although some improved, others worsened, and by 12 months after treatment approximately 30% of the cancer patients had some sexual dysfunction. In relation to the sexual response cycle, diminution of sexual excitement was pronounced for women with benign disease, but was more severe and distressing for women with cancer, possibly due to significant coital and postcoital pain, premature menopause, treatment side effects, or a combination. Signs and symptoms of estrogen deficiency were significant in both the benign and malignant groups at 4 and 8 months, but had resolved for the benign group by 12 months.

■ Regarding psychosocial issues, Auchincloss (1995) found that gynecologic cancer survivors have difficulty in forming support groups to help deal with survivor problems and stresses, in part because of the relative rarity of each individual disease. This results in difficulties with depression, energy level, occupational functioning, relationships, and a sense of well-being.

■ The following are appropriate general quality-of-life instruments:

1. Functional Assessment of Cancer Therapy (FACT-G) (Cella, Tulsky, & Gray, 1993)—A measurement system of self-report and 33-item scale of quality of life for people with cancer. The general version has been validated in English and has been used extensively in the United States.

2. European Organization for Research and Treatment of Cancer (EORTC) QLQ-C30 (Aaronson et al., 1993)—A 36-item questionnaire for assessing the quality of life of cancer patients participating in international clinical trials. It has been validated and used extensively in a wide range of cancer clinical trials in Europe and throughout the world.

■ In addition to evaluating long-term survivors of gynecologic cancer, it is important to evaluate the quality of life of patients with overall short life spans. Included in this population are women diagnosed with ovarian cancer. These women tend to have protracted courses of treatment, followed by short periods of disease control. The disease has a profound effect on physical function as well as social and psychosexual functioning. Studies of women with ovarian cancer have focused on descriptive information, assessment, or comparison of treatment alternatives, evaluation of programs or interventions, and facilitation of communication with patients (Bezjak, 1999). Since radiation therapy is used in a limited number of patients, the impact of this therapy on quality of life has not been well documented.

REFERENCES

Aaronson, N. K., Ahmedzai, S., Bergman, B., Bullinger, M., Cull, A., Duez, N. J., Filiberti, A., Flechtner, H., Fleishman, S. B., de Haes, J. C. J. M., Kaasa, S., Klee, M., Osoba, D., Razavi, D., Rofe, P. B., Schraub, S., Sneeuw, K., Sullivan, M., & Takeda, F. (1993). The European Organization for Research and Treatment of Cancer QLQ-C30; A quality-of-life instrument for use in international clinical trials in oncology. *Journal of the National Cancer Institute* 85(5), 365–376.

American Cancer Society. (1997). *Cancer facts and figures—1997* (ACS Publication No. 5008-97). Atlanta: American Cancer Society.

American Cancer Society. (1998). *Cancer facts and figures—1998* (ACS Publication No. 5008-98). (pp. 7–31). Atlanta: American Cancer Society.

American College of Obstetrics and Gynecology. (1996). Guidelines for women's health care (Rev. ed.). Washington, DC: American College of Obstetrics and Gynecology.

American College of Obstetrics and Gynecology. (1997). *Routine cancer screening. Tech. Bull. No. 185.* Washington, DC: American College of Obstetrics and Gynecology.

American College of Physicians. (1992). Guidelines for counseling post-menopausal women about preventive hormone therapy. *Annals of Internal Medicine, 117*(12), 1038–1041.

Andersen, B. L., Anderson, B., & deProsse, C. (1989a). Controlled prospective longitudinal study of women with cancer: I. Sexual functioning outcomes. *Journal of Consulting and Clinical Psychology, 57*(6), 683–691.

Andersen, B. L., Anderson, B., & deProsse, C. (1989b). Controlled prospective longitudinal study of women with cancer: II. Psychological outcomes. *Journal of Consulting and Clinical Psychology, 57*(6), 692–697.

Andersen, B., & Lutgendorf, S. (1997). Quality of life in gynecologic cancer survivors. *CA: Cancer Journal for Clinicians, 47*(4), 218–225.

Auchincloss, S. S. (1995). After treatment. Psychosocial issues in gynecologic cancer survivorship. *Cancer, 76*(10 Suppl): 2117–2124.

Barton, S. E., Maddox, P. H., Jenkins, D., Edwards, R., Cuzick, J., & Singer, A. (1988). Effect of smoking on cervical epithelial immunity: A mechanism for neoplastic change (letter). *Lancet, 2*(8612), 652–654.

Bezjak, A. (1998). Quality of life in women with cancer. In J. J. Kavanagh, S. E. Singletary, N. Einhorn, & A. D. DePetrillo (Eds.), *Cancer in women.* Malden, MA: Blackwell Science.

Blake, P., Lambert, H., & Crawford, R. (1998). *Gynecological oncology. A guide to clinical management* (pp. 98–121). Oxford: Oxford University Press.

Brader, K. R., Morris, M., Levenback, C., Levy, L., Lucas, K. R., & Gershenson, D. M. (1998). Chemotherapy for cervical carcinoma: Factors determining response and implications for clinical trial design. *Journal of Clinical Oncology, 16*(5), 1879–1884.

Bruner, D. W., Lanciano, R., Keegan, M., Corn, B., Martin, E., & Hanks, G. E. (1993). Vaginal stenosis and sexual function following intracavitary radiation for the treatment of cervical and endometrial carcinoma. *International Journal of Radiation Oncology, Biology, Physics*, 27(4), 825–830.

Burger, M. P., Hollema, H., Emanuels, A. G., Krans, M., Pras, E., & Bouma, J. (1995). The importance of the groin node status for the survival of T_1 and T_2 vulva carcinoma patients. *Gynecologic Oncology*, 57(3), 327–334.

Cella, D. F., Tulsky, D. S., & Gray, G. (1993). The Functional Assessment of Cancer Therapy Scale: Development and Validation of the General Measure. *Journal of Clinical Oncology*, 11(3), 570–579.

Chao, K. S. C., Perez, C. A., & Brady, L. W. (1999). *Radiation Oncology: Management Decisions*. Philadelphia: Lippincott-Raven.

Claus, E. B., Schildkraut, J. M., Thompson, W. D., & Risch, N. J. (1996). The genetic attributable risk of breast and ovarian cancer. *Cancer*, 77(11), 2318–2324.

Counter, S. F., Froese, D. P., & Hart, M. J. (1999). Prospective evaluation of formalin therapy for radiation proctitis. *American Journal of Surgery*, 177(5), 396–398.

Decruze, S. B., Guthrie, D., & Magnani, R. (1999). Prevention of vaginal stenosis in patients following vaginal brachytherapy. *Clinical Oncology (Royal College of Radiologists)* 11(1), 46–48.

de Hullu, J. A., Doting, E., Piers, D. A., Hollema, H., Aalders, J. G., Koops, H. S., Boonstra, H., & van-der-Zee, A. G. (1998). Sentinel lymph node identification with technetium-99m-labeled nanocolloid in squamous cell cancer of the vulva. *Journal of Nuclear Medicine*, 39(8), 1381–1385.

Figge, D. C., Tamimi, H. K., & Greer, B. E. (1985). Lymphatic spread in carcinoma of the vulva. *American Journal of Obstetrics and Gynecology* 152(4), 387–394.

Fish, L. S., & Lewis, B. E. (1999) Quality of life issues in the management of ovarian cancer. *Seminars on Oncology*, 26(Suppl. 1): 32–39.

Fyles, A. W., Dembo, A. J., & Bush, R. S. (1992). Analysis of complications in patients treated with abdomino-pelvic radiation therapy for ovarian carcinoma. *International Journal of Radiation Oncology, Biology, Physics*, 22(5), 847–851.

Grady, D., Gebretsadik, T., Kerlikowske, K., Ernster, V. & Petitti, D. (1995). Hormone replacement therapy and endometrial cancer risk: A meta-analysis. *Obstetrics and Gynecology*, 85(2), 304–313.

Greenlee, R. T., Murray, T., Bolden, S., & Wingo, P. A. (2000). Cancer statistics, 2000. *CA Cancer Journal for Clinicians*, 50(1), 7–33.

Grigsby, P. W., Roberts, H. L., & Perez, C. A. (1995). Femoral neck fracture following groin irradiation. *International Journal of Radiation Oncology, Biology, Physics*, 32(1), 63–67.

Henriksson, R., Franzen, L., & Littbrand, B. (1992). Effects of sucralfate on acute and late bowel discomfort following radiotherapy of pelvic cancer. *Journal of Clinical Oncology* 10(6), 969–975.

Holcomb, K., Maiman, M., Dimaio, T., & Gates, J. (1998). Rapid progression to invasive cervix cancer in a woman infected with the human immunodeficiency virus. *Obstetrics and Gynecology*, 91(5, Pt. 2), 848–850.

Homesley, H. D. (1986). GOG Report: Radiation therapy versus pelvic node resection for carcinoma of the vulva with positive groin nodes. *Obstetrics and Gynecology*, 68(6), 733–740.

International Agency for Research on Cancer. (1995). IARC monographs on the evaluation of the carcinogenic risks to humans. (Vol. 64). *Human papilloma viruses.* Lyon, France: International Agency for Research on Cancer.

Keys, H. (1993). Gynecologic Oncology Group randomized trials of combined therapy for vulvar cancer. *Cancer*, 71 (Suppl. 4), 1691–1696.

Keys, H. M., Bundy, B. N., Stehman, F. B., Muderspach, L. I., Chafe, W. E., Suggs, C. L. 3rd, Walker, J. L., & Gersell, D. (1999). Cisplatin, radiation, and adjuvant hysterectomy compared with radiation and adjuvant hysterectomy for bulky stage IB cervical carcinoma. *New England Journal of Medicine*, 340(15), 1154–1161.

Kochhar, R., Sriram, P. V., & Sharma, S. C. (1999). Natural history of late radiation proctosigmoiditis treated with topical sucralfate suspension. *Digestive Diseases and Sciences*, 44(5), 973–978.

Kosary, C. L., Reis, L. A. G., Miller, B. A., Hankey, B. F., Harras, A., & Edwards, B. K. (Eds.). (1995). SEER *Cancer Statistics Review, 1973–1992: Tables and graphs.* (NIH Publication No. 96–2789). Bethesda, MD: National Cancer Institute.

Kuçera, I I., & Vavra, N. (1991). Primary carcinoma of the vagina. Clinical and histopathological variables associated with survival. *Gynecologic Oncology*, 40(1), 12–16.

Lanciano, R. M., & Corn, B. W. (1998). Gynecologic cancer. In L. R. Coia & D. J. Moylan (Eds.), *Introduction to clinical radiation oncology* (pp. 317–350). Madison, WI: Medical Physics Publishing.

Magrina, J. F. (1993). Therapy for urologic complications secondary to irradiation of gynecologic malignancies. *European Journal of Gynecology and Oncology*, 14(4), 265–273.

Magrina, J. F., Gonzalez-Bosquet, J., Weaver, A. L., Gaffey, T. A., Webb, M. J., Podratz, K. C., & Cornella, J. L. (1998). Primary squamous cell cancer of the vulva: Radical versus modified radical vulvar surgery. *Gynecologic Oncology*, 71(1), 116–121.

Maker, A. P. & Trope, C. G. (1992). Gynecologic malignancy and surgery: From quantity to quality of life. *Current Opinion in Obstetrics and Gynecology*, 4(3), 419–429.

Mathews, R., Rajan, N., & Josefson, L. (1999). Hyperbaric oxygen therapy for radiation induced hemorrhagic cystitis. *Journal of Urology*, 161(2), 435–437.

Monk, B. J., Burger, R. A., Lin, F., Parham, G., Vasilev, S. A., & Wilczynski, S. P. (1995). Prognostic significance of human papilloma virus DNA in vulvar cancer. *Obstetrics and Gynecology*, 85(5, Pt. 1), 709–715.

Montana, G. S., & Fowler, W. C. (1989). Carcinoma of the cervix: Analysis of bladder and rectal radiation dose and complications. *International Journal of Radiation Oncology, Biology, Physics*, 16(1), 95–100.

Morris, M., Eifel, P. J., Lu, J., Grigsby, P. W., Levenback, C., Stevens, R. E., Rotman, M., Gershenson, D. M., & Mutch, D. G. (1999). Pelvic radiation with concurrent chemotherapy compared with pelvic and para-aortic radiation for high-risk cervical cancer. *New England Journal of Medicine*, 340(15): 1198–2000.

National Cancer Institute. (1998). *Surveillance, epidemiology, and end results program*, 1998. Bethesda, MD: National Cancer Institute.

National Cancer Institute (1999a). *Cervical cancer: Background information*. Accessed on 9/10/99: http://cancertrials.nci.nih.gov/NC.../TrialInfo/News/cervcan/ccbgd.html.

National Cancer Institute. (1999b). NCI *Common Toxicity Criteria (CTC) Version 2 with the Radiation Therapy Oncology Group (RTOG) and European Organization for Research and Treatment of Cancer (EORTC) Acute Effects Criteria*. Bethesda, MD: National Cancer Institute.

National Institutes of Health Consensus Conference. (1995). Ovarian cancer: Screening, treatment, and follow-up. *JAMA*, 273(6), 491–497.

Nordin, A. J. (1994). Primary carcinoma of the fallopian tube: A 20-year literature review. *Obstetrical and Gynecological Survey*, 49(5), 349–361.

Oncology Nursing Society—Radiation Therapy Special Interest Group Documentation Project Core Committee. (1994). *Radiation Therapy Patient Care Record: A tool for documenting nursing care*. Pittsburgh, PA: Oncology Nursing Society.

Origoni, M., Sideri, M., Garsia, S., Carinelli, S. G., & Ferrari, A. G. (1992). Prognostic value of pathological patterns of lymph node positivity in squamous cell carcinoma of the vulva. Stage III and IVA FIGO. *Gynecologic Oncology*, 45(3), 313–316.

Ozols, R. F. (1997). Update of NCCN Ovarian Cancer Practice Guidelines. *Oncology*, 11(11A), 95–105.

Parazzini, F., La Vecchia, C., Garsia, S., Negri, E., Sideri, M., Rognoni, M. T., & Origoni, M. (1993). Determinants of invasive vulvar cancer risk: An Italian case-control study. *Gynecologic Oncology*, 48(1), 50–55.

Parkin, D. M., Pisani, P., & Ferlay, J. (1993). Estimates of the worldwide incidence of eighteen major cancers in 1985. *International Journal of Cancer*, 54(4), 594–606.

Parsons, G. L. (1986). Successful management of radiation cystitis with sodium pentosanpolysulfate. *Journal of Urology*, 136(4), 813–814.

Pinto, A., Fidalgo, P., Cravo, M., Midoes, J., Chaves, P., Rosa, J., dos-Anjos-Brito, M., & Leitao, C. N. (1999). Short chain fatty acids are effective in short-term treatment of chronic radiation proctitis: Randomized, double-blind, controlled trial. *Diseases of the Colon and Rectum*, 42(6), 788–795.

Rabkin, C. S., Biggar, R. J., Melbye, M., & Curtis, R. E. (1992). Second primary cancers following anal and cervical carcinoma: Evidence of shared etiologic factors. *American Journal of Epidemiology*, 136(1), 54–58.

Robinson, J. W., Faris, P. D., & Scott, C. B. (1999). Psychoeducational group increases vaginal dilation for younger women and reduces sexual fears for women of all ages with gynecological carcinoma treated with radiotherapy. *International Journal of Radiation Oncology, Biology, Physics*, 44(3), 497–506.

Rose, P. G., Bundy, B. N., Watkins, E. B., Thigpen, J. T., Deppe, G., Maiman, M. A., Clarke-Pearson, D. L., & Insalaco, S. (1999). Concurrent cisplatin-based chemoradiation improves progression-free and overall survival in advanced cervical cancer: Results of a randomized Gynecologic Oncology Group study. *New England Journal of Medicine*, 34(15), 1144–1153.

Seltzer, V. L. (1999). Ovarian cancer. In B. S. Kramer, J. K. Gohagan, & P. C. Prorok (Eds.), *Cancer screening: Theory and practice*, (pp. 431–440.). New York: Marcel Dekker.

Shepherd, J., Sideri, M., Benedet, J., Maisonneuve, P., Pecorelli, S., Odicino, F., & Creasman, W. (1998). Carcinoma of the vulva. *Journal of Epidemiology and Biostatistics*, 3(1), 111–127.

Sturgeon, S. R., Brinton, L. A., Devesa, S. S., & Kurman, R. J. (1992). In situ and invasive vulvar cancer incidence trends (1973 to 1987). *American Journal of Obstetrics and Gynecology*, 166(5), 1482–1485.

Sturgeon, S. R., Curtis, R. E., Johnson, K., Ries, L., & Brinton, L. A. (1996). Second primary cancers after vulvar and vaginal cancers. *American Journal of Obstetrics and Gynecology*, 174(3), 929–933.

Swaroop, V. S., & Gostout, C. J. (1998). Endoscopic treatment of chronic radiation proctopathy. *Journal of Clinical Gastroenterology*, 27(1), 36–40.

Terada, K. Y., Coel, M. N., Ko, P., & Wong, J. H. (1998). Combined use of intraoperative lymphatic mapping and lymphoscintigraphy in the management of squamous cell cancer of the vulva. *Gynecologic Oncology*, 70(1), 65–69.

Walker, J. L. & Nuñez, E. R. (1999). Endometrial cancer. In B. S. Kramer, J. K. Gohagan & P. C. Prorok (Eds.), *Cancer screening* (pp. 531–556). New York: Marcel Dekker.

Wang, C. J., Leung, S. W., Chen, H. C., Sun, L. M., Fang, F. M., Huang, E. Y., Hsiung, C. Y., & Changchien, C. C. (1998). The correlation of acute toxicity and late rectal injury in radiotherapy for cervical carcinoma: Evidence suggestive of consequential late effect (CQLE). *International Journal of Radiation Oncology, Biology, Physics*, 40(1), 85–91.

Whitney, C. W., Sause, W., Bundy, B. N., Malfetano, J. H., Hannigan, E. V., Fowler, W. C., Jr; Clarke-Pearson, D. L., & Liao, S. Y. (1999). A randomized comparison of fluorouracil plus cisplatin versus hydroxyurea as an adjunct to radiation therapy in stages IIB-IVA carcinoma of the cervix with negative para-aortic lymph nodes. *Journal of Clinical Oncology*, 17(5), 1339–1348.

Williams, J. A., Jr., Clarke, D., Dennis, W. A., Dennis, E. J., 3rd, & Smith, S. T. (1992). The treatment of pelvic soft tissue radiation necrosis with hyperbaric oxygen. *American Journal of Obstetrics and Gynecology*, 167(2), 412–415.

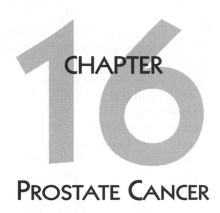

CHAPTER 16

PROSTATE CANCER

Deborah Watkins Bruner
Gerald E. Hanks

PROBLEM

The American Cancer Society predicted that 180,400 new cases of prostate cancer would be diagnosed in 2000, and approximately 37,000 men would die of the disease (Greenlee, Murray, Bolden, & Wingo, 2000). The cumulative lifetime risk of developing prostate cancer is approximately 6.25%, and the cumulative risk of death from prostate cancer is 2% (Rietbergen, Hoedemaeker, Kruger, Kirkels, & Schroder, 1999).

ASSESSMENT

RISK FACTORS

- Age is the primary risk factor for prostate cancer. Although prevalence is difficult to quantify with this disease, it has been estimated that prevalence may be as high as 40% between 50 and 69 years of age with rising prevalence each decade reaching almost 100% after age 80 (Gerard & Frank-Stromborg, 1998; Parker, Tong, Bolden, & Wingo, 1997).
- Family history and a genetic predisposition have been documented as risk factors for developing prostate cancer (Gronberg, Damber, & Damber, 1996; Isaacs, Kiemeney, Baffoe-Bonnie, Beaty, & Walsh, 1995; Schaid, McDonnell,

Blute, & Thibodeau, 1998). However, this accounts for only about 9% of all prostate cancers, but more than 40% of early-onset disease (Carter et al., 1993).

- The increased risk associated with family history has been found for all ages, but it is more pronounced in younger men before age 65 (Gronberg et al., 1996).
- For men at high risk it is not only their own age at the time of screening but the age of onset of prostate cancer of their first-degree relatives that is of concern (Carter et al., 1993). For example, if a brother is diagnosed before age 62 years, the remaining brothers have a four times higher relative risk of developing malignancy (Huncharek & Muscat, 1995).

■ Race or ethnicity has also been associated with increased risk of prostate cancer. African American men have the highest incidence of and mortality from prostate cancer in the world (Brawley & Thompson, 1996).

- African American men have a 9.6% risk of being diagnosed with prostate cancer and a 3% risk of dying of the disease as compared with a 5.2% risk of diagnosis and a 1.4% risk of dying from the disease for White men in the United States (Morton, 1994).
- African American men have about a 73% 5-year survival as compared with an 89% 5-year survival for White men (Parker et al., 1997). Additionally, the proportion of Black men diagnosed with metastatic disease is higher as compared with White men (Steele, Osteen, Winchester, Murphy, & Menck, 1994).

■ In addition to ethnicity, family history, and age, it has become clear that there are lifestyle risk factors associated with the development of prostate cancer. Several studies have demonstrated an association between animal fat intake, particularly red meat, and risk of developing prostate cancer (Giovannucci et al., 1993; Whittemore et al., 1995). Weaker associations have been found with the use of tobacco in which a significant increase in relative risk (RR = 1.31) has been reported and may be dose-dependent in the development of prostate cancer (Coughlin, Neaton, & Sengupta, 1996).

SCREENING AND DIAGNOSTIC TESTS

The American Cancer Society's prostate cancer screening guidelines recommend that annual prostate-specific antigen (PSA) testing and digital rectal examination (DRE) begin at age 50 years for men with a life expectancy *of at least* 10 years, or age 45 years for men with a strong family history, or men who are African American (von Eschenbach, Ho, Murphy, Cunningham, & Lins, 1997). Recommendations from the Mayo Clinic for screening men at high risk for prostate cancer include annual DRE and PSA beginning at age 40 (Cupp & Oesterling, 1993). However, others have suggested that baseline screenings for men at high risk for prostate cancer begin at age 35 (Bruner et al., 1999a; Crawford & DeAntoni, 1995). Screening, diagnostic workup, and staging are delineated in the National Comprehensive Cancer Network (NCCN) oncology practice guidelines (Baker, 1996).

- ■ Digital Rectal Examination (DRE) The positive predictive value of the DRE is low and studies have shown that the DRE alone has a limited ability to detect pathologically localized cancers (Littrup, Lee, & Mettlin, 1992). Yet the DRE remains a standard part of screening and follow-up for prostate cancer (Schroder, 1999).
- ■ Prostate-Specific Antigen (PSA) PSA is a glycoprotein produced in the prostate and was initially used as an indicator of disease progression. Some elevations in PSA may be as a result of benign conditions of the prostate such as benign prostatic hypertrophy (BPH). Since the positive predictive value of the PSA has increased with improved technology, the test is routinely used in screening.
  - It has been reported that the positive predictive value of the PSA increases to 66% for values limited to 2.1 to 4.0 ng/ml. It has been suggested that a prostate cancer screening program should include DRE and PSA at 4.0 ng/ml, which should produce an estimated sensitivity for the PSA + DRE combination of 83% (66% + 17%) (Littrup et al., 1992).
  - Assays to measure several molecular forms of PSA that exist in the serum, including free PSA, PSA complexed to alpha$_1$-antichymotrypsin (bound), and total PSA have helped to further increase the positive predictive value of the PSA. Free PSA ≤ 22% in men with normal DREs and total PSA of between 4 and 10 ng/ml are associated with 90% sensitivity of detecting cancer and 29% avoidance of unnecessary prostate biopsies (Catalona et al., 1998).
  - In addition, other developments to enhance either the sensitivity or specificity of the PSA have been reported including age-specific PSA values, PSA velocity or the rate of

change over time (three PSA values over 2 years), and PSA density, the ratio between prostatic volume and serum PSA (requires a transrectal ultrasound) (Pannek & Partin, 1997).

■ Ultrasound, CT-guided biopsy, MRI with endorectal coil, and/or bone scan can all be used to determine extent of disease in men with a PSA > 10 or Gleason score ≥ 7.

STAGING

The AJCC staging system is included in Table 16–1. AJCC rules allow for changing stage based on imaging results, however this is controversial. Current consensus dictates that staging by palpation is still the preferred method.

In prostate cancer, a pathologic grading system is usually added to the staging system and together they are highly correlated with survival and metastatic outcomes. Histopathologic grading is based on the Gleason system, which identifies both the major and minor predominant prostate cancer cell patterns. Both are scored on a scale of 1 (well differentiated) to 5 (poorly differentiated). The major and minor pattern scores are summed for a total Gleason score (Gleason, 1977).

OUTCOMES MANAGEMENT

THERAPIES

Radiation Therapy

Radiation therapy is most effective with clinically localized disease and is the treatment of choice with locally advanced disease. Radiation therapy can be delivered by standard external-beam radiation therapy, three-dimensional conformal radiation therapy (3D-CRT), intensity-modulated radiation therapy (IMRT), permanent interstitial seed implantation, or a combination.

■ Standard external-beam therapy historically delivers 65 to 70 gray (Gy) to the prostate, periprostatic tissues, and lymph nodes over 6 to 7 weeks. However, this method is becoming outdated with the dramatic improvements in 5-year cure rates of 15% to 40% seen with escalating doses used in conformal radiation therapy.

TABLE 16–1   TNM STAGING OF PROSTRATE CANCER

Primary Tumor (T) (male and female)

T_X	Primary tumor cannot be assessed
T_0	No evidence of primary tumor
T_a	Noninvasive papillary, polypoid, or verrucous carcinoma
T_{is}	Carcinoma in situ
T_1	Tumor invades subepithelial connective tissue
T_2	Tumor invades any of the following: corpus spongiosum, prostate, periurethral muscle
T_3	Tumor invades any of the following: corpus cavernosum, beyond prostatic capsule, anterior vagina, bladder neck
T_4	Tumor invades other adjacent organs

Stage Grouping of Prostate Cancer

Stage 0_a	T_a	N_0	M_0
Stage 0_{is}	T_{is}	N_0	M_0
	T_{is} pu	N_0	M_0
	T_{is} pd	N_0	M_0
Stage I	T_1	N_0	M_0
Stage II	T_2	N_0	M_0
Stage III	T_1	N_1	M_0
	T_2	N_1	M_0
	T_3	N_0	M_0
	T_3	N_1	M_0
Stage IV	T_4	N_0	M_0
	T_4	N_1	M_0
	Any T	N_2	M_0
	Any T	Any N	M_1

From the AJCC *Cancer Staging Manual* (5th ed.). Copyright 1997 by Lippincott-Raven. Adapted with permission of the publisher.

- ■ Conformal radiation therapy uses CT images to enhance treatment planning. This allows for more precise localization of the target tissue and better-designed blocks that conform to the prostate and spare normal tissue (Beard et al., 1997).
  - A recent analysis of 5-year outcomes with 3D-CRT showed a no biochemical evidence of disease (bNED) rate of 35% at 70 Gy and 75% at 76 Gy for PSA 10 to 19.9 ng/mL and a bNED of 10% at 70 Gy and 32% at 76 Gy for PSA > 20ng/mL. No dose response was seen for PSA < 10 ng/mL (Hanks et al., 1998).

- The Patterns of Care Study have documented an unfortunately slow diffusion of this technology into practice across the United States, with 20% of institutions surveyed using 3D conformal therapy in 1994 and 40% in 1998 (G. E. Hanks, personal communication, January 2000).

■ A new complexity of treatment under recent investigation that may have an incremental response benefit over 3D conformal therapy is intensity-modulated radiation therapy (IMRT). This technique allows for dose escalation (≥ 81 Gy) while satisfying normal tissue constraints for rectal and bladder walls, and in preliminary studies has shown promise (Reinstein et al., 1998).

■ Interstitial implants use radioactive seeds, introduced transperineally under transrectal ultrasonography, to provide a predictable dose of radiation to a confined area. This technique places the radioactive source in close proximity to the tumor, thus sparing nearby healthy tissue (Davis, 1998). The short half-life allows for permanent implantation. Interstitial implants can be used alone or, although somewhat controversial, used in combination with external-beam radiation therapy.

- Early reports of morbidity postimplant have been relatively low, however the accuracy of these reports has been questioned recently (Hanks, 2000).

- The American Brachytherapy Society (ABS) has developed recommendations for the clinical quality assurance and guidelines for appropriate patient selection and dose reporting of permanent transperineal prostate brachytherapy with ^{125}I or [103]Pd. Recommendations for treatment volume, dose, dose distribution, and postimplant seed distribution are included. The ABS states that patients with a high probability of organ-confined disease are appropriately treated with brachytherapy alone. Brachytherapy candidates with a significant risk of extraprostatic extension should be treated with supplemental external-beam radiation therapy (Nag, Beyer, Friedland, Grimm, & Nath, 1999). The issue of implant training or certification is not addressed in the ABS recommendations, however it is of concern and is included in many residency programs.

Surgery

Radical prostatectomy, used for clinically localized disease, is the surgical removal of the prostate gland and seminal vesicles, usually with a lymph node dissection to rule out micrometastasis. During a classic radical prostatectomy the neurovascular bundles controlling erection are transected, which often leads to impotence. This has led to the development of a nerve-sparing prostatectomy that is attempted when the lesion is small and potency is an issue (Brendler & Walsh, 1992; Walsh, 1988).

■ The nerve-sparing prostatectomy has revolutionized the acceptability of the prostatectomy, although studies consistently show that radiation is superior for the preservation of potency and continence.

A concern with surgery is that approximately 30% to 50% of patients thought to have localized adenocarcinoma of the prostate gland are found at radical prostatectomy to have extracapsular disease or positive surgical margins. Recent studies have shown that adjuvant radiation therapy in patients with poor prognostic factors (e.g., positive surgical margins, rising PSA after prostatectomy) can improve disease-free survival 20% to 50% depending on subgroup. In addition, morbidity is acceptable with adjuvant radiation therapy (Petrovich et al., 1999; Pisansky et al., 2000).

Hormone Therapy

Because prostate cancer is androgen dependent it often responds to androgen deprivation therapy (ADT). ADT consists of either a bilateral orchiectomy or an antiandrogen alone or in combination with a luteinizing hormone releasing hormone (LH-RH) analogue, which blocks adrenal androgens.

■ Initially ADT was the treatment reserved for metastatic disease. Antiandrogens are now being used in multiple clinical trials as neoadjuvant therapy in earlier stages of disease prior to either surgery or radiation therapy in an effort to shrink the prostate, and hopefully the tumor, for better local control.

■ In an effort to improve survival, one study incorporated hormone therapy during radiation therapy followed by 3 years of an LH-RH agonist. Local control, disease-free survival, and overall survival improved nearly 20% at 5 years (Bolla et al., 1997).

■ RTOG 85-31 evaluated the effect of immediate androgen suppression (LH-RH agonist), in conjunction with standard external-beam irradiation versus radiation alone in a group of pathologically staged lymph node-positive patients with adenocarcinoma of the prostate (n = 173). With a median follow-up of 4.9 years, estimated 5-year progression-free survival with PSA < 1.5 ng/mL was 55% for the patients who received radiation plus immediate LH-RH agonist versus 11% for the patients who received radiation alone with the addition of hormones at relapse (p = 0.0001). Estimated absolute survival at 5 years for the radiation and LH-RH group was 73% versus 65% for the radiation alone group who received androgen suppression at relapse. Estimated disease-specific survival at 5 years was 82% for the radiation and immediate LH-RH agonist group and 77% for the radiation alone group (Lawton et al., 1997).

■ These two studies have established guidelines for practice for T_3, T_4, and Gleason 8-10 disease. Patients with cancer of the prostate with extension to the pelvic lymph nodes (pN^+ or clinical stage D_1) should be seriously considered for external-beam radiation therapy plus immediate androgen suppression over radiation alone with hormonal manipulation at the time of relapse (Lawton et al., 1997). A survival benefit may require long-term adjuvant hormonal therapy (Roach, 1999).

■ While studies show that the pathologic staging of tumors following ADT treatment is improved compared with surgical controls, the PSA disease-free survival rates are similar (Fair et al., 1997). Without improvements in outcome, the present state of the art does not support the use of neoadjuvant ADT prior to surgery.

■ Side effects of ADT include an 80% to 100% risk of impotence (Bruner, Hanlon, Nicolaou, & Hanks, 1997; Schover, 1993), and hot flushes that occur in about half of the men treated. A recent study of bone mineral density (BMD) in men treated with ADT found osteopenia and osteoporosis to be common in men with prostate cancer before initiating ADT. Five to eight men (63%) who had not received ADT and twenty-one to twenty-four men (88%) who had received ADT for more than 1 year fulfilled the criteria for osteopenia or osteoporosis at one or more sites. However, men on ADT for more than 1 year had significantly lower BMD in the lumbar spine than men who had not started treatment (p < 0.05). Both ADT and the duration of ADT were significantly associated with the loss of BMD. The authors estimated that it would take 48 months of ADT to develop BMD criteria for osteopenia in the lumbar spine for a man with average BMD at the initiation of therapy (Wei et al., 1999).

Multimodality Therapy

Androgen insensitive metastatic disease has been treated promisingly with varying combinations of estramustine, etoposide, vinblastine, doxorubicin, paclitaxel, docetaxel, and suramin. An in vivo synergism has been reported to yield higher cytotoxicity when combinations of the drugs are used than when any of the drugs are used alone. Toxicities associated with theses chemotherapeutic agents include myelosuppresion (e.g., neutropenia, leukopenia); gastrointestinal symptoms (e.g., anorexia, stomatitis, diarrhea, epigastric pain); neurotoxicity (polyneuropathy), hypocalcemia and hypophosphatemia, alopecia, fatigue, and allergic skin rash (Arah, Dixon, Horti, & Figg, 1999; Culine et al., 1998; Kreis et al., 1999; Pienta & Smith, 1997).

Gene Therapy

Gene therapy used alone or as adjuvant therapy is under study in prostate cancer. The rationale for gene therapy is that it may make it possible to treat localized and systemic disease effectively and simultaneously. In situ gene therapy research in which viral vectors have been used to transduce specific genes that generate cytotoxic activity and/or systemic immunity to the cancer has offered hope for significantly reducing prostate cancer mortality, but these studies are still in their infancy (Thompson, 1999).

Guidelines for the appropriate type and timing of prostate cancer therapies for initial and salvage treatments are further delineated in the NCCN oncology practice guidelines (Baker, 1996; Bruner et al., 1995; Logothetis & Millikan, 1999; Millikan & Logothetis, 1997).

Symptom Management

Bladder, bowel, sexual, and fatigue outcomes may be poorer than necessary because of the lack of standard therapies to treat the side effects after radiation therapy. To improve outcomes, a combination of medical *and* behavioral interventions are necessary (Bruner, Bucholtz, Iwamoto, & Strohl, 1998a), but few health care professionals in radiation therapy are well trained in the behavioral interventions and counseling required. This stresses the need for a multidisciplinary approach to the improvement of outcomes after prostate cancer therapy.

Urinary stress incontinence has been treated effectively with behavioral therapies including:

■ Fluid spacing, bowel regulation, adjustment of medications, and timed voiding (Pickett, Watkins Bruner, Joseph, & Burggraf, 2000).

■ Strengthening support muscles with pelvic floor muscle exercises helps to decrease urinary stress incontinence, however, the patient needs to be motivated and continue exercises throughout his life or the positive benefit will be lost (Burgio, Stutzman, & Engel, 1989).

■ Biofeedback can be very helpful in improving symptoms; however, success is dependent on the intensity of the program, patient motivation, the severity of the problem, and the skill of the provider (Jackson, Emerson, Johnston, Wilson, Morales, 1996). In one study, patients treated with a verbal behavioral program reported 56.6% improvement in continence (Meaglia, Joseph, Chang, & Schmidt, 1990).

Urge incontinence, leakage of urine due to detrusor instability or a noncompliant bladder, can be treated with medication:

■ Anticholinergic agents (e.g., oxybutynin and tolterodine) act at postganglionic parasympathetic cholinergic receptor sites on the detrusor muscle, reducing the strength of detrusor contraction instability.

• Tricyclic antidepressants (e.g., imipramine) have anticholinergic effects, block presynaptic uptake of amine neurotransmitters, and directly inhibit detrusor muscle instability (Sullivan & Abrams, 1999).

• Although anticholinergics have proven to be effective, many patients dislike the side effects of dry mouth and constipation.

■ New antimuscarinic agents such as tolterodine are now available with fewer side effects. Tolterodine has recently been approved as therapy in patients with overactive bladder who have symptoms of urinary frequency, urgency, or urge incontinence. It acts by muscarinic receptor blockade in the bladder wall and detrusor muscle (Abrams, Greeman, Anderstrom, & Mattiasson, 1998; Guay, 1999).

SEXUAL FUNCTION

Pharmacologic and nonpharmacologic interventions that can restore voluntary erectile function for sexual intercourse have been available for years but have gained little attention from physicians and patients alike, probably because of inconvenience and cost. The American Urologic Association (AUA) Clinical Guidelines Panel on Erectile Dysfunction recently published recommendations based on the treatment outcomes data on men with organic (versus psychological) erectile dysfunction. The panel reviewed published outcomes for five treatment alternatives including vacuum constriction devices, intracavernous vasoactive injections, penile prosthesis implants, venous and arterial surgery, and oral drug therapy with yohimbine. The panel concluded that only the first three alternatives had acceptable outcomes in terms of return to intercourse, patient satisfaction, and partner satisfaction (Montague et al., 1996). An extensive discussion of these interventions is discussed in Chapter 26, "Maintenance of Body Image and Sexual Function."

The AUA undertook their review prior to FDA approval of the now-popular drug Sildenafil, a recently approved vasoactive oral agent for the treatment of erectile dysfunction. The drug has demonstrated significant improvement in erectile dysfunction in patients treated with radical prostatectomies. At the end of one long-term study, 88% of patients reported that Sildenafil improved their erections. Across all trials, Sildenafil improved erections in 43% of radical prostatectomy patients compared with 15% with placebo (Boolell, Gepi-Attee, Gingell, & Allen, 1996). Large clinical trials evaluating the use of this drug in patients treated with radiation therapy have yet to be conducted, although the Radiation Therapy Oncology Group (RTOG) has recently approved a protocol to study the effects of Sildenafil in men treated with radiotherapy for prostate cancer.

BOWEL SYMPTOMS

- Mild rectal bleeding may be treated with stool softeners, steroid enemas, and anti-inflammatory drugs such as corticosteroids administered either systemically or topically.
- Sucralfate enemas have been used successfully to treat radiation-induced rectal bleeding that had been unresponsive to steroid enemas (Stockdale & Biswas, 1997).
- Rectal urgency can be treated successfully with "bulking agents" such as Metamucil or medications such as loperamide or diphenoxylate (Crook, Esche, & Futter, 1996) (Pickett et al., 2000).
- Management of radiation enteritis includes assessment of height and weight, change in eating habits, amount of

residue in the diet, and signs of dehydration such as poor skin turgor, serum electrolyte imbalance, increased weakness, or fatigue (NCI/PDQ Physician Statement, 1997).

■ Medical management includes antidiarrheal agents such as the following:
  • Diphenoxylate atropine 1 to 2 tablets po q 4 hr
  • Loperamide hydrochloride 4 mg po q 4 hr initially, then 2 mg po after each loose stool
  • Kaolin-pectat 30 to 60 cc po after each loose bowel movement
  • Paragoric 5 cc po qid prn
  • Anticholinergic agents such as Donnatal (combination of atropine sulfate, hyoscyamine sulfate, phenobarbital, and scopolamine hydrobromide), 1 to 2 tablets q 4 hr prn [Pickett et al., 2000]

■ Dietary management includes encouraging:
  • Clear fluids and broth
  • Eight glasses of water per day
  • Easily digested foods such as rice, bananas, applesauce, pasta, and baked, boiled, or mashed potatoes
  • Eating small, frequent meals
  • Eating food at room temperature

■ Foods that should be avoided include:
  • Dairy products
  • Greasy, fatty, spicy, or fried foods, and rich pastries
  • Raw vegetables, fresh and dried fruits, and prune juice
  • Whole-grain breads and cereals, nuts, and seeds
  • Alcohol and tobacco
  • Caffeine including coffee, tea, and soft drinks with caffeine, and chocolate (Pickett et al., 2000)

OUTCOMES MEASURES

Measurement and quantification of side effects and outcomes are essential before any interventions can be initiated and can be shown to directly affect appropriate outcomes (Goluboff, Chang, Olsson, & Kaplan, 1995).

Follow-up after prostate cancer therapy includes regularly scheduled physician examination, DRE and PSA, as previously described, with additional testing such as CT scans or bone scans as symptoms indicate. Patients on ADT require periodic liver function tests and studies of bone mineral density.

Documented discrepancies in physician versus patient self-report of therapy-related morbidity support guidelines requiring patient self-assessment questionnaires or patient interviews to be used to assess factors that impact quality of life after prostate cancer therapy (Bruner et al., 1995; Bruner et al., 1998b). Changes from pre-illness baseline are the critical outcome measure. A review of nine prostate-specific QOL instruments has recently been reported (Sommers & Ramsey, 1999). More importantly, a recent study documented that several interviewer-administered QOL instruments tested in low-income patients were able to provide valid and reliable information even in busy clinical settings (Sharp et al., 1999).

Urinary outcomes should include assessment of frequency, urgency, dysuria, nocturia, obstructive symptoms, and urge or stress incontinence. Urinalysis and urine cultures should be done for fever, pain, hematuria, or cloudy urine. Instruments that measure the impact that these symptoms have on quality of life include:

- American Urologic Association (AUA) Symptom Problem Index (SPI)/Benign Prostatic Hyperplasia Impact Index (BPHII). The SPI is a 7-item, Likert-type questionnaire (rated on a 0 to 4 scale) designed to assess the difficulty patients experience with their urinary symptoms. The BPHII is a 4-item scale that measures how much patients' urinary symptoms affect various domains of health including discomfort, worry, distress, and daily activities. Both indices have demonstrated acceptable reliability and validity (Barry et al., 1995). The symptoms measured by these instruments are similar to those reported after therapy for prostate cancer with either surgery or radiation therapy, and the instrument is being used in prostate cancer trials.

- The UCLA Prostate Cancer Index with its disease-targeted measures of function and bother in the three domains of sexual, urinary, and bowel function has demonstrated good psychometric properties and, in at least one study, appeared to be well understood and easily completed (Litwin et al., 1998).

- The Joseph Continence Assessment Tool (JCAT) is an instrument developed to assess urinary continence (Joseph, 1992). It is a biopsychosocial checklist that includes the assessment of chronic disease/disorders, medications, nutrition, fluid intake, elimination (bowel and bladder), sensory abilities, skin integrity, exercise/rest pattern, functional capabilities, neurologic abilities, and the endrocrine system. In addition, the individual's role function, self-concept, interdependence, behavior, and feelings as well as their goal in returning to continence are also addressed.

■ Functional Alterations due to Changes in Elimination (FACE), is an experimental instrument being piloted in two National Clinical Trial Groups, the Radiation Therapy Oncology Group and Gynecologic Oncology Group. FACE is an expansion of CUF (Changes in Urinary Function) developed by Bruner et al. (1994). CUF was developed specifically to assess symptoms related to prostate and bladder cancer therapies and their impact on quality of life. FACE is a 15-item, Likert-type, self-rating scale divided into two subscales, one assessing urinary function and one assessing bowel function. The questionnaire was designed to measure the construct of intrusion on daily functioning caused by changes in elimination as measured by these two subscales. Dimensions of intrusion include control, fear, anxiety, sexual activity/body image, and incontinence.

■ A self-assessment questionnaire using a linear-analog scale for evaluating urinary and intestinal late side effects after pelvic radiotherapy in patients with prostate cancer has also been developed (Widmark, Fransson, & Tavelin, 1994).

The impact that radiation therapy (with or without ADT) has on men's sexual function should be assessed by first obtaining a detailed sexual history. This includes:

■ Previous frequency of activity
■ Problems with arousal or orgasm
■ Conditions (e.g., diabetes) or medications (e.g., antihypertensives, antidepressants) that may interfere with sexual function

Measures of sexual function and intimacy are discussed in depth in Chapter 26, "Maintenance of Body Image and Sexual Function" as well as elsewhere (Bruner & Iwamato, 1999). One measure that has been used extensively in the Radiation Therapy Oncology Group (RTOG) to measure sexual functioning after treatment for prostate cancer is the Sexual Adjustment Questionnaire (SAQ).

■ The SAQ was originally developed by Waterhouse and Metcalfe (1986). The questionnaire rated most responses on a five-point patient self-rating scale, with a higher score indicating a higher level of sexual adjustment. The SAQ has been modified by the RTOG and is a 16-item questionnaire that assesses five domains including desire, activity, arousal, orgasm, and satisfaction. Validity and reliability are acceptable (Bruner et al., 1998b).

Additional outcomes that impact QOL after prostate cancer therapy such as fatigue or anxiety can be measured with symptom checklists or with measures that incorporate the multidimensional outcomes of interest.

- Functional Assessment Cancer Therapy-Prostate (FACT-P), developed by Cella et al. (1993) is an instrument designed to assess the multidimensional aspects of QOL including physical well-being, social/family well-being, emotional well-being, functional well-being, treatment satisfaction, and prostate cancer specific concerns. FACT-P includes 13 "Additional Concerns" developed to address prostate cancer specific symptoms that may impact quality of life. The psychometric properties of the instrument have been well established (Esper et al., 1997).

- The European Organization for Research and Treatment of Cancer (EORTC) has developed and tested several health-related quality-of-life scales that have shown validity and reliability in the prostate cancer setting including the Core Quality of Life Questionnaire (QLQ-C30); a trial-specific quality-of-life module (QLM-P14); and the Prostate Cancer Specific Quality of Life Instrument (PROSQOLI), a measure of health-related quality of life (HRQL) that was designed to be an outcome measure for clinical trials in advanced hormone-resistant prostate cancer (Stockler, Osoba, Corey, Goodwin, & Tannock, 1999).

EXPECTED OUTCOMES

Early Patterns of Care Surveys documented a doubling of serious morbidity when radiation therapy dose to the prostate exceeded 70 Gy with conventional therapy (Hanks, Teshima, & Pajak, 1997). However, several recent technical advances in radiation therapy as previously discussed, such as conformal therapy and IMRT, more precisely target the tumor and result in decreased exposure of healthy surrounding tissue.

Acute urinary symptoms such as frequency, dysuria, and hematuria resulting from radiation therapy at standard doses of 65 to 70 Gy have been reported at about 17% (Beard et al., 1997).

- Late urinary effects occurring longer than 6 months after conventional radiation therapy that are considered to be serious ($\geq$ grade 3) include bladder contracture (2–32%), cystitis (2–15%), bleeding (1–7%), incontinence (1–10%), and fistual formation (1–7%) (Marks, Carroll, Dugan, & Anscher, 1995).
- Late intestinal effects have been reported to occur at a median of 8 to 12 months, but have also been reported years after conventional radiation therapy. The most common late side effects include frequent and urgent stools, although bleeding and abdominal and rectal pain may also be present (Coia, Myerson, & Tepper, 1995).

SURVIVAL

A recent multi-institutional series reported actuarial 5-year survival in 1,765 men after treatment for stage T_{1b}, T_{1c}, and T_2 tumors treated in the PSA era between 1988 and 1995 with radical external-beam radiation (Shipley et al., 1999). Approximately 60% of patients were > 70 years and about one-quarter had initial PSA values of 20 ng/mL or higher. Follow-up ranged from 2 to 9 years.

- Overall survival was 85.0% (95% confidence interval [CI], 82.5–87.6%)
- Disease-specific survival was 95.1% (95% CI, 94.0–96.2%)
- Freedom from biochemical failure was 65.8% (95% CI, 62.8–68.0%)

The PSA failure-free rates after treatment for patients presenting with a PSA of less than 10 ng/mL were

- 5-years—77.8% (95% CI, 74.5–81.3%)
- 7-years—72.9% (95% CI, 67.9–78.2%)
- Disease-specific survival was 63.5% minimum and 96% maximum (Shipley et al., 1999)

Comparatively, 5-year survival data after radical prostatectomy in 1,620 men with stage T_{1c} versus T_{2a} or T_{2b} prostate cancer, treated between 1988 and1998 with radical retropubic prostatectomy with a mean age of 62 years have recently been reported (Ramos, Carvalhal, Smith, Mager, & Catalona, 1999).

- 5-year recurrence-free survival rate was 85% for T_{1c}, 83% for T_{2a}, and 72% for T_{2b}.
- 5-year disease-specific survival rate was 100% for the T_{1c} and T_{2a} groups, and 97% for the T_{2b} group (Ramos et al., 1999).
- In a study of the impact of margin status on the survival outcome of 5,467 surgical patients with otherwise organ-confined disease, 5-year progression-free survival to the combined endpoint of clinical and/or PSA progression (≤ 0.2 ng/mL) was 86% for stage pT_2N_0, and 70% for stage pT_3N_0 (Blute et al., 1998).
- Surveillance, for carefully selected candidates, also had relatively high 5-year overall survival at 67% minimum and 92% maximum, and for disease-specific survival, 89% minimum and 99% maximum (Middleton, Smith, Melzer, & Hamilton, 1986).

QUALITY-OF-LIFE

Quality-of-life outcome studies after treatment for localized prostate cancer have focused mainly on incontinence and impotence, although other symptoms are recognized to impact QOL including diarrhea, proctitis, and fatigue.

- Incontinence after radiation therapy, documented using patient self-report, has been reported in 2% to 15% of men compared with 35% to 52% of men receiving radical prostatectomy (Schrader-Bogen, Kjellberg, McPherson, & Murray, 1997; Talcott et al., 1998; Yarbro & Ferrans, 1998).
- The impact of bowel and bladder symptoms on QOL in 120 prostate cancer patients (mean age 68 years; range 52–82) treated with 3D-CRT alone was recently reported. Bowel and bladder QOL measures for these patients were compared with that of the normal population of men with a similar age distribution. Eighty percent of the prostate cancer patients reported overall satisfaction with bowel and bladder functioning. There was no significant difference in the other bladder symptoms caused by men treated with radiotherapy as compared with men without cancer (Hanlon, Bruner, & Hanks, 1999).
- Impotence after radiation therapy has been reported in 50% to 67% of men compared with 70% to 98% of men receiving radical prostatectomy (Schrader-Bogen et al., 1997; Talcott et al., 1998; Yarbro & Ferrans, 1998).

- Sixty-two percent of men treated with radiation therapy and 69% of men treated with surgery have reported dissatisfaction with posttreatment sexual function (Schrader-Bogen et al., 1997).
- However, in contrast to surgical series, a recent study of 67 men aged 65 years or less treated with 3D conformal radiation therapy for clinically localized prostate between April 1989 and December 1993, demonstrated high and durable rates of posttreatment potency preservation. At 3 years, potency was 73% for treated patients and 85% for controls, and at 5.6 years the potency preservation rate was 59% for treated patients and 78% for controls (Wurzer, Nicolaou, Hanlon, Bruner, & Hanks, 1999).
- In a separate retrospective study of 3D-CRT for prostate cancer on sexual function and related quality of life, 60 patients (median age 72.3 years) who were potent prior to treatment were surveyed. Following 3D-CRT, 37 of 60 patients (62%) retained sexual function sufficient for intercourse. However, intercourse at least once per month was reduced from 71% to 40%, whereas intercourse less than once per year increased from 12% to 35%. After treatment, 25% of patients reported that the change in sexual dysfunction negatively affected their relationship or resulted in poor self-esteem. This negative effect on relationships or poor self-esteem was associated with impotence following treatment ($p < 0.01$). Patients who had partners and satisfactory sexual function prior to treatment appeared to be at a higher risk of having a negatively affected relationship or losing self-esteem if they become impotent posttreatment ($p < 0.05$) (Roach, Chinn, Holland, & Clarke, 1996).
- The assumption appears to be that morbidity following neoadjuvant hormones would level off at the percent of morbidity conferred by the primary therapy (surgery or radiation therapy) alone once the hormones are discontinued, however preliminary data does not support this. One report found that men treated with radiation therapy plus ADT were significantly inferior to both the radiation therapy alone and the control group, even after hormones were discontinued, in all areas of sexual function measured including sexual arousal, function, and frequency.

Posttreatment potency rates for the radiation therapy alone group and the RT/ADT group were 67% and 41%, respectively (Bruner et al., 1997).

In addition, fatigue following radiation therapy for prostate cancer has been reported in up to 65% of patients by the end of treatment and shown to persist in up to 14% of patients by 3 months posttreatment (Greenberg, Gray, Mannix, Eisenthal, & Carey, 1993; King, Nail, Kreamer, Strohl, & Jojnson, 1985).

Interestingly, although radiotherapy causes site-specific decrements in quality of life, patients have actually reported better global QOL as compared to men without prostate cancer (Bruner et al., 1999b).

BOWEL SYMPTOMS

Patients experiencing radiation-induced proctitis, or inflammation of the rectum, may report mucoid rectal discharge, rectal pain, and rectal bleeding.

- Diarrhea and abdominal discomfort have been reported in up to 49% of men receiving greater than or equal to 70 Gy, however less than 1% of these symptoms are reported as severe ($\geq$ grade 3) (Jonler et al., 1994; Lawton et al., 1991).
- In a study of the impact of bowel and bladder symptoms on QOL in 120 prostate cancer patients (mean age 68 years) treated with 3D-CRT alone compared with a normal population of men with a similar age distribution, patients did have more very small to moderate bother from bowel dysfunction than the normal population (59% vs. 33%), yet no patients reported bowel dysfunction bother as a big problem (Hanlon et al., 1999).
- With brachytherapy 3% of prostate cancer patients may develop rectal ulcerations causing pain and bleeding with bowel movements. Rectal ulceration may occur up to 2.5 years after the implant and last 4 to 6 months. Rectal ulceration has been successfully treated with laser surgery (Whittington et al., 1997).
- Acute radiation enteritis results from the cytotoxic effect of radiation therapy on rapidly proliferating epithelial cells resulting in diarrhea, abdominal cramping, and rectal urgency (Pickett et al., 2000).

Follow-Up

NCCN guidelines recommend:

- For men treated with curative intent, PSA should be checked every 6 months for the first 5 years and then annually; DRE should be conducted annually.
- For men treated with locally advanced or metastatic disease, history, physical, DRE, and PSA are suggested every 3 months.
- For men treated with antiandrogens, liver enzymes should be monitored monthly for 3 months. Bone scans are only recommended when symptoms are reported or there are two consecutive rises in the PSA (Logothetis & Millikan, 1999).

References

Abrams, P., Greeman, R., Anderstrom, C., & Mattiasson, A. (1998). Tolterodine, a new antimuscarinic agent: As effective but better tolerated than oxybutynin in patients with an overactive bladder. *British Journal of Urology*, 81(6), 801–810.

Arah, I. N., Dixon, S. C., Horti, J., & Figg, W. D. (1999). Enhanced activity of estramustine, vinblastine, etoposide, and suramin in prostate carcinoma. *Neoplasma*, 46(2), 117–123.

Baker, L. (1996). NCCN prostate cancer practice guidelines. NCCN *Proceedings*, 10(Suppl. 11) 265–288.

Barry, M., Fowler, F., O'Leary, M., Bruskewitz, R., Holtgrewe, H., Mebust, W., & American Urologic Association. (1995). Measuring disease-specific health status in men with benign prostatic hyperplasia. *Medical Care*, 33(4), AS145–AS155.

Beard, C., Propert, K. J., Rieker, P., Clark, J., Kaplan, I., Kantoff, P., & Talcott, J. (1997). Complications after treatment with external-beam irradiation in early-stage prostate cancer patients: A prospective multiinstitutional outcomes study. *Journal of Clinical Oncology*, 15, 223–229.

Blute, M. L., Bostwick, D. G., Seay, T. M., Martin, S. K., Slezak, J. M., Bergstrath, E. J., & Sincke, H. (1998). Pathologic classification of prostate carcinoma: The impact of margin status. *Cancer*, 82(5), 902–908.

Bolla, M., Gonzales, D., Warde, P., Dubois, J. B., Mirimanoff, R. O., Storme, G., Bernier, J., Kuten, A., Sternberg, C., Gil, T., Collette, L., & Pierart, M. (1997). Improved survival in patients with locally advanced prostate cancer treated with radiotherapy and goserelin. *New England Journal of Medicine*, 337(5), 295–300.

Boolell, M., Gepi-Attee, S., Gingell, J. C., & Allen, M. J. (1996). Sildenafil, a novel effective oral therapy for male erectile dysfunction. *British Journal of Urology*, 78, 257–261.

Brawley, O. W., & Thompson, I. M. (1996). The chemoprevention of prostate cancer and the Prostate Cancer Prevention Trial. *Cancer Treatment and Research*, 88, 189–200.

Brendler, C. B., & Walsh, P. C. (1992). The role of radical prostatectomy in the treatment of prostate cancer. CA: *Cancer Journal for Clinicians*, 42, 212–222.

Bruner, D. W., Baffoe-Bonnie, A., Miller, S., Diefenbach, M., Tricoli, J. V., Daly, M., Pinover, W., Campbell-Grumet, S., Stofey, J., Ross, E., Raysor, S., Balshem, A., Malick, J., Mirchandani, I., Engstrom, P., & Hanks, G. E. (1999a). Prostate cancer risk assessment program: A model for early detection of prostate cancer. *Oncology*, 13(3), 325–334.

Bruner, D. W., Bucholtz, J., Iwamoto, R., & Strohl, R. (1998a). *Manual for radiation oncology nursing practice and education* (2nd ed.). Pittsburgh, PA: Oncology Nursing Press.

Bruner, D. W., Hanlon, A., Nicolaou, N., & Hanks, G. (1997). Sexual function after radiotherapy ± androgen deprivation for clinically localized prostate cancer in younger men (age 50–65). *Oncology Nursing Forum*, 24(2), 327.

Bruner, D. W., & Iwamato, R. (1999). Altered sexuality. In S. Groenwald, M. Frogge, M. Goodman, & C. Yarbro (Eds.), *Cancer symptom management* (2nd ed.). Boston: Jones & Bartlett.

Bruner, D. W., Ross, E., Raysor, S., Hanlon, A. L., Grumet, S., & Hanks, G. (1999b). Men treated with radiotherapy have better global quality of life outcomes despite decrements in site-specific quality of life domains than men at increased risk but without prostate cancer [Abstract]. *International Journal of Radiation Oncology, Biology, Physics*, 45(Suppl. 2), 432.

Bruner, D. W., Scott, C., Byhardt, R., Coughlin, C., Friedland, J., & DelRowe, J. (1994). *Changes in Urinary Function (CUF): Pilot data on the development and validation of a measure of the intrusion of quality of life caused by changes in urinary function after cancer therapy.* Paper presented at the Drug Information Association 2nd Symposium on Quality of Life Evaluation, Charleston, SC.

Bruner, D. W., Scott, C., Lawton, C., DelRowe, J., Rotman, M., Buswell, L., Beard, C., & Cella, D. (1995). RTOG's first quality of life study—RTOG 90-20: A phase II trial of external beam radiation with etanidazole for locally advanced prostate cancer. *International Journal of Radiation Oncology, Biology, Physics*, 33(4), 901–906.

Bruner, D. W., Scott, C., McGowan, D., Lawton, C., Hanks, G., Prestidge, B., Gaspar, L., Gore, E., & Asbell, S. (1998b). Validation of the Sexual Adjustment Questionnaire (SAQ) in prostate cancer patients enrolled on Radiation Therapy Oncology Group (RTOG) studies 90-20 and 94-08 [Abstract]. *International Journal of Radiation Oncology, Biology, Physics*, 42(Suppl. 1), 202 (Abstract No. 156).

Bruner, D. W., Scott, C. B., McGowan, D., Lawton, C., Hanks, G., Prestidge, B., Han, S., Gore, E., & Asbell, S. (1998). The RTOG modified sexual adjustment questionnaire: Psychometric testing in the prostate cancer population. *International Journal of Radiation Oncology, Biology, Physics*, 42(1), 202.

Burgio, K. L., Stutzman, R. E., & Engel, B. T. (1989). Behavioral training for post-prostatectomy urinary incontinence. *Journal of Urology*, 141, 303–306.

Carter, B. S., Bova, G. S., Beaty, T. H., Steinberg, G. D., Childs, B., Isaacs, W. B., & Walsh, P. C. (1993). Hereditary prostate cancer: Epidemiologic and clinical features. *Journal of Urology*, 150, 797–802.

Catalona, W. J., Partin, A. W., Slawin, K. M., Brawer, M. K., Flanigan, R. C., Patel, A., Richie, J. P., deKernion, J. B., Walsh, P. C., Scardino, P. T., Lange, P. H., Subong, E. N. P., Parson, R. E., Gasior, G. H., Loveland, K. G., & Southwick, P. C. (1998). Use of the percentage of free prostate-specific antigen to enhance differentiation of prostate cancer from benign prostatic disease. *Journal of the American Medical Association*, 279(19), 1542–1547.

Cella, D. F., Tulsky, D., Gray, G., Sarafian, B., Linn, E., Bonomi, A., Silberman, M., Yellen, S., Winicour, P., Brannon, J., Eckberg, K., Lloyd, S., Purl, S., Blendowski, L., Goodman, M., Barnicle, M., Stewart, I., McHall, M., Bonomi, P., Kaplan, E., Taylor, S., IV., Thomas, C., Jr., & Harris, J. (1993). The Functional Assessment Cancer Therapy Scale: Development and validation of the general measure. *Clinical Oncology*, 11, 570–579.

Coia, L. R., Myerson, R. J., & Tepper, J. E. (1995). Late effects of radiation therapy on the gastrointestinal tract. *International Journal of Radiation Oncology, Biology, Physics*, 31(5), 1213–1236.

Coughlin, S. S., Neaton, J. D., & Sengupta, A. (1996). Cigarette smoking as a predictor of death from prostate cancer in 348,874 men screened for the Multiple Risk Factor Intervention Trial. *American Journal of Epidemiology*, 143(10), 1002–1006.

Crawford, E. D., & DeAntoni, E. P. (1995, April). *Prostate Cancer Awareness Week demonstrates continued value to early detection strategies*. Paper presented at the Conference Proceedings of the American Urological Association, Las Vegas.

Crook, J., Esche, B., & Futter, N. (1996). Effect of pelvic radiotherapy for prostate cancer on bowel, bladder and sexual function: The patient's perspective. *Urology*, 47, 387–394.

Culine, S., Kattan, J., Zanetta, S., Theodore, C., Fizazi, K., & Droz, J. P. (1998). Evaluation of estramustine phosphate combined with weekly doxorubicin in patients with androgen-independent prostate cancer. *American Journal of Clinical Oncology*, 21(5), 470–474.

Cupp, M. R., & Oesterling, J. E. (1993). Prostate-specific antigen, digital rectal examination, and transrectal ultrasonography: Their roles in diagnosing early prostate cancer. *Mayo Clinic Proceedings*, 68(3), 297–306.

Davis, D. L. (1998). Prostate cancer treatment with radioactive seed implantation. *Association of Operating Room Nurses Journal*, 68(1), 18, 21–23, 26–30.

Esper, P., Mo, F., Chodak, G., Sinner, M., Cella, D., & Pienta, K. J. (1997). Measuring quality of life in men with prostate cancer using the Functional Assessment of Cancer Therapy-Prostate instrument. *Urology*, 50(6), 920–928.

Fair, W. R., Cookson, M. S., Stroumbakis, N., Cohen, D., A.G., A., Want, Y., Russo, P., Soloway, S. M., Sogani, P., Sheinfeld, J., Herr, H., Dalgabni, G., Begg, C. B., Heston, W. D., & Reuter, V. E. (1997). The indications, rationale, and results of neoadjuvant androgen deprivation in the treatment of prostatic cancer: Memorial Sloan-Kettering Cancer Center results. *Urology*, 49(Suppl. 3A), 46–55.

Gerard, M. J., & Frank-Stromborg, M. (1998). Screening for prostate cancer in asymptomatic men: Clinical, legal, and ethical implications. *Oncology Nursing Forum*, 25(9), 1561–1569.

Giovannucci, E., Rimm, E. B., Colditz, G. A., Stampfer, M. J., Ascherio, A., Chute, C. C., & Willett, W. C. (1993). A prospective study of dietary fat and risk of prostate cancer. *Journal of the National Cancer Institute*, 85(19), 1571–1579.

Gleason, D. F. (1977). The Veteran's Administration Cooperative Urologic Research Group: Histologic grading and clinical staging of prostate carcinoma. In M. Tannenbaum (Ed.), *Urologic Pathology: The prostate* (pp. 171–198). Philadelphia: Lea & Febiger.

Goluboff, E. T., Chang, D. T., Olsson, C. A., & Kaplan, S. A. (1995). Urodynamics and the etiology of post-prostatectomy urinary incontinence: The initial Columbia experience. *Journal of Urology*, 153(3, Pt. 2), 1034–1037.

Greenberg, D. B., Gray, J. L., Mannix, C. M., Eisenthal, S., & Carey, M. (1993). Treatment-related fatigue and serum interleukin-1 levels in patients during external beam irradiation for prostate cancer. *Journal of Pain and Symptom Management*, 8, 196–200.

Greenlee, R. T., Murray, T., Bolden, S., & Wingo, P. A. (2000). Cancer statistics, 2000. *CA: Cancer Journal for Clinicians*, 50(1), 7–33.

Gronberg, H., Damber, L., & Damber, J. E. (1996). Familial prostate cancer in Sweden: A nationwide register cohort study. *Cancer*, 77(1), 138–143.

Guay, D. R. (1999). Tolterodine, a new antimuscarinic drug for treatment of bladder overactivity. *Pharmacotherapy*, 19(3), 267–280.

Hanks, G. E. (2000). The case for external beam treatment of early stage prostate cancer. *Urology*, 55(3), 301–305.

Hanks, G. E., Hanlon, A. L., Schultheiss, T. E., Pinover, W. H., Movsas, B., Epstein, B. E., & Hunt, M. A. (1998). Dose-escalation with 3D conformal treatment: Five year outcomes, treatment optimization, and future directions. *International Journal of Radiation Oncology, Biology, Physics*, 41(3), 501–510.

Hanks, G. E., Teshima, T., & Pajak, T. (1997). 20 Years of progress in radiation oncology: Prostate cancer. *Seminars in Radiation Oncology*, 7(2), 114–120.

Hanlon, A. L., Bruner, D. W., & Hanks, G. E. (1999). Long term quality of life study in prostate cancer patients treated with three-dimensional conformal radiation therapy: Bowel and bladder quality of life symptoms are similar to that of the normal population [Abstract]. *International Journal of Radiation Oncology, Biology, Physics,* 45(Suppl. 2), 240.

Huncharek, M., & Muscat, J. (1995). Genetic characteristics of prostate cancer. *Cancer Epidemiology, Biomarkers and Prevention,* 4, 681–687.

Isaacs, S. D., Kiemeney, L. A., Baffoe-Bonnie, A., Beaty, T. H., & Walsh, P. C. (1995). Risk of cancer in relatives of prostate cancer probands. *Journal of the National Cancer Institute,* 87(13), 991–996.

Jackson, J., Emerson, L., Johnston, B., Wilson, J., & Morales, A. (1996). Biofeedback: A noninvasive treatment for incontinence after radical proptatectomy. *Urologic Nursing,* 16(2), 50–54.

Jonler, M., Ritter, M. A., Brinkmann, R., Messing, E. M., Rhodes, P. R., & Bruskewitz, R. C. (1994). Sequelae of definitive radiation therapy for prostate cancer localized to the pelvis. *Urology,* 44(6), 876–882.

Joseph, A. C. (1992). Joseph continence assessment tool. *Urologic Nursing,* 12(4), 144–146.

King, K. B., Nail, L. M., Kreamer, K., Strohl, R. A., & Jojnson, J. E. (1985). Patients' description for the experience of receiving radiation therapy. *Oncology Nursing Forum,* 12(4), 55–61.

Kreis, W., Budman, D. R., Fetten, J., Gonzales, A. L., Barile, B., & Vinciguerra, V. (1999). Phase I trial of the combination of daily estramustine phosphate and intermittent docetaxel in patients with metastatic hormone refractory prostate carcinoma. *Annals of Oncology,* 10(1), 33–38.

Lawton, C. A., Winter, K., Byhardt, R., Sause, W. T., Hanks, G. E., Russell, A. H., Rotman, M., Porter, A., McGowan, D. G., DelRowe, J. D., & Pilepich, M. V. (1997). Androgen suppression plus radiation versus radiation alone for patients with D_1 (pN^+) adenocarcinoma of the prostate (results based on a national prospective randomized trial, RTOG 85-31). Radiation Therapy Oncology Group. *International Journal of Radiation Oncology, Biology, Physics,* 38(5), 931–939.

Lawton, C. A., Won, M., Pilepich, M. V., Asbell, S. O., Shipley, W. U., Hanks, G. E., Cox, J. D., Perez, C. A., Sause, W. T., Doggett, S. R. L., & Rubin, P. (1991). Long-term treatment sequelae following external beam irradiation for adenocarcinoma of the prostate: Analysis of RTOG studies 7506 and 7706. *International Journal of Radiation Oncology, Biology, Physics,* 21(4), 935–939.

Littrup, P., Lee, F., & Mettlin, C. (1992). Prostate cancer screening: Implications for the future. *Cancer,* 42, 198–211.

Litwin, M. S., Hays, R. D., Fink, A., Ganz, P. A., Leake, B., & Brook, R. H. (1998). The UCLA Prostate Cancer Index: Development, reliability, and validity of a health-related quality of life measure. *Medical Care,* 36(7), 1002–1012.

Logothetis, C. J., & Millikan, R. (1999). Update: NCCN practice guidelines for the treatment of prostate cancer. *Oncology,* 13(11A), 118–132.

Marks, L. B., Carroll, P. R., Dugan, T. C., & Anscher, M. S. (1995). The response of the urinary bladder, urethra, and ureter to radiation and chemotherapy. *International Journal of Radiation Oncology, Biology, Physics,* 31(5), 1257–1280.

Meaglia, J., Joseph, A. C., Chang, M. K., & Schmidt, J. (1990). Post-prostectomy urinary incontinence: Response to behavioral training. *Journal of Urology*, 144, 674–676.

Middleton, R. G., Smith, J. A., Jr., Melzer, R. B., & Hamilton, P. E. (1986). Patient survival and local recurrence rate following radical prostatectomy for prostatic carcinoma. *Journal of Urology*, 136(2), 422–424.

Millikan, R., & Logothetis, C. (1997). Update of the NCCN guidelines for treatment of prostate cancer. *NCCN Proceedings*, 11(11A), 180–193.

Montague, D. K., Barada, J. H., Belker, A. M., Levine, L. A., Nadig, P. W., Roehrborn, C. G., Sharlip, I. D., & Bennett, A. H. (1996). Clinical guidelines panel on erectile dysfunction: Summary report on the treatment of organic erectile dysfunction. *Journal of Urology*, 156, 2007–2011.

Morton, R. (1994). Racial differences in adenocarcinoma of the prostate in North American men. *Urology*, 44(5), 637–645.

Nag, S., Beyer, D., Friedland, J., Grimm, P., & Nath, R. (1999). American Brachytherapy Society (ABS) recommends for transperineal permanent brachytherapy of prostate cancer. *International Journal of Radiation Oncology, Biology, Physics*, 44(4), 789–799.

NCI/PDQ Physician Statement. (1997). *Radiation enteritis*. Available: http://oncolink.upenn.edu/pdg_html/3/engl/304093-2.html 9/7/99.

Pannek, J., & Partin, A. W. (1997). Prostate-specific antigen: What's new in 1997. *Oncology*, 11(9), 1273–1282.

Parker, S., Tong, T., Bolden, S., & Wingo, P. A. (1997). Cancer statistics, 1997. *CA A Cancer Journal for Clinicians*, 47(1), 5–27.

Petrovich, Z., Lieskovsky, G., Langholz, B., Bochner, B., Formenti, S., Streeter, O., & Skinner, D. G. (1999). Comparison of outcomes of radical prostatectomy with and without adjuvant pelvic irradiation in patients with pathologic stage C (T_3N_0) adenocarcinoma of the prostate. *American Journal of Clinical Oncology*, 22(4), 323–331.

Pickett, M., Watkins Bruner, D., Joseph, A., & Burggraf, V. (2000). Prostate cancer elder alert (Part II). Living with treatment choices and outcomes. *Journal of Gerontological Nursing*, 26(2), 22–34.

Pienta, K. J., & Smith, D. C. (1997). Paclitaxel, estramustine, and etoposide in the treatment of hormone-refractory prostate cancer. *Seminars in Oncology*, 24(5) (Suppl. 15), S1572–S1577.

Pisansky, T. M., Kozelsky, T. F., Myers, R. P., Hillman, D. W., Blute, M. L., Buskirk, S. J., Cheville, J. C., Ferrigni, R. G., & Schild, S. E. (2000). Radiotherapy for isolated serum prostate-specific antigen elevation after prostatectomy for prostate cancer. *Journal of Urology*, 163, 845–850.

Ramos, C. G., Carvalhal, G. F., Smith, D. S., Mager, D. E., & Catalona, W. J. (1999). Clinical and pathological characteristics, and recurrence rates of stage T_{1c} versus T_{2a} or T_{2b} prostate cancer. *Journal of Urology*, 161(5), 1525–1529.

Reinstein, L. E., Wang, X. H., Burman, C. M., Chen, Z., Mohan, R., Kutcher, G., Leibel, S. A., & Fuks, Z. A. (1998). A feasibility study of automated inverse treatment planning for cancer of the prostate. *International Journal of Radiation Oncology, Biology, Physics*, 40(1), 207–214.

Rietbergen, J. B., Hoedemaeker, R. F., Kruger, A. E., Kirkels, W. J., & Schroder, F. H. (1999). The changing pattern of prostate cancer at the time of diagnosis: Characteristics of screen detected prostate cancer in a population based screening study. *Journal of Urology*, 161(4), 1192–1198.

Roach, M., III. (1999). Current status of androgen suppression and radiotherapy for patients with prostate cancer. *Journal of Steroids, Biochemistry and Molecular Biology*, 69(1–6), 239–245.

Roach, M., III., Chinn, D. M., Holland, J., & Clarke, M. A. (1996). A pilot survey of sexual function and quality of life following 3D conformal radiotherapy for clinically localized prostate cancer. *International Journal of Radiation Therapy Oncology, Biology, Physics*, 35(5), 869–874.

Schaid, D. J., McDonnell, S. K., Blute, M. L., & Thibodeau, S. N. (1998). Evidence for autosomal dominant inheritance of prostate cancer. *American Journal of Human Genetics*, 62, 1425–1438.

Schover, L. R. (1993). Sexual rehabilitation after treatment for prostate cancer. *Cancer*, 72(Suppl. 3), 1024–1030.

Schrader-Bogen, C. L., Kjellberg, J. L., McPherson, C. P., & Murray, C. L. (1997). Quality of life and treatment outcomes: Prostate carcinoma patients' perspectives after prostatectomy or radiation. *Cancer*, 79(10), 1977–1986.

Schröder, F. H. (1999). Lest we abandon digital rectal examination as a screening test for prostate cancer. *Journal of the National Cancer Institute*, 91(15), 1331–1332.

Sharp, L. K., Knight, S. J., Nadler, R., Albers, M., Moran, E., Kuzel, T., Sharifi, R., & Bennett, C. (1999). Quality of life in low-income patients with metastatic cancer: Divergent and convergent validity of three instruments. *Quality of Life Research*, 8(5), 461–470.

Shipley, W. U., Thames, H. D., Sandler, H. M., Hanks, G. E., Zietman, A. L., Perez, C. A., Kuban, D. A., Hancock, S. L., & Smith, C. D. (1999). Radiation therapy for clinically localized prostate cancer: A multi-institutional pooled analysis. *Journal of the American Medical Association*, 281(17), 1598–1604.

Sommers, S. D., & Ramsey, S. D. (1999). A review of quality-of-life evaluations in prostate cancer. *Pharmoeconomics*, 16(2), 124–140.

Steele, G., Osteen, R., Winchester, D. P., Murphy, G., & Menck, H. R. (1994). Clinical highlights from the National Cancer Data Base. *CA: Cancer Journal for Clinicians*, 44, 71–80.

Stockdale, A. D., & Biswas, A. (1997). Case report: Long-term control of radiation proctitis following treatment with sucralfate enemas. *British Journal of Surgery*, 84(3), 379.

Stockler, M. R., Osoba, D., Corey, P., Goodwin, P. J., & Tannock, I. F. (1999). Convergent, discriminitive, and predictive validity of the Prostate Cancer Specific Quality of Life Instrument (PROSQOLI) assessment and comparison with analogous scales from the EORTC QLQ-C30 and a trial-specific module. European Organization for Research and Treatment of Cancer. Core Quality of Life Questionnaire. *Journal of Clinical Epidemiology*, 52(7), 653–666.

Sullivan, J., & Abrams, P. (1999). Pharmacological management of incontinence. *European Urology*, 36(Suppl. 1), 89–95.

Talcott, J. A., Rieker, P., Clark, J. A., Propert, K. J., Weeks, J. C., Beard, C. J., Wishnow, K. I., Kaplan, I., Loughlin, K. R., Richie, J. P., & Kantoff, P. W. (1998). Patient-reported symptoms after primary therapy for early prostate cancer: Results of a prospective cohort study. *Journal of Clinical Oncology*, 16(1), 275–283.

Thompson, T. C. (1999). In situ gene therapy for prostate cancer. *Oncology Research*, 11(1), 1–8.

von Eschenbach, A., Ho, R., Murphy, G. P., Cunningham, M., & Lins, N. (1997). American Cancer Society guidelines for the early detection of prostate cancer: Update, June 10, 1997. *Cancer*, 80(9), 1805–1807.

Walsh, P. C. (1988). Nerve sparing radical prostatectomy for early stage prostate cancer. *Seminars in Oncology*, 15(4), 351–358.

Waterhouse, J., & Metcalfe, M. C. (1986). Development of the sexual adjustment questionnaire. *Oncology Nursing Forum*, 13(3), 53–59.

Wei, J. T., Gross, M., Jaffe, C. A., Gravlin, K., Lahaie, M., Faerber, G. J., & Cooney, K. (1999). Androgen deprivation therapy for prostate cancer results in significant loss of bone density. *Urology*, 54(4), 607–611.

Whittemore, A. S., Kolonel, L. N., Wu, A. H., John, E. M., Gallagher, R. P., Howe, G. R., Burch, J. D., Hankin, J., Dreon, D. M., West, D. W., Teh, C.-Z., & Paffenbarger, R. S., Jr. (1995). Prostate cancer in relation to diet, physical activity, and body size in blacks, whites and Asians in the United States and Canada. *Journal of the National Cancer Institute*, 87(9), 652–661.

Whittington, R., Malkowicz, S. B., Machtay, M., Van Arsdalen, K., Barnes, M. M., Broderick, G. A., & Wein, A. J. (1997). The use of combined radiation therapy and hormonal therapy in the management of lymph node-positive prostate cancer. *International Journal of Radiation Oncology, Biology, Physics*, 39(3), 673–680.

Widmark, A., Fransson, P., & Tavelin, B. (1994). Self-assessment questionnaire for evaluating urinary and intestinal late side effects after pelvic radiotherapy in patients with prostate cancer compared with an age-matched control population. *Cancer*, 74(9), 2520–2532.

Wurzer, J., Nicolaou, N., Hanlon, A., Bruner, D. W., & Hanks, G. (1999). Long term durability of potency preservation in younger prostate cancer patients following 3D conformal radiation therapy [Abstract]. *International Journal of Radiation Oncology, Biology, Physics*, 45(Suppl. 2), 169.

Yarbro, C. H., & Ferrans, C. E. (1998). Quality of life of patients with prostate cancer treated with surgery or radiation therapy. *Oncology Nursing Forum*, 25(4), 685–693.

Nonmelanoma Skin Cancer

Marilyn L. Haas, PhD, ANP-C
J. Battle Haslam, MD

PROBLEM

Skin cancers account for approximately one-third of all cancers diagnosed in the United States (Chao, Perez, & Brady, 1999). Skin cancers are generally divided into two groups: nonmelanoma (basal cell carcinoma and squamous cell carcinoma) and malignant melanoma. The American Cancer Society estimates that 900,000 to 1.2 million new cases of nonmelanoma skin cancers will be diagnosed each year (ACS, 1999). Historically, nonmelanoma skin cancers affect more men than women. Approximately 77% of all skin cancers are basal cell carcinomas, 20% are squamous cell carcinomas, and 3% are malignant melanoma/rare skin cancers. The ratio of basal cell carcinoma to squamous cell carcinoma is 10:1 in women and 5:1 in men (Maguire, 1997). Typically, basal cell carcinoma

- Is diagnosed in individuals over the age of 40, however this type of skin cancer is becoming more common in younger individuals in their 20's (Gale & Charette, 1994).
- Occurs primarily in individuals exposed to prolonged or intense sunlight, especially White individuals with light eyes, light hair, and fair complexions (so-called "Scotch-Irish" complexion). Rarely do dark-skinned individuals develop this type of skin cancer.

In comparison, squamous cell carcinoma

■ Increases with age and is seen more in older individuals (mean age 68 years for men and 73 years for women).

■ Occurs primarily where skin is exposed to high levels of ambient ultraviolet B radiation.

■ Is responsible for most of the deaths (Preston & Stern, 1992).

The frequency of nonmelanomas varies geographically. Demographic statistics reveal higher rates in southern United States in comparison with northern United States (143 individuals per 100,000 vs. 25 individuals per 100,000) (American Joint Committee on Cancer, 1998). Although nonmelanoma skin cancers are very common, they tend to remain localized and account for less than 0.1% of patient deaths due to cancer.

ASSESSMENT

RISK FACTORS

Factors that place a patient at high risk of developing nonmelanoma skin cancers include:

■ Excessive exposure to ultraviolet radiation (UVR) from the sun. The maximal exposure rate is intensified during 11 A.M. and 3 P.M. and in geographic regions close to the equator. People with outdoor occupations, such as commercial fishing and farming, that involve high exposure to ultraviolet B light are placed at higher risk.

■ Physical attributes—The so-called "Scotch-Irish" complexion with fair skin, blue or green eyes, blonde or red hair, and sun-induced freckles, or those who easily burn are at higher risk.

■ Race—Nonmelanoma skin cancer is rare in African Americans, Asians, and Hispanics. Reasons for this may be due to increased protection of the skin afforded by melanin or other genetically determined differences (Preston & Stern, 1992).

■ Genetic disorders—People with xeroderma pigmentosa (genetic disorder of DNA repair resulting in inability to fix UVR damage) or albinism are at increased risk. Also, ultraviolet radiation induces mutation of $p53$ tumor-suppressor genes (Preston & Stern, 1992).

TABLE 17–1   FACTORS ASSOCIATED WITH INCREASED
RISK OF DEVELOPING SKIN CANCERS

Older age	Scotch-Irish complexion
Gender (male)	Red, blond, or light brown hair
Chronically irritated/infected skin	Blue or green eyes
Sunburned skin	Chemical exposure
Freckling	Immunosuppressed individual

■ Precursor lesions—Actinic keratoses need close supervision because these lesions can quickly turn into nonmelanoma skin cancers. Atypical, bleeding, or changing moles are also suspicious.

■ Chemical exposure—Carcinogens, such as coal tar, arsenic, shale, paraffin or creosote oil, or petroleum lubricating oil predispose individuals to develop lesions.

■ Immunosuppressed individuals—Organ transplants and HIV individuals carry a higher risk.

■ Chronically infected, chronically irritated, or previously burned skin is also at high risk.

A summary of factors associated with increased risk of developing skin cancer is located in Table 17–1.

PREVENTION/SCREENING AND PRESENTING SYMPTOMS

Since there is a strong correlation between excessive sunlight (UVR) and the development of nonmelanoma skin cancers, prevention is the key. Education regarding sun exposure and other risk factors should be stressed. Patients should be informed about the importance of regular sunscreen use. The lifetime incidence of developing nonmelanoma lesions could decrease 78% if individuals would utilize sunscreen (SPF15 or higher) during childhood and adolescence (Maguire, 1997). Annual screening is extremely important for those individuals at high risk.

Basal cell carcinoma is a malignant neoplasm of the skin arising from the basal cells of the epidermis and its appendages. The characteristics include slow-growing lesions that occasionally cause extensive tissue destruction if left untreated, however metastases are rare. In comparison, squamous cell carcinomas are malignant tumors of the keratinizing cells of the epidermis. This cancer type is typically more aggressive than basal cell carcinomas with higher rates of metastasis to regional lymph nodes and distant sites.

DIAGNOSTIC WORKUP

A complete body assessment is also needed after obtaining the patient's risk factors and history. Physical examination should focus on the changes in the normal appearance of the skin. Recognition of nonmelanoma skin cancers is critical. The clinical manifestations of nonmelanoma skin cancers are:

- ■ Basal cell carcinomas—Typically elevated lesions with umbilicated, ulcerated centers with waxy or pearly borders, and moderately firm.
- ■ Squamous cell carcinomas—Appearance varies from an elevated nodular mass to a punched out ulcerated lesion or a scaly, opaque, and possibly fungal-appearing lesion. While recognition is the first step in suspecting the diagnosis, biopsies are required to make the final diagnosis. Different biopsy methods can be employed: incisional, shave, or punch biopsies. Microscopic verification is necessary to determine the histological type. Lesions are graded by the American Joint Committee on Cancer (1998) as follows:

     G_1 (well differentiated)
     G_2 (moderately differentiated)
     G_3 (poorly differentiated)
     G_4 (undifferentiated)

Common sites of occurrence for basal cell carcinomas are nose, eyelids, cheeks, and sun-exposed trunk. Metastases are rare ($< 0.1\%$) (Guthrie, 1999). Common sites for squamous cell carcinomas are head and hands. Metastases can occur to the regional lymph nodes (2%) (Guthrie, 1999). If nodes are enlarged and metastatic spread is suspected, a computerized tomography study (CT scan) can be ordered to rule out regional involvement and a biopsy done to confirm involvement. If regional spread to lymph nodes is confirmed, then distant metastatic workup with chest x-ray, live function tests, and other indicated studies are needed. The clinical and pathological staging system is the same for basal cell carcinoma and squamous cell carcinoma (Table 17–2). The stage grouping is identified in Table 17–3.

TABLE 17-2   TNM STAGING OF BASAL CELL AND SQUAMOUS CELL CARCINOMA OF THE SKIN (EXCLUDING EYELID, VULVA, AND PENIS)

Primary Tumor (T)	Description
T_x	Primary tumor cannot be assessed
T_0	No evidence of primary tumor
T_{is}	Carcinoma in situ
T_1	Tumor $\leq$ 2 cm in greatest dimension
T_2	Tumor $>$ 2 cm in greatest dimension, but no $>$ 5 cm in greatest dimension
T_3	Tumor $>$ 5 cm in greatest dimension
T_4	Tumor invades deep extradermal structures (i.e., cartilage, skeletal muscle, or bone)
Regional Lymph Nodes (N)	
N_x	Regional lymph nodes cannot be assessed
N_0	No regional lymph node metastasis
N_1	Regional lymph node metastasis
Distant Metastasis (M)	
M_x	Distant metastasis cannot be assessed
M_0	No distant metastasis
M_1	Distant metastasis

Used with the permission of the American Joint Committee on Cancer (AJCC®), Chicago, Illinois. The original source for this material is the AJCC® Cancer Staging Manual, 5th edition (1997) published by Lippincott-Raven Publishers, Philadelphia, Pennsylvania.

TABLE 17-3   STAGE GROUPING FOR BASAL CELL AND SQUAMOUS CELL CARCINOMA

Stage 0	T_{is}	N_0	M_0
Stage I	T_1	N_0	M_0
Stage II	T_2	N_0	M_0
	T_3	N_0	M_0
Stage III	T_4	N_0	M_0
	Any T	N_1	M_0
Stage IV	Any T	Any N	M_1

Used with the permission of the American Joint Committee on Cancer (AJCC®), Chicago, Illinois. The original source for this material is the AJCC® Cancer Staging Manual, 5th edition (1997) published by Lippincott-Raven Publishers, Philadelphia, Pennsylvania.

OUTCOMES MEASURES

Although large numbers of individuals are being diagnosed with nonmelanoma skin cancers, very little emphasis has been given to this population in regard to outcomes other than tracking single local control rates. Since cure rates are high, few if any research studies focus on outcomes measures for skin lesions. Subjective cosmetic ratings (excellent, good, fair, and poor) are reported by radiation oncologists. Generic quality-of-life instruments that could be applied to this population would include Quality of Life Index, Functional Living Index, Functional Assessment of Cancer Therapy Scale, or Medical Outcomes Short Form 36. Since disfigurement from the lesion and/or treatment can be emotional, psychological measures could be investigated.

OUTCOMES MANAGEMENT

The goal of therapy is to completely eliminate the lesion while conserving normal structure and function, and yielding a good cosmetic result. Fortunately, many skin carcinomas are diagnosed early and are cured with surgery alone. Surgeries can include curettage and electrosurgery, cryosurgery, Mohs surgery, or laser surgery. However, radiation therapy can often play a role in treatment either definitively or adjuvant after surgery if high risk of local recurrence is suspected after excision. Certain factors are considered when deciding if radiation therapy would be appropriate. These include:

- Lesions deemed technically inoperable because of extent or location (nose, eyelid, lip, and canthus) would lead to an unacceptable cosmetic result with surgery.
- Poor surgical risk due to age or comorbidity illnesses.
- Recurrent disease, positive surgical margins, perineural invasion, and Merkel's cells histology are often indications for postoperative radiation therapy.
- Young age, lesions on the palms or soles, and lesions arising in chronically infected areas are contraindications to radiation therapy (Wilder & Margolis, 1998).

Radiation doses are individualized and vary according to the tumor size, location, and depth. Most skin cancers are treated with low-energy x-rays or electrons. Both offer the advantage of rapid dose falloff, thus sparing the underlying normal tissue. Typically for either of the nonmelanoma skin cancers, radiation treatments are delivered in 2 to 3 Gy fractions with total doses of 40 to 70 Gy (NCCN, 1999).

Possible short- and long-term complications of radiation for skin cancers may include:

- Brisk skin reactions—Moderate to severe erythema with or without moist desquamation that can lead to scarring.
- Cutaneous necrosis—Incidence of soft tissue necrosis is 3% (Chao et al., 1999).
- Chronic radiation dermatitis is rare.
- Chronic posttreatment changes could include hyperpigmentation, hypopigmentation, telangiectasia, and fibrosis.

EXPECTED OUTCOMES

The overall cure rate for nonmelanoma skin cancers is directly related to the stage of the disease and the type of treatment employed. Prognosis for both nonmelanoma skin cancers is very favorable. Approximately 90% to 95% of basal cell carcinomas and 75% to 80% of squamous cell carcinomas are cured (Friedman, Rigel, Nossa, & Dorf, 1995). Approximately 95% of all recurrences and metastases occur within a 5-year period (Maguire, 1997).

Little is researched on the effect of skin cancers on people's lives. One study by Blackford and colleagues reports that having basal cell carcinoma had very little impact on people's lives in regard to quality of life (Blackford, Roberts, Salek, & Finlay, 1996). They speculate that this may be the reason why people do not seek medical attention in early stages, and recommend that public health education is needed for early recognition.

High-risk patients need lifelong follow-up and examinations. Those patients who have been diagnosed and treated need close surveillance for the next 5 years. Patients with basal cell carcinomas should be clinically examined every 6 months for 5 years. Thereafter, the patient can be examined for recurrent tumor or new primary tumors on an annual basis. The National Cancer Institute reports 36% of patients who develop a basal cell carcinoma will develop a second primary basal cell carcinoma within the next 5 years (Brady, Binnick, & Fitzpatrick, 1987). Patients diagnosed with squamous cell carcinomas need closer surveillance because of the higher risk of local recurrence and potential for metastases. Patients should be reexamined every 3 months for the first several years and then followed indefinitely at 6-month intervals (Brady et al., 1987).

REFERENCES

American Cancer Society. (1999). *Cancer facts and figures.* New York: American Cancer Society.

American Joint Committee on Cancer. (1998). *AJCC cancer staging handbook.* I. Fleming, J. Cooper, D. Henson, R. Huter, B. Kennedy, G. Murphy, B. O'Sullivan, L. Sobin, & J. Yarbro (Eds.). Philadelphia: Lippincott-Raven.

Blackford, S., Roberts, D., Salek, M., & Finlay, A. (1996). Basal cell carcinomas cause little handicap. *Quality of Life Research,* 5(2), 191–194.

Brady, L., Binnick, S., & Fitzpatrick, P. (1987). Skin cancer. In C. Perez & L. Brady (Eds.), *Principles and practices of radiation oncology.* Philadelphia: J. B. Lippincott.

Chao, K., Perez, C., & Brady, L. (1999). *Radiation oncology: Management decisions.* Philadelphia: Lippincott-Raven.

Friedman, R., Rigel, D., Nossa, R., & Dorf, R. (1995). Basal cell and squamous cell carcinoma of the skin. In G. Murphy, W. Lawrence, & R. Lenhard (Eds.), *American Cancer Society textbook of clinical oncology.* Atlanta, GA: American Cancer Society.

Gale, D., & Charette, J. (1994). *Oncology nursing care plans.* El Paso, TX: Skidmore-Roth.

Guthrie, T. (1999). Squamous cell and basal cell carcinoma of the skin. In J. Foley, J. Vose, & J. Armitage (Eds.), *Current therapy in cancer.* Philadelphia: W. B. Saunders.

Maguire, A. (1997). Skin cancers. In C. Varricchio, M. Pierce, C. Walker, & T. Ades (Eds.), *A cancer source book for nurses.* Sudbury, MA: Jones & Bartlett.

National Comprehensive Cancer Network. (1999). Nonmelanoma skin cancer: Basal cell carcinoma and squamous cell carcinoma, Version 1.01. Chair Stanley Miller, MD, Co-presenters Richard Cheney, MD, Joseph Kusiak, MD. Presented at NCCN Practice Guidelines and Outcomes Data in Oncology at Fort Lauderdale, Florida Feb 26–March 2.

Preston, D., & Stern, R. (1992). Nonmelanoma cancers of the skin. *The New England Journal of Medicine,* 327 (23), 1649–1662.

Wilder, R., & Margolis, L. (1998). Skin cancer. In S. Leibel & T. Phillips (Eds.), *Textbook of radiation oncology.* Philadelphia: W. B. Saunders.

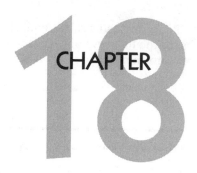

CHAPTER 18

SOFT TISSUE SARCOMAS

Kellie Wolk, RN, BSN
Robert A. Zlotecki, MD, PhD

PROBLEM

- Sarcomas are a group of varied and complex diseases. They can arise within any musculoskeletal connective tissue of the body and are typically segmented into two categories: sarcomas of the soft tissue and sarcomas of the bone. Another distinction is between tumors of children and tumors of the adult population. Because of the diversity of this tumor, this chapter will focus only on soft tissue sarcomas in adults arising within the extremities or retroperitoneum.
- Soft tissue sarcomas are malignant tumors that develop from fat, muscle, nerve sheath, joint spaces, blood vessels, or deep fibrous connective tissues.
- Soft tissue sarcomas are relatively rare tumors, accounting for less than 1% of all tumors (Demetri et al., 1998; Enzinger & Weiss, 1995). The American Cancer Society (ACS) estimated that 8,100 new cases of soft tissue sarcomas would be diagnosed in the year 2000, with approximately 4,600 related deaths (Greenlee, Murray, Bolden, & Wingo, 2000).
- Extremity and superficial trunk sarcomas account for 60% of all soft tissue sarcomas (Pisters, Fein, Casper, & Somls, 1999). Retroperitoneal sarcomas account for 15% of all soft tissue sarcomas (Pisters, Fein, Casper, Somls, 1999).
- There is a geographically similar distribution and incidence worldwide (Enzinger & Weiss, 1995). Age distribution in

adults: < 40 years = 20.7%, 40 to 60 years = 27.6%, > 60 years = 51.8% (Pisters et al., 1999). The female to male ratio is 1.0:1.1 (Pisters et al., 1999).

RISK FACTORS

FAMILY HISTORY

■ A family history of certain inherited conditions increases a person's risk of developing soft tissue sarcomas (Table 18–1).

CHEMICAL EXPOSURE

■ Exposure to various chemicals (in specific occupations or situations) has been linked with the development of soft tissue sarcoma. These include the phenoxyacetic acids (forestry and agricultural workers), chlorophenols (sawmill workers), Thorotrast® (diagnostic x-ray workers), vinyl chloride (vinyl chloride workers), and arsenic (vineyard workers) (Pisters, 1999). In an evaluation of occupational risks, Hoppin and colleagues associated herbicide use, chlorophenol

TABLE 18–1 HEREDITARY NEOPLASTIC SYNDROMES

Hereditary neoplasms of sarcoma-like conditions
   Gardner's syndrome
   Chemodectoma
   Retinoblastoma
   Pheochromocytoma and medullary thyroid carcinoma
Preneoplastic conditions (hamartomatous syndromes)
   Neurofibromatosis
   Tuberous sclerosis
   von Hippel-Lindau syndrome
   Mutliple exostoses
   Peutz-Jeghers syndrome

Reprinted with permission from T. K. Das Gupta and P. K. Chaudhun. (1998). *Tumors of the Soft Tissues* (2nd ed.). Stamford, CT: Appleton & Lange.

exposure, and cutting oil exposure with malignant fibrohistiocytic sarcoma (Hoppin et al., 1999). Their analysis also
suggested that occupational risk factors for sarcoma are not
uniform across all histologic subtypes.

Radiation

- Radiation exposure has been related to the development of
  sarcomas. However, considering the frequency of radiotherapy, radiation-induced soft tissue sarcomas are still rare, and
  the benefit of radiation in the treatment of malignant neoplasms outweighs the risk of developing sarcomas.
- Approximately 0.01% of cancer patients treated with radiation who survive more than 5 years may develop a sarcoma
  of either bone or soft tissue (Enzinger & Weiss, 1995). This is
  a late lifetime risk with time of occurrence generally 10 to 20
  years after radiation exposure.

Chemotherapy

- Soft tissue sarcomas have been reported after previous exposure to alkylating chemotherapy agents (such as cyclophosphamide, melphalan, procarbazine, nitrosoureas,
  and chlorambucil). The relative risk appears to increase with
  cumulative drug exposure (Pisters et al., 1999).

Damage to Lymphatic Drainage

- Sarcomas can develop in parts of the body where lymphatic
  drainage has been disrupted congenitally or by surgery or radiation. This can be noted in women who have Stewart-
  Treves syndrome or chronic lymphedema after radical mastectomy and/or axillary radiotherapy.

Injury

- There is no clear causal relationship between injury and the
  development of sarcoma. Most often, trauma to an area
  brings awareness to the underlying problem. Rare examples
  of soft tissue sarcomas have arisen in postsurgical scar tissue, thermal or acid burns, in fracture sites, and in the vicinity of foreign body implants (Enzinger & Weiss, 1995).

ASSESSMENT

- Currently, there are no recommended guidelines for screening for sarcomas. However, patients who have previously received radiation therapy usually have follow-up evaluations during which careful examination of the treated area may lead to early diagnosis of radiation-induced sarcoma.
- Patients may initially present with a new enlarging mass. Often there are no complaints of pain, but pain may occur about one-third of the time. Retroperitoneal sarcomas may also present secondary to complaints of bowel obstruction or bleeding, but most complaints are nonspecific.
- NCCN Sarcoma Practice Guidelines (1998) recommend that the first consideration for patients who are suspected of having sarcomas is to have them evaluated by a multidisciplinary team before diagnostic testing (Demetri et al., 1998). The team should consist of surgical, medical, and radiation oncologists skilled in the management of sarcomas. A diagnostic radiologist and a pathologist experienced at diagnosing histologic subtypes and grading of sarcomas are also essential.
- Initial evaluation should include the following:
  1. Complete medical history and physical exam are essential to gather information on presenting symptoms, risk factors, and other medical conditions. The palpable mass should be evaluated for size, mobility, depth, and involvement of other structures (such as bone, nerves, or organs).
  2. Imaging studies should include:
     a. Magnetic resonance imaging (MRI) is the imaging study of choice for evaluation of a soft tissue mass in the extremity and superficial trunk. Whereas both CT and MRI permit comparable assessment of tumor size and depth, only MRI enhances the contrast between tumor and muscle and between tumor and adjacent neurovascular structures. Standard CT is usually sufficient to assess retroperitoneal sarcomas.
     b. CT scan of the chest should be performed to complete the staging workup because sarcomas of the extremities have a high risk of metastasis to the lung. Overall, at diagnosis, approximately 10% of patients have demonstrable metastatic disease (Demetri et al., 1998).

      c. Bone scan is indicated to assess for both invasion of adjacent bone structures and distant bony metastasis.

      d. Plain radiographic films of the primary lesion are considered optional.

3. Suspected soft tissue tumors of the extremities require a carefully planned biopsy to confirm the diagnosis of sarcoma. Several forms of biopsy may be performed depending on the location and size of the mass. These include such as a needle aspiration biopsy, core-needle biopsy, and incisional biopsy. The incisional biopsy must always be performed in the direction of the muscle compartment, i.e. the long axis of the extremity; never in a transverse orientation. The routine use of an excisional biopsy procedure is to be discouraged. Biopsy of retroperitoneal masses is controversial. It may be considered if other malignancies are suspected.

■ Pathologic classification of the biopsy should include histologic subtyping and grading, precise location of the origin of the tumor, size of primary lesion, and involvement or compromise of neurovascular or adjacent bony structures.

- *Malignant fibrous histiocytoma* (MFH) arises from fibrohistiocytic tissue. It is the most common malignant soft tissue sarcoma found in the arms or legs. This sarcoma is most common in older adults. It also can occur in the retroperitoneum.

- *Angiosarcomas* are malignant tumors that can develop either from blood vessels (hemangiosarcomas) or from lymph vessels (lymphangiosarcomas).

- *Fibrosarcoma* is cancer of the fibrous tissue, usually occurring in the arms, legs, or trunk.

- *Hemangiopericytoma* is a sarcoma of perivascular tissue. Perivascular cells help control the amount of blood flowing through veins. It most often develops in the legs, pelvis, and retroperitoneum.

- *Liposarcoma* is a malignant tumor that develops from fat tissue. Liposarcomas can grow anywhere in the body, but are most common in the retroperitoneum.

- *Leiomyosarcoma* is a malignant tumor of involuntary muscle tissue. Leiomyosarcoma is therefore most common in the retroperitoneum, but may also develop in the deep soft tissues of the extremities.

- Malignant peripheral nerve sheath tumors are malignant tumors of the cells that surround a nerve. They are also called malignant schwannomas, neurofibrosarcomas, or neurogenic sarcomas.
- Rhabdomyosarcoma is a malignant tumor of skeletal muscle and is most common in the extremities. Although it is more common in children, it does affect adults and therefore is included here.
- Synovial sarcoma is a malignant tumor of the soft tissue around a joint, not actually arising from the synovium or joint space. It is most common in young adults.

■ Hematogenous metastases are the most common, with lung being the frequent first site of metastasis. Sarcomas can also invade locally into muscle, skin, nerve, and bone.

■ Histologic grade and tumor size are important prognostic factors and are the primary determinants of clinical stage. Nodal status and distant metastasis are not factors of stage I, II, or III disease. Patients who present with evidence of metastasis or nodal involvement are classified as stage IV (Pisters, Fein, Casper, & Somls, 1996). See Table 18–2 for the AJCC staging system for soft tissue sarcomas.

OUTCOMES MANAGEMENT

■ Shifts in treatment have taken place over the past decade, from single modality treatment involving radical surgery to sophisticated limb salvage strategies combined with radiation therapy and protocol-administered chemotherapy (Pollock, Karnell, Menck, & Winchester, 1996). The National Cancer Data Base report on soft tissue sarcoma (Pollock et al., 1996) found that limb-sparing procedures were now standard. However, in a stage subset analysis, many stage II and stage III patients were undertreated because of a lack of multimodality therapy usage. They concluded that the use of a pretreatment multimodality planning conference would increase the likelihood that stage-appropriate combinations of surgery, chemotherapy, and radiation therapy would be used and would result in the possibility of improved overall and disease-free survival in the future.

TABLE 18–2   AJCC STAGING OF SOFT TISSUE SARCOMAS

Primary Tumor

T_X Primary tumor cannot be assessed
T_0 No evidence of primary tumor
T_1 Tumor 5 cm or less in greatest dimension
T_{1a} superficial tumor
T_{1b} deep tumor
T_2 Tumor more than 5 cm in greatest dimension
T_{2a} superficial tumor
T_{2b} deep tumor

Regional Lymph Nodes

N_X Regional lymph nodes cannot be assessed
N_0 No regional lymph node metastasis
N_1 Regional lymph node metastasis

Distant Metastasis

M_X Distant metastasis cannot be assessed
M_0 No distant metastasis
M_1 Distant metastasis

Histopathologic Grade

G_X Grade cannot be assessed
G_1 Well differentiated
G_2 Moderately differentiated
G_3 Poorly differentiated
G_4 Undifferentiated

Stage I

A (low grade, small, superficial and deep)	G_{1-2}	T_{1a-1}	N_0	M_0
B (low grade, large, superficial)	G_{1-2}	T_{2a}	N_0	M_0

Stage II

A (low grade, large, deep)	G_{1-2}	T_{2b}	N_0	M_0
B (high grade, small, superficial, deep)	G_{3-4}	T_{1a-1b}	N_0	M_0
C (high grade, large, superficial)	G_{3-4}	T_{2a}	N_0	M_0

Stage III (high grade, large, deep) G_{3-4} T_{2b} N_0 M_0

Stage IV (any metastasis)   Any G   Any T N_1 M_0

Any G   Any T N_0 M_1

From I. D. Fleming, J. S. Cooper, D. E. Henson, et al. (1998). AJCC *Cancer Staging Handbook* (5th ed.). Philadelphia: Lippincott-Raven.
Used with the permission of the American Joint Committee on Cancer (AJCC®), Chicago, Illinois. The original source for this material is the AJCC® Cancer Staging Manual, 5th edition (1997) published by Lippincott-Raven Publishers, Philadelphia, Pennsylvania.

SURGERY

■ The goal of surgery is to obtain optimal margins for local control while maximizing function, ideally sparing the limb. Changes in patterns of treatment have been identified, with wide local excision increasing threefold over a 5-year period of time to 45.2% of patients by 1993, whereas amputation had decreased from 35.5% to 11.1% of patients (Pollock et al., 1996). Intralesional excision, marginal excision, wide local excision, radical excision, and amputation are the types of surgical procedures used. Limb salvage has been achieved with sarcoma by means of compartmental resection, soft-tissue reconstruction, and adjuvant therapy without increased rates of local recurrence, metastasis, or mortality (Serletti, Carras, O'Keefe, & Rosier, 1998). Limb salvage procedures have encouraged the development of composite, one-stage reconstructions that employ microvascular surgical techniques with a combination of autologous tissues, bone allografts, and endoprosthetic devices in an effort to improve functional outcome. The complications of limb salvage continue to decrease while the durability of the reconstructions continues to increase (Terek, 1997).

RADIATION

■ The inclusion of adjuvant radiation therapy in the treatment of sarcomas is primarily for high-grade lesions in an attempt to improve functional and cosmetic outcomes and to reduce the risk of late complications of high-dose radiotherapy alone (Chao, Perez, & Brady, 1999). Two types of adjuvant radiation therapy are available to treat sarcomas: external-beam radiation and brachytherapy. Rosenberg et al. (1982) established the use of radiation in a National Cancer Institute (NCI) prospective randomized trial of amputation alone versus wide local excision plus external-beam radiation. The trial showed that high rates of local control could be achieved, thus avoiding amputation. Yang et al. (1998) in a study of limb-sparing surgery with or without postoperative external-beam radiation found a highly significant decrease ($p = 0.0028$) in the probability of local recurrence with radiation, but no difference in overall survival. In low-grade lesions, there was also a lower probability of local failure ($p = 0.016$) in patients receiving radiation, without a difference in overall survival. For extremity sarcomas typically a total dose of 50 to 74 Gy is delivered to the site using fractions of 1.2 Gy twice daily or 1.8 to 2.0 Gy once daily. For retroperitoneal sarcomas the total dose is restricted to 45 to 54 Gy because of the tolerance limits of sensitive abdominal organs.

■ Brachytherapy is the delivery of radiation to a specific site inside a patient. It has the advantages of treating complex areas (with less exposure to normal tissues and organs) and of reducing the time commitment to treatment. This procedure generally requires intraoperative placement of the radioactive sources. Ideal patients are those with intermediate- or high-grade tumors amenable to en bloc resection (Crownover & Marks, 1999). Harrison et al. (1993) compared surgery alone versus surgery plus brachytherapy for either high- or low-grade sarcomas. They found that high-grade tumors treated with brachytherapy had 5-year local control rates of 90% compared with rates of 60% to 70% with resection alone.

CHEMOTHERAPY

■ The systemic administration of chemotherapeutic agents allows for treatment of disease that has spread to distant sites. Chemotherapy for soft tissue sarcoma typically uses a combination of several anticancer drugs. The most commonly used drugs are ifosfamide and doxorubicin. Sometimes other drugs such as dacarbazine, methotrexate, vincristine, cisplatin, paclitaxel, and others are added in combination. Intra-arterial doxorubicin-based concurrent chemoradiation treatment strategies are evolving to improve local control rates (Pisters et al., 1999).

TREATMENT APPROACH BY STAGE

Stage I

■ Surgery is a potential first treatment choice for tumors at this stage. Radiation therapy is beneficial at this stage in two instances. Preoperative radiation can be used to reduce tumor volume and increase the success of removing a previously unresectable lesion. Postoperative radiotherapy can be used if adequate margins could not be obtained during surgical resection. Radiation can be considered as an alternative to surgery if the tumor is considered inoperable because of involvement of critical structures or if the patient cannot tolerate the surgical procedure because of other health conditions. Radiation therapy alone is most often not effective for cure of soft tissue sarcoma.

Stage II
■ Preoperative radiotherapy should strongly be considered to facilitate complete surgical resection. Otherwise, postoperative radiotherapy may be required.

Stage III
■ Surgery with a definite request for radiation therapy either pre- or postoperatively because of the increased chance of tumor recurrence with surgery alone. Chemotherapy may be considered at this stage.

Stage IV
■ Metastasis to distant sites is the limiting factor affecting treatment outcomes at this stage. Surgery to remove the primary tumor plus radiation therapy is the treatment of choice. Amputation may be required if complete surgical removal is not possible. Surgical removal of all metastases if possible. If surgery is unable to accomplish complete removal of the primary tumor and all metastases, palliative radiation and/or chemotherapy is recommended.

TOXICITY OF TREATMENT
■ The patient can experience side effects based on the type of treatment and location of the tumor. Surgery carries the risk of infection, scarring, nerve damage, pain, bleeding, and edema. Chemotherapy has systemic effects such as nausea/vomiting, weight loss, alopecia, fatigue, neuropathy, or organ toxicity. Radiation therapy has effects that are confined to the local treatment area and progress slowly throughout the course of treatment. Outcomes of radiation therapy can be divided into acute side effects and latent/chronic side effects. Management options for these symptoms are as follows:

Acute Toxicities
1. Pain—Patients who begin treatment with pain from previous surgery or injury or secondary to the tumor compressing

nearby structures, (primarily the neuro-vascular bundles), can be successfully managed with medications. Patients often report general aching and muscle spasms in the treatment field secondary to tissue inflammation as the treatment progresses. This is managed with the use of nonsteroidal anti-inflammatory drugs (NSAID) and muscle relaxants and can range to the use of long-acting narcotics for more chronic, lasting pain. Refer to Chapter 20, "Maintenance of Comfort (Pain and Fatigue)" for further recommendations.

2. Skin reactions—The skin will gradually develop a dry desquamation and pigment change between weeks 2 and 3 after the start of radiation therapy. Initial skin care includes the use of a moisturizer (aloe/vitamin E) after daily treatments. Skin changes may progress to erythema or moist desquamation depending on the area treated. For management options refer to Chapter 21, "Sustained Integrity of Protective Mechanisms (Skin, Oral, Immune System)."

3. Edema—Monitor extremities for swelling, especially in postoperative patients. Drainage of the extremity might be compromised secondary to surgery or damage to lymph vessels. Edema can also be exacerbated by radiation and will contribute to the discomfort a patient feels. It is recommended that the patient elevates the extremity daily above the level of the heart to promote drainage. A compression stocking may also be appropriate. Massage to the affected area should be reserved for postoperative patients only.

4. Neuropathy—May exist from the location of the tumor in relation to nerve structure, or as a side effect of surgery or chemotherapy. It may be aggravated by the inflammation from radiation and needs to be monitored closely.

5. Fatigue—An estimated 72% to 99% of all cancer patients experience fatigue (ONS, 1998). Many factors contribute to the development of fatigue including the disease process itself and the treatments utilized. Acute effects of fatigue usually occur between 2 and 3 weeks after the start of radiation and may last for 3 months after completion. Patient limitations as a result of fatigue can range from mild to severe. Monitoring and intervention are necessary to minimize negative effects on patients' quality of life and to promote compliance with treatment. Refer to Chapter 20 for specific interventions on fatigue management.

6. Anorexia—Patients who receive radiation to the abdomen for a retroperitoneal mass can experience a loss of appetite. An

estimated 15% to 25% of patients with cancer have anorexia at the time of diagnosis (ONS, 1998). Close monitoring of weight at least weekly during treatment is recommended. Immediate dietary counseling should be instituted for patients with weight loss of 5% to 10% of their usual body weight.

7. Nausea and vomiting—Occurs in 50% of patients receiving radiation therapy to the abdomen (ONS, 1998). It can occur after the first treatment, be intermittent or continuous, and last several days after the completion of therapy. Management with antiemetics should be instituted 1 hour prior to the first radiation treatment and monitored closely for effectiveness. The goal is to prevent weight loss, dehydration, and interruption of treatment. Collaboration with the dietary team is crucial especially for patients already compromised.

8. Gastrointestinal—Disruption of bowel function is an expected short-term side effect of radiation to the abdomen and pelvis. Patients may have constipation from narcotic use and need to be regulated with an appropriate stool softener or laxative. If the radiation treatment field includes the pelvis, then generally about the third week of treatment, diarrhea can be an expected side effect. Patients should be monitored for frequency and consistency of stools, rectal discomfort, rectal bleeding, pain, and signs of dehydration. Management with dietary modifications and antidiarrheals should be initiated and monitored. See Chapter 23 for specific recommendations.

9. Acute bladder symptoms can begin between the second and third week of treatment to the pelvis and can include pain or burning with urination, increased frequency of urination, hesitancy, urgency, or increased nocturia. Management includes urinary tract analgesics, antispasmodics, and antihypertensives (i.e., terazosin) to improve urinary flow and decrease symptoms. See Chapter 23 for specific recommendations.

Late and Chronic Toxicities

1. Fibrosis—The formation of scar tissue secondary to surgery with or without radiation therapy alone. Fibrosis may cause discomfort in the treatment site and permanent loss of range of motion (ROM) of an extremity. Encouraging patients to begin a regular daily stretching program immediately after surgery and during and after the course of radiation is vital to maximizing the patient's functional status. A physical therapist can initiate a program.

2. Edema—Damage to lymph vessels may compromise drainage from an extremity and lead to chronic edema. Such chronic states can increase risk of infection, cause pain, alter body image, and decrease ROM. See Chapter 11 on management of lymphedema.

3. Bone fracture—Damage may occur to bones from original tumor destruction or from resection of bone or the periosteum or secondary to radiation. Bones may have a greater risk of fracture because of limited healing capacity and may have increased risk of infection.

4. Skin—Latent skin reactions are classified as occurring 6 or more months after radiation begins and include fibrosis, atrophy, ulceration, pigment changes, thinning, and telangiectasia (ONS, 1998).

EXPECTED OUTCOMES

■ The expected outcomes when treating for cure are achieving local control and reducing the risk of metastasis while maintaining optimal functioning for the patient and promoting the maximum disease-free survival.

OUTCOMES MEASURES

SURVEILLANCE

■ Follow-up evaluation by the treatment team is recommended every 3 to 4 months for 2 to 3 years, then every 6 months for 5 years, then on an annual basis or prn. Follow-up is to evaluate local recurrence and distant metastasis, and to monitor side effects of treatment. Recurrence is most common in the first 2 to 3 years after treatment (Demetri, 1998). Hence close follow-up is crucial. The following procedures should be included:

1. Complete history and physical examination

2. Chest x-ray every 6 to 12 months or CT scan because of the high risk of pulmonary metastasis. In 75% of patients with primary tumors of an extremity, the predominant site of first recurrence is the lung (Demetri et al., 1998; Enzinger

& Weiss, 1995). Whooley and colleagues found that chest x-ray imaging was a cost-effective strategy for follow-up of patients with high-grade extremity soft tissue sarcomas (Whooley, Mooney, Gibbs, & Kraybill, 1999).

3. Primary site imaging—Imaging with CT scan or MRI·on an annual basis was found to be an ineffective strategy for detecting recurrence. However, certain patient characteristics such as body habitus, previous radiation therapy, and location of the primary tumor site may require the use of imaging for adequate clinical assessment (Whooley et al., 1999).

4. Laboratory blood studies have been found to be ineffective strategies for detecting recurrence (Whooley et al., 1999).

■ The NCI Common Toxicity Criteria (CTC) Version 2 with the Radiation Therapy Oncology Group (RTOG) and European Organization for Research and Treatment of Cancer (EORTC) Acute Effects Criteria instrument provides a scale for many different organ systems and some symptoms (NCI, 1999). It is a very useful tool for grading severity of acute effects of radiation therapy in all sites.

■ The Radiation Therapy Patient Care Record: A Tool for Documenting Nursing Care (ONS, 1994) provides a tool for weekly assessment and grading of severity of acute effects of radiation therapy in all sites.

PROGNOSIS AND RECURRENCE

■ Improvements have taken place in soft tissue sarcoma patient survivorship and quality of life over the past 20 years, with overall 5-year survival currently at approximately 50–65% (Pollock et al., 1996). Many factors must be considered in the survival data including histology, grade of tumor, stage of disease, and treatment approaches.

■ A key factor in determining overall patient survival is whether distant metastasis has occurred by the time of presentation. At diagnosis, approximately 10% of patients have demonstrable disease (Demetri et al., 1998).

■ In patients with sarcomas of the extremity, about 90% of treatment failures are ultimately due to pulmonary metastasis.

■ In patients with truncal or retroperitoneal sarcomas, 50% fail at the local site (Demetri et al., 1998).

QUALITY OF LIFE

Currently there is not a tool developed specifically to evaluate a patient's quality of life after treatment for sarcoma with multimodality therapy. However, several studies have recently published functional outcome results after multimodality therapy for soft tissue sarcomas of the limb. Although these data are focused on surgical intervention, they give some insight into the complications that occur.

Amputation versus Limb-Sparing Multimodality Therapy

■ In one of the earliest evaluations of quality of life in patients with soft tissue sarcoma, Sugarbaker and colleagues found minimal differences between a group of individuals treated with amputation and a group treated with limb-sparing surgery and postoperative radiation with or without chemotherapy. Sexual function was significantly decreased in patients who underwent limb-sparing multimodality therapy, probably related to a protracted course of treatment (Sugarbaker, Barofsky, Rosenberg, & Gianola, 1982).

■ In a matched case-controlled study, Davis, Devlin, Griffin, Wunder, & Bell (1999) evaluated the differences in physical disability and handicap experienced by patients with lower extremity sarcoma who required amputation for the primary tumor compared with those treated with limb-sparing surgery. They found a trend toward increased disability for those in the amputation group with significantly higher levels of handicap.

Limb-Sparing Procedures with Reconstruction

■ Zunino and Johnston (1998) evaluated the functional and subjective condition of individuals during a 2-year postoperative period, evaluating the nature and frequency of complications after surgical procedures. They found that during the first 6 months, most patients have a poor functional and subjective condition that progressively improves throughout the first and second year. There was a high rate of complications during this period (46%), most frequently related to proximal femur and proximal tibia sites, and they were primarily a mechanical dysfunction of the reconstructive system.

■ Similar findings were reported by Ham, Schraffordt-Koops, Veth, van-Horn, Molenage, & Hoekstra (1998) in an evaluation of 32 patients with primary bone sarcomas of the femur or proximal tibia who had undergone endoprosthetic procedures. They found that these reconstructions gave satisfying functional results in most patients after long-term survival (median survival = 10 years). Endoprosthetic-related complications occurred in 41%; most complications were mechanical failures. Proximal tibial and distal femoral endoprosthesis were found to be particularly at risk for complications requiring additional surgical procedures.

■ Serletti, Carras, O'Keefe, & Rosier (1998) evaluated the functional outcome of 20 patients with sarcoma after soft-tissue reconstruction for limb salvage. Patients were examined for range of motion, deformity, stability, pain level, strength, functional activity, and emotional acceptance. Using the Musculoskeletal Tumor Society Scale (MSTSS), 45% achieved an overall rating of excellent, 25% a rating of good, and 30% a rating of fair. There were no differences in the results obtained comparing upper versus lower extremity, immediate versus delayed reconstruction, or reconstructions performed with a free flap versus a pedicle flap (Enneking, Dunham, Gebhardt, Malawar, & Pritchard, 1993).

Radiation Therapy with Limb-Sparing Procedures

■ Yang et al. (1998) evaluated quality of life in a randomized prospective study assessing postoperative radiation therapy after limb-sparing resection of extremity sarcomas. They found that radiotherapy resulted in compromized limb strength, edema, and range of motion, but these deficits were often transient and had few measurable effects on activities of daily living or global quality of life. Similar findings were identified by Robinson et al. (1991). Doses in excess of 60 Gy resulted in increased fibrosis and a worse functional outcome.

■ Karasek, Constine, & Rosier (1992) evaluated the functional outcome of patients treated with surgery and irradiation. They found a direct relationship between volume irradiated to at least 55 Gy and functional score, strength, fibrosis, and skin changes. Total dose independent of volume was significantly associated with skin changes. Increasing maximum dose was associated with fibrosis and skin changes. In patients in whom a portion of the joint was included in the treatment field, neither range of motion nor functional score was correlated with joint dose. Edema and functional score were not related to either the volume or percent of limb spared.

Instruments available to measure quality of life as well as functional outcomes in this population include:

1. Functional Assessment of Cancer Therapy (FACT-G) (Cella, Tulsky, & Gray, 1993)—Measurement system of self-report, 33-item scale of quality of life for people with cancer. The general version has been validated in English and has been used extensively in the United States.
2. European Organization for Research and Treatment of Cancer (EORTC) QLQ-C30 (Aaronson et al., 1993)—A 36-item questionnaire for assessing the quality of life of cancer patients participating in international clinical trials. It has been validated and used extensively in a wide range of cancer clinical trials in Europe and throughout the world.
3. The Toronto Extremity Salvage Score (TESS) (Davis et al., 1996; Davis et al., 1999)—Measure of functional status for patients with lower extremity sarcoma. It recently has been found to be a reliable and efficient measure for evaluating patients (Davis et al., 1999).
4. Musculoskeletal Tumor Society Scale (MSTSS) (Enneking et al., 1993)—Standardized system of reporting end results of various surgical alternatives after limb salvage and ablative procedures for musculoskeletal tumors.

RESEARCH

■ There has been much progress in understanding how certain changes in the DNA of soft tissue cells cause sarcomas to develop. This information is already being applied to new tests for diagnosis and classification of sarcomas. It is hoped that this information will soon lead to new strategies for treating these cancers.

■ Experimental treatments are being tested that boost patients' immune reaction to fight soft tissue sarcomas more effectively. Active immunotherapy through vaccines causes the immune system to recognize the abnormal surface antigens in sarcomas and kill these cells. Passive immunotherapy uses antibodies made in the laboratory to seek out sarcoma cells that contain certain abnormal cancer cell proteins. Toxins or radioactive agents can be attached to these antibodies so that the cell-killing chemicals or radiation are targeted specifically to the cancer cells and do not attack the healthy cells of the body.

■ New chemotherapy protocols are being developed that test new drugs, varying dosages, and methods of administration for the treatment of soft tissue sarcomas.

■ New radiation administration techniques are also being developed and currently include use of intraoperative radiation therapy for abdominal and retroperitoneal sarcomas.

REFERENCES

Aaronson, N. K., Ahmedzai, S., Bergman, B., Bullinger, M., Cull, A., Duez, N. J., Filiberti, A., Flechtner, H., Fleishman, S. B., de Haes, J. C.J. M., Kaasa, S., Klee, M., Osoba, D., Razavi, D., Rofe, P. B., Schraub, S., Sneeuw, K., Sullivan, M., & Takeda, F. (1993). The European Organization for Research and Treatment of Cancer QLQ-C30; A quality-of-life instrument for use in international clinical trials in oncology. *Journal of the National Cancer Institute*, 85(5), 365–376.

Cella, D. F., Tulsky, D. S., & Gray, G. (1993). The Functional Assessment of Cancer Therapy Scale: Development and validation of the general measure. *Journal of Clinical Oncology*, 11(3), 570–579.

Chao, K. S. C., Perez, C. A., & Brady, L. W. (1999). *Radiation oncology: Management decisions.* Philadelphia: Lippincott-Raven.

Crownover, R. L., & Marks, K. E. (1999). Adjuvant brachytherapy in the treatment of soft-tissue sarcomas. *Hematology/Oncology Clinics of North America*, 13(3), 595–607.

Das Gupta, T. K. & Chaudhun, P. K. (1998). *Tumors of the soft tissues* (2nd ed.). Stamford, CT: Appleton & Lange.

Davis, A. M., Bell, R. S., Bradley, E. M., Yoshida, K., & Williams, J. I. (1999). Evaluating functional outcome in patients with lower extremity sarcoma. *Clinical Orthopedics and Related Research*, 358, 90–100.

Davis, A. M., Devlin, M., Griffin, A. M., Wunder, J. S., & Bell, R. S. (1999). Functional outcome in amputation versus limb sparing of patients with lower extremity sarcoma: A matched case-control study. *Archives of Physical Medicine and Rehabilitation*, 80(6), 615–618.

Davis, A. M., Wright, J. G., Williams, J. I., Bombardier, C., Griffin, A., & Bell, R. S. (1996). Development of a measure of physical function for patients with bone and soft tissue sarcoma. *Quality of Life Research*, 5(5), 508–516.

Demetri, G. D., Pollock, R., Baker, L., Balcerzak, S., Casper, E., Conrad, C., Fein, D., Hutchinson, R., Schupak, K., Spiro, I., & Wagman, L. (1998). NCCN sarcoma practice guidelines. *Oncology*, 12(7A), 183–218.

Enneking, W. F., Dunham, W., Gebhardt, M. C., Malawar, M., & Pritchard, D. J. (1993). A system for the functional evaluation of reconstructive procedures after surgical treatment of tumors of the musculoskeletal system. *Clinical Orthopedics and Related Research*, 286, 241–246.

Enzinger, F. M., & Weiss, S. W. (1995). *Soft tissue sarcomas*, (3rd ed.). St. Louis: Mosby.

Greenlee, R. T., Murray, T., Bolden, S., & Wingo, P. A. (2000). *Cancer statistics, 2000.* CA: *Cancer Journal for Clinicians*, 50(1), 7–33.

Ham, S. J., Schraffordt-Koops, H., Veth, R. P., van-Horn, J. R., Molenaar, W. M., & Hockstra, H. J. (1998). Limb salvage surgery for primary bone sarcoma of the lower extremities: Long term consequences of endo-prosthetic reconstruction. *Annals of Surgical Oncology*, 5(5), 423–436.

Harrison, L. B., Franzese, F., Gaynor, J. J., Brennan, M. F. (1993). Long-term results of a prospective randomized trial of adjuvant brachytherapy in the management of completely resected soft tissue sarcomas of the extremity and superficial trunk. *International Journal of Radiation Oncology, Biology, Physics*, 27(2), 259–265.

Hoppin, J. A., Tolbert, P. E., Flanders, W. D., Zhang, R. H., Daniels, D. S., Ragsdale, B. D., & Brann, E. A. (1999). Occupational risk factors for sarcoma subtypes. *Epidemiology*, 10(3), 300–306.

Karasek, K., Constine, L. S., & Rosier, R. (1992). Sarcoma therapy: Functional outcome and relationship to treatment parameters. *International Journal of Radiation, Oncology, Biology, Physics*, 24(4).

National Cancer Institute. (1999). *NCI Common Toxicity Criteria (CTC) Version 2 with the Radiation Therapy Oncology Group (RTOG) and European Organization for Research and Treatment of Cancer (EORTC) Acute Effects Criteria.* Bethesda, MD: National Cancer Institute.

Oncology Nursing Society. (1998). *Manual for radiation oncology nursing practice and education.* Pittsburgh, PA: Oncology Nursing Society.

Oncology Nursing Society—Radiation Therapy Special Interest Group Documentation Project Core Committee. (1994). *Radiation Therapy Patient Care Record: A tool for documenting nursing care.* Pittsburgh, PA: Oncology Nursing Society.

Pisters, P. W. (1999). Chemoradiation treatment strategies for localized sarcoma: Conventional and investigational approaches. *Seminars in Surgical Oncology*, 17(1), 66–71.

Pisters, P. W., Fein, D. A., Casper, E. S., & Somls, G. (1996). *Cancer management: A multidisciplinary approach: Medical surgical, and radiation oncology* (3rd ed.). Huntington, NY: PRR Inc.

Pisters, P. W., Fein, D. A., Casper, E. S., & Somls, G. (1999). *Cancer management: A multidisciplinary approach: Medical, surgical, and radiation oncology* (4th ed.). Huntington, NY: PRR Inc.

Pollock, R. E., Karnell, L. H., Menck, H. R., & Winchester, D. P. (1996). The National Cancer Data Base report on soft tissue sarcoma. *Cancer*, 78(10), 2247–2257.

Robinson, M. H., Spruce, L., Eeles, R., Fryatt, I., Harmer, C. L., Thomas, J. M., & Westbury, G. (1991). Limb function following conservation tretment of adult soft tissue sarcoma. *European Journal of Cancer*, 27(12), 1567–1574.

Rosenberg, S. A., Tepper, J., Glatstein, E., Costa, J., Baker, A., Brennan, M., DeMoss, E. V., Seipp, C., Sindelar, W. F., Sugarbaker, P., & Wesley, R. (1982). The treatment of soft-tissue sarcomas of the extremities: prospective randomized evaluations of (1) limb-sparing surgery plus radiation therapy compared with amputation and (2) the role of adjuvant chemotherapy. *Annals of Surgery*, 196(3), 305–315.

Serletti, J. M., Carras, A. J., O'Keefe, R. J., & Rosier, R. N. (1998). Functional outcome after soft-tissue reconstruction for limb salvage after sarcoma surgery. *Plastic and Reconstructive Surgery*, 102(5), 1576–1583.

Sugarbaker, P. H., Barofsky, I., Rosenberg, S. A., & Gianola, F. J. (1982). Quality of life assessment of patients in extremity sarcoma clinical trials. *Surgery*, 91(1), 17–23.

Terek, R. M. (1997). Sarcoma of bone. *Medical Health Rhode Island*, 80(1), 19–25.

Whooley, B. P., Mooney, M. M., Gibbs, J. F., & Kraybill, W. G. (1999). Effective follow-up strategies in soft tissue sarcoma. *Seminars in Surgical Oncology*, 17(1), 83–87.

Yang, J. C., Chang, A. E., Baker, A. R., Sindelar, W. F., Danforth, D. N., Topalian, S. I., DeLancy, T., Glatstein, E., Steinberg, S. M., Merino, M. J., & Rosenberg, S. A. (1998). Randomized prospective benefit of adjuvant radiation therapy in the treatment of soft tissue sarcomas of the extremity. *Journal of Clinical Oncology*, 16(1), 197–203.

Zunino, J. H., & Johnston, J. O. (1998). Early results of lower limb surgery for osteogenic sarcoma of bone. *Orthopedics*, 21(1), 47–50.

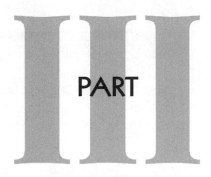

PART

PATIENT RELATED OUTCOMES

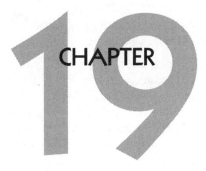

CHAPTER 19

INCREASED KNOWLEDGE

Marilyn L. Haas, PhD, ANP-C
J. Battle Haslam, MD

PROBLEM

Although cancer still remains the second leading cause of death, the National Center for Health Statistics and the National Cancer Institute Surveillance, Epidemiology, and End Results (SEER) reports the incidence of cancer has declined slightly over the past several years in the United States (Landis, Murray, Bolden, & Wingo, 1999). The American Cancer Society estimated that 1.2 million new cases of invasive cancer would be diagnosed in 1999 and approximately 552,000 people would die of this disease (American Cancer Society, 2000). Among the standard treatment modalities (surgery, chemotherapy, and radiation), approximately 60% of patients will receive radiation therapy sometime during the course of their disease (Iwamoto, 1997). Surprisingly, many patients are unfamiliar with radiation as a treatment option.

Patients experience many feelings when they are first informed they have cancer. Reactions may include anger, fear, guilt, anxiety, withdrawal, depression, hopelessness, and/or powerlessness (Brotzman & Robertson, 1998). Lack of knowledge about the disease process and available treatment options only compounds these feelings. Therefore, it is extremely important to provide information to the patients and family members as quickly as possible and in terminology they can understand in order for them to regain a sense of control over their lives. This will eventually promote understanding, cooperation, and higher compliance with treatments. Barriers that may impede a patient's understanding about his or her disease and/or care include the following:

- Lack of Prevention Information or Early Detection Services—Cancer screening and early detection is an extremely important factor in the survival of patients (Smart, Mettlin, Tabar, & Eyre, 1997). While survival rates are better for those patients diagnosed with early-stage cancers rather than those with advanced cancers, many individuals still do not seek screening. Possible reasons may include lack of knowledge or understanding of the benefits of preventive measures, forgetfulness, sexual embarrassment, economic issues, low priority, or lack of preventive health care coverage.
- Cultural and Social Factors—For many decades there has been a stigma attached to the word "cancer." Individuals and society associate "cancer" with the five **D's: d**eath sentence, **d**isability, **d**isfigurement, **d**ependency, and/or **d**isruption of close relationships (Holland, 1997). Also, the meaning of cancer varies among different age groups. Young adults deal with the decreasing family role, sterility, and impotence. Middle-aged adults fear disruption in job performance and achievements, while older individuals deal with increasing isolation, and decreasing financial security. Social class also impacts on coping skills. Typically, individuals from a lower socioeconomic background tend to have poorer coping mechanisms and more difficulty dealing with the diagnosis/treatment (Tavani et al., 1999).
- Highly Charged Emotional Status—Fear of the unknown or high anxiety can affect the decision process or course of treatment. Some patients may have an irrational fear of radiation and are afraid to receive large doses of radiation (Yarbro, 1997). Other patients may have mixed emotions regarding the possible body image alterations (i.e., alopecia, skin changes, or weight loss) and may choose not to have the treatments. Highly anxious or nervous patients may become noncompliant because of their feelings. Worrying about treatment failure or recurrence breaks down the patient's ability to cope (Gale & Charette, 1994). Other emotions such as denial, confusion, anger, guilt, or grief may also break down communication lines.
- Unproven Alternative Cancer Methods—Historically, when traditional medicine proved unable to provide a cure, individ-

uals turned toward nontraditional methods (Holland, 1997). Many unscientific methods/treatments flourished because individuals were vulnerable and searching for a cure. Other motivators can include fear, desire for self-control, antiestablishment beliefs, or social pressures from family and friends (Groenwald, Frogge, Goodman, & Yarbro, 1995). Some individuals elect to utilize nontraditional methods hoping to enhance the body's defenses. Unfortunately, many patients receive conflicting information and become confused.

ASSESSMENT

Understanding what the patient knows about his or her disease, belief system, and overall perception of health is especially important to assess during the initial consult. A comprehensive medical history should be obtained from the patient and family members. It should include the following information.

- Age—Individuals over 65 years of age are ten times more likely to develop cancer (Groenwald et al., 1995). This is as a result of the aging process and prolonged exposure to carcinogenic agents.
- Race—Racial background becomes an important risk factor in the development of some cancers. Although for the first decade since statistics have been tracked and cancer rates have declined in the United States overall, African American males continue to have a higher incidence of many cancers, are diagnosed at less favorable stages, and have uniformly lower survival than their Caucasian counterparts (American Cancer Society; Cummingham, 1997).
- Educational Level—While cancer can strike any individual, those with minimal education tend to present with more advanced cancers. Also, a patient's learning needs and his or her readiness to learn become important to assess (Bruner, Bucholtz, Iwamoto, & Strohl, 1998).
- Cultural and Socioeconomic Background—Some lifestyle choices are associated with developing certain cancers (e.g., homosexuality or promiscuity) (Lacey et al., 1999; Saunders, 1999). Lower socioeconomic status is associated with some cancers. Cultural factors cause differences in incidence and mortality.

■ Health Habits—Certain health habits have shown a strong association with developing cancer and place patients at high risk for this disease. Cancer of the lung is the number-one killer of men and women. Tobacco use contributes to 30% of cancer deaths and cigarette smoking causes 90% of lung cancers (Groenwald et al., 1995). Occupational exposure to carcinogens is related primarily to lung cancers and accounts for 4% to 9% of cancer deaths. Alcohol is associated with cancers of the oral cavity, pharynx, larynx, esophagus, and liver. Alcohol contributes to 3% of cancer deaths (Groenwald et al., 1995). Improper nutrition contributes to 20% to 70% of cancer deaths (Groenwald et al., 1995). Research has shown that a high-fat diet may increase the risk of breast, colon, prostate, and ovarian cancers. Ultraviolet exposure increases the risk of developing skin cancers. The use of unopposed estrogens increases the risk of endometrial, breast, and ovarian cancers. Also, there is a strong association between the number of sexual partners and the development of cervical cancers.

■ Health Screening History—Early detection enhances curability. Annual assessment and appropriate diagnostic testing/laboratory workup of the breast, cervix, colon/rectum, oral, prostate, skin, and testicle are important. According to the American Cancer Society (1997) and most professional medical societies (Smart et al., 1997), recommended general guidelines are as follows:

Breast: Monthly self-breast examinations. Beginning at age 40, mammography is encouraged every year.

Cervix: Annual Pap smear and pelvic examination should be done on all women who are sexually active or at least 18 years of age.

Colon/Rectum: Beginning at age 50, annual fecal occult blood testing should be performed with colonoscopy every 3 to 5 years.

Oral: Visual oral examination and palpation of the tongue, floor of mouth, salivary glands, and lymph nodes of the neck should be a part of every routine examination.

Prostate: Men over 50 should have an annual digital rectal examination and a prostate-specific antigen blood test.

Skin: Examination of the skin should be a part of every routine physical examination. Fair-skinned individuals should check themselves frequently for any suspicious moles.

Testicular: Monthly self-examination. Clinical examination should be performed at every annual physician visit.

■ Family History—Individuals may be genetically predisposed to developing cancer. Increased genetic risk has been documented with significant family histories of breast cancers, hereditary retinoblastoma, familial polyposis coli, ovarian, colon, and pancreatic cancers.

■ Overall Health Perception—Provides an insight into how the patient is managing and coping with the disease. Positive attitudes influence recovery periods. Feelings of hopelessness generate despair, thus affecting appetite, energy level, sleeping, and sexual activity.

■ Utilization of Complementary Therapies—Patients have found relief of some symptoms by utilizing acupuncture, herbal medicines, hypnosis, biofeedback, massage, progressive muscle relaxation, meditation, or visualization.

■ Knowledge of Advance Directives—While medical providers may not wish to discuss with the patient a living will immediately, at some point during the treatment phase the discussion should be initiated.

EXPECTED OUTCOMES

In outcomes research, clinical outcomes are measurable end points whose assessments lead to improvements in quality of life. Today, health care providers and patients can look beyond disease-free survival end points and consider their quality of life as an important outcome. With the explosion of information on the Internet, patients are asking more questions and becoming more knowledgeable about their disease process. Patients are receiving more in-depth, concise information regarding their disease and treatment. The National Comprehensive Cancer Network (1999) in conjunction with the American Cancer Society published the first state-of-the-art cancer treatment guideline booklet for breast cancer patients, *Breast Cancer Treatment Guidelines for Patients*. This is intended to inform patients about the disease process, staging, standard workup, surgical options, and treatment guidelines utilizing layman's language. As

consumers of health care, patients are becoming more knowledgeable about treatment options and what to expect during their course
of treatment. With this information in hand they can make better informed end-of-life decisions and deal with survivorship issues. The
American Cancer Society called attention to cancer survivors' needs
and offered *The Cancer Survivor's Bill of Rights* (Springarn, 1988). Health
care providers should recognize that

1. Survivor's have the right to assurance of lifelong medical care.
2. In their personal lives, survivors have the right to the pursuit
   of happiness.
3. In the workplace, survivors have the right to equal job opportunities.
4. Since health insurance coverage is an overriding survivorship
   concern, every effort should be made to ensure all survivors
   adequate health insurance, whether public or private.

Outcomes Measures

Cancer remains a significant health care problem in the United
States. One possible way to lower the incidence of cancer is to inform patients of associated cancer risk factors—predisposing factors
and environmental/lifestyle factors. Knowledge can be a powerful
tool. For health conscious patients, cancer risk assessments can be
very useful. Identification of risk factors can contribute to better understanding of the disease process, thus modifying patients' high
risk behaviors (Mahon, 1998). Several mathematical models exists
to predict the risk of developing cancer. The "Risk Disk," referred to
as the Breast Cancer Risk Assessment Tool for Health Care
Providers, from the National Cancer Institute (NCI) was modified after the Gail model to predict the risk of developing breast cancer
(Gail, Brinton, & Byar, 1989). This program is available to any clinician free of charge from NCI to utilize in clinical practice to assist in
increasing the patient's awareness. Information regarding functional
status, well-being, and other health outcomes is important data for
the clinician. Various tools are available to administer to the patients to ascertain this information and incorporate into patient
care. The Short Form 36 Health Survey (SF-36) from the Medical Outcomes Study is a generic instrument that measures eight subcate-
gories: physical functioning, role-physical, bodily pain, general

health, vitality, social functioning, role-emotional, and mental health (Ware, 1993). The Functional Assessment of Cancer Therapy (FACT) is a cancer-specific instrument that measures physical, social, family, emotional, and functional well-being and the quality of the relationship with the physician (Weitzner et al., 1995).

OUTCOMES MANAGEMENT

Shortly after being diagnosed with cancer, patients are faced with making immediate treatment decisions. Unfortunately, patients may not have had time to adjust or process the information. For most patients, radiation therapy is often one of the initial treatment options. Health care providers must quickly focus on preparing the patient both physically and psychologically. Patients should be given the following information: •

- Diagnosis/Prognosis—Information regarding the disease and the prognosis should be clearly presented to the patient. Full disclosure should be given at the time of diagnosis. Competent patients have the right to know and to decide what is best for them.
- Appropriate Radiation Therapy Modalities—Patients should understand the goals and purpose of teletherapy and/or brachytherapy. Information regarding the risks and benefits and possible side effects should be explained prior to obtaining informed consent. Patients should be given specific treatment information: simulation, setups, tattoos, blocks/shielding, scheduling, and side effects (Bruner et al., 1998).
- Clinical trial is a controlled, experimental study designed to evaluate the potential value of treatment/therapies in human subjects. Today, clinical trials are recognized as the best method of developing and evaluating improved standards of care for cancer patients. However, accrual of patients into these studies is low. Less than 3% of all eligible individuals enter into a clinical trial (Benson et al., 1991). At participating institutions, appropriate individuals meeting enrollment criteria should be given the information and asked to consider a clinical trial as a treatment option.
- Complementary Therapies—Disclosure of alternative treatments is controversial. However, psychological and behavioral

methods are considered and utilized in mainstream medicine. Support groups have become an integral part of cancer therapy. Visual imagery, relaxation, and music therapy are endorsed for receptive patients to assist with symptom management and enhance quality of life (Ezzone, Baker, Rosselet, & Terepka, 1998). Patients in a randomized trial using guided imagery who received relaxation training were more relaxed, had reduced emotional suppression, and an improved quality of life during treatment (Walker et al., 1999).

■ Advance directives is a statement made by an individual outlining his or her wishes regarding medical interventions should a time ever come when the individual is no longer able to communicate his or her wishes. The underlying prerequisite of advance directives is informed consent. Patients have the right to determine what can and cannot be done to their bodies (Lynch & Edwards, 1998). Patients can carry out their advance directives through oral instructions, a living will, durable power of attorney for health care decisions, or a combination of a living will and durable power of attorney. Advantages to having advance directives are that the patient's end-of-life medical wishes are clearly identified, caregivers can direct the medical care consistent with the patient's wishes, and family members will not be burdened with making life and death decisions. Nevertheless, many patients remain reluctant to file advance directives. Common reasons cited are procrastination, apathy, general discomfort with the topic, family inability to discuss death/dying, or the medical system's failure to inform the patient about the need for such a document.

RESOURCES

Available resources are plentiful from the American Cancer Society and other site-specific support groups. National organizations are extremely helpful places to begin researching. Individuals can locate information quickly and easily on the Internet. Possible sites include:

http://www.cancer.org (American Cancer Society)
http://www.moffitt.usf.edu (H. Lee Moffitt Cancer Center and Research Institute)

http://nccn.org (National Comprehensive Cancer Network—NCCN)

http://www.nccn.org/patient_guidelines (NCCN patient guidelines)

REFERENCES

American Cancer Society. (1997). *American Cancer Society's guidelines for the early detection of cancer.* New York: American Cancer Society.

American Cancer Society. (2000). *Cancer facts and figures.* New York: Lippincott, Williams & Wilkins.

Benson, A., Pregler, J., Bean, J., Rademaker, A., Eshler, B., & Anderson, K. (1991). Oncologists' reluctance to accrue patients onto clinical trials: An Illinois cancer center study. *Journal of Clinical Oncology, 9* (11), 2067–2075.

Brotzman, G., & Robertson, R. (1998). Role of the primary care physician after the diagnosis of cancer. *Primary Care, 25* (2), 401–406.

Bruner, D., Bucholtz, J., Iwamoto, R., & Strohl, R. (1998). *Manual for radiation oncology nursing practice and education* (2nd ed.). Pittsburgh, PA: Oncology Nursing Press.

Cummingham, M. (1997). Giving life to numbers. CA: *Cancer Journal for Clinicians, 47* (1), 3–4.

Ezzone, S., Baker, C., Rosselet, R., & Terepka, E. (1998). Music as an adjunct to antiemetic therapy. *Oncology Nursing Forum, 25* (9), 1551–1556.

Gail, M., Brinton, L., & Byar, D. (1989). Projecting individualized probabilities of developing breast cancer for white females who are being examined annually. *Journal of the National Cancer Institute, 81,* 1879–1886.

Gale, D., & Charette, J. (1994). *Oncology nursing care plans.* El Paso, TX: Skidmore-Roth.

Groenwald, S., Frogge, M., Goodman, M., & Yarbro, C. (1995). *A clinical guide to cancer nursing.* Boston: Jones & Bartlett.

Holland, J. (1997). Principles of psycho-oncology. In J. Holland, R. Bast, D. Morton, E. Frei, R. Kafe, & R. Weichselbaum (Eds.), *Cancer medicine.* Baltimore, MD: Williams & Wilkins.

Iwamoto, R. (1997). Radiation therapy. In C. Varricchio, M. Pierce, C. Walker, & T. Ades (Eds.). *A cancer source book for nurses.* Atlanta, GA: American Cancer Society.

Lacey, H., Wilson, G., Tilston, P., Wilkins, E., Bailey, A., Corbitt, G., & Green, P. (1999). A study of anal intraepithelial neoplasia in HIV positive homosexual men. *Sexually Transmitted Infections, 3,* 172–177.

Landis, S., Murray, T., Bolden, S., & Wingo, P. (1999). Cancer statistics, 1999. CA: *Cancer Journal For Clinicians, 49* (1), 8–31.

Lynch, J., & Edwards, S. (1998). Advance directives. *Oncology Issues, 13* (2), 31–32.

Mahon, S. (1998). Cancer risk assessment: Conceptual considerations for clinical practice. *Oncology Nursing Forum*, 25 (9), 1535–1547.

National Comprehensive Cancer Network. (1999). *Breast cancer treatment guidelines for patients*. New York: National Comprehensive Cancer Network (NCCN) and American Cancer Society.

Saunders, J. (1999). Health problems of lesbian women. *Nursing Clinics of North America*, 34 (2), 381–391.

Smart, C., Mettlin, C., Tabar, L., & Eyre, H. (1997). Cancer screening and early detection. In J. Holland, R. Bast, D. Morton, E. Frei, R. Kafe, & R. Weichselbaum (Eds.), *Cancer medicine*. Baltimore, MD: Williams & Wilkins.

Springarn, N. (1988). *The cancer survivor's bill of rights*. Atlanta, GA: American Cancer Society.

Tavani, A., Fioretti, R., Franceschi, S., Gallus, S., Negri, E., Montella, M., Conti, E., & La Vecchia, C. (1999). Education, socioeconomic status and risk of cancer of the colon and rectum. *International Journal of Epidemiology*, 28 (3), 380–385.

Walker, L., Walker, M., Ogston, K., Heys, S., Ah-See, A., Miller, I., Hutcheon, A., Sarkar, T., & Eremin, O. (1999). Psychological, clinical and pathological effects of relaxation training and guided imagery during primary chemotherapy. *British Journal of Cancer*, 80 (1–2), 262–268.

Ware, J. (1993). *SF-36 Health Survey: Manual and interpretation guide*. Boston: The Health Institute, New England Medical Center.

Weitzner, M., Meyers, C., Gelke, C., Byrne, K., Cella, D., & Levin, V. (1995). The Functional Assessment of Cancer Therapy (FACT) Scale. Development of a brain subscale and revalidation of the general version (FACT-G) in patients with primary brain tumors. *Cancer*, 75 (5), 1151–1161.

Yarbro, C. (1997). Principles of oncology nursing. In J. Holland, R. Bast, D. Morton, E. Frei, R. Kafe, & R. Weichselbaum (Eds.), *Cancer medicine*. Baltimore, MD: Williams & Wilkins.

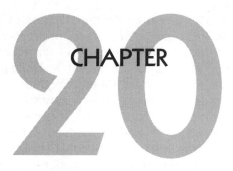

CHAPTER 20

MAINTENANCE OF COMFORT (FATIGUE AND PAIN)

Giselle J. Moore, ARNP, MSN
Cherylle Hayes, MD

PROBLEM

Fatigue and pain are two common problems that patients receiving radiation therapy may experience before, during, and after the treatment. They are both multifactorial symptoms that can affect the patient's ability to tolerate radiation therapy and can directly affect the patient's quality of life.

FATIGUE

■ Fatigue is a complex problem for which there is no general definition that applies to every situation. It is a subjective state of overwhelming, sustained exhaustion and decreased capacity for physical and mental work that is not relieved by rest (Cella, Passik, Jacobsen, & Breitbart, 1998). Common descriptive terms include tiredness, weariness, sleepiness, weakness, exhaustion, lack of energy, lethargy, malaise, inability to concentrate, asthenia, boredom, lack of motivation, decreased mental status, and depression.

■ Fatigue is a universal symptom of illness and often the first indication of some abnormal process in the body. Pain, easy fatigue, and anorexia are consistently among the 10 most prevalent symptoms of advanced cancer in most disease sites (Donnelly & Walsh, 1995).

■ Fatigue may precipitate a deterioration of psychological, physical, and social activities resulting in increased discomfort and decreased efficiency. It is a force that affects all dimensions of quality of life rather than being just an isolated symptom (Ferrell, Grant, Dean, Funk & Ly, 1996).

■ Fatigue has been identified as the most prevalent and disturbing symptom of cancer and its treatment (Winningham et al., 1994). Cancer-related fatigue has recently been accepted as a diagnosis in the International Classification of Disease 10th Revision—Clinical Modification. Cancer treatment–related fatigue differs from the fatigue experienced by healthy people in severity (higher), persistence (longer), and efficacy of sleep (fatigue persists on rising). The majority of patients receiving radiation therapy experience cumulative fatigue or fatigue that increases over time regardless of treatment site (Graydon, 1994; Greenberg, Sawicka, Eisenthal, & Ross, 1992; Haylock & Hart, 1979).

■ Factors that affect the level of fatigue among cancer patients include female gender, presence of metastatic disease, and poor performance status. Pater, Zee, Palmer, Johnston & Osoba, (1997) found that older patients have less fatigue, as do patients with breast cancer, while patients with ovarian and lung cancer experience greater fatigue. They also found that patients with well-controlled emesis showed significantly less increase in fatigue after receiving chemotherapy.

■ The exact etiology of fatigue related to radiotherapy is unknown. A number of actual or potential causes of fatigue have been identified. They include the accumulation of byproducts due to radiation-induced cellular breakdown, malnutrition, anemia, pharmacological side effects, pain, anxiety, and depression. Smets, Visser, Carssen, Frijda, Oosterveld & de-Haes (1998c) found that, at pretreatment, physical condition explained most of an individual's fatigue, whereas after treatment both the patient's physical condition and perception of burden contributed to the fatigue. In addition, when radiation is combined with other modalities such as chemotherapy and/or surgery, the effects may be intensified.

■ There does not appear to be a relationship between radiation dose and degree of radiation-induced fatigue. King, Nail, Kreamer, Strohl & Johnson (1985) interviewed 96 subjects weekly during the radiation therapy course and then monthly for 3 months after. The patient population included those receiving radiation for cure or control, rather than palliation, to the chest, head and neck, bladder, prostate, or pelvis (gynecologic malignancies). Most patients reported fatigue at some point during the evaluation period. Patients receiving radiation to the chest had the highest incidence (93%), followed by pelvis (72%), head and neck (68%), and prostate and bladder (65%). The peak incidence occurred in most groups from the third week through the end of treatment and was reported as continuous during the last 2 weeks. Greenberg, Sawicka, Gisenthal & Ross (1992) in a study of women receiving breast irradiation found that fatigue did not increase linearly with cumulative radiation dose over time. They found that fatigue dropped from the first to second week and then rose in the third week. The cumulative effects reached a plateau in the fourth week that was maintained during the remaining weeks of treatment.

- Patients who receive cranial irradiation may have a higher incidence of significant fatigue due to *somnolence syndrome*, which is excessive sleepiness, drowsiness, lethargy, and anorexia. Somnolence syndrome is a clinical manifestation of subacute effects of cranial irradiation related to transient demyelination mediated by radiation injury to oligodendrocytes or through alterations in capillary permeability. It usually occurs within 10 weeks of completion of treatment. It is a self-limiting process, but some patients benefit from steroids to reduce the clinical manifestations. Faithfull and Brada (1998) in a time series analysis identified a cyclical pattern to the symptoms with a period of drowsiness and fatigue occurring from day 11 to day 21 and from day 31 to day 35 after radiotherapy. The principal symptoms were excessive drowsiness, feeling clumsy, an inability to concentrate, lethargy, mental slowness, and fatigue. Patients treated with accelerated fractionation compared with more conventional fractionation experienced more severe drowsiness and fatigue, although there was no difference in the pattern or the incidence of symptoms. The unexplained and overwhelming nature of the symptoms was a cause of patient anxiety.

- Controversy exists regarding the role of the traditional "weekend" break and fatigue. Haylock and Hart (1979) performed daily evaluations on 30 patients receiving localized radiotherapy. Fatigue scores were consistently lower on

Sundays correlating with the weekend break from treatment. Greenberg et al. (1992) found that with the apparent cumulative fatigue there was no reduction on weekends. Different measures of fatigue could have accounted for the differences in outcomes.

■ Radiation therapy–induced fatigue does take several weeks to months to resolve after treatment. Greenberg et al. (1992) reported that the fatigue had diminished in most patients within 3 weeks after treatment. King et al. (1985) found that the fatigue appeared to persist through the third month after treatment in a substantial number of patients (14–46%). Smets (1998) evaluated 250 patients before and within 2 weeks of radiotherapy with curative intent. They found that after treatment 46% of the patients reported fatigue among the three symptoms that caused them the most distress. Significant associations were found between posttreatment fatigue and diagnosis, physical distress, functional disability, quality of sleep, psychological distress, and depression. No association was found between fatigue and treatment or personality characteristics. In a multivariate analysis, the intensity of pretreatment fatigue was the best predictor of fatigue after treatment. The degree of functional disability and impaired quality of sleep were found to explain 38% of the variance in fatigue before starting radiotherapy.

■ Patients often report persistent fatigue 6 months or more after completing treatment. Smets et al. (1998b) followed the patients from the previous study for 9 months after treatment and performed a reevaluation on 154 patients. Findings indicated that fatigue in disease-free cancer patients did not differ significantly from fatigue in the general population. However, for 34% of the patients, fatigue after treatment was worse than anticipated, 39% listed fatigue as one of the three symptoms causing them the most distress, 26% of patients worried about their fatigue, and patients' overall quality of life was negatively related to fatigue ($r = -0.46$). Fatigue in disease-free patients was significantly associated with gender, physical distress, pain rating, sleep quality, functional disability, psychological distress, and depression, but not with medical or treatment-related variables. The degree of fatigue, functional disability, and pain before radiotherapy were the best predictors of fatigue at 9-month follow-up, explaining 30%, 3%, and 4% of the variance, respectively.

■ Hodgkin's disease survivors may be more fatigued than the general population. Fobair, Hoppe, Broom, Cox, Varghese & Spiegel (1986) evaluated 403 long-term survivors of Hodgkin's disease. Median time since treatment was 9 years. Thirty-seven percent reported unsatisfactory return of energy level and an additional 63% reported that energy levels did not return to satisfactory levels for 12 to 16 months after treatment. Depression, combined modality therapy for advanced disease, and age over 30 appeared to be important variables in long-term fatigue. Loge and colleagues conducted a similar study and found that survivors of Hodgkin's disease had significantly higher levels of fatigue than did the controls. Fatigue among the survivors equaled that of the controls in poorest health. Again, no significant associations were found between treatment characteristics and fatigue (Loge, Abrahamsen, Ekeberg, & Kaasa, 1999).

■ The relationship between fatigue and quality of life is significant and linear (Cella, 1997; Yellen, Cella, Webster, Blendowski & Kaplan, 1997). Fatigue has the most impact on the physical and functional domains of quality of life, a modest effect on emotional well-being, and little effect on social well-being (Cella, 1997; Yellen et al., 1997). In a study of women interviewed 7 weeks after breast-conservation surgery followed by radiotherapy, the women reported few or no changes in their usual activities, no significant emotional distress, and few other symptoms with the exception of some persistent fatigue (Graydon, 1994). Those who experienced the most fatigue had the most symptoms and the poorest level of functioning. Similar findings were reported by Hann, Garovoy, Finkelstein, Jacobsen, Azzarello, & Fields (1999) in women undergoing autologous stem cell transplantation for breast cancer. They found that these women reported significantly more frequent fatigue and more severe fatigue than women with no cancer history. The fatigue had a greater significant impact on daily functioning and ultimately on quality of life.

■ In patients with advanced disease and those receiving palliative care, Stone, Hardy, and Broadley (1999) found fatigue in 75% of patients interviewed. The severity of the fatigue was unrelated to age, sex, diagnosis, presence or site of metastases, anemia, dose of opiate or steroid, hematologic or biochemical indices (except urea), nutritional status, voluntary muscle function, or mood. Multivariate analysis found that fatigue severity was significantly associated with pain and dyspnea scores.

■ Fatigue may also affect family caregivers of cancer patients (impacting care and support). Jensen and Given (1991) found no relationship between severity of fatigue experienced by the caregiver of the cancer patient and the caregiver's age, employment status, the number of hours of daily caregiving, or the duration of the caregiving. However, a significant relationship was found between fatigue and the impact of care on the daily schedule. The more the caregiver's schedule was a burden, the more fatigue was experienced, negatively impacting the ability to care for the patient.

■ Fatigue, in the form of exhaustion of physical, emotional, spiritual, financial, familial, communal, and other resources, increases risk of suicide in cancer patients (Breitbart, 1987).

■ Barriers to available treatment for fatigue may be patient-related and/or physician-related (Cella, Passik, Jacobsen, & Breitbart, 1998). Underreporting and underestimation of fatigue are the two most common reasons given for not addressing fatigue.

ASSESSMENT—FATIGUE

Fatigue may be an acute, subacute or chronic problem for patients treated with radiation therapy. A comprehensive medical history and physical examination are necessary to evaluate the specific cause(s) and severity of the fatigue.

MEDICAL HISTORY

■ The medical history should include a characterization of the fatigue:
1. Patient description of symptoms of fatigue and degree to which fatigue interferes with activities of daily living
2. Onset, location, and quantification of symptoms
3. Presence of sleep disturbances—disruption of sleep/rest cycle can cause chronic lethargy (Cella et al., 1998)
4. Presence of anorexia or barriers to adequate nutritional intake

5. Current medications
6. Role of underlying disease and treatments in fatigue: symptoms such as pain, nausea, and shortness of breath place compensatory demands on the patient resulting in energy depletion (Cella et al., 1998)
7. Comorbid conditions
8. Mental illness

PHYSICAL EXAMINATION

■ A thorough physical examination including all vital signs should be obtained. In the evaluation of acute and subacute fatigue, special attention should be paid to changes in mental status, evidence of dehydration, pallor, and miosis. In the chronic setting, attention should focus on evidence of chronic disease including changes in skin and hair texture and quality, chcilosis, pallor of gums, and evidence of malnutrition.

LABORATORY AND RADIOLOGY STUDIES

■ Laboratory and radiology studies may be performed depending on clinical manifestations and physical findings.
1. Complete blood count including hemoglobin and white blood cell count for evidence of bone marrow suppression, particularly anemia
2. Serum electrolytes including sodium, potassium, calcium, and magnesium for evidence of electrolyte imbalance
3. Serum glucose: hypo- or hyperglycemia
4. Serum BUN, creatinine, and liver enzymes: renal or liver dysfunction
5. TSH: hypothyroidism
6. Toxicology levels for evidence of barbiturates, sedatives, or narcotic analgesics
7. Chest x-ray to evaluate for pleural effusions, infiltrates, or tumor that may affect efficiency of oxygenation
8. CT scan: site specific to evaluate for evidence of disease progression
9. MRI of the brain to evaluate for brain metastases

DIFFERENTIAL DIAGNOSIS OF FATIGUE

ACUTE FATIGUE OR DROWSINESS (ONSET < 24 HOURS)

- Respiratory depression or sedation due to medications prescribed to manage side effects (such as analgesics, antiemetics, antidepressants, anticonvulsants, and hypnotics)
- Increased intracranial pressure resulting from cerebral edema or hemorrhage
- Septicemia
- Hypoglycemia
- Acute hypercapnia resulting from respiratory compromise from tumor compression of bronchi, pleural effusion, or pulmonary emboli
- Hypercalcemia resulting from bone metastasis or paraneoplastic syndrome
- Bleeding from a tumor, surgical wound, or gastric ulcer (with subsequent anemia)
- Hyponatremia (SIADH)

SUBACUTE FATIGUE (> 1 WEEK)

- Radiation-induced fatigue
- Anemia due to combined modality therapy or large volume of bone marrow in radiation field
- Pharmaceuticals given for side effect management (including analgesics, antiemetics, antidepressants, anticonvulsants, and hypnotics)
- Poor quality of sleep or insomnia
- Uncontrolled pain
- Hypoadrenalism resulting from rapid tapering of corticosteroids
- Hypoglycemia resulting from poor nutritional intake or cachexia
- Liver or renal failure resulting from metastatic disease or disease progression
- Advanced disease with significant tumor burden
- Altered metabolism (including hyponatremia, hypokalemia, hypercalcemia)
- Paraneoplastic syndromes (such as Eaton-Lambert and other myopathies)

CHRONIC OR INDOLENT FATIGUE (> 3 MONTHS)

- Advanced disease with significant tumor burden
- Anemia due to disease progression with bone marrow involvement or significant combined-modality treatment
- Chronic infection despite antimicrobial therapy
- Cachexia
- Depression
- Pharmaceuticals given for side effect management (including analgesics, antiemetics, antidepressants, anticonvulsants, and hypnotics)
- Poor quality of sleep or insomnia
- Prolonged immobilization and/or lack of exercise
- Anxiety and/or uncontrolled personal stress
- Hypothyroidism
- Chronic fatigue syndrome

EXPECTED OUTCOMES

MAINTENANCE OF PREILLNESS LEVELS OF COMFORT AND FUNCTION

- Fatigue is the most common side effect of cancer and its treatment and therefore should be expected. However, early assessment and intervention can reduce the impact of fatigue on a patient's ability to function and quality of life.
- Patients who present with symptoms of depression (including fatigue with or without other precipitating factors) need to be referred to clinical psychology or psychiatry for treatment.

OUTCOMES MEASURES

It is difficult to measure a multidimensional concept such as fatigue. It may be influenced by a number of factors including the timing of the assessment, the patient's culture, the patient's developmental stage, medications, stage of disease, comorbid disease, and course of treatment. A number of self-report instruments are available to measure fatigue in cancer patients:

- *Rhoten Fatigue Scale* (Rhoton, 1982): Developed as a subjective rating scale to quantify fatigue
- *Piper Fatigue Self-Report Scale* (PFS) (Piper, Lindsey, & Dodd, 1989): Scale that measures four dimensions of subjective fatigue: temporal, affective, sensory, and severity
- *Multidimensional Fatigue Inventory* (MFI) (Smets, Garssen, Bonk, & DeHaes, 1995): Scale to assess fatigue in five dimensions: general fatigue, physical fatigue, mental fatigue, reduced motivation, and reduced activity
- *Functional Assessment of Cancer Therapy with Fatigue Module* (FACT-F) (Cella, 1997): FACT general quality-of-life measurement with a module that contains 13 items specifically measuring fatigue
- *Functional Assessment of Cancer Therapy with Anemia Module* (FACT-An) (Cella, 1997): FACT general quality-of-life measurement questionnaire with seven items addressing concerns related to anemia, but unrelated to fatigue
- *Schwartz Cancer Fatigue Scale* (Schwartz, 1998): A 28-item measure to assess the effect of interventions to treat and manage cancer-related fatigue
- *Brief Fatigue Inventory* (BFI) (Mendoza et al., 1999): Rapid assessment of fatigue severity for use in both clinical screening and clinical trials

A number of other measurement tools are available that include fatigue as a single item or as a subscale embedded within a side effects or symptom checklist or quality-of-life evaluation. One of the most frequently used instruments is the monopolar version of the *Profile of Mood States* (Spiegel, Bloom, & Yalom, 1981).

OUTCOMES MANAGEMENT

The complexity of fatigue experienced by cancer patients makes it difficult to manage. The National Cancer Care Network has published guidelines for management of fatigue (Cella, Pasik, Jacobsen & Breitbart, 1998) that are very applicable in the radiation oncology setting.

EDUCATE PATIENT AND FAMILY

- Fatigue is an expected side effect of radiation therapy. Patients and families who understand this are able to prepare for this side effect and can develop self-care fatigue interventions to reduce its impact on daily activities and quality of life.

1. Maintain adequate fluid hydration and nutrition
2. Stress-reduction activities:
   a. Avoid environmental effects such as temperature extremes, loud noise, large crowds of people.
   b. Initiate periods of relaxation, meditation, yoga.
3. Modify activities:
   a. Develop a plan that encourages activities during the time of day when patients report having the least fatigue.
   b. Sleep and exercise have been identified as the most effective strategies to relieve fatigue (Graydon, Bubela, Irvine, & Vincent, 1995).
   c. Prioritize, delegate, and pace activities.
   d. Encourage short rest periods after major activities.
   e. Encourage rest periods (30 to 45 minutes) during the day.

DIFFERENTIATE FATIGUE FROM DEPRESSION

■ If depressive symptoms are present as well as fatigue, patients should be referred to an appropriate provider (psychologist or psychiatrist) for further evaluation and treatment.

ADDRESS REVERSIBLE CAUSES

Anemia

1. Transfuse with packed red blood cells.
2. Erythropoietin supplementation: Controlled clinical trials have shown that r-HuEPO increases hemoglobin and hematocrit levels and reduces the need for transfusions in patients with cancer-related anemia. These controlled trials have suggested that the improvements in hemoglobin are associated with increases in energy level, functional status, and overall quality of life (Glaspy & Cavill, 1999). However, only 50% of patients respond adequately to usual doses of r-HuEPO. The most common cause of inadequate response to r-HuEPO is functional iron deficiency.

Hypokalemia

1. Determine underlying cause and correct it.
2. Potassium replacement.

Hypercalcemia

1. Oral or intravenous fluid hydration depending on severity.
2. Loop diuretic after hydration to enhance calcium excretion.
3. Administer drugs that inhibit bone resorption or increase bone formation (biphosphonates, mithramycin, calcitonin).

Pharmaceutical Sedation

1. Consider reduction of drug dose or alternative drug to reduce sedative effects. If a specific drug is necessary, consider giving it before bedtime.
2. A trial of methylphenadate 5 to 20 mg twice to three times a day (30 to 45 minutes before meals) may reduce narcotic analgesic sedation.

Insomnia

1. Determine the cause of the sleep disturbance.
2. Consider sedative/hypnotic medication.
3. Develop routine of relaxation techniques before bedtime including yoga, meditation, hot bath, or a soothing beverage.
4. Avoid caffeine products 6 hours before bedtime.
5. Reduce stimulation (do not exercise before bedtime).
6. Encourage routine bedtime and rising time.
7. Avoid large volumes of food or fluid before bedtime.
8. Avoid alcohol consumption.

Anorexia/Cachexia

1. Evaluate nutritional intake.
2. Treat symptoms that are affecting the ability to eat (e.g., dysphagia, mucositis, pain).
3. Consider appetite stimulants including dexamethasone 1 to 2 mg qd or megestrol 800 mg qd. Bruera et al. (1998) found a significant improvement in two or three factors measured by the Piper Fatigue Scale and in the overall fatigue score for patients receiving megestrol acetate 160 mg three times a day for 10 days.

Sepsis

1. Appropriate antimicrobial therapy.
2. Consider hospitalization for intravenous antimicrobial therapy and fluid support.

Prolonged Immobilization and/or Lack of Exercise

1. Consider physical therapy three times a week.

2. Initiate low-impact exercise program (e.g., walking for 30 minutes a day). Dimeo et al. (1999) evaluated patients receiving high-dose chemotherapy followed by autologous peripheral blood stem cell transplantation. The patients followed an exercise program during hospitalization (consisting of biking on an ergometer in the supine position, following an interval training pattern for 30 minutes daily). By the time of hospital discharge, fatigue and somatic complaints had increased significantly in the control group but not in the training group. Furthermore, by the time of hospital discharge, the training group had a significant improvement in several scores of psychological distress. Mock et al. (1997) evaluated women participating in a walking exercise program during radiation therapy for breast cancer. The exercise group scored significantly higher than the control group on physical functioning and symptom intensity (particularly fatigue, anxiety, and difficulty sleeping).

3. Exercise prescriptions should include five basic criteria: status of the individual, type of exercise, and intensity, frequency, and duration of the exercise (Winningham, 1996).

Endocrine Imbalance (Hypothyroid or Hypoadrenal)

1. Replacement therapy with appropriate hormone or steroid.

TREAT SYMPTOMS OF COMORBID DISEASE

■ Patients with comorbid disease should be referred to their primary care physician or specialist for management of disease symptoms or adjustment in medications.

PAIN

■ Pain may be defined as an "unpleasant sensory and emotional experience associated with actual or potential tissue damage, or described in terms of such damage" (Merskey, 1986). Individuals with cancer can experience acute, intermittent, or chronic pain from their disease (61%), related to the disease debility (such as muscle spasm)(12%), related to diagnostic procedures or treatments (5%), or from preexisting conditions (22%) (Twycross & Fairfield, 1982).

■ Moderate to severe pain occurs in 30% of individuals with cancer who are receiving treatment and in 50% to 90% of patients with advanced disease. The severity of pain is not in linear relation to the amount of tissue damage (Waller & Caroline, 1996).

■ Pain related to cancer can be categorized (based on its pathophysiologic mechanisms) into somatic, visceral, or neuropathic pain. Each type of pain has unique etiologies and distinct clinical features, and responds to different types of therapeutic interventions (Miaskowski, 1998). Patients may experience one or more types of pain at any one time.

■ A number of factors influence an individual's perception of pain (including age, gender, fatigue, depression, anger, fear, anxiety, feelings of helplessness and hopelessness, and duration of uncontrolled pain).

■ Pain as a direct result of radiation therapy may be acute or chronic. Acute pain follows injury to the body and generally disappears when the bodily injury heals. Radiation-induced acute pain is pain that develops during a course of radiation treatment and lasts less than 3 months after treatment is completed. Chronic pain follows an injury to the body that results in significant soft tissue and/or nerve damage that does not completely heal. Radiation-induced chronic pain is defined as pain that does not resolve within 3 months after treatment or occurs in relationship to the late effects of radiation therapy.

■ Acute radiation-induced pain may result from localized skin reaction, mucosal reaction, soft tissue edema, cerebral edema, and/or tumor swelling. The pain corresponds directly with the amount of thermal tissue injury and/or local tissue swelling. In addition to localized skin reactions in most treatment sites, specific pain related to treatment sites may include the following:

• Cranial irradiation: headaches, otalgia, orbital mucosal irritation, external auditory canal irritation
• Head and neck irradiation: sinus inflammation, oropharyngeal mucositis, otalgia, esophagitis that may result in severe dysphagia
• Chest: esophagitis, dysphagia, pneumonitis, costrocondritis
• Breast: breast edema
• Abdomen: intestinal cramping, vomiting-induced esophagitis, enteritis, proctitis
• Pelvis: intestinal cramping, enteritis, proctitis, vaginitis, tenesmus

- Extremity: lymphedema or local tissue swelling
- Bone: may experience an initial "pain flare" because of tumor swelling during first 24 to 48 hours after initiation of radiation treatment

■ Despite clinician recognition of radiation-induced pain, very little research has been conducted to evaluate pain as a specific entity of radiation, or the efficacy of specific pain-management protocols in radiation-induced acute or chronic pain. Currently, the evaluation of pain is often a single question in a list of symptoms or side effects.

■ Weissman, Janjan, and Buyhardt (1989) found that despite the use of analgesics/anesthetics for oral mucositis that developed during radiation therapy for head and neck cancer, patients rated the pain as moderate or severe on 37% of treatment days. The pain was constant or present throughout most of the day on 58% of treatment days. Eating and sleeping disturbances related to pain occurred on 55% and 34% of treatment days, respectively. Eight patients had greater than 2 kg weight loss. In a similar study, Epstein and Stewart (1993) found that pain related to radiation therapy for head and neck cancer increased through the course of treatment and in some patients continued for 6 to12 months.

■ Jonler, Ritter, Brunkman, Messing, Rhodes, & Bruskewitz (1994) evaluated sequelae of definitive radiation to the pelvis for prostate cancer. Forty-nine percent of patients described abdominal pain, diarrhea, or abdominal cramping during or after radiation and 31% of all patients still had some intestinal symptoms at the follow-up evaluation 14 to 60 months later.

■ Postradiation pain syndromes include plexopathies, chronic radiation myelopathy, chronic enteritis and proctitis, burning perineum syndrome, and osteoradionecrosis. In addition, skin, joint, and soft tissue fibrosis may decrease range of motion and cause pain with stretching or movement. In a retrospective review of 145 patients who underwent limb-sparing surgery and radiation for a primary soft tissue sarcoma, long-term treatment complications included edema (19%), contracture (20%), moderate to severe decrease in range of motion (32%), and 7% reported pain that required narcotic analgesics 1 year after completing all treatment. (Rosenberg & Glatstein, 1991).

■ A number of procedures used to treat patients with radiation therapy can cause some degree of discomfort or pain. These procedures include immobilization device placement (head fixation ring for stereotactic radiosurgery), placement of HDR and LDR devices, and endocavitary contact radiation therapy.

■ The quality of life of cancer patients with pain is significantly worse than that of cancer patients without pain (Ferrell, Cohen, Rhiner, & Rozek, 1991). It can have an effect on all four domains of quality of life (physical, psychological, social, and spiritual). The effects may include decreased functional capacity, increased anxiety, fear, or depression, loss of control, diminished social relationships, increased caregiver burden, and increased suffering.

■ Ninety percent of all cancer pain can be managed effectively by means of noninvasive pharmacologic and nonpharmacologic interventions (Agency for Health Care Policy & Research, 1994). Unfortunately, a significant number of patients with cancer have undertreated pain. Common reasons for undertreatment of pain are problems related to health care professionals, patients, and the health care system. They include access to care, minority status, age, debility, female gender, history of substance abuse, patient underreporting, noncompliance with recommendations, patient fear of medications and side effects, clinician attitude and knowledge, low priority given to cancer pain treatment, inadequate reimbursement, and federal regulations of controlled substances.

■ Yeager, Miaskowski, Dibble, and Wallhagan, (1997) evaluated the differences in pain knowledge for cancer patients with and without pain. They found that patients with cancer-related pain knew significantly more about pain and its management than pain-free patients ($p < 0.004$). However, in both groups, mean knowledge scores were below 60%. Older patients with cancer-related pain had less knowledge about pain than younger patients ($p < 0.0001$). In addition, patients with cancer pain who had more education and those with higher reported pain intensity scores had more knowledge about pain and pain management. Women with cancer pain had more knowledge than men. This study suggests that oncology patients with and without pain need more education about pain and effective management strategies.

■ Breakthrough pain is a significant problem in patients with cancer-related pain. Portenoy and Hagen (1990) surveyed patients with cancer pain and found that 64% reported breakthrough pain (transient flares of severe or excruciating pain). Fifty-one different types of pain were described, and the characteristics were extremely varied. Forty-three percent of the pain described was paroxysmal in onset—the remainder more gradual. The duration varied from seconds to hours. Twenty-nine percent of the pain described was related to the fixed opioid dose, occurring solely at the end of the dosing interval. Precipitated pain occurred in 55% of patients, brought on by action of the patient (sudden movement) or a nonvolitional precipitant (such as flatulence).

ASSESSMENT—PAIN

■ Pain may be an acute, subacute, or chronic problem for patients treated with radiation therapy. Effective pain management involves a detailed pain assessment at each new report of pain, at regular intervals after the initiation of radiation therapy, and at a suitable interval after pharmacologic or nonpharmacologic intervention. A comprehensive medical history incorporating a tool such as the *Initial Pain Assessment Tool* developed by McCaffery and Beebe (1989) and a physical examination are necessary to evaluate the specific cause(s) of the pain.

MEDICAL HISTORY

■ Characterization of the pain
1. Patient description of symptoms of pain
2. Onset, location, and quantification of symptoms
3. Presence of aggravating and relieving factors
4. Cognitive response to the pain
■ Presence of comorbid disease with associated pain syndromes
■ Presence of depressive symptoms, anxiety, and/or fear
■ Current medications

PHYSICAL EXAMINATION

■ Examine the site of pain and evaluate common referral patterns
■ Perform pertinent neurologic evaluation

LABORATORY AND RADIOLOGY

■ Perform appropriate studies based on clinical manifestations and physical findings

Laboratory
1. Tumor markers: evidence of recurrent or progressive disease

Radiology and Other Studies
1. Skeletal plain film x-rays: suspicion of bone metastasis or pathologic fracture; superior in imaging lytic lesions
2. Bone scan: suspicion of bone metastasis
3. MRI: suspicion of bone metastasis or nerve compression by soft tissue mass; superior in imaging the CNS especially the brain and spinal cord
4. CT scan: particularly useful to evaluate soft tissue and bone for evidence of progressive disease
5. Ultrasonography: evidence of deep vein thrombosis (DVT); may be useful in characterizing a mass (solid, cystic, or fluid-filled)
6. Electromyography: evidence of neurologic deficit
7. Somatosensory testing: evidence of neurologic deficit

CLASSIFICATION OF PAIN BY PATHOPHYSIOLOGIC MECHANISM

Somatic Pain
■ Results from the activation of nociceptors in cutaneous and deep tissues
■ Common causes include the following:
1. Radiation-induced skin desquamation
2. Mucositis
3. Bone metastasis
4. Pathologic fracture
5. Spinal cord compression
6. Surgery
7. Tissue inflammation/infection/necrosis
■ Characteristics include the following:
1. Dull, aching, throbbing, or gnawing pain
2. Well-localized pain
3. Pain may increase with movement or stress
4. Pain improves with splinting or application of heat and cold

■ Additional physical findings may include the following:
1. Muscle spasms

Visceral Pain

■ Results from damage to organs innervated by the sympathetic nervous system.
■ The major mechanism for visceral pain in cancer patients includes abnormal distention or contraction of a hollow viscera, rapid capsular stretch, ischemia of a visceral muscle, and tissue necrosis.
■ Common causes include the following:
1. Acute ischemia
2. Chemical irritation
3. Distention of the capsule of a solid viscus
4. Gastrointestinal malignancies
5. Hepatic metastasis
6. Bacterial peritonitis
7. Inflammation of the parietal peritoneum
8. Obstruction of a hollow viscus
9. Omental metastasis
10. Thrombosis or engorgement of splenic and renal veins
11. Volvulus of the small intestine
■ Characteristics include the following:
1. Deep, cramping, dull, aching, pressure-like pain
2. Poorly localized pain
■ Additional physical findings may include the following:
1. Tachycardia, tachypnea, and hypertension
2. Autonomic symptoms such as nausea, vomiting, and diaphoresis
3. Abdominal distention or bloating

Neuropathic Pain

■ Pain that is initiated or caused by a primary lesion of dysfunction in the nervous system; tumor compression or infiltration or damage from surgery, radiation, or chemotherapy. There are three types of neuropathic pain.
• *Deafferentation* pain follows the distribution of a spinal nerve root (dermatome).
• *Neuropathy or neuralgia* is pain in an area supplied by a peripheral nerve.
• *Sympathetically maintained* pain is pain that follows along the same distribution as the arterial supply.

■ Common characteristics include the following:
1. Superficial burning, stinging, tingling, numbing pain
2. Electric shock-like component
3. Maybe localized to the site of neural injury or referred distally depending on the nerve distribution or dermatome
4. Increased pain sensation when touched by clothes, bedding, water, or extremes in temperature

■ Common causes include the following:
1. Bone or soft tissue metastasis, especially to the base of skull, pelvis, or vertebrae
2. Leptomeningeal disease
3. Postherpatic neuralgia
4. Radiation-induced damage to peripheral nerves (neuroplexopathy)
5. Surgical procedures that damage peripheral nerves (mastectomy, limb amputation, radical neck dissection, thoracotomy). Sist, Miner, and Lema (1999) evaluated postradical neck pain syndrome and found that all patients had at least one type of neuropathic pain: spontaneous, continuous burning pain (81%), shooting pain (69%), and/or allodynia (88%). Neuropathic pain sites were within the distribution of the superficial cervical plexus (SCP). Regional myofascial pain was also common (72%).
6. Chemotherapy agents (vinca alkaloids, platinum-based agents, taxanes)

■ Additional physical findings may include the following:
1. Muscle atrophy
2. Autonomic changes
3. Trophic changes in the skin and hair loss (smooth and fine skin)
4. Loss of reflexes
5. Dysesthesia

EXPECTED OUTCOMES

MAINTENANCE OF SATISFACTORY LEVEL OF COMFORT AND FUNCTION

■ Cost-effective pain control with the use of nonopioid and opioid analgesics in combination with adjuvant medications should be available for all cancer patients. Early comprehensive pain assessment and evidence-based analgesic decision-making processes do enhance usual pain outcomes and should be implemented in every practice. Du Pen et al. (1999) compared a multilevel treatment algorithm based on the Agency for Health Care Policy and Research Guidelines for Cancer Pain with standard-practice pain and symptom management therapies used by community oncologists. The patients randomized to the pain algorithm group achieved a statistically significant reduction in usual pain intensity, measured as slope scores, when compared with standard community practice ($p < .02$).

■ Patients who present with symptoms of depression or anxiety, or display drug-seeking behaviors with or without other precipitating factors need to be referred to clinical psychology or psychiatry for evaluation and treatment.

■ Side effects of analgesia are kept to a minimum including a normal bowel-elimination pattern.

OUTCOMES MEASURES

UNIDIMENSIONAL MEASURES

These are simple tools that allow the patient to quickly describe the intensity of pain he or she is experiencing at any point in time.

■ *Numeric Rating Scale*: A 0 to 10 numeric pain intensity scale
■ *Visual Analog Scale*: A 10-cm line that extends from "no pain" to "pain as bad as it could possibly be"
■ *Simple Descriptive Pain Intensity Scale*: Scale with 6 points describing degrees of pain from "no pain" to "worst pain possible"

MULTIDIMENSIONAL MEASURES

A number of multidimensional instruments have been developed to measure pain and its impact on quality of life. It is important to use an instrument that is easy for the patient to read and answer and that captures the information required.

■ *Short-Form McGill Pain Questionnaire* (SF-MPQ): Multiple descriptors to evaluate the sensory and affective component of pain (Melzack, 1987)

■ *Brief Pain Inventory* (BPI): Measures location, quality, and the effect pain has on various aspects of a patient's life (Cleeland, 1985; Daut, Cleeland, & Flannery, 1983)

OUTCOMES MANAGEMENT

An individualized detailed plan for pain management (involving the use of appropriate pharmacological and nonpharmacological interventions) should be developed for each patient based on the comprehensive assessment. The plan should include the following steps (McCaffery & Pasero, 1999):

TREATMENT PLAN

■ The treatment plan should include specific goals related to pain intensity, activities, and minimizing side effects. In radiation oncology, acute pain management should be part of the radiation therapy care map. Patients with chronic pain issues should be referred to a physician or to a team of specialists that provides comprehensive pain management.

MULTIMODALITY BALANCED ANALGESIA

■ Use different modalities in an attempt to decrease potential side effects and to improve satisfaction with treatment.

SELECTION OF PHARMACOLOGIC AGENTS

■ Selection should be based on the following factors:
   1. Diagnosis, condition, or procedure
   2. Current or expected pain intensity
   3. Age
   4. Known drug allergies or previous reaction to an opioid
   5. Presence of major organ failure (renal, hepatic, and/or respiratory)
   6. Presence of comorbid disease
   7. Potential metabolite accumulation
   8. Potential interactions with concurrent medications

SELECTION OF AVAILABLE ROUTES OF ADMINISTRATION AND FORMULATION

■ Pharmacologic agents may be given via oral, rectal, subcutaneous, intramuscular, inhalation, nasal, buccal and transdermal routes as well as through invasive procedures such as intravenous, intrathecal and epidural routes. When pharmacologic agents are recommended, the World Health Organization (WHO) 3-step approach is recommended (Canadian Society of Palliative Care Physicians & the Canadian Association of Radiation Oncologists, 1998). The oral route should be the first choice for opioid administration. If the oral route fails, transdermal or rectal administration should be considered. When parenteral administration is necessary, the intravenous or subcutaneous routes can be used according to circumstances. Intramuscular administration of opioids is not recommended.

PATIENT PREFERENCE

■ Compliance with treatment requires that the patient feels comfortable with the treatment plan and is able to take medications as prescribed. Some patients may prefer treatment that has minimal side effects despite only moderate pain control while others may have an aversion to certain drugs or routes of administration. Patient and family ability to adhere to the regimen should also be taken into consideration.

DOSING AND DOSE TITRATION

■ Careful observation and titration are required when switching from one opioid to another, particularly when the patient is already receiving a high dose. After initiating morphine or making any change of dose or route of administration, the dose should be evaluated after 24 hours. Other considerations include:

1. Previous dosing requirements and relative analgesic potencies when initiating treatment
2. Use of pain intensity and equianalgesic chart to determine initial dose, and then titrate until adequate analgesia is achieved or dose-limiting side effects are encountered

3. Use appropriate dosing schedules
4. When a dose is safe, but additional analgesia is desired, titrate upward by 25% for mild increase, 50% for moderate increase, and 100% for considerable increase in pain
5. Provide rescue doses for breakthrough pain (immediate release formulas)
6. Consider patient-controlled analgesia systems (PCA)

TREATMENT OF SIDE EFFECTS

- Be aware of prevalence and impact of side effects.
- Use a preventive approach in the management of side effects, particularly constipation.
- Prevent respiratory depression by monitoring sedation levels in opioid-naive patients.
- Advise patient and family about which side effects are likely to subside.

REPETITIVE EVALUATION

- Evaluate the treatment plan on the basis of the specific goals identified (including pain intensity, pain side effects and activity levels) on an ongoing basis.
- Make necessary modifications to treatment plan.

TAPERING AND CESSATION OF TREATMENT

- Decrease in accordance with decreased pain ratings.
- Be aware of potential for withdrawal syndrome and need for tapering schedule for patients who have been receiving opioid therapy for more than a few days.
- Use equianalgesic dosing to determine appropriate decreases in doses.

PHARMACOLOGIC INTERVENTIONS

NONOPIOID ANALGESICS

Facts

1. All nonopioid analgesics have a ceiling effect after a certain dose.

2. Addition of a nonopioid analgesic to an opioid may have a dose-sparing effect and may permit a lower dose of the opioid.

Categories of Nonopioid Analgesics

1. Nonsteroidal anti-inflammatory drugs (NSAIDs): These agents have both a peripheral effect on inflammation and a role in attenuating central pain pathways.
2. Acetaminophen.

OPIOID ANALGESICS

Facts

1. Includes all drugs with morphine-like actions on endogenous opioid receptors.
2. Opioid analgesics have no ceiling effect.

Categories of Opioid Analgesics

1. Full agonists include morphine, hydromorphone, codeine, oxycodone, hydrocodone, methadone, levorphanol, and fentanyl. Payne, Mathias, Pasta, Wanke, Williams & Mahmoud (1998) found that patients who received transdermal fentanyl were more satisfied overall with their pain medication than were those who received sustained-release oral forms of morphine. They also experienced a significantly lower frequency and impact of pain medication side effects.
2. Partial agonists include buprenorphine.
3. Mixed agonist-antagonists include butorphanol, dezocine, nalbuphine, and pentazocine.

LOCAL ANESTHETICS

Facts

1. Commonly used for oropharyngeal mucositis and localized tissue inflammation (anus)
2. May be used as alternative therapy for neuropathic pain when opioids, antidepressants, and anticonvulsants are not effective

Categories of Local Anesthetics

1. Topical agents including benzocaine, viscous lidocaine, diclonine, and tetracaine.
2. Antiarrhythmic agents including mexiletine, tocainide, flecainide, and lidocaine.

3. Lidocaine-prilocaine cream and amethocaine gel provide topical anesthetic for procedures such as vascular access device puncture. Amethocaine gel requires a shorter application time for skin anesthesia. In a trial of the two products, Bishai, Taddio, and Bar-Oz (1999) found no significant difference in mean pain assessments between the two products.

ADJUVANT ANALGESICS

Facts
1. Drugs that were developed for clinical indications other than pain relief

Categories
1. Tricyclic and nontricyclic antidepressants
2. Anticonvulsants
3. Phenothiazines
4. Corticosteroids
5. Antihistamines
6. Amphetamines
7. Biphosphonates
8. Antimicrobials

NEUROLOGIC AND ANESTHETIC PROCEDURES

Facts
1. Helpful in treating well-localized somatic or visceral pain
2. Not helpful for deafferentation pain

Types of Procedures
1. *Trigger point injection*: for localized myofascial pain with identifiable trigger point. Defalque (1982) found that repeated injections of alcohol into the trigger point in operative scars provided a simple, safe, and effective treatment with permanent cure or marked improvement in 91% of patients with painful trigger points in surgical scars.
2. *Continuous epidural infusion*: for unilateral and bilateral lumbosacral pain or midline perineal pain.
3. *Nerve blocks*: including peripheral, epidural, intrathecal, and autonomic procedures.
4. *Neuroablation procedures*: interrupt specific nerve tracts including rhizotomy, cordotomy, and myelotomy.
5. *Neurostimulating procedures*.

OTHER PROCEDURES

Chemotherapy and Hormonal Therapy

1. May reduce tumor volume

Administration of Biphosphonates

1. Pamidronate for bone metastasis to reduce pain

Physical Modalities

1. *Cutaneous stimulation* is an alternative noninvasive method for controlling pain (based on the Gate Control Theory) that involves stimulating the skin and underlying tissues in order to moderate or relieve pain (Mobily, Herr, & Nicholson, 1994). These interventions are easily performed, inexpensive, and noninjurious to the patient when used properly. They easily can be taught to the patient and/or the family.

2. *Soft tissue techniques*: including massage therapy, myofascial release, vibration therapy, and manual lymphatic drainage (MLD). Johansson, Albertsson, Ingavar, and Ekdahl (1999) examined the effects of low stretch compression bandaging (CB) alone or in combination with MLD for women with arm lymphedema after treatment for breast cancer. They found that the CB with MLD showed decreased pain ($p < 0.03$) as compared to CB alone.

3. *Electrotherapy*: including transcutaneous electrical nerve stimulation (TENS).

4. *Acupuncture*: He, Friedrick, Ertan, Muller & Schmidt (1999) evaluated the use of acupuncture for pain relief and movement improvement after ablation and axillary lymphadenectomy for patients with breast cancer. They found significantly a higher maximum abduction angle without pain at the first treatment immediately after acupuncture. In addition, there was a statistically significant difference ($p < 0.01$) in the appearance of pain in the surgical wound in the rest position on the fifth postoperative day in the acupuncture group compared with the control group. However, there was no difference in pain on the seventh postoperative day or at the time of discharge. Pain with arm movement was also significantly less in the acupuncture group on day 5 ($p < 0.01$) with significant improvement in abduction angle without pain.

5. *Exercise and physical therapy*.

Psychosocial Interventions

1. *Psychotherapy*
2. *Relaxation techniques*: including guided imagery and hypnosis

3. *Cognitive and behavioral therapies*: including art and music therapy, distraction, biofeedback, and support groups

RADIATION THERAPY

- Approximately one-half of prescribed radiotherapy is given for palliation of symptoms due to incurable cancer (Hoegler, 1997). Palliative radiation therapy provides good pain relief by reducing tumor volume in a local site. Unfortunately, there is often a delay in referral for palliative radiation therapy. Wirth et al. (1998) found that the median duration of symptoms before prescription of radiation therapy was 4 weeks. Some of the causes of delay were "diagnostic uncertainty," other treatment offered, "patient-related delay," language difficulty, and unexplained delay.
- The skeleton is the most common organ to be affected by metastatic cancer (Coleman, 1997). Tumors arising from breast, prostate, thyroid, lung and kidney possess a special propensity to spread to bone. Bone pain is the most common complication of metastatic bone disease resulting from structural damage, periosteal irritation, and nerve entrapment. Recent evidence suggests that pain caused by bone metastasis may also be related to the rate of bone resorption (Coleman, 1997). Hypercalcemia and pathologic fracture are also late complications associated with bone metastasis.
- The choice of treatment (total dose, fraction size, and overall length of course of treatment) depends on a number of factors including performance status, extent of metastatic disease, length of disease-free interval (as appropriate), status of the primary tumor, the specific site(s) requiring therapy and potential late effects, and patient preference.
  1. *Painful bone metastasis*: Ninety percent of patients with symptomatic bone metastases obtain some pain relief with a low-dose, brief course of radiotherapy (Hoegler, 1997). Common treatment plans consist of 30 Gy in 10 fractions, 20 Gy in 5 fractions, or 8 Gy in a single fraction. Three single-dose regimens of radiation were evaluated by Jeremic et al. (1998). The findings seemed to confirm that 8 Gy could be considered as probably the "lowest" optimal single fraction of radiation therapy in the treatment of painful bone metastasis. Single fractions of 4 to

6 Gy achieved results in some specific cases. In another study, Nielsen, Bentzen, Sandberg, Gadeberg & Timothy (1998) compared the effects of 8 Gy × 1 with 5 Gy × 4. They found that the degree of pain relief did not differ between the two groups. At 4 weeks the difference in pain relief was 6% and at 8 weeks the difference was 13%. In addition, there was no significant difference in the duration of pain relief, the number of new painful sites, or the need for reirradiation.

2. *Spinal cord compression* is considered a medical emergency due to the propensity for patients to have potentially permanent neurologic deficits. A common treatment plan is 30 Gy in 10 fractions. Maranzano et al. (1998) evaluated two different schedules of treatment for patients with spinal cord compression in prostate cancer. The first was a split-course regimen of 5 Gy in 2 fractions, followed by a 4 day rest, and then 3 Gy in 5 fractions. The second was a short-course regimen of 8 Gy in 1 fraction, followed by a 7 day rest, and then 8 Gy in 1 fraction. Back pain total response was 82%. Effectiveness of radiation therapy on motor and bladder capacity was conditioned by pretreatment status of patients. All patients who were walking before treatment maintained the function, whereas 46% with motor impairment regained the ability to walk. All patients able to void at presentation preserved the capacity, whereas 38% with sphincter dysfunction no longer needed an indwelling catheter.

3. *Painful chest tumor*: Pain or dysphagia may be related to obstruction of the bronchus, erosion into the mediastinum or pleura, or extension into the ribs. Common treatment plans include 20 Gy in 5 fractions or 30 Gy in 10 fractions.

4. *Painful skin or soft tissue lesion* is dependent on histology of the tumor. Lymphoma may respond to a relatively low dose (4 to 8 Gy) given in a single fraction, whereas other solid tumors may require a higher dose (30 Gy) in 5 to 10 fractions.

■ Treatment may be given using the following methods:

1. Local external-beam irradiation: For local lesions that require a small field to treat.

2. Hemibody irradiation: For multiple bone metastases.

3. Radiopharmaceuticals: Strontium-89 has been shown to relieve pain due to bone metastasis and delay development of new painful sites (Hoegler, 1997). It has also been associated with myelosuppression.

REFERENCES

Agency for Health Care Policy and Research. (1994). *Management of cancer pain. Clinical Practice Guidelines, No. 9.* (AHCPR Publication No. 94-0592). Rockville, MD: U.S. Department of Health and Human Services, Public Health Service.

Bishai, R., Taddio, A., & Bar-Oz, B. (1999). Relative efficacy of amethocaine gel and lidocaine-prilocaine cream for Port-a-Cath puncture in children. *Pediatrics, 104*(3), e31.

Breitbart, W. (1987). Suicide in cancer patients. *Oncology, 1*(2), 49–54.

Bruera, E., Ernst, S., Hagen, N., et al. (1998). Effectiveness of megestrol acetate in patients with advanced cancer: A randomized, double-blind, crossover study. *Cancer Prevention and Control, 2*(2), 74–78.

Canadian Society of Palliative Care Physicians and Canadian Association of Radiation Oncologists. The Steering Committee on Clinical Practice Guidelines for the Care and Treatment of Breast Cancer (1998). The management of chronic pain in patients with breast cancer. *Canadian Medical Association Journal, 158*(Suppl. 3), S71–81.

Cella, D. (1997). The Functional Assessment of Cancer Therapy—Anemia (FACT-An) Scale: A new tool for the assessment of outcomes in cancer anemia and fatigue. *Seminars in Hematology, 34*(3 Suppl. 2), 13–19.

Cella, D., Passik, S., Jacobsen, P., & Breitbart, W. (1998). Progress toward guidelines for the management of fatigue. *Oncology, 12*(11A), 369–377.

Cleeland, C. S. (1985). Measurement and prevalence of pain in cancer. *Seminars in Oncology Nursing, 1*(2), 87–92.

Coleman, R. E. (1997). Skeletal complications of malignancy. *Cancer, 80*(Suppl. 8), 1588–1594.

Daut, R. L., Cleeland, C., & Flannery, R. C. (1983). Development of the Wisconsin Brief Pain Questionnaire to assess pain in cancer and other disease. *Pain, 17*(2), 197–210.

Defalque, R. J. (1982). Painful trigger points in surgical scars. *Anesthesia and Analgesia, 61*(6), 518–520.

Dimeo, F. C., Stieglitz, R. D., Novelli-Fischer, U., et al. (1999). Effects of physical activity on fatigue and psychological status of cancer patients during chemotherapy. *Cancer, 85*(10), 2273–2277.

Donnelly, S., & Walsh, D. (1995). The symptoms of advanced cancer. *Seminars in Oncology, 22*(2 Suppl. 3), 67–72.

Du Pen, S. L., Du Pen, A. R., Polissar, N., Hansberry, J., Kraybill, B. M., Stillman, M., Panke, J., Everly, R., & Syrjala, K. (1999). Implementing guidelines for cancer pain management: Results of a randomized controlled clinical trial. *Journal of Clinical Oncology, 17*(1), 361–367.

Epstein, J. B., & Stewart, K. H. (1993). Radiation therapy and pain in patients with head and neck cancer. *European Journal of Cancer. Part B, Oral Oncology, 29B*(3), 191–199.

Faithfull, S., & Brada, M. (1998). Somnolence syndrome in adults following cranial irradiation for primary brain tumors. *Clinical Oncology (Royal College of Radiologists), 10*(4), 250–254.

Ferrell, B. R., Grant, M., Dean, G. E., Funk, B., & Ly, J. (1996). "Bone tired": The experience of fatigue and its impact on quality of life. Oncology Nursing Forum, 23(10), 1539–1547.

Ferrell, B. R., Cohen, M. Z., Rhiner, M., & Rozek, A. (1991). Pain as a metaphor for illness. Part II: Family caregivers' management of pain. Oncology Nursing Forum, 18(8), 1303–1309.

Fobair, P., Hoppe, R. T., Bloom J., Cox, R., Varghese, A., & Spiegel, D. (1986). Psychosocial problems among survivors of Hodgkin's disease. Journal of Clinical Oncology, 4(5), 805–814.

Glaspy, J., & Cavill, I. (1999). Role of iron in optimizing responses of anemic cancer patients to erythropoietin. Oncology, 13(4), 461–488.

Graydon, J. E. (1994). Women with breast cancer: Their quality of life following a course of radiation therapy. Journal of Advanced Nursing, 19(4), 617–622.

Graydon, J. E., Bubela, N., Irvine, D., & Vincent, L. (1995). Fatigue-reducing strategies used by patients receiving treatment for cancer. Cancer Nursing, 18(1), 23–28.

Greenberg, D. B., Sawicka, J., Eisenthal, S., & Ross, D. (1992). Fatigue syndrome due to localized radiation. Journal of Pain and Symptom Management, 7(1), 38–45.

Hann, D. M., Garovoy, N., Finkelstein, B., Jacobsen, P. B., Azzarello, L. M., & Fields, K. K. (1999). Fatigue and quality of life in breast cancer patients undergoing autologous stem cell transplantation: A longitudinal comparative study. Journal of Pain and Symptom Management, 17(5), 311–319.

Haylock, P. J., & Hart, L. K. (1979). Fatigue in patients receiving localized radiation. Cancer Nursing, 2(6), 461–467.

He, J. P., Friedrick, M., Ertan, A. K., Muller, K., & Schmidt, W. (1999). Pain-relief and movement improvement by acupuncture after ablation and axillary lymphadenectomy in patients with mammary cancer. Clinical and Experimental Obstetrics and Gynecology, 26(2), 81–84.

Hoegler, D. (1997). Radiotherapy for palliation of symptoms in incurable cancer. Current Problems in Cancer, 21(3), 129–183.

Jensen, S. & Given, B. A. (1991). Fatigue affecting family caregivers of cancer patients. Cancer Nursing, 14(4), 181–187.

Jeremic, B., Shibamoto, Y., Acimovic, L., Milisavljevic, S., Nikolic, N., Aleksandrovic, J., & Igrutinovic, I. (1998). A randomized trial of three single-dose radiation therapy regimens in the treatment of metastatic bone pain. International Journal of Radiation Oncology, Biology, Physics, 42(1), 161–167.

Johansson, K., Albertsson, M., Ingavar, C., & Ekdahl, C. (1999). Effects of compression bandaging with or without manual lymph drainage treatment in patients with postoperative arm lymphedema. Lymphology, 32(3), 103–110.

Jonler, M., Ritter, M. A., Brinkmann, R., Messing, E. M., Rhodes, P. R., & Bruskewitz, R. C. (1994). Sequelae of definitive radiation therapy for prostate cancer localized to the pelvis. Urology, 44(6), 876–882.

King, K. B., Nail, L. M., Kreamer, K., Strohl, R. A., & Johnson, J. E. (1985). Patients' descriptions of the experience of receiving radiation therapy. *Oncology Nursing Forum*, 12(4), 55–61.

Loge, J. H., Abrahamsen, A. F., Ekeberg, O., & Kaasa, S. (1999). Hodgkin's disease survivors more fatigued than the general population. *Journal of Clinical Oncology*, 17(1), 253–261.

Maranzano, E., Latini, P., Beneventi, S., Marafioti, L., Piro, F., Perrucci, E., & Lupattelli, M. (1998). Comparison of two different radiotherapy schedules for spinal cord compression in prostate cancer. *Tumori*, 84(4), 472–477.

McCaffery, M., & Beebe, A. (1989). *Pain: Clinical manual for nursing practice*. St. Louis: Mosby.

McCaffery, M., & Pasero, C. (1999). *Pain: Clinical manual*. St. Louis: Mosby.

Melzack, R. (1987). The short-form McGill Pain Questionnaire. *Pain*, 30(2), 191–197.

Mendoza, T. R., Wang, X. S., Cleeland, C. S., Morrissey, M., Johnson, B. A., Wendt, J. K., & Huber, S. L. (1999). The rapid assessment of fatigue severity in cancer patients: Use of the Brief Fatigue Inventory. *Cancer*, 85(5), 1186–1196.

Merskey, H. (Ed.). (1986). Classification of chronic pain: Description of chronic pain syndromes and definition of pain terms. *Pain* (Suppl. 3), S1–226.

Miaskowski, C. (1998). Pain management: Somatic, visceral and neuropathic. In C. C. Chernecky & B. J. Berger (Eds.), *Advanced and critical care oncology nursing* (pp. 476–489). Philadelphia: W. B. Saunders.

Mobily, P. R., Herr, K. A., & Nicholson, A. C. (1994). Validation of cutaneous stimulation interventions for pain management. *International Journal of Nursing Studies*, 31(6), 533–544.

Mock, V., Dow, K. H., Meares, C. J., Grimm, P. M., Dienemann, J. A., Haisfield-Wolfe, M. E., Quitasol, W., Mitchell, S., Chakravarthy, A., & Gage, I. (1997). Effects of exercise on fatigue, physical functioning, and emotional distress during radiation therapy for breast cancer. *Oncology Nursing Forum*, 24(6), 991–1000.

Nielsen, O. S., Bentzen, S. M., Sandberg, E., Gadeberg, C. C., & Timothy, A. R. (1998). Randomized trial of single dose versus fractionated palliative radiotherapy of bone metastases. *Radiotherapy Oncology*, 47(3), 233–240.

Pater, J. L., Zee, B., Palmer, M., Johnston, D., & Osoba, D. (1997). Fatigue in patients with cancer: Results with National Cancer Institute of Canada Clinical Trials Group studies employing the EORTC QLQ-C30. *Supportive Care in Cancer*, 5(5), 410–413.

Payne, R., Mathias, S. D., Pasta, D. J., Wanke, L. A., Williams, R., & Mahmoud, R. (1998). Quality of life and cancer pain: Satisfaction and side effects with transdermal fentanyl versus oral morphine. *Journal of Clinical Oncology*, 16(4), 1588–1593.

Piper, B. F., Lindsey, A. M., & Dodd, M. J. (1998a). Development of an instrument to measure the subjective dimension of fatigue. In

S. G. Funk, E. M. Turnquist, M. T. Champagne, L. A. Copp, & R. A. Wiese (Eds.), *Key aspects of comfort: Management of pain, fatigue and nausea* (pp. 199–208). New York: Springer-Verlag.

Portenoy, R. K., & Hagen, N. A. (1990). Breakthrough pain: Definition, prevalence and characteristics. *Pain*, 41(3), 273–281.

Rhoten, D. (1982). Fatigue and the postsurgical patient. In C. M. Norris (Ed.), *Concept clarification in nursing*, (pp. 277–300). Rockville, MD: Aspen.

Rosenberg, S. A., & Glatstein, E. J. (1991). Acute and long-term effects on limb function of combined modality limb sparing therapy for extremity soft tissue sarcoma. *International Journal of Radiation Oncology, Biology, Physics*, 21(6), 1493–1499.

Schwartz, A. L. (1998). The Schwartz Cancer Fatigue Scale: Testing reliability and validity. *Oncology Nursing Forum*, 25(4), 711–717.

Sist, T., Miner, M., & Lema, M. (1999). Characteristics of postradical neck pain syndrome: A report of 25 cases. *Journal of Pain and Symptom Management*, 18(2), 95–102.

Smets, E. M., Garssen, B., Bonk, B. & DeHaes, J. C. (1995). The multidimensional fatigue inventory (MFI). Psychometric quality of an instrument to assess fatigue. *Journal of Psychosomatic Research*, 39(3), 315–325.

Smets, E. M., Visser, M. R., Garssen, B., Frijda, N. H., Oosterveld, P., & de-Haes, J. C. (1998). Understanding the level of fatigue in cancer patients undergoing radiotherapy. *Journal of Psychosomatic Research*, 45(3), 277–293.

Smets, E. M., Visser, M. R., Willems-Groot, A. F., Garssen, B., Oldenburger, F., van-Tienhoven, G., & de-Haes, J. C. (1998). Fatigue and radiotherapy: (A) experience in patients undergoing treatment. *British Journal of Cancer*, 78(7), 899–906.

Smets, E. M., Visser, M. R., & Willems-Groot, A. F., Garssen, B., Schuster-Uitterhoeve, A. L., & de-Haes, J. C. (1998). Fatigue and radiotherapy: (B) experience in patients 9 months following treatment. *British Journal of Cancer*, 78(7), 907–912.

Spiegel, D., Bloom, J. R., & Yalom, E. (1981). Group support for patients with metastatic disease. *Archives of General Psychiatry*, 38(5), 527–533.

Stone, P., Hardy, J., Broadley, K., Tookman, A. J., Kurowska, A., & A'Hern, R. (1999). Fatigue in advanced cancer: A prospective controlled cross-sectional study. *British Journal of Cancer*, 79(9-10), 1479–1486.

Twycross, R. G. & Fairfield, S. (1982). Pain in far advanced cancer. *Pain*, 14(3), 303–310.

Waller, A., & Caroline, N. L. (1996). *Handbook of palliative care in cancer*. Boston: Butterworth & Heinemann.

Weissman, D. E., Janjan, N., & Byhardt, R. W. (1989). Assessment of pain during head and neck irradiation. *Journal of Pain and Symptom Management*, 4(2), 90–95.

Winningham, M. L., Nail, L. M., Barton Burke, M., Brophy, L., Cimprich, B., Jones, L. S., Pickard-Holley, S., Rhodes, V., St-Pierre, B., Beck, S. Glass, E. C., Mock, V. L., Mooney, K. H., & Piper, B. (1994). Fatigue and the cancer experience: The state of the knowledge. *Oncology Nursing Forum*, 21(1), 23–35.

Winningham, M. L. (1996). Fatigue. In S. L. Groenwald, M. H. Frogge, M. Goodman, & C. H. Yarbro (Eds.), *Cancer symptom management*, (pp. 42–58). Boston: Jones & Bartlett.

Wirth, A., Smith, J. G., Ball, D. L., Mameghan, H., Corry, J., Bernshaw, D. L., & Drummond, R. M. (1998). Symptom duration and delay in referral for palliative radiotherapy in cancer patients: A pilot study. *Medical Journal of Australia*, 169(1), 32–36.

Yeager, K. A., Miaskowski, C., Dibble, S. & Wallhagan, M. (1997). Differences in pain knowledge in cancer patients with and without pain. *Cancer Practice*, 5(1), 39–45.

Yellen, S., Cella, D., Webster, K., et al. (1997). Measuring fatigue and other anemia-related symptoms with the Functional Assessment of Cancer Therapy (FACT) measuring system. *Journal of Pain and Symptom Management*, 13(2), 63–74.

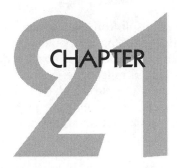

CHAPTER 21

SUSTAINED INTEGRITY OF PROTECTIVE MECHANISMS (SKIN, ORAL, IMMUNE SYSTEM)

Giselle J. Moore-Higgs, ARNP, MSN
Robert J. Amdur, MD

PROBLEM

Radiation therapy has a direct cellular effect on the human body's protective mechanisms including the skin, mucous membranes, and immune system. The mature cells of these three body systems originate from a rapidly reproducing differentiated stem cell, which increases the radiosensitivity of the three systems. In healthy tissue, radiation elicits the inflammatory response with histamine and serotonin release and an increase in tissue perfusion allowing infiltration of the treatment area by leukocytes. The result is a localized tissue response that alters the ability of the system to maintain protective mechanisms both acutely and chronically.

SKIN

■ In human skin, ionizing radiation affects the rapidly dividing cells of the epidermis, hair follicles, and sebaceous glands and follows a predictive pattern of acute and late skin reactions. These reactions are normal and expected side effects of treatment, since the radiation must enter and in some instances exit through the skin in order to reach the target volume.

■ Skin reactions result from the depletion of actively proliferating cells in a renewing cell population. The time course of
development of gross changes and the dose level at which
they are produced reflect the evolution, time course, and
dose response of population changes in component populations of the epidermis, dermis, and microvasculature. The
evolution reflects a continuous remodeling of these populations (Archambeau, Pezner, & Wasserman, 1995).

■ Radiation-induced skin reactions can be classified as acute
or late. Acute skin reactions depend more on time-dose factors than on the total dose delivered. The acute sequence
occurs during the first 70 days after irradiation at absorbed
doses of 5 to 20 Gy single-dose fractions or during and after
30 to 60 Gy multifraction schedules (Archambeau, 1987).
The acute reactions manifest as erythema, hyperpigmentation, and dry desquamation, and may proceed to moist
desquamation.

■ Temporary and partial hair loss occurs at skin doses of approximately 30 Gy. Complete and permanent hair loss can
occur at skin doses of 55 Gy. Hair regrowth usually resumes
at 8 to 9 weeks after completion of treatment, usually at a
slower rate of growth. New hair return continues for up to 1
year (McDonald, 1992).

■ A time period of varying length, during which the skin appears "normal," follows the acute reaction. Then, after as
much as several years, late effect changes of scaling, finer
hair, atrophy, telangiectasia, pigmentation changes, subcutaneous fibrosis, and necrosis occur (Archambeau et al.,
1995).

■ The dose schedules that produce late reactions are similar to
those that produce acute reactions. However, while total dose
is critical in determining the severity, late effects are more severe after dose schedules using fractions of 2.5 to 3.0 Gy or
higher, than after dose schedules using 1.8 to 2.0 Gy daily
(Archambeau et al., 1995). The severity of an acute skin reaction does not necessarily predict the severity of late changes
(Arcangeli, Friedman, & Paoluzi, 1974).

■ In addition to time-dose-volume relationships, a number of
treatment-related factors influence the onset, duration, and
intensity of skin reactions.

 • Appositional skin found in the axilla, inframammary area,
   groin, perineum, and other tissue folds results in in-

creased moisture, warmth, and friction, which results in increased skin reactions. This is also true for skin in tangential fields or glancing fields that receive a higher skin dose than those perpendicular to the radiation beam.

- Some types of skin tolerate radiation better than others. The scalp has the greatest tolerance for radiation, followed in decreasing order by the face, neck, trunk, ears, groin, and extremities (Dutreix, 1986).
- Cells that are in G and M phases are the most radiosensitive, while cells in S phase are most resistant. Radiosensitivity is greater in oxygenated cells than in hypoxic cells.
- The quality of radiation affects the severity of the skin reaction and is related to the amount of energy absorbed by the skin. The electron beam is superficially penetrating and delivers high doses to the skin resulting in an increased incidence of severe skin reactions. The photon beam penetrates deeply into the body tissue and is more skin-sparing. The application of a tissue-equivalent material or bolus increases the skin dose and correlates with a more severe skin reaction.

■ Other non-treatment-related factors include integrity of skin at initiation of treatment, age, nutritional status, presence of comorbid disease, previous radiation therapy in the same field, prior exposure to some chemotherapy agents, and patient compliance with recommendations for daily skin care.

■ In current treatment practices, the most common sites for severe skin reaction with moist desquamation are the ear, neck, axilla, inframammary fold, perineum, and groin. If the reaction is severe, a treatment break may be necessary to allow the skin to begin healing before completing the recommended total dose (resulting in a compromised treatment).

■ In addition to visible skin changes, acute skin reactions can cause discomfort including pruritus and varying degrees of somatic pain. If the reaction develops into moist desquamation, the pain may increase and the risk of superficial skin infection increases. Late reactions can also cause discomfort including skin fibrosis, pruritus, and an increased vulnerability to injury (bruises and breaks in skin integrity). Occasionally, the damage to microcirculation results in tissue necrosis and ulceration. Lost of elasticity of the skin may affect range of motion, resulting in persistent discomfort and (in some cases) lymphedema.

MUCOUS MEMBRANES

- Mucous membranes are the transitions between the external and internal environment that line the vagina, oral cavity, respiratory tract, and the genital urinary tract. Radiation therapy can cause both acute and late injury to these tissues and their supporting structures.

- Acute radiation injury in the mucous membranes (known as mucositis) develops from cellular destruction with an inflammatory response that is similar to that described in the skin including capillary engorgement, edema, and leukocytic infiltration. The duration and intensity of the inflammatory response depends on the site of radiation, the total dose, the depth of penetration, and the number and frequency of treatments. The response usually begins 1 to 2 weeks after initiation of the radiation (approximately 20 Gy) and persists for several weeks after treatment is complete.

- Radiation to the head and neck region can result in mucositis in the oral cavity, nasal cavity, sinuses, oropharynx, larynx, esophagus, and tracheostomy sites. In the oral cavity, mucositis (stomatitis) is associated with hypogeusia and xerostomia. Mucositis results in dysphagia and pain that in turn results in poor nutritional intake and weight loss.

- Patients who receive high-dose radioiodine (I-131) for thyroid cancer also experience salivary gland impairment, generally caused by free radicals (Bohuslavizki, et al., 1999).

- Radiation to the pelvis results in cystitis, urethritis, vaginitis, and proctitis. The symptoms include urgency, hesitancy, dysuria, vaginal discharge, dyspareunia, rectal pain, and tenesmus.

- Secondary complications can include *Candida albicans*, bacterial infections, and hemorrhage. These complications are more common in patients who are immunocompromised or who have thrombocytopenia.

- In patients with HIV disease there appears to be a decrease in normal tissue tolerance. These patients may develop skin reactions and mucositis much earlier than average. Watkins, Findlay, Gelmann, Lane & Zabell (1987) evaluated patients with AIDS and Kaposi's sarcoma requiring oropharyngeal irradiation or total skin electron treatment. The degree of mucositis occurred at doses much lower than expected based on normal tissue tolerances seen in other patient populations. Presence or absence of candidiasis was not a factor, nor was the immune status based on T_4 counts. Kao, Devine, and Mirza (1999) also compared patients with HIV to patients with HIV and Kaposi's sarcoma who required radiation therapy to the oral cavity or oropharynx. The findings revealed that patients with non-Kaposi's tumors had fewer acute reactions and significantly less weight loss than did patients with Kaposi's sarcoma. Although infection with HIV is not a contraindication when aggressive radiation therapy is needed, patients should be selected carefully based on the status of HIV infection and related comorbid illnesses.

- Late effects that correspond with radiation to mucous membranes include xerostomia, hypogeusia, dental caries, dysphagia, odynophagia, osteoradionecrosis, vaginal dryness, dyspareunia, dysuria, and tenesmus. These complications can affect an individual's quality of life in many ways.

IMMUNE SYSTEM

- The elements of the blood and bone marrow including the precursor cells of the three main hematopoietic lines (erythroblasts, myeloblasts, and megakaryoblasts) respond to radiation by progressively decreasing in number because of destruction of the stem cells. The neutropenia seen in the first week results from cessation of production and rapid turnover of these cells. This is followed in 2 to 3 weeks by thrombocytopenia and in 2 to 3 months by anemia. Recovery is related to the degree of initial response and generally begins with regeneration of the depleted stem cells (Rubin, Constine, & Nelson, 1992).

- The degree of bone marrow suppression related to radiation depends on volume of bone marrow included in the treatment field and on previous exposure to chemotherapy. Patient populations at risk for development of significant bone marrow suppression are those treated with a TBI field, whole-abdomen field, mantle field, extended mantle field, PANS and spleen field, TLI field, craniospinal field, or large pelvic field that includes the iliac crest and/or fossa.

- Patients whose neutrophil count declines rapidly are at increased risk of infection and sepsis. More than half of all infections in neutropenic patients are attributed to colonization of organisms acquired from the local environment.

- ■ Immunocompromised patients are susceptible to opportunistic infections and to organisms that usually cause minimal infection (including the herpesvirus).
- ■ Secondary infections including *Candida albicans*, *Candida tropicalis*, cytomegalovirus, and aspergillus are common in severely immunocompromised patients.
- ■ The duration of the hypoplasia that results in irradiated bone marrow appears to be directly related to the total dose of radiation given. The majority of patients have full recovery or near full recovery within 12 months of treatment. Patients who have had adjuvant chemotherapy may have chronic hypoplasia.

ASSESSMENT

SKIN

- ■ An evaluation of the skin should be performed before initiation of treatment to identify any factors that may increase the skin reaction.
- ■ A careful visual examination of the skin within the treatment fields (including exit sites) should be performed once a week during treatment and during regular follow-up examinations.
- ■ The following grading systems for early and late effects of radiation on skin have been developed:
  - • National Cancer Institute's Common Toxicity Criteria, Version 2.0, with Radiation Therapy Oncology Group (RTOG) and European Organization for Research and Treatment of Cancer (EORTC) Acute Effects Criteria (NCI, 1999)—Instrument that provides a scale for many different organ systems and some symptoms.
  - • The Oncology Nursing Society Radiation Oncology Documentation Tool (ONS, 1994)—Instrument to assist health care professionals in monitoring patients and accurately documenting the care delivered.

MUCOUS MEMBRANES

- ■ A visual evaluation of the oral mucosa should be performed before initiation of treatment to identify existing infection and any factors that may increase the mucosal reaction including use of tobacco or alcohol, dentures, and/or evidence of oropharyngeal infection.

■ A visual evaluation of the vaginal mucosa should be performed before initiation of treatment to identify existing infection and any factors that may increase the mucosal reaction including evidence of vaginal infection.

■ A careful visual examination of the oral mucosa should be performed once a week during treatment and on regular follow-up examinations. Several tools are available to assess the acute oral complications of radiotherapy.

- Oral Assessment System (Sonis et al., 1999)—New scoring system that has shown high interobserver reproducibility and response over time, and measures those elements deemed to be associated with mucositis.
- National Cancer Institute's Common Toxicity Criteria, Version 2.0, with Radiation Therapy Oncology Group (RTOG) and European Organization for Research and Treatment of Cancer (EORTC) Acute Effects Criteria (NCI, 1999).
- The Oncology Nursing Society Radiation Oncology Documentation Tool (ONS, 1994).

■ Assessment of symptoms such as urethritis, cystitis, vaginitis, and proctitis should be performed each week during treatment and during regular follow-up examinations.

- National Cancer Institute's Common Toxicity Criteria, Version 2.0, with Radiation Therapy Oncology Group (RTOG) and European Organization for Research and Treatment of Cancer (EORTC) Acute Effects Criteria (NCI, 1999).
- The Oncology Nursing Society Radiation Oncology Documentation Tool (ONS, 1994).

IMMUNE SYSTEM

■ An evaluation of the immune system should be performed before initiation of treatment to identify any factors that may increase the risk of radiation-induced neutropenia, thrombocytopenia, and/or anemia. The evaluation should include the following:

- Medical history and physical examination looking for evidence of local or systemic infection and to assess for history of recent fevers, chills, or night sweats

- Medications including current drugs and previous use of steroids, chemotherapy agents, and over-the-counter vitamin and herbal preparations
- Laboratory studies including a culture of any suspicious lesions that may resemble an infectious process and a CBC with differential

■ The immune system should be evaluated weekly during radiation therapy.

- Appropriate examination of the treatment site.
- Laboratory studies including a CBC with differential should be performed at least weekly on patients who are at high risk for neutropenia, thrombocytopenia, and/or anemia.
- Culture of any suspicious lesions that resemble an infectious process.
- Grading systems for early and late effects of radiation on the immune system have been developed. They are the same as those used for the skin and mucous membranes.
- National Cancer Institute's Common Toxicity Criteria, Version 2.0, with Radiation Therapy Oncology Group (RTOG) and European Organization for Research and Treatment of Cancer (EORTC) Acute Effects Criteria (NCI, 1999).
- The Oncology Nursing Society Radiation Oncology Documentation Tool (ONS, 1994).

EXPECTED OUTCOMES

MAINTAIN INTEGRITY OF SKIN, MUCOUS MEMBRANES, AND IMMUNE SYSTEM AND LEVEL OF COMFORT AND FUNCTION

■ Bone marrow suppression and reactions of the skin and mucous membranes are expected side effects of radiation therapy. Early identification and careful planning (to diminish factors that may increase the reaction) can reduce the impact of these injuries (to the body's protective mechanisms) on a patient's ability to function and on quality of life. In addition, appropriate management of the clinical manifestations of these reactions will improve the patient's level of comfort and function.

OUTCOMES MEASURES

The following instruments may be used to evaluate the impact of skin reactions, mucous membrane reactions, and bone marrow suppression on quality of life.

- EORTC QLQ-C30 Version 2.0 with appropriate site-specific module (Aaronson et al., 1993)—Integrated system for assessing QOL of cancer patients participating in international clinical trials. The current version is a 30-item instrument that has been used extensively.
- FACT-G with appropriate site specific module (Cella, Tulsky & Gray, 1993)—Thirty-three-item general cancer quality-of-life measure for evaluating patients receiving cancer treatment. Specific modules have been developed for a number of sites that complement the general instrument.

OUTCOMES MANAGEMENT

The following provides an overview of management options for specific symptoms. The *Manual for Radiation Oncology Nursing Practice and Education* provides another useful clinical resource (ONS, 1998).

SKIN

Reduce Risk Factors for Skin Reaction

Identify factors that may increase the skin reaction and take measures to reduce the impact of each factor.

- Special positioning devices to reduce appositional skin folds.
- Shield skin surrounding the treatment field, particularly sensitive areas such as the eye.
- Delay treatment until surgical wound has completed healing process.
- Confirm drug/dose of adjuvant chemotherapy to avoid treatment with drugs that may cause a radiation recall effect.
- Nutritional evaluation by dietician.
- Evaluation by internist to maximize stability of comorbid disease.
- Educate patient and family to promote compliance with the following skin care protocol:

- Explain expected skin reaction and pattern of alopecia.
- Avoid applying skin care products (perfume, deodorant, body powders, and lotions) in treatment field.
- If departmental protocol includes use of a product to reduce symptoms of skin reaction, discuss appropriate cleansing and use of product. Provide schedule of appropriate times to perform skin care that do not conflict with treatment time.
- Wash gently with mild soap and water, rinse thoroughly with tepid water, and dry with gentle patting motions using a soft towel. Frosch and Kligman (1979) rated soaps in terms of irritant qualities and found that Dove® soap was the only one classified as mild. Patients treated to the scalp should use a mild shampoo, such as baby shampoo, and let hair dry naturally. Hair dryers should be avoided. Campbell and Illingworth (1992) conducted a randomized controlled trial to determine whether patients should wash the skin within the treatment field during and shortly after radiation therapy. The findings suggested that patients using a mild soap and water to cleanse the skin each day did not change the skin reactions in treatment fields receiving up to 40 Gy. This study has not been repeated nor has it been conducted for patients receiving higher doses of radiotherapy.
- Teach patients to minimize skin trauma by reducing friction to the skin. Patients should avoid tight clothing, clothing that increases skin moisture (nylon), and they should use an electric razor.
- Avoid sun exposure and temperature extremes.
- Maintain adequate nutritional and fluid intake.
- Identify signs and symptoms of skin reaction and infection to report.
- ■ If the skin integrity is compromised by the presence of tumor in the treatment field, a plan should be initated for minimizing further trauma and irritation, preventing infection, absorbing exudate, and decreasing odor. The plan should take into consideration the planned dose of treatment to the surrounding skin and should avoid dressings that will compromise the intact skin (including tape, moisturizers, and lotions).

Management of Acute Skin Reactions

A number of products have been used to prevent and treat acute skin reactions. These products include hydrous lanolin, Aquaphor®,

Eucerin®, aloe gel, A&D ointment®, topical steroids, and moisturizing lotion. Few randomized trials have been performed to evaluate the efficacy of these different products in either the prevention or treatment of acute skin reactions. Most of the information available is anecdotal based on experience. However, the following is a review of data available on some of these products:

1. Aloe Vera Gel: Pilot data and clinical experience show that aloe vera gel may help to prevent radiation therapy–induced dermatitis. In two Phase III randomized trials conducted on women receiving breast or chest wall irradiation, there was no difference in skin dermatitis scores among the group using a placebo gel, the no-treatment group, and the group using aloe gel (Williams et al., 1996). In fact, aloe gel has been found to delay the healing of wounds left open to heal by second intention (Schmidt & Greenspoon, 1991). The gel may provide some relief of symptoms associated with radiation-induced dermatitis, but will not prevent it and should be used with caution in areas of moist desquamation as it may delay healing.

2. Azelastine: This is an oral antiallergic agent. In mice, radiation-induced acute skin reactions were significantly less prominent in the group treated with azelastine than in the control group (Murakami et al., 1997). However, no clinical data on humans has been reported.

3. Topical Steroids: Potera, Lookingbill, and Stryker (1982) evaluated the effectiveness of 0.2% hydrocortisone valerate versus placebo in reducing acute radiation dermatitis. No statistically significant difference was found between the 0.2% hydrocortisone valerate and the placebo in the acute skin response, the symptoms of radiation dermatitis, or late skin effects (3 mo). In another study, 1% hydrocortisone cream was compared with 0.05% clobetasone butyrate cream (Glees, Mameghan-Zadeh, & Sparkes, 1979). The cream was applied starting at 20 Gy. The majority of patients using either cream derived benefit in its soothing effect. However, a significant difference was seen in the intensity of skin reactions. Patients using clobetasone butyrate developed more severe reactions. Topical steroid creams may soothe symptoms associated with acute skin reactions, but should not be used to prevent these reactions. They should not be used if infection is suspected or present in the skin.

4. Hydrocolloid dressings: These dressings provide moderate absorption and hydrate the wound by interacting with the wound fluid to form a gel-like substance. Margolin, Brennan, Denman, LaChapelle, Weckbach & Aron (1990) found that these dressings provide pain relief and timely healing (average 13 days).

5. Bepanthen cream®: Compared with a group of patients who received no topical ointment in a prospective study of 86 patients (Lokkevik et al., 1996). The study did not find any benefit for ameliorating radiation-induced skin reactions.

6. Sucralfate cream: Delaney, Fisher, Hook, and Barton (1997) evaluated the use of sucralfate cream in the management of moist desquamation during radiotherapy. Patients were randomized to receive sorbolene alone or 10% sucralfate in sorbolene cream. Despite a small accrual of patients, the two groups did not differ significantly in time to healing or pain relief. Further studies are needed to completely evaluate this approach.

7. Hyaluronic acid cream: Evaluated in a randomized, double-blind, placebo-controlled study (Liguori, Guillemin, Pesce, Mirimanoff & Bernier, 1997). Acute radiation-induced dermatitis was significantly higher in the placebo group than in the group using a hyaluronic acid cream. In addition, the cream appeared to delay slightly the onset of reactions (from week 1 to week 2) in this group.

■ **Pruritus**
  • Cleanse with tepid water per department policy
  • Dry cornstarch
  • Apply oatmeal colloidal soap to the affected area for 5 to 10 minutes and then rinse
  • Apply oatmeal colloidal lotion after treatment and before bed
  • Apply pure aloe gel after treatment and before bed
  • Apply mild topical steroid once a day

■ **Dry Desquamation and Alopecia**
  • Same procedures as with pruritus
  • Apply an approved unscented moisturizer after treatment and before bed

■ **Moist Desquamation**
The treatment of moist desquamation has changed as a result of the research available on wound healing. Current wound healing policy is to support the wound with protective dressing and moisture rather

than to leave the wound to air dry. A number of different types of wound dressings have been tried. Several key factors must be considered before selecting a wound care plan for an individual patient. They are as follows:

1. Size and site of the wound
2. Presence of infection
3. Radiation treatment plan
4. Ability of the patient to comply with a wound care plan, which includes the following:
   a. Cleanse the wound
      - Tepid water
      - A mild cleanser (Dove®)
   b. Small bleeding points can be controlled with silver nitrate sticks
   c. Apply wound care products
      - For patients who are continuing with treatment, use a product that absorbs and does not provide a "bolus" effect. For example, hydroactive gels (95% water with 5% gel-forming polymers).
      - For patients who are not continuing with treatment, use a product that provides moisture with or without an antibacterial or antifungal effect. For example, silver sulfadiazine (effective against gram-positive and gram-negative organisms and *Candida albicans*).
   d. Apply protective dressing
      - A nonstick absorbent dressing should be applied (i.e., Exu-dry® or telfa pad).
      - Hydrocolloid, occlusive, and moisture-vapor-permeable dressings can be used. However, they must be removed before daily treatment and therefore may cause more desquamation and pain.
   e. Treat infection if present
   f. Control pain with appropriate medication
   g. If tumor is present in the wound, a chronic wound care program should be initiated that includes cleansing the wound, debridement, controlling bleeding, controlling odor, protecting the wound from further damage, and controlling pain.
      - Metronidazole 0.8% gel, charcoal dressings, a suspension of aluminum hydroxide/magnesium hydroxide, or yogurt may be applied to the wound to reduce the odor (Waller & Caroline, 1996).

- Silver nitrate sticks or a sucralfate paste (1 g sucralfate tablet crushed in 2 to 3 mL of hydrogel) may reduce oozing sites of blood (Waller & Caroline, 1996).
- If dressings become stuck to the wound, soak them off with normal saline.
- Aluminum hydroxide/magnesium hydroxide suspension or yogurt applied to an ulcerated area will often relieve burning sensations (Waller & Caroline, 1996).

Management of Late Skin Reactions

The late skin reactions progress slowly and subclinically from 6 months to many years later. Each patient needs an individualized plan to improve skin texture and elasticity as well as to reduce risks for trauma. If skin breakdown or necrosis occurs, a local recurrence of the cancer should be ruled out before referral to a chronic wound care specialist.

Skin Texture and Elasticity

- Apply moisturizing lotion that includes vitamin E or aloe vera gel to the treatment field at least once a day.
- Avoid exposure to the sun or generously apply an appropriate sunscreen and repeat during sun exposure (minimum of 15 SPF).
- Initiate physical therapy with gentle massage or myofascial release to increase elasticity and to reduce fibrosis and scar formation.

Reduce Risk for Trauma

- Avoid activities that increase risk of skin break or bruising.
- Avoid scratching, the use of adhesive tape, and other activities that increase skin friction.
- Avoid temperature extremes including hot water bottles, heating pads, ice packs, and use of sunlamps.
- Avoid activities that increase risk of lymphedema.
- Immediately report to the physician any skin changes or injury.

Mucous Membranes

Reduce Risk Factors for Mucositis

Identify factors that may increase mucositis and take measures to reduce the impact of each factor.

Oral Cavity

- ■ Oral oncology (dental) evaluation to identify teeth that are in poor condition within the planned treatment field. Panorex x-ray films to identify other tooth or bone abnormalities (tooth remnants under the gum). Repair or remove teeth outside the treatment field that are in poor condition to reduce the risk of further inflammation or infection. Poor fitting dentures should not be used and new ones should be made after treatment side effects have healed.

- Develop buccal lingual guards. Metal restorations such as full gold crowns and dental implants can cause radiation scatter with a dose enhancement of adjacent tissues.
- Delay treatment until surgical wound has completed healing process.
- Nutritional evaluation by dietician.
- Evaluation by internist to maximize stability of comorbid disease.
- Educate the patient and family to promote compliance with mucous membrane protocol.
  - Explain expected oral mucous membrane reaction including xerostomia and hypogeusia.
  - If departmental protocol includes use of a product to reduce symptoms of oral mucosa reaction, discuss appropriate cleansing and use of product. Provide schedule of appropriate times to perform oral care that do not conflict with treatment time.
  - Teach patients to minimize oral mucosa trauma. Use soft toothbrush and avoid commercial mouthwashes that contain alcohol.
  - Maintain adequate nutritional and fluid intake. Avoid tobacco and ETOH use.
  - Identify signs and symptoms of oral mucositis and infection to report.

Bladder, Urethra, Vagina, and Rectum

- Delay treatment until any surgical wound has completed the healing process.
- Nutritional evaluation by dietician.
- Evaluation by internist to maximize stability of comorbid disease.
- Educate the patient and family to promote compliance with mucous membrane protocol.
  - Explain expected mucous membrane reactions in the bladder, urethra, rectum and vagina.
  - Maintain adequate nutritional and fluid intake.
  - Identify signs and symptoms of mucositis and infection to report.

Management of Acute Oral Mucositis

■ A number of products have been used to prevent and treat acute oral mucositis. A few randomized trials have been performed to evaluate the efficacy of these different products in either the prevention or treatment of acute reactions. However, the data are conflicting.

Dietary Recommendations

• Avoid food temperature extremes
• Avoid spicy foods
• Choose soft and moist foods
• Eat small frequent meals
• Drink dietary liquid supplements or high-calorie milk-shakes

Pharmaceutical Recommendations

• Sucralfate suspension 5 to 10 mL: Swish and swallow four times a day. The data regarding the use of sucralfate suspension to prevent radiation-induced mucositis has been mixed. Lievens et al. (1998) found no clinical evidence indicating that the oral intake of sucralfate reduced the acute radiation-induced side effects. Cengiz and colleagues found that sucralfate significantly lowered the degree of mucositis with no serious side effects (Cenzig, Ozyar, Ozturk, Akyol, Atahan, & Hayran, 1999).
• Topical oral medications include the following:
    • Xylocaine viscous 2% solution 15 mL: swish and spit every 3 hours as needed.
    • Tetracaine 4% lollipops (made by compounding pharmacy) as needed.
    • Oral capsaicin, active ingredient in chili peppers, desensitizes some neurons and has provided moderate pain relief when applied to a skin surface. Berger et al. (1995) found that oral capsaicin in a candy (taffy) vehicle produced substantial pain reduction in 11 patients with oral mucositis, but the relief was not complete and was only temporary. Further investigations are needed to find a more suitable method of using this natural product.
    • Orabase® solution applied to the lesion as needed.
    • Analgesic oral mixture—departmental preference.
• Systemic pain medication.
• Treat oral infection with appropriate antimicrobial agent. In a recent study, Oguchi and colleagues (1998) evaluated

a mucosa-adhesive water-soluble polymer film (AD film®) containing anesthetics and antibiotics for the treatment of acute radiation-induced oral mucositis. They found that the product alleviated pain, maintained oral feeding opportunity, and prevented secondary oral infections. No further studies have confirmed these findings to date.

- Chlorhexidine mouthwash should be avoided. Foote, Loprinzi, and Frank (1994) found that chlorhexidine was detrimental during radiation therapy to the oral cavity, and that it increased mucositis and toxicity (including mouthwash-induced discomfort, taste alteration, and teeth staining).

- Bubley and colleagues evaluated the use of prophylactic acyclovir. In a double-blind prospective trial of patients receiving radiation with chemotherapy for head and neck tumors, they found that although the frequency of culture-positive herpes simplex virus was low in the untreated group, it was significantly lower (zero) in the acyclovir-treated group (Bubley, Chapman, Chapman, Crumpaeker, & Schnipper, 1989). However, there were no differences in the frequency or type of mouth lesions experienced between the two groups.

- Antibiotic pastilles have also been evaluated in two studies (Okuno et al., 1997; Symonds et al., 1996). In both studies, patients were found to have some benefit in reducing mucositis, but the evidence was not compelling to recommend this as a standard treatment.

- Low-energy He/Ne laser: A simple atraumatic technique for the prevention and treatment of mucositis of various origins. In a trial using this therapy in patients to receive radiation therapy for head and neck cancer, Grade III mucositis occurred in 7.6% with the laser treatment compared with 35.2% of patients not treated (Bensadoun et al., 1999). The frequency of severe pain was 1.9% in the laser treatment group compared with 23.8% in the non-treatment group. Further evaluation is necessary to confirm these findings and to develop appropriate protocols in which to use this promising method.

- Treatment of irradiation-induced mucositis with growth factors (rhGM-CSF) is another promising approach. Wagner, Alfrink, Haus, and Matt (1999) evaluated 32 patients with locally advanced head and neck cancer. Sixteen patients received rhGM-CSF for 5 days starting after a radiation dose of 20 Gy. When compared with controls, the patients on rhGM-CSF showed decreased severity of oral mucositis and a statistically significant reduction in pain.

Patient Education
- Mouth care procedure every 4 hours
- Remove dentures
- Symptoms of infection to report

Management of Late Oral Mucosal Changes
- ■ Management of late oral mucosal changes depends on specific symptoms and evidence of tissue infection and/or necrosis.

Dental caries
- Scrupulous oral hygiene.
- If teeth present, appointment with oral oncology within 4 to 6 weeks of treatment to initiate dental caries prevention with 1% sodium fluoride gel. The gel should be used in custom vinyl vacuform mouth guards each evening for 5 minutes for the life of the natural teeth. Use of fluoride during radiation has been associated with colonization by *Candida albicans* (Epstein, Chin, Jacobson, Rishiraj & Le 1998).
- Regular dental evaluations.
- Dietary restrictions.

Xerostomia
- Stimulate salivary flow
  - Crushed ice
  - Sugar-free lemon drops or gum
  - Treatment with pilocarpine 5 to 7.5 mg three times a day has been associated with a clinically significant increase of salivary flow from the palatal glands, but not from the parotid glands (Niedermeier, Matthaeus, Meyer, Staar, Muller & Schulze, 1998). Manifestations and treatment of xerostomia and associated oral effects are secondary to head and neck radiation therapy.
- Oral Balance gel® (saliva substitute based on polyglycerylmethacrylate, lactoperoxidase, and glucose oxidase) has been found to diminish the sensation of oral dryness and to improve oral function in patients with severe xerostomia (Regelink, Vissink, Reintsema, & Nauta, 1998).
- Biotene® oral care products include toothpaste, chewing gum, and oral moisturizer

- Replace lost secretions
  - Carboxymethyl cellulose preparations
  - Mucin-based preparations
  - Treat dehydration
- Consider use of radioprotectors
  - Amifostine has recently been evaluated in protection of salivary gland function in high-dose radioiodine therapy. Bohuslavizki and colleagues (1999) found that parenchymal damage in salivary glands was reduced significantly by amifostine ($p < 0.01$) in a group of 8 patients treated with amifostine as compared with 9 control patients.

Halitosis
- Avoid tobacco use
- Scrupulous daily mouth care
- Treat infection
- Sugar-free mint candy or gum

Soft Tissue Necrosis
- Promote optimum caloric and protein intake
- Tetracycline 250 mg PO qid times 4 weeks
- Pentoxifylline 400 mg tid times 8 weeks

Osteoradionecrosis
- Result of radiation therapy to maxilla and mandible. Patients present with frank soft tissue necrosis with bone exposure or may report persistent tooth or jaw pain. Treatment includes surgical resection of necrotic tissue and bone, antibiotics, and on occasion hyperbaric oxygenation to promote healing.

Management of Acute Bladder, Urethral, Vaginal, Rectal Mucositis

General
- Encourage adequate fluid intake
- Dietary modification may be necessary to manage diarrhea

Pharmacologic
- Avoid medications that increase fluid output or increase diarrhea
- Treat infection with appropriate antimicrobial

- Bladder spasms:
  Imipramine 10 to 20 mg PO qhs
  Amitriptyline 25 to 50 mg PO qhs
  Oxybutynin 5 mg PO tid
- Diarrhea:
  Loperamide HCL 4 mg PO then 2 mg PO after each
  loose stool
  Diphenoxylate HCL 2.5 to 5 mg PO qid
- Tenesmus:
  Chlorpromazine 12.5 mg q 4 to 8 hours
  Belladonna 2 mg PR
  Betamethasone cream +/− 2% lidocaine gel applied to
  perirectal tissue (Waller & Caroline, 1996)
- Proctosigmoiditis:
  Kochhar, Sriram, Sharma, Goel, & Patel (1999) reported on
  the use of topical sucralfate in controlling bleeding from
  proctosigmoiditis. All patients were treated with 20 mL
  of 10% rectal sucralfate suspension enemas twice a day
  until bleeding stopped. A good response at 4 weeks was
  found in 76.9% of patients, increasing to 92.3% at 16
  weeks. Over a median of 45.5 months, 70.8% had no recurrences of bleeding. All recurrences responded to a
  short-term reinstitution of treatment. However, this
  treatment is not recommended to prevent acute radiation proctitis (O'Brien, Franklin, & Dear, 1997).
- Vaginitis:
  Baking soda douche
  Vaginal moisturizer

Management of Late Effects of Bladder, Urethra, Vagina, and Rectal Mucosa

■ The late effects of radiation to the bladder, urethra, vagina, and rectal mucosa include persistent urgency and frequency of uri- nation, urinary incontinence, atrophic vaginitis, bowel inconti- nence, and tenesmus. These side effects are managed sympto- matically. However, on occasion tissue necrosis may occur that results in fistulae formation that requires surgical intervention.

IMMUNE SYSTEM

Reduce Risk Factors for Bone Marrow Suppression

■ Potential factors for increasing the risk of immunosuppres- sion should be identified and measures taken to reduce the impact of each factor.

- Adequate hematologic status should be attained before the initiation of radiation therapy.
- Nutritional evaluation by dietician.
- Evaluation by internist to maximize stability of comorbid disease including infections.
- Educate patient and family to promote compliance with recommendations to reduce exposure to infection.
- Maintain adequate nutritional and fluid intake.
- Identify signs and symptoms of infection to report.

Management of Acute and Late Bone Marrow Suppression

■ The care of patients who develop neutropenia, thrombocytopenia, and anemia should be individualized based on age, previous chemotherapy, current point in radiation treatment, and symptoms expressed. The patient may require hospitalization, antimicrobial therapy, and hematopoietic supplementation. Late bone marrow suppression may indicate another underlying hematologic disease process and should be evaluated with appropriate bone marrow studies.

- Recombinant human erythropoietin (r-HuEPO)—Several clinical trials have addressed the safety and efficacy of r-HuEPO in patients receiving radiation therapy. Dusenbery et al. (1994) conducted an open-label study that examined the efficacy of r-HuEPO in reversing the anemia of cervical cancer patients undergoing radiation therapy. In r-HuEPO-treated patients, the mean hemoglobin level rose from 10.3 ± 1.0 g/dL to 13.2 ± 1.3 g/dL by the completion of treatment. The difference in the hemoglobin response was statistically significant between the r-HuEPO group and the two control groups. Minor, transient discomfort associated with the subcutaneous administration was reported by the majority of patients. Similiar increases in hemoglobin levels have been found in other patient populations including concomitant treatment (Lavey & Dempsey, 1993; Vijayakumar et al., 1993).
- Filgrastim (r-metHuG-CSF) has been studied for its potential to reduce radiation-induced oropharyngeal mucositis as well as to reduce neutropenia. Schneider (1999) randomized patients receiving external-beam irradiation for head and neck malignancies to receive subcutaneous injections of either filgrastim or placebo beginning on day 1 of radiation and continuing daily throughout treatment. Study medication was titrated to keep the neutrophil

count between $10 \times 10^9/L$ and $30 \times 10^9/L$. Weekly evaluation of the buccal mucosa, hard palate, and posterior pharyngeal wall were conducted using two different scales and the most severe score per week was used in the data analysis. No statistically significant between-group differences were seen in the mean worst scores across time. At almost all time points, however, the worst mean scores were lower in patients treated with filgrastim compared with those in patients treated with placebo, and the number of severe (grade 3) mucositis scores was significantly lower in the filgrastim-treated group.

Fyles and colleagues evaluated 16 patients with ovarian cancer who had previously received chemotherapy and were receiving whole-abdominal radiation therapy. The patients received filgrastim for neutrophil counts $< 2 \times 10^9/L$ (Fyles, Manchul, Levin, Robertson, Sturgeon, & Tsuji, 1998). Fourteen patients received a mean of 2.9 courses of filgrastim (mean duration of 4.1 days), with no treatment interruptions because of neutropenia. The majority of neutrophil counts were maintained above the target range of $2 \times 10^9/L$ during treatment. Thrombocytopenia requiring interruption was seen in six patients and required platelet transfusions in one. In comparison with a control group who did not receive filgrastim, there was no reduction in treatment interruptions due to neutropenia. Although the filgrastim prevented neutropenia, there was no clear benefit found in this patient population since thrombocytopenia was the dose-limiting toxicity rather than neutropenia.

References

Aaronson, N. K., Ahmedzai, S., Bergman, B., Bullinger, M., Cull, A., Duez, N. J., Filiberti, A., Flechtner, H., Fleishman, S. B., de Haes, J. C. J. M., Kaasa, S., Klee, M., Osoba, D., Razavi, D., Rofe, P. B., Schraub, S., Sneeuw, K., Sullivan, M., & Takeda, F. (1993). The European Organization for Research and Treatment of Cancer QLQ-C30: A quality-of-life instrument for use in international clinical trials in oncology. *Journal of the National Cancer Institute*, 85(5), 365–376.

Arcangeli, G., Friedman, M., & Paoluzi, R. (1974). A quantitative study of late radiation—affect on normal skin and subcutaneous tissues in human beings. *British Journal of Radiology*, 47(553), 44–50.

Archambeau, J. O. (1987). Relative radiation sensitivity of the integumentary system dose response of the epidermal, microvascular, and dermal populations. In J. Lett & K. Altman (Eds.), *Advances in radiation biology*, (Vol. 12, pp. 147–203). San Diego, CA: Academic Press.

Archambeau, J. O., Pezner, R., & Wasserman, T. (1995). Pathophysiology of irradiated skin and breast. *Internatiional Journal of Radiation Oncology, Biology, Physics*, 31(5), 1171–1185.

Bensadoun, R. J., Franquin, J. C., Ciais, G., Darcourt, V., Schubert, M. M., Viot., M., Dejou, J., Tardieu, C., Benezery, K., Nguyen, T. D., Laudoyer, Y., Dassonville, O., Poissonnet, G., Vallicioni, J., Thyss, A., Hamdi, M., Chauvel, P., & Demard, F. (1999). Low-energy He/Ne laser in the prevention of radiation-induced mucositis. A multicenter phase III randomized study in patients with head and neck cancer. *Supportive Care in Cancer*, 7(4), 244–252.

Berger, A., Henderson, M., Nadoolman, W., Duffy, V., Cooper, D., Saberski, L., & Bartoshuk, L. (1995). Oral capsaicin provides temporary relief for oral mucositis pain secondary to chemotherapy/radiation therapy. *Journal of Pain and Symptom Management*, 10(3), 243–248.

Bohuslavizki, K. H., Klutmann, S., Bleckmann, C., Brenner, W., Lassmann, S., Mester, J., Henze, E., & Clausen, M. (1999). Salivary gland protection by amifostine in high-dose radioiodine therapy of differentiated thyroid cancer. *Strahlentherapie und Onkologie*, 175(2), 57–61.

Bubley, G. J., Chapman, B., Chapman, S. K., Crumpacker, C. S., & Schnipper, L. E. (1989). Effect of acyclovir on radiation- and chemotherapy-induced mouth lesions. *Antimicrobial Agents and Chemotherapy*, 3(6), 862–865.

Campbell, I. R., & Illingworth, M. H. (1992). Can patients wash during radiotherapy to the breast or chest wall? A randomized controlled trial. *Clinical Oncology (Royal College of Radiologists)*, 4(2), 78–82.

Cella, D. F., Tulsky, D. S., Gray, G., (1993). The Functional Assessment of Cancer Therapy scale: Development and validation of the general measure. *Journal of Clinical Oncology*, 11(3), 570–579.

Cengiz, M., Ozyar, E., Ozturk, D., Akyol, F., Atahan, I. L., & Hayran, M. (1999). Sucralfate in the prevention of radiation-induced oral mucositis. *Journal of Clinical Gastroenterology*, 28(1), 40–43.

Delaney, G., Fisher, R., Hook, C., & Barton, M. (1997). Sucralfate cream in the management of moist desquamation during radiotherapy. *Australasian Radiology*, 41(3), 270–275.

Dusenbery, K. E., McGuire, W. A., Holt, P. J., Carson, L. F., Fowler, J. M., Twiggs, L. B., & Potish, R. A. (1994). Erythropoietin increases hemoglobin during radiation therapy for cervical cancer. *International Journal of Radiation Oncology, Biology, Physics*, 29(5), 1079–1084.

Dutreix, J. (1986). Human skin: Early and late reactions in relation to dose and its time distribution. *British Journal of Radiology*, 19(Suppl.), 22–28.

Epstein, J. B., Chin, E. A., Jacobson, J. J., Rishiraj, B., & Le, N. (1998). The relationships among fluoride, cariogenic oral flora, and salivary flow rate during radiation therapy. *Oral Surgery Oral Medicine Oral Pathology Oral Radiology Endodontics*, 86(3), 286–292.

Foote, R. L., Loprinzi, C. L., & Frank, A. R. (1994). Randomized trial of a chlorhexidine mouthwash for alleviation of radiation-induced mucositis. *Journal of Clinical Oncology*, 12(12), 2630–2633.

Frosch, P., & Kligman, A. (1979). The soap chamber: A new method for assessing the irritancy of soaps. *Journal of the American Academy of Dermatology*, 1(1), 35–41.

Fyles, A. W., Manchul, L., Levin, W., Robertson, J. M., Sturgeon, J., & Tsuji, D. (1998). Effect of filgrastim (G-CSF) during chemotherapy and abdomino-pelvic radiation therapy in patients with ovarian carcinoma. *International Journal of Radiation Oncology, Biology, Physics*, 41(4), 843–847.

Glees, J. P., Mameghan-Zadeh, H., & Sparkes, C. G. (1979). Effectiveness of topical steroids in the control of radiation dermatitis: A randomized trial using 1% hydrocortisone cream and 0.05% clobetasone butyrate (Eumovate). *Clinical Radiology*, 30(4), 397–403.

Kao, G. D., Devine, P., & Mirza, N. (1999). Oral cavity and oropharyngeal tumors in human immunodeficiency virus-positive patients: Acute response to radiation therapy. *Archives of Otolaryngology Head and Neck Surgery*, 125(8), 873–876.

Kochhar, R., Sriram, P. V., Sharma, S. C., Goel, R. C., Patel, F. (1999). Natural history of late radiation proctosigmoiditis treated with sucralfate suspension. *Digestive Diseases and Sciences*, 44(5), 973–978.

Lavey, R. S. & Dempsey, W. H. (1993). Erythropoietin increases hemoglobin in cancer patients during radiation therapy. *International Journal of Radiation Oncology, Biology, Physics*, 27(5), 1147–1152.

Lievens, Y., Haustermans, K., Van-den-Weyngaert, D., Van-den-Bogaert, W., Scalliet, P., Hutsebaut, L., Fowler, J., & Lambin, P. (1998). Does sucralfate reduce the acute side-effects in head and neck cancer treated with radiotherapy? A double-blind randomized trial. *Radiotherapy Oncology*, 47(2), 149–153.

Liguori, V., Guillemin, C., Pesce, G. F., Mirimanoff, R. O., & Bernier, J. (1997). Double-blind, randomized clinical study comparing hyaluronic acid cream to placebo in patients treated with radiotherapy. *Radiotherapy and Oncology*, 42(2), 155–161.

Lokkevik, E., Skovlund, E., Reitan, J. B., Hannisdal, E., & Tanum, G. (1996). Skin treatment with Bepanthen cream versus no cream during radiotherapy—A randomized controlled trial. *Acta Oncologica*, 35(8), 1021–1026.

Margolin, S., Breneman, J., Denman, D., LaChapelle, P., Weckbach, L., & Aron, B. S. (1990). Management of radiation-induced moist skin desquamation using hydrocolloid dressing. *Cancer Nursing*, 13(2), 71–80.

McDonald, A. (1992). Altered protective mechanisms. In K. Hassey Dow & L. J. Hilderley (Eds.), *Nursing care in radiation oncology*. Philadelphia: W. B. Saunders.

Murakami, R., Baba, Y., Nishimura, R., Furusawa, M., Yokoyama, T., Yamashita, Y., Takahashi, M., Yamashita, N., & Ono, T. (1997). The effect of azelastine on acute radiation dermatitis in mice models. *International Journal of Radiation Oncology, Biology, Physics*, 37(4), 907–911.

National Cancer Institute. (1999). *National Cancer Institute's Common Toxicity Criteria, Version 2.0, with Radiation Therapy Oncology Group (RTOG) and Eu-*

ropean Organization for Research and Treatment of Cancer (EORTC) Acute Effects Criteria. Bethesda, MD: National Cancer Institute.

Niedermeier, W., Matthaeus, C., Meyer, C., Staar, S., Muller, R. P., & Schulze, H. J. (1998). Radiation-induced hyposalivation and its treatment with oral pilocarpine. Oral Surgery Oral Medicine Oral Pathology Oral Radiology Endodontics, 86(5), 541–549.

O'Brien, P. C., Franklin, C. I., Dear, K. B. Hamilton, C. C., Poulsen, M., Joseph, D. J., Spry, N., & Denham, J. W. (1997). A phase III double-blind randomized study of rectal sucralfate suspension in the prevention of acute radiation proctitis. Radiotherapy Oncology, 45(2), 117–123.

Oguchi, M., Shikama, N., Sasaki, S., Gomi, K., Katsuyama, Y., Ohta, S., Hori, M., Takei, K., Arakawa, K., & Sone, S. (1998). Mucosa-adhesive water-soluble polymer film for treatment of acute radiation-induced oral mucositis. International Journal of Radiation Oncology, Biology, Physics, 15(40), 1033–1037.

Okuno, S. H., Foote, R. L., Loprinzi, C. L., Gulavita, S., Sloan, J. A., Earle, J., Novotny, P. J., Burk, M., & Frank, A. R. (1997). A randomized trial of a nonabsorbable antibiotic lozenge given to alleviate radiation-induced mucositis. Cancer, 79(11), 2193–2199.

Oncology Nursing Society. (1994). Radiation Therapy Patient Care Record. A tool for documenting nursing care. Pittsburgh, PA: Oncology Nursing Society.

Oncology Nursing Society. (1998). Manual for radiation oncology nursing practice and education. Pittsburgh: Oncology Nursing Press.

Potera, M. E., Lookingbill, D. P., & Stryker, J. A. (1982). Prophylaxis of radiation dermatitis with a topical cortisone cream. Radiology, 143(3), 775–777.

Regelink, G., Vissink, A., Reintsema, H., & Nauta, J. M. (1998). Efficacy of synthetic polymer saliva substitute in reducing oral complaints of patients suffering from irradiation-induced xerostomia. Quintessence International, 29(6), 383–388.

Rubin, P., Constine, L. S., Nelson, D. F. (1992). In C. A. Perez & L. W. Brady (Eds.), Principles and practice of radiation oncology, (2nd ed. pp. 124–161). Philadelphia: Lippincott.

Schmidt, J. M., & Greenspoon, J. S. (1991). Aloe vera dermal wound gel is associated with a delay in wound healing. Obstetrics and Gynecology, 78(1), 115–117.

Schneider, S. B., Nishimura, R. D., Zimmerman, R. P., Tran, L., Shiplacoff, J., Tormey, M., Contreras, R., & Juillard, G. F. (1999). Filgrastim (r-metHuG-CSF) and its potential use in the reduction of radiation-induced oropharyngeal mucositis: An interim look at a randomized, double-blind placebo-controlled trial. Cytokines Cellular Molecular Therapy, 5(3), 175–180.

Sonis, S. T., Eilers, J. P., Epstein, J. B., LeVeque, F. G., Liggett, W. H., Jr., Mulagha, M. T., Peterson, D. E., Rose, A. H., Schubert, M. M., Spijkervet, F. K. & Wittes, J. P. (1999). Validation of a new scoring system for the assessment of clinical trial research of oral mucositis induced by radiation or chemotherapy. Mucositis Study Group. Cancer, 85(10), 2103–2113.

Symonds, R. P., McIlroy, P., Khorrami, J., Paul, J., Pyper, E., Alcock, S. R., McCallum, I., Speekenbrink, A. B., McMurray, A., Lindemann, E., & Thomas, M. (1996). The reduction of radiation mucositis by selective decontamination antibiotic pastilles: A placebo-controlled double-blind trial. *British Journal of Cancer, 74*(2), 312–317.

Vijayakumar, S., Roach, M., Wara, W., Chan, S. K., Ewing, C., Rubin, S., Sutton, H., Halpern, H., Awan, A., & Houghton, A. (1993). Effect of subcutaneous recombinant human erythropoietin in cancer patients receiving radiotherapy: Preliminary results of a randomized, open-labeled, phase II trial. *International Journal of Radiation Oncology, Biology, Physics, 26*(4), 721–729.

Wagner, W., Alfrink, M., Haus, U., & Matt, J. (1999). Treatment of irradiation-induced mucositis with growth factors (rhGM-CSF) in patients with head and neck cancer. *Anticancer Research, 19*(1B), 799–803.

Waller, A., & Caroline, N. L. (1996). *Handbook of palliative care in cancer.* Boston: Butterworth-Heinemann.

Watkins, E. B., Findlay, P., Gelmann, E., Lane, H. C., & Zabell, A. (1987). Enhanced mucosal reactions in AIDS patients receiving oropharyngeal irradiation. *International Journal of Radiation Oncology, Biology, Physics, 13*(9), 1403–1408.

Williams, M. S., Burk, M., Loprinzi, C. L., Hill, M., Schomberg, P. J., Nearhood, K., O'Fallon, J. R., Laurie, J. A., Shanahan, T. G., Moore, R. L., Urias, R. E., Kuske, R. R. (1996). Phase III double-blind evaluation of an aloe vera gel as a prophylactic agent for radiation-induced skin toxicity. *International Journal of Radiation Oncology, Biology, Physics, 36*(2), 345–349.

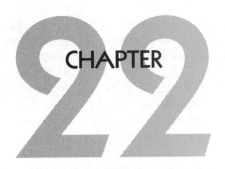

CHAPTER

ADEQUATE NUTRITIONAL INTAKE

Marilyn L. Haas, PhD, ANP-C
J. Dattle Haslam, MD

PROBLEM

Nutritional status during radiation therapy becomes an important issue for cancer patients. Since radiation therapy affects normal healthy cells along with the cancer cells, good nutrition is needed to repair the body's healthy cells. Poor nutritional intake can result from poor tolerance of the specific anatomical site being irradiated (oral cavity, esophagus), magnitude of the radiation dose, addition of concurrent chemotherapy, carbohydrate metabolic disturbances (glucose intolerance and insulin resistance), or simply psychological distress. Poor nutrition may lead to clinical malnutrition that can eventually contribute to cancer cachexia. Prevalence of reported malnutrition is high among cancer patients (Ottery, 1994a). Approximately one-third to two-thirds of hospitalized cancer patients experience cachexia. Eventually, malnutrition affects quality of life and survival rates (Rivadeneira, Evoy, Fahey, Lieberman, & Daly, 1998). The side effects from radiation therapy that may interfere with nutrition include the following:

■ Anorexia is the most common symptom patients experience (Weihofen & Marino, 1998). Loss of appetite is probably multifactorial. Possible reasons would include early satiety, development of food aversions, malaise, depression, pain, bloating, and/or constipation.

■ Nausea and vomiting add to the nutritional deficiency and are
   probably the most distressing quality-of-life issues for cancer
   patients. Radiation-induced nausea is site-dependent and
   dose-related (John, 1998). The Italian Group for Antiemetic
   Research in Radiotherapy (1999) conducted a prospective observation multicenter trial and found that 37% of their patients experienced nausea, 17% vomited, and 38% experienced both nausea and vomiting. The group identified three
   significant prognostic factors relating to radiation-induced
   emesis: previous chemotherapy, field size, and irradiated site
   (upper abdomen). While chemotherapeutic agents increase
   the radiosensitivity of cancer cells, combined-modality treatment can cause gastrointestinal distress.
■ Taste Alterations—Patients may experience ageusia (little
   or no sense of taste) or dysgeusia (metallic, bitter, too salty,
   or too sweet tasting) (Lutz & Przytulski, 1997).
■ Inflammation/Infected Mucous Membranes—Mucosal membranes of the upper aerodigestive and gastrointestinal tracts
   are very sensitive to cancer treatments because these cells
   also reproduce very rapidly. Temporary damage from radiation therapy can lead to oral and throat pain, thickening of secretions, dysphagia, or odynophagia. Stomatitis, pharyngitis,
   and esophagitis inhibit oral intake, thus compounding nutritional deficiencies and delaying healing.
■ Xerostomia—High doses of radiation can lead to atrophy of
   the salivary glands, thus diminishing saliva and increasing
   acidity. Dryness of the mouth from salivary gland dysfunction affects the mechanical process of eating, dental care,
   and quality of life.
■ Postradiation Fibrosis—Late effects of irradiation can occur
   3 to 6 months or even years after treatments (Archambeau,
   Pezner, & Wasserman, 1995). Slow-progressing fibrosis can
   cause strictures and long-term swallowing difficulties.
■ Superinfections—Radiation therapy can predispose patients to infections by suppressing the immune system
   (Skipper, Szeluga, & Groenwald, 1995). Oral candidiasis is
   very common among cancer patients, especially when the
   patient is taking oral steroids .
■ Diarrhea—Pelvic radiation may cause damage to the bowel,
   thus affecting nutritional absorption. Radiation enteritis may
   cause acute or chronic loose stools/diarrhea. Concomitant
   chemotherapy may exacerbate radiation-induced diarrhea.

ASSESSMENT

A comprehensive nutritional review should be obtained prior to radiation treatments to establish the patient's baseline status. History, physical examination, and laboratory findings are all important assessments. Information includes the following:

■ Body Weight—Unexplained decrease in body weight is one of the nonspecific general signs and symptoms of cancer (American Cancer Society, 1999). Unintentional weight loss of 10 pounds or more within the past 6 months is considered a nutritional risk factor (DeWys et al., 1980). Weight loss is an important prognostic factor in cancer patients.

■ Cultural/Ethnic Differences—Inquire about the patient's cultural background and dietary preferences. Be aware of any cultural or religious eating patterns and make recommendations accordingly.

■ 24-Hour Dietary Recall—When patients are able to recall all the food including snacks and fluid taken within the last 24 hours, a general idea of eating habits can be ascertained. Inadequate intake of calories, fluid, and protein can be identified and suggestions for improvement can be recommended.

■ Laboratory Data—Serum prealbumin and retinal binding globulin are the first to show a decrease when patients experience nutritional difficulties, since these proteins have short lives (0.5 and 2.0 days, respectively). Transferrin and albumin concentrations drop after longer periods of nutritional deficiency (8.0 and 20.0 days, respectively). If dehydration is a problem, electrolytes and blood counts are important indicators of the patient's fluid status.

■ Measures of Malnutrition—A patient is considered to be malnourished if two of the following three measures are found: weight loss of 10% or more of body weight, serum albumin is less than 3.4 g/dL, or serum transferrin is less than 190 mg/dL (Daly and Shinkwin, 1995).

■ Dietary supplements are herbal products, botanical preparations and megadoses of vitamins or minerals. These should be taken with caution and may inhibit oral intake and nutritional status by causing diarrhea, constipation, nausea, vomiting, anorexia, or nutrient malabsorption. Also, dietary supplements may interfere with some medications.

- ■ Physical Examination—May reveal muscle wasting (easily assessed by measuring midarm muscle circumference and making a comparison prior to nutritional deficiency), loss of muscle strength, depletion of fat stores, and dehydration signs.

EXPECTED OUTCOMES

The aim of nutritional support with cancer patients is to prevent or reverse the cachexia of malignancy, thus offering a higher quality of life. Initiation of nutritional support begins immediately to ensure adequate oral intake. It is reasonable to expect patients not to regain weight quickly as tissue loss responds slowly to treatment. While minimizing weight loss is a priority, adequate hydration is essential throughout treatments. Oral nutrition and supplements are the preferred routes. However, other methods may need to be employed to assist patients with their nutritional needs, (i.e., enterally or intravenously). Esophagostomy or gastrostomy/jejunostomy tube feedings are preferred and are kept until the patient can safely resume oral feedings. Enteral formulas are selected based on digestibility of nutrients, osmolality, viscosity, rate of delivery, and nutritional completeness (Wilkes & Yemma, 1997). When patients are unable to take foods/fluids orally and enteral feedings are not an option, total parenteral nutrition is an alternative. Hyperalimentation provides macronutrients, vitamins, minerals, trace elements with dextrose, and amino acid solutions. If weight can be stabilized, then euvolemic state is restored, electrolyte abnormalities are corrected, and essential laboratory values are improved—serum protein, albumin, and folic acid (Chernecky & Berger, 1998).

OUTCOMES MEASURES

Food becomes therapy for cancer patients undergoing treatments. For the clinician, following the patient's weight during radiation therapy is the quickest measure of adequate nutritional intake. While dietary assessments should be performed on all cancer patients, dietary consults provide additional resources for the patients. A multidisciplinary approach by the registered dietitian, radiation oncologist, midlevel practitioner, nurse, patient, and his or her family members is critical to having a successful outcome of maintaining weight throughout treatment. Medical nutrition therapy provided by a registered dietitian is essential in treating cancer patients. All medical staff should take an active role in supporting a patient's effort to maintain good nutrition. Available nutritional assessment tools are as follows:

- Visual Analogue Scale is a generic rating instrument (0 to 100 mm linear scale) that patients can use to rate their nutritional status (Grant, Padilla, & Rhiner, 1991).
- Subjective Global Assessment (SGA) tool is a universal nutritional screening tool that reviews weight changes, dietary intake, gastrointestinal symptoms, functional impairment, and physical examination (Bowers & Dols, 1996; Ottery, 1994b).

Gastrostomy tubes should be considered in appropriate patients prior to beginning treatments, before the patient reaches the point of limited oral intake. Ongoing assessments, counseling, and intervention are needed throughout treatment. Finally, when individuals can maintain or gain weight, they will have more energy, accelerate the healing process, lessen their risk for developing infections, increase therapy tolerance, and improve their overall comfort.

OUTCOMES MANAGEMENT

The most important aspect of physical well-being is the ability to eat and have an appetite (Padilla et al., 1983). Nutritional management involves both the patient and his or her caregiver. Patient teaching and daily reinforcement are required to support the patient through therapy. The following guidelines may assist patients in dealing with their nutritional problems:

- Good Oral Hygiene—Meticulous mouth care before and after meals is essential to stimulate the appetite and assist in the mechanical process of eating. Isotonic saline alone or combined with soda bicarbonate is recommended (Iwamoto, 1997). Use of commercial saliva substitutes may assist with the xerostomia such as Salivart Synthetic Saliva® (Gebauer Company, Cleveland, OH). The palliative effects on oral dryness may be alleviated with topical agents such as Biotene's Oralbalance Gel® or Toothpaste® (Laclede Professional

Products, Gardena, CA) (Epstein, Emerton, Le, & Stevenson-Moore, 1999).

■ Meal Times—Encourage patients to eat whether they are hungry or not. Remember food is therapy. Small, frequent meals should be served in a pleasant environment.

■ Inverted Food Pyramid—When a patients develops cancer and undergoes therapy, the body's nutritional needs are different. The typical food pyramid does not apply (Figure 22–1). More fats and proteins are required to restore the body (Bristol-Meyers Squibb, 1998). Simple formulas to assist in determining caloric and protein needs include the following:

Minimum daily caloric needs:
Normal weight: weight (kg) × 25 cal/kg
Decreased weight: weight (kg) × 30–35 cal/kg
Minimum daily protein needs:
Normal weight: weight (kg) × 1.2 protein/kg
Decrease weight: weight (kg) × 1.5–2 g protein/kg

Recipes with peanut butter, eggs, cheese, ice creams, buttered beans, and real mayonnaise can provide the extra

FIGURE 22–1   EATING RIGHT WITH CANCER

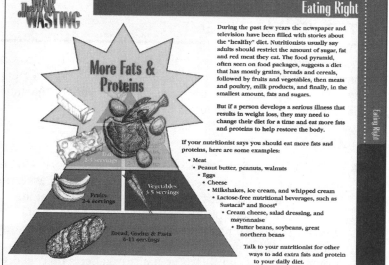

From Briston-Meyers Squibb. (1998). *Understanding Nutritional Needs During Illness: The War on Wasting.* Bristol-Meyers Squibb Oncology/Immunology. Princeton, NJ.

fats/proteins. Maximize protein intake by suggesting creative recipes using powdered/liquid egg whites (with cooked food only) or extra dry milk added to shakes, gravies, casseroles, or soups.

■ Nutritional Supplements—Various products on the market can easily be purchased at local grocery stores or through the mail directly from the manufacturer. Products that may be helpful to maintain adequate caloric intake in light of anorexia and nausea/vomiting are identified in Table 22–1.

■ Appetite Stimulants—Sometimes it is necessary to add drug therapy to increase the patient's appetite. Drug therapy may include appetite stimulants: megestrol acetate, steroids, and growth hormones. Megestrol acetate (Megace, Mead Johnson Oncology Products of Bristol-Meyers Squibb, Princeton, NJ) has impacted appetite, body weight, and quality of life for cancer patients (Bruera et al., 1998).

■ Zinc or Multivitamin Supplements—Administration of oral zinc sulfate helps prevent and even correct taste abnormalities in cancer patients receiving head and neck external radiotherapy (Ripamonti et al., 1998). According to these researchers, initiating zinc sulfate at the beginning of therapy can lessen hypogeusia (reduction in taste sensitivity), ageusia (absence of taste sensation), or dysgeusia (distortion of normal taste). Multivitamin supplements containing no more than 100% of the RDI for any particular nutrient may be used to prevent or correct any micronutrient deficiency. Vitamin supplements containing herb or botanical compounds are not advised.

■ Tube Feedings—Intensive nutritional support should be considered before the patient reaches a level of dehydration, or malnutrition becomes an issue. Typically, when support is anticipated for 6 weeks or longer, gastrostomy or jejunostomy feedings are preferred instead of nasogastric tube feedings.

■ Antiemetics—Resolve the patient's nausea first with the assistance of medications prior to eating any foods. Helpful antiemetics for cancer patients include lorazepam (Ativan®, Wyeth-Ayerst, Philadelphia, PA), dronabinol (Marinol®, Roxane Laboratories, Columbus, OH), or promethazine (Phenergan®, Wyeth-Ayerst, Philadelphia, PA). If the nausea is significant, encourage long-acting antiemetics around the clock—prochlorperazine (Compazine Spansules®, SmithKline Beecham Pharmaceuticals, Philadelphia, PA).

TABLE 22-1 NUTRITIONAL SUPPLEMENTS AVAILABLE OVER-THE-COUNTER

Product	Company	Calories/Protein	Description
Advera®	Ross Products Division of Abbott Laboratories, Columbus, OH	303 calories/8 oz. 14.2 g protein	Beneficial for patients with mucositis or stomatitis. Specialized peptides for easier absorption, allowing healing of the alimentary tract
Boost®	Mead Johnson & Company, Evansville, IN	240 calories/8oz. 10 g protein	Lactose-free
Boost Plus®	Mead Johnson & Company, Evansville, IN	360 calories/8oz. 14 g protein	Concentrated calories
Carnation Instant Breakfast®	Nestle USA-Beverage Division, Glendale, CA	280 calories/8 oz. 12 g protein with whole milk	Lactose-containing, plus mineral/vitamins
Ensure®	Ross Products Division of Abbott Laboratories, Columbus, OH	253 calories/8 oz. 11 g protein	Hyperosmolar solution, containing no fiber
Ensure Plus®	Ross Products Division of Abbott Laboratories, Columbus, OH	355 calories/8 oz. 13 g protein	Concentrated hyperosmolar solution, containing no fiber. Best used when limited volume is required
Jevity®	Ross Products Division of Abbott Laboratories, Columbus, OH	250 calories/8 oz. 10 g protein	Good for short- or long-term tube feedings. Isotonic, fiber-fortified, high-nitrogen liquid
Nestle Sweet Success®	Nestle USA-Beverage Division, Glendale, CA	250 calories/8oz. 11 g protein with whole milk	Lactose-containing, plus minerals/vitamins
NuBasic®	Nestle USA-Beverage Division, Glendale, CA	250 calories/8 oz. 8.75 g protein	Isomolar drinks, Lactose- and gluten-free
NuBasic Soup®	Nestle USA-Beverage Division, Glendale, CA	250 calories per packet/ 8.75 g protein	Chicken and tomato flavors available

NuBasics Coffee®	Nestle USA-Beverage Division, Glendale, CA	125 calories per packet, 8 g protein	Decaffeinated and instant available
NutraShakes®	Nutra/Balance Products, Inc., Indianapolis, IN	200 calories/4 oz. 6 g protein	Dairy and non-dairy drinks, lactose-free
Resource®	Sandoz Nutritional Corporation	250 calories/8 oz. 9 g protein	Lactose-free
Sustacal®	Mead Johnson & Company, Evansville, IN	240 calories/8 oz. 10 g protein	Lactose-free
Sustacal Plus®	Mead Johnson & Company, Evansville, IN	360 calories/8 oz. 14 g protein	Lactose-free
Scandishake®	Scandiapharm, Birmingham, AL	440 calories/8 oz. 1 g protein	Lactose and lactose-free

Note. This table is not inclusive of all available products.

■ Complementary Therapies—Relaxation and massage may
   assist the patients in coping and increase their desire to eat.
   Music can be utilized as a diversional adjunct intervention
   to minimize symptoms (Ezzone, Baker, Rosselet, & Terepka,
   1998). Acupuncture, as complementary therapy, has been
   shown to increase salivary flow postradiation (Blom, Davidson, & Angmar-Mansson, 1993).

RESOURCES

There are readily available resources for health professionals and
patients. Printed nutritional materials can be obtained through the
American Cancer Society, the National Cancer Institute, and companies that supply nutritional supplements. A toll-free telephone nutritional hotline is available from the American Institute for Cancer
Research (1-800-843-8114). The Internet also provides easy access to
instructional information. Possible sites include http://cancernet.
nci.nih.gov and http://rex.nci.nih.gov.

REFERENCES

American Cancer Society. (1999). *Signs and symptoms of cancer*. Atlanta, GA:
   American Cancer Society.
Archambeau, J., Pezner, R., & Wasserman, T. (1995). Pathophysiology of ir-
   radiated skin and breast. *International Journal of Radiation Oncology, Biol-
   ogy, Physics*, 31, 1171–1185.
Blom, M., Davidson, I., & Angmar-Mansson, B. (1993). Acupuncture treat-
   ment of xerostomia caused by irradiation of the head and neck region:
   Case reports. *Journal of Oral Rehabilitation*, 20(5), 492–494.
Bowers, J., & Dols, C. (1996). Subjective Global Assessment in HIV-infected
   patients. *Journal of the Association of Nurses in AIDS Care*, 7(4), 83–89.
Bristol-Myers Squibb. (1998). *The War on Wasting*. Bristol-Myers Squibb
   Oncology/Immunology. Princeton, NJ.
Bruera, E., Ernst, S., Hagen, N., Spachynski, K., Belzile, M., Hanson, J., Sum-
   mers, N., Brown, B., Dulude, H., & Gallant, G. (1998). Effectiveness of
   megestrol acetate in patients with advanced cancer: A randomized,
   double-blind, crossover study. *Cancer Prevention Control*, 2(2), 74–78.
Chernecky, C., & Berger, B. (1998). *Advanced and critical care oncology nursing*.
   Philadelphia: W. B. Saunders.
Daly, H., & Shinkwin, M. (1995). Nutrition and the cancer patient. In G.
   Murphy, W. Lawrence, & R. Lenhard (Eds.), *American Cancer Society textbook of clinical oncology*. Atlanta, GA: American Cancer Society.

DeWys, W., Begg, C, Lavin, P., Band, P., Bennett, J., Bertino, J., Cohen, M., Douglass, H.,Engstrom, P., Ezdinli, E., Horton, J., Johnson, G., Moertel, C., Oken, M., Perlia, C., Rosenbaum, C., Silverstein, M., Skeel, R., Sponzo, R., & Tormey, D. (1980). Prognostic effect of weight loss prior to chemotherapy in cancer patients. Eastern Cooperative Oncology Group. *American Journal of Medicine*, 69, 491–497.

Epstein, J., Emerton, S., Le, N., & Stevenson-Moore. (1999). A double-blind crossover trial of Oral Balance Gel and Biotene Toothpaste versus placebo in patients with xerostomia following radiation therapy. *Oral Oncology*, 35(2), 132–137.

Ezzone, S., Baker, C., Rosselet, R., & Terepka, E. (1998). Music as an adjunct to antiemetic therapy. *Oncology Nursing Forum*, 25(9), 1551–1556.

Grant, M., Padilla, G., & Rhiner, M. (1991). *Patterns of anorexia in cancer patients: Maintaining nutritional status in patients with cancer*. Atlanta, GA: American Cancer Society.

Italian Group for Antiemetic Research in Radiotherapy. (1999). Radiation-induced emesis: A prospective observational multicenter Italian trial. *International Journal of Radiation Oncology, Biology, and Physics*, 44(3), 619–625.

Iwamoto, R. (1997). Cancers of the head and neck. In K. Dow, J. Bucholtz, R. Iwamoto, V. Fieler, & L. Hilderley (Eds.), *Nursing care in radiation oncology*. Philadelphia: W. B. Saunders.

John, M. (1998). Radiotherapy and chemotherapy. In S. Leibel, & T. Phillips (Eds.), *Textbook of radiation oncology*. Philadelphia: W. B. Saunders.

Lutz, C., & Przytulski, K. (1997). *Nutrition and diet therapy*. Philadelphia: F. A. Davis.

Ottery, F. (1994a). Rethinking nutritional support of the cancer patient: The new field of nutritional oncology. *Seminars in Oncology*, 21, 770.

Ottery, F. (1994b). Oncology patient-generated Subjective Global Assessment (SGA) of nutritional status. *Nutritional Oncology*, 1(2), 9.

Padilla, G., Preasant, C., Grant, M., Metter, G., Lipsett, J., & Heide, F. (1983). Quality of life index for patients with cancer. *Research in Nursing Health*, 6,117–126.

Ripamonti, C., Zecca, E., Brunelli, C., Fulfaro, F., Villa, S., Balzarini, A., Bombardieri, E., & DeConno, F. (1998). A randomized, controlled clinical trial to evaluate the effects of zincsulfate on cancer patients with taste alterations caused by head and neck irradiation. *Cancer*, 82(10), 1938–1945.

Rivadeneira, D., Evoy, D., Fahey, T., Lieberman, M., & Daly, J. (1998). Nutritional support of the cancer patient. *CA: Cancer Journal For Clinicians*, 48 (2), 69–80.

Skipper, A., Szeluga, D., & Groenwald, S. (1995). Nutritional disturbances. In S. Groenwald, M. Frogge, M. Goodman, & C. Yarbo (Eds.). *Cancer nursing: Principles and practice*. Boston: Jones & Bartlett.

Weihofen, D. & Marino, C. (1998). *The cancer survival cookbook*. New York: John Wiley and Sons.

Wilkes, G., & Yemma, T. (1997). Nutritional support. In C. Varricchio, M. Pierce, C. Walker, & T. Ades (Eds.), *A cancer source book for nurses*. (7th ed.). Atlanta, GA: American Cancer Society.

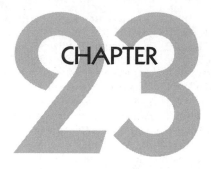

CHAPTER

23

MAINTENANCE OF NORMAL ELIMINATION

Constance Engelking RN, MS, OCN
Carmel Sauerland RN, MSN, AOCN

PROBLEM

Altered bowel elimination and bladder elimination commonly occur in patients undergoing abdominopelvic, lower thoracic, and lumbosacral irradiation. Abdominopelvic radiation is used to treat genitourinary, gynecologic, and gastrointestinal cancers. Thoracic and lumbosacral radiation, which exerts local effects on the organs and tissues contained within the abdominal field, is used in the treatment of spinal tumors and cord compression. Primary elimination problems encountered by patients undergoing abdominopelvic radiation include diarrhea, cystitis, and incontinence. Other related symptoms include nephritis, urethritis, dysuria, hematuria, tenesmus, and proctitis. The character of the particular bowel and/or bladder alteration accompanying the symptoms and the intensity of resulting clinical problems range from mild to severe depending on radiation dose rate, field location and size, treatment protocol (i.e., concurrent chemotherapy) and techniques, presence of related comorbid conditions, and other host factors. In addition to physical symptomatology, alterations in bowel and urinary elimination are also associated with the psychosocial issues related to interpersonal relationships, body image, and sexuality.

ALTERED BOWEL ELIMINATION

Diarrhea

■ Two principal mechanisms ensure the balanced transport of intestinal fluid and electrolytes: *secretion*, which takes place in the crypt cells and *absorption*, which occurs in the enterocytes lining the intestinal villi. Deviations in one or both of these mechanisms disrupt the ratio between intestinal secretion and absorption. Diarrhea results when the total secretion of fluid and electrolytes overwhelms the absorptive capacity of the bowel (Chang, 1992; Engelking, 1998a; Mercadante, 1996).

■ Cancer-related diarrhea is a complex and multifactorial problem that occurs in response to an array of causative factors specifically associated with malignant disease and its treatment and is categorized according to six discrete pathophysiologic mechanisms (Table 23–1). Among those, acute radiation-induced diarrhea is classified as "exudative syndrome" (Engelking, 1998a; Mercadante, 1996). Other types of diarrhea experienced by patients following radiation therapy are osmotic, malabsorptive, and dysmotility-associated diarrhea. Accurate categorization of the underlying cause of and mechanism responsible for producing diarrhea is essential to defining appropriate treatment (Engelking, 1998b).

■ Exudative diarrhea is typified by the discharge of mucus, serum proteins, and blood in the bowel lumen produced by disruptions in the integrity of the intestinal mucosa that occur in response to inflammation and ulceration. Specific morphologic changes in the intestinal mucosa include sloughing of the epithelial surface and shortening of the villi with a subsequent reduction in the total surface area of denuded mucosa available for the absorption of fluid and electrolytes, thus leading to decreased absorptive capacity (Bruner, Bucholtz, Iwamoto, & Strohl, 1998; Mercadante, 1996). Acute radiation-induced enterocolitis is a result of crypt stem cell depletion. In contrast, late or chronic enteritis is produced by atrophy of the mucosa (Mercadante, 1996).

■ Malabsorption of fats, carbohydrates and protein each play a role in the production of postradiation diarrhea. Fat malabsorption reduces bile salt absorption in the terminal

TABLE 23–1   PATHOPHYSIOLOGIC MECHANISMS, ETIOLOGIES, AND CLINICAL MANIFESTATIONS
ASSOCIATED WITH CANCER-RELATED DIARRHEA

Type	Pathophysiologic Mechanisms	Etiologies	Clinical Manifestations
Osmotic	Mechanical disturbance Characterized by large volume influx of fluid and electrolytes into intestinal lumen that overwhelms absorptive capacity of bowel Osmotic forces responsible for drawing substrates across the intestinal epithelium are interrupted by direct contact with hyperosmolar stimuli	Ingestion of hyperosmolar preparations and substances • Nonabsorbable solutes (e.g., sorbitol, magnesium-based antacids) • Enteral feeding solutions Intestinal hemorrhage • Intraluminal blood gets as osmotic substance	Large volume, watery stools that resolve with withdrawal of causative agent
Malabsorptive	Combined disturbance of mechanical and biochemical mechanisms responsible for mediating absorptive processes Secondary to factors that alter luminal and mucosal integrity and nature. Reduction in available mucosa or membrane permeability disrupts enterohepatic circulation of bile salts; unabsorbed osmotically-active substances then can enter colon, exerting direct bowel stimulatory effects	Enzyme deficiencies that prevent complete digestion of fats • Lactose intolerance • Pancreatic insufficiency secondary to obstruction by cancer or pancreatectomy Morphologic/structural changes resulting in decreased absorptive capacity • Surgical resection of intestine Mucosal changes that alter membrane permeability	Large volume, foul-smelling steatorrhea-type stools
Exudative	Characterized by discharge of mucus, serum protein, blood into bowel Results from inflammation, ulceration of the bowel mucosa	Radiation to bowel mucosa; incidence and severity are dose-dependent. Acute effects are caused by depletion of crypt stem cells. Late or chronic radiation enteritis secondary to mucosol atrophy and fibrosis	Variable volume ($<$ 1,000 cc/day) but high frequency stools ($>$ 6 stools/day); associated with hypoalbuminemia, anemia from cumulative protein, blood loss

Type	Pathophysiology	Etiology	Clinical manifestations
Secretory	Primary biochemical disturbance with mechanical responses. Characterized by intestinal hypersecretion stimulated by an array of endogenous mediators that exert primary effect on intestinal transport of water and electrolytes, resulting in accumulation of intestinal fluids	Endocrine tumors can produce excessive quantities of peptide secretogogues. • VIPoma, carcinoid gastrinoma, insulinoma, glucagonoma Enterotoxin-producing pathogens irritate bowel wall, stimulating intestinal secretion. Associated with antibiotic-induced change in microbial flora that permits growth of C. difficile	Large volume, water stools (> 1,000 cc/day) that persist despite fasting; osmolality equals plasma concentration
Dysmotility-associated	Mechanical disturbance characterized by deranged intestinal motility resulting in rapid transit of stool through small/large intestine. Peristaltic dysfunction (enhancement of suppression) in response to alternations in variety of mechanical stretch or neural stimuli	Clinical problems (e.g., irritable bowel syndrome, narcotic withdrawal syndrome) External factors such as ingestion of peristaltic stimulants (food, fluid or medication) or psychoneuroimmunologic effects of stress, anxiety, and fear	Frequent small semi-solid/liquid stools of variable volume and frequency
Chemotherapy-induced	Combined mechanical and biochemical disturbances stimulated by chemotherapeutic effects on bowel mucosa. Characterized by cascade of events, mitotic arrest of intestinal epithelial crypt cells, followed by superficial necrosis and extensive inflammation of bowel wall, resulting in production of mucosa, submucosal factors (leukotrienes, cytokines, free radicals) that subsequently stimulate oversecretion of intestinal water and electrolytes Destruction of brush border enzymes responsible for carbohydrate and protein digestion further adds to excess gut-wall secretion	Chemotherapy-induced gut wall toxicity. Although many agents are associated with diarrhea, most common include • Fluoropyrimidines (e.g., 5-fluorouracil) • Topoisomerase inhibitors (e.g., CPT-11)	Frequent watery to semi-solid stools with onset occurring within 24–96 hours postchemotherapy administration

Based on information from Cascinu, 1995a; Martz, 1996; Mercandante, 1995; Wadler, Benson, Engelking, et al., 1998.

ileum, thus leading to the inhibition of water reabsorption and heightened peristalsis. Combined, these alterations further intensify the severity of diarrhea (Bruner et al., 1998; Mercadante, 1996).

■ High-frequency (> 6 bowel movements/day), variable volume (< 1,000 mL/day) stools with hypoalbuminemia and anemia secondary to cumulative protein and blood loss characterize exudative syndrome. Because albumin is the plasma protein essential to the maintenance of colloid osmotic pressure, albumin levels of 2.5 g/dL or less produce intestinal wall edema, which further disrupts the absorptive process (Burns & Jairath, 1994; Engelking, 1998a; Mercadante, 1995).

■ Diarrhea (acute) is the most common symptom following pelvic irradiation. Reported incidence of peri- and posttreatment diarrhea in patients undergoing abdominoperineal radiation is 20% to 49% (Rutledge & Engelking, 1998). Incidence and severity are directly related to the radiation dose rate and the volume of bowel in the radiation field. Whole abdomen and full pelvis fields are most associated with diarrhea (McCarthy, 1992).

• Concurrent treatment with chemotherapeutic agents known to produce gastrointestinal effects (i.e., fluoropyrimidines, topoisomerase inhibitors) (Engelking, 1998b) and comorbidities such as a history of colitis, ileitis, irritable bowel syndrome, or previous abdominal surgeries heighten the risk of diarrhea occurrence and severity as well as the likelihood that symptoms will occur at lower dose rates (McCarthy, 1996).

• Onset of diarrhea has been described as variable but generally begins following a total dose in the range of 15 to 30 Gy. Patients receiving 35 to 50 Gy develop injury to the small intestine resulting in severe diarrhea that may be unresponsive to dietary and pharmacological interventions (Cascinu, 1995; McCarthy, 1992; Mercadante, 1995). In prostate cancer for example, grade 1 to 2 diarrhea accompanied by abdominal pain and cramping have been reported in up to 49% of patients receiving up to 70 Gy (Jonler et al., 1994; Lawton et al., 1991). In cervical cancer management, a 15% to 25% incidence of severe small intestine injury occurs with 50 to 55 Gy administered to para-aortic nodes and pelvis (Perez et al., 1991).

- Chronic ischemic radiation enteritis, occurring in 5% to 15% of patients undergoing abdominoperineal radiation, has a median onset of 8 to 12 months and can occur as late as 15 years post radiation. This late effect is the result of mucosal atrophy, fibrosis, and vascular insufficiency secondary to damaged endothelial cells in the blood vessels and connective tissues. These changes ultimately produce osmotic and/or malabsorptive types of diarrhea (see Table 23–1) (Cascinu, 1995; Engelking, 1998b; Levy, 1992; Martz, 1996; Sedgwick, Howard, & Ferguson, 1994). The dose-limiting structure in the use of abdominopelvic radiation is the small intestine because it is the most sensitive to late radiation effects (Bruner et al., 1998).
- Overall morbidities associated with neoadjuvant and adjuvant chemoradiotherapy in patients treated for rectal cancer are significant and include small bowel obstruction (5–10%), radiation enteritis (4%) and rectal stricture formation (5%) (Ooi, Tjandra, & Green, 1999).
  - In one study, 100 patients with B_2 and C stage rectal carcinoma treated with postoperative adjuvant chemoradiotherapy were surveyed 2 to 5 years after treatment to profile the pattern of long-term effects on bowel function. The telephone survey revealed that the chemoradiotherapy group had more frequent bowel activity and symptoms than did the group not receiving radiation including bowel movements per day (median 7 vs. median 2, $p <$ 0.001), clustering of bowel movements (42% vs. 3%, $p <$ 0.001), nighttime movements (46% vs. 14%, $p < 0.001$), fecal incontinence (17% vs. 0%, $p < 0.001$), wore an incontinent pad (41% vs. 10%, $p < 0.001$), and were unable to defer defecation for more than 15 minutes (78% vs. 19%, $p <$ 0.001). In addition, the treated group had stool of liquid consistency, regularly used antidiarrheal medications, had perianal skin irritations, were unable to differentiate stool form gas, and needed to repeat defecation within 30 minutes of a bowel movement (Kollmorgen et al., 1994).
  - In another study of 171 patients who had undergone curative high-dose (5 × 5 Gy) preoperative radiotherapy, fecal incontinence, urgency, and emptying difficulties were all significantly higher in the treated group at least 5 years posttreatment. Further, 30% of the treated group reported experiencing impaired social life secondary to bowel

dysfunction versus 10% of patients undergoing surgery alone (Dahlberg, Glimelius, Graf, & Pahlman, 1998).

■ The effects of pelvic radiotherapy on bowel, bladder, and sexual functioning in patients treated for prostate cancer were evaluated by means of a confidential questionnaire ($n = 192$). Moderate changes in bowel function were reported by 25% of respondents while 11% reported severe changes. The most frequent complication related to bowel function noted by respondents was rectal urgency (20%). No correlation between technical factors such as treatment volumes and total dose rate and symptom severity could be documented (Crook, Esche, & Futter, 1996).

■ Diarrhea produces a spectrum of physiologic and psychosocial consequences that may be life-threatening and can significantly impair quality of life.

• Physical complications of uncontrolled diarrhea include dehydration, fluid and electrolyte imbalances, malnutrition and wasting, abdominal cramping, pain and discomfort, proctitis, fecal incontinence, disrupted skin integrity and subsequent infection in the anal and perianal regions, intestinal hemorrhage, and impaired immune function.

• Quality-of-life consequences include but are not limited to sleep-wake pattern disturbances, diminished self-esteem, altered body image, isolation and disruption of roles and interpersonal relationships, altered sexual functioning, fear and anxiety, and loss of personal control (Engelking, Wickham, & Iwamoto, 1996; Engelking, 1998a; Jensen, 1997).

■ Though it may be life-threatening and can significantly impair quality of life, cancer-related diarrhea has received relatively limited attention in the oncology nursing community. Among 1,288 nurses surveyed about their clinical practice experiences with disease and treatment-related diarrhea, radiation oncology nurses perceived radiation therapy as being more influential as a cause of diarrhea in their patients than did nurses from all other practice settings ($n = 93$, $p < 0.001$). This finding suggests that oncology nurses who care for patients undergoing radiation therapy but who do not specialize in the field may need further education regarding the problem of radiation-induced diarrhea in their patients and the impact of combined modality therapy (Rutledge & Engelking, 1998).

ASSESSMENT—ALTERED BOWEL ELIMINATION

Diarrhea is defined as an increase in one or more of the following parameters: stool weight (> 200 g), stool water content (> 75%), and frequency (> 3 episodes or 300 cc/day). Since bowel patterns can vary among individuals, some authors suggest that the definition be expanded to indicate that in order to be classified as diarrhea, stool losses must be significant enough to constitute a change in the patient's normal bowel habits (Fruto, 1994; Martz, 1996; Mercadante, 1995).

Diarrhea is a complex and multifactorial clinical consequence of radiation therapy that may be acute or chronic in nature and that is heightened in patients who undergo multimodal therapies or who are experiencing comorbid conditions. A comprehensive physical history to ascertain risk for occurrence and project severity coupled with establishment of a clear picture of the current clinical presentation are essential to the development of an effective diarrhea management plan (Engelking, 1998b).

MEDICAL HISTORY

The medical history is comprised of parameters that profile the patient's normal and altered bowel elimination pattern including:

Risk Factors

■ Preexisting bowel conditions (e.g., irritable or inflammatory bowel syndromes such as colitis, diverticulosis, lactose intolerance)

■ Previous abdominopelvic surgery—Bowel resection with or without diversion (How much resected? Which segment of the intestine?)

■ Presence of abdominal or gastrointestinal tumor associated with hormonal hypersecretion (e.g., VIPoma), gastric enzyme production, or impairment of bowel function (e.g., colorectal or other abdominal tumor), specific tumor locations (i.e., primary and metastatic sites)

■ Past and proposed therapeutic interventions for cancer management to ascertain those that might induce or exaggerate diarrhea (e.g., concurrent chemoradiotherapy with fluoropyrimidines or topoisomerase inhibitor, use of diarrhea inducing cytoprotectants, chemotherapy and radiation dosage levels, radiation field size and location)

■ Anticipated plan for supportive care plan that may induce or exaggerate diarrhea (e.g., total parenteral nutrition, antibiotic therapy)

■ Past/current pattern of using laxatives and other over-the-counter medications including use of herbal remedies and botanicals

■ History of recent travel outside of the country or family members with diarrhea

Clinical Manifestations

■ Recent change in pattern of bowel function, stool frequency, or character (e.g., frequency, amount, character, time of day, incontinence)

■ Onset and duration of diarrhea, response to home remedies or prescribed medication/treatment plan, aggravating and alleviating factors

■ Presence/character of associated abdominal pain or cramping (intermittent or continuous and intensity)

■ Presence of other associated or coexisting signs and symptoms (e.g., fever, flatus, incontinence, urgency, nocturnal stool, dehydration)

Physical Examination

Baseline Data

• Usual bowel elimination pattern and stool character (e.g., defecation frequency and timing, stool consistency)

• Dietary pattern and habits (e.g., eating schedule and food types)

• Fluid intake pattern (e.g., volume and schedule)

Examination

• Vital signs (e.g., in addition to TPR, orthostatic blood pressures)

• Auscultation for bowel sounds (e.g., normal, hyperactive, or absent), abdominal palpation and rectal examination to rule out fecal impaction and obstruction

• Determination of hydration status (e.g., thirst level, vein filling and emptying times, skin turgor and resiliency, degree of mucosal moisture, intake and output comparisons, urine specific gravity and osmolality, weight)

• Visual inspection of stool for consistency, color, odor, presence of blood, mucus, or pus

- Visual inspection of perianal or peristomal areas to identify disruptions in skin integrity or presence of hemor-
  rhoids, proctitis, or tenesmus.

Laboratory and Diagnostic Evaluations
These evaluations should be employed from least to most invasive
testing with a primary focus on utilizing objective measures to distinguish between infectious and noninfectious etiologies for diarrhea.

- ■ Complete blood count to rule out infection and determine
  the impact of bleeding.
- ■ Serum chemistry profile to determine electrolyte abnormalities and establish the existence of dehydration and protein/
  calorie malnutrition (e.g., hypoalbuminemia).
- ■ Stool analyses to rule out infectious causes (e.g., blood, fecal leukocytes, bacteria such as *clostridium difficile*, ova, and
  parasites).
- ■ Radiographic examination—Endoscopic exploration and
  biopsy are more invasive and are therefore reserved for clinical situations in which diarrhea is persistent and refractory
  to antidiarrheal interventions or to rule out conditions requiring tissue diagnosis.

Differential Diagnoses
Parameters useful in determining whether diarrhea is acute or
chronic are not well established, although these categories are associated with time dimensions, relief patterns, severity, impact on
functionality and quality of life as well as patient population.

EXPECTED OUTCOMES

RESTORATION/MAINTENANCE OF NORMAL BOWEL ELIMINATION PATTERN

- ■ Diarrhea is a common side effect that can be anticipated in
  patients undergoing abdominopelvic radiation therapy.
  Recognition of risk for occurrence and early intervention
  can oftentimes minimize severity and occasionally prevent
  occurrence.
- ■ Empowering patients to identify and self-manage the
  problem of diarrhea by providing anticipatory guidance

and information places them in a position of control and promotes early intervention, thus facilitating prevention of secondary complications that may be more serious and can delay anticancer treatment.

OUTCOMES MEASURES

The multifactorial nature of diarrhea and the tendency of patients to underreport its occurrence produce numerous challenges to accurate measurement of the experience and the impact of diarrhea management interventions. Existing instruments tend to be simple, superficial, and unidimensional, neither taking into account the broad impact of this clinical problem on the physical and psychosocial well-being of the patient nor targeting the evaluation to a patient's unique characteristics, which typically determine the feasibility of available management approaches and have bearing on overall outcomes. Defining the experience, distinguishing among causative factors, and determining whether it is an acute or chronic phenomenon are the most difficult challenges to outcomes measurement. A limited number of instruments that rely heavily on patient self-report and clinician interpretation are available to measure diarrhea in patients with cancer.

- ■ *National Cancer Institute Common Toxicity Criteria for Grading Severity of Diarrhea* (NCI, 1998; Wadler et al., 1998)—A four-point grading scale measuring number of loose stools per day and accompanying symptoms.
- ■ *Diarrhea Self-Report Questionnaire* (Mertz et al., 1995)—A three-part self-report questionnaire addressing stool form (consistency) with pictorial grading across six categories, stool frequency, and diarrhea morbidity grading from the patient's perspective and including a scoring technique.
- ■ *Bowel Movement Consistency Schema* (Pearson, 1996)—Continence history instrument that includes a 10-point pictorial scale representing a range of stool consistency graphics from "watery" to "hard and dry."
- ■ *Incontinence Scoring System* (Rothenberger, 1989)—A scoring schema addressing the type and frequency of incontinent episodes as well as the impact of incontinence on lifestyle.
- ■ *Functional Alterations due to Changes in Elimination* (FACE) (Bruner et al., 1994)—A 15-item Likert self-rating scale de-

signed to measure the construct of intrusion on daily functioning caused by changes in elimination as measured by
two subscales (changes in urinary function and changes in
bowel function).

■ *Cognitive Scale for Functional Bowel Disorders* (Toner et al.,
1998)—A 25-item scale examining psychosocial factors associated with functional bowel disorders.

A number of other measurement tools that include diarrhea
and/or its accompanying symptoms are available and include the *Dehydration Scale* and *Scale for Grading Graft versus Host Disease* in patients
who have undergone bone marrow transplantation (for certain subpopulations total body irradiation is a component of the conditioning
regimen). In addition, a variety of outcomes measures such as the
FACT-D, a modification of the FACT-G (Cella et al., 1993), are available
to measure quality-of-life dimensions of the diarrhea experience.

OUTCOMES MANAGEMENT

A wide spectrum of traditional pharmacologic and nonpharmacologic interventions are available to manage radiation-induced diarrhea. Some newer approaches involving novel applications of traditional drugs, pretreatment prophylaxis, multiagent combination
regimens, and innovative supportive care strategies are also reported. However, definitive scientific evidence to support many of
these management approaches and practice standards is lacking. In
the absence of data, anecdotal observations have led to integration
of these interventions into routine clinical care rendering them
state-of-the-art management (Engelking, 1998b).

PHARMACOLOGIC INTERVENTIONS

Absorbents/Adsorbents

■ Common over-the-counter antidiarrheal agents.
■ Control diarrhea mechanically by forming stool bulk, absorbing water, producing a protective barrier between luminal contents and intestinal wall.
■ Difficult to ingest, thus create uncomfortable bloating
sensations.
■ Have limited efficacy in controlling persistent or moderate
to severe diarrhea.

Agent Categories
- Absorbents (e.g., psyllium derivatives, mucilloid preparations)
- Adsorbents (e.g., kaolin and pectate, bismuth subsalicylate, activated charcoal)

Anticholinergics
■ Act as local antispasmodics, temporarily reducing both gastric secretion and intestinal motility. Exert antispasmodic effects on the gut.

■ Unpleasant side effects that may overlap coexisting symptoms, especially blurred vision, urinary retention, and drying of the mucosal membranes. Encourage prescribing clinicians to seek alternatives to this class of antidiarrheals.

Agent Categories
- Atropine sulfate
- Belladonna preparations (e.g., Donnatal)

Opioid Preparations
■ Act by binding to opiate receptors in the smooth muscle of both small and large intestine to increase tone and decrease motility, resulting in enhanced fluid absorption.

■ Traditionally prescribed opioids are associated with undesirable side effects including sedation and constipation and are therefore reserved for special clinical situations (e.g., refractory diarrhea or patients with advanced disease who are experiencing pain or other symptoms that would be amendable to opioid therapy).

■ Current gold standard and most commonly prescribed opioids include diphenoxylate and loperamide because they are highly effective yet have a limited side effect profile. Both are now available as over-the-counter preparations.

Agent Categories
- Traditional agents (tincture of opium, paregoric, codeine)
- Newer agents (loperamide, diphenoxylate)

Other Antidiarrheal Agents
■ Agents from a variety of drug classes have been employed to manage radiation-induced diarrhea including antisecretory synthetic somatostatin analogue (octreotide), nonsteroidal anti-inflammatories, ammonium resins, glucocorticoids, and thiols. Many of these pharmacologic interventions are under investigation.

- The passage of unreabsorbed bile salts into the colon is known to induce water and electrolyte secretion subsequently promoting the occurrence of diarrhea. Cholestyramine, an ammonium resin, minimizes choleric diarrhea by binding bile salts in the terminal ileum before they pass through to the colon (Cascinu, 1995; McCarthy, 1992).
- Selected prostaglandin fractions thought to cause diarrhea may be blocked by salicylates such as aspirin. A small pilot study at the Royal Marsden Hospital demonstrated that 12 of 15 women with unresponsive diarrhea secondary to pelvic irradiation experienced clinical improvement after treatment with aspirin (Mennie, Dally, 1973).
- Glucocorticoids exert an antisecretory action subsequent to synthesis on intracellular proteins that inhibit the action of certain enzymes and block the release of transmitter substances that stimulate secretagogues implicated in diarrhea production following bowel wall injury (Cascinu, 1995).
- Thiols such as glutathione may protect cells from the toxic effects of free radicals ". . . generated by the interaction between ionizing radiation and intercellular water react with DNA to impair cellular replication, transcription and protein synthesis, events associated with transient mucosal atrophy" (Cascinu, 1995, p. 39). Administering glutathione just prior to radiation in one small clinical trial appeared to reduce the incidence of diarrhea by 24% in treated patients (DeMaria, Falchi, & Venturino, 1992).
- Sucralfate has been shown to be effective in ameliorating diarrhea during pelvic irradiation but recent conflicting data has raised questions about its use.
  - In one double-blind randomized trial, dose granules of sucralfate or placebo were administered 2 weeks postirradiation and continued for a 6-week period. Patients receiving sucralfate experienced fewer problems with acute and chronic bowel distress and had lower loperamide consumption than did the placebo group without adverse effects (Henriksson, Fanzen, & Littbrand, 1992).
  - In contrast, the results of another randomized study of patients receiving pelvic radiation indicated that moderate to severe diarrhea was experienced with significantly greater frequency in the sucralfate-treated group ($n = 123$, 53% vs. 41%), experienced more fecal incontinence (34% vs. 16%) and required protective clothing more often (23% vs. 8%).

In addition, the occurrence and severity of nausea and vomiting were higher in those who were treated with sucralfate (Martenson et al., 2000). More study will be necessary to resolve the debate.

Nonpharmacologic Interventions

Drug therapy alone is rarely sufficient to completely ameliorate the problem of radiation-induced diarrhea. Rather, to achieve the primary expected outcome of bowel elimination pattern restoration and maintenance while at the same time providing for patient safety, comfort, and dignity, a variety of supportive care interventions can be employed as an adjunct to drug therapy.

- ■ Fluid and electrolyte supplementation to maintain homeostasis when diarrhea is severe enough to produce significant fluid loss (>1 L unreplaced) and the patient is exhibiting indicators of electrolyte imbalance (especially hypokalemia and hypomagnesemia).
  - *Oral rehydration solutions* (e.g., Pedialyte, Gatorade)—If patient is exhibiting indicators of obstruction (e.g., vomiting, toxic fluid volume deficit) or cannot tolerate high-volume intake of glucose-electrolyte solutions, replace with parenteral fluids. If patient is replacing orally, recommend that he or she vary the type of fluids ingested to avoid water toxicity.
  - *Dietary modifications* directed at stopping diarrhea or, when that is not feasible, reducing its severity. Primary nutritional interventions are modifications to render the diet low in residue (avoidance of fresh raw vegetables, dried legumes, whole-grain breads and cereals, nuts, high-fat spreads or dressings, fried or fatty meats, candied fruits or coconut), low or lactose-free, high in foods that will build stool consistency (rice, pectin-containing foods), and to eliminate bowel irritants (caffeine containing food and fluids). One randomized trial evaluated the health-related quality-of-life effects of a low-fat, lactose diet on women undergoing pelvic radiotherapy for gynecologic malignancy ($n = 143$) utilizing the 36-item EORTC Core Quality of Life Questionnaire. Findings revealed that fewer women in the intervention group experienced diarrhea than in the control group (23% vs. 48%, $p < 0.01$) without

interfering with emotional and social functioning (Bye, Ose, & Kaasa, 1995).

- Modification of enteral supplements and tube-feeding formulas is necessary when other nutritional alternatives are not appropriate for the patient. Lactose-free sisotonic formula with dilution to at least 75 mOsm is recommended. Adding fiber content to the formula and rate titration are other options for controlling diarrhea (Burns & Jairath, 1994).
- Elemental diets and bowel rest with parenteral nutrition are strategies generally reserved for severe refractory diarrhea that are currently under investigation. In one small study, however, 17 patients with gynecologic cancer were accrued to a study evaluating the effect of prophylactic elemental supplements (ES) during treatment with pelvic radiotherapy. Of these patients, 76.5% complied with the ES regimen. Those who did not comply with the regimen experienced higher grade diarrhea of longer duration (Craighead & Young, 1998).

PATIENT EDUCATION

Since diarrhea is primarily a self-managed problem, patient/family education underlies the success of any diarrhea management plan.

- Make patients and at-home caregivers aware of symptoms that may indicate life-threatening complications including sepsis, obstruction, dehydration, and electrolyte abnormalities. Red flag symptoms to emphasize include fever, excessive thirst, dizziness, palpitations, severe abdominal cramping with rectal spasm, bloody stools, and diarrhea that does not respond to interventions within 12 hours.
- Recognize the tendency for patients to underreport and stress the importance of reporting occurrence and character of diarrhea, self-care interventions employed at home, and their efficacy in diarrhea control. Suggest the use of a diary or symptom log that includes cues for self-assessment.
- Instruct patients/family members on dietary modification, skin care strategies and, use of over-the-counter medications and prescription drugs, when and how to seek professional help.

ALTERED URINARY ELIMINATION

Urinary Frequency

■ Urinary frequency is described as voiding at frequent intervals as a result of cystitis or bladder irritation that produces a sense of bladder fullness even in the absence of a full bladder or at low bladder volumes (Coe, 1991). Frequency also occurs when bladder capacity is reduced.

■ *Cystitis* is the most common acute genitourinary symptom experienced within the first 6 months of radiation therapy to the lower pelvic area. The onset of cystitis occurs during the third to fourth week of treatment with resolution generally within a few months of the treatment completion. Chronic cystitis occurs between 6 and 18 months posttreatment and can lead to significant reductions in bladder capacity, hematuria, and possibly hemorrhagic cystitis.

■ Cystitis is an inflammation of the bladder wall lining. The mucosal lining of the bladder is especially sensitive to the effects of radiation with inflammation generally beginning at doses of 30 Gy. Late effects are seen in patients receiving a total radiation dose in the range of 65 to 70 Gy over a 7- to 8-week treatment period (McCarthy, 1992). The risk for significant inflammation is higher when the patient is receiving concurrent bladder-irritating cytotoxic agents. As with most acute reactions to radiation, the effect is believed to be on cell renewal tissues. However, Dorr, Eckhardt, Ehme, and Koi (1998) found when examining the bladders of mice for acute radiation-induced changes in urinary bladder function that the changes were not reflective of urothelial denudation but impairment of urothelial cell function exhibited by changes in protein expression. The successful use of acetylsalicylic acid (ASA) to treat cell function changes suggests that prostaglandins are involved in the response. Further exploration of the possible role of ASA in the treatment of bladder irritation is underway.

■ In addition to frequency, cystitis can present with an array of other distressing symptoms including dysuria, urgency, hematuria, and may produce urinary incontinence. Patients may experience one or any combination of these symptoms.

■ *Hematuria* is usually described as painless blood in the urine. Although relatively rare, it can be a traumatizing symptom for the patient. It is seen during radiation therapy to the pelvis for cervical, ovarian, and prostate cancers and to the bladder for bladder cancer. Hematuria may be a symptom of infection in the bladder or hemorrhagic cystitis and should be investigated. Hematuria can present as a late side effect of radiation therapy due to interstitial fibrosis of the bladder following high-dose radiation therapy. Interstitial fibrosis leads to dilated blood vessels with thin walls that can rupture easily.

■ *Hemorrhagic cystitis* is a variation of cystitis that occurs late and is considered a serious side effect of radiation therapy. As radiation techniques become more targeted and tissue sparing, this problem is becoming less common. When radiation doses to the bladder were higher than today, hemorrhagic cystitis occurred in approximately 20% of the patients. High doses of radiation to the bladder can result in tissue fibrosis and subsequent mucosal ulceration of the bladder wall. Today, the use of small radiation fractions and changes in technology have made this side effect very rare. However, certain patient subpopulations remain at risk for this problem including women treated for cervical cancer stage IB (Ogino et al., 1995).

■ *Bladder capacity* can be reduced depending on the treatment dose rate and field leading to increased urinary frequency. In one small pilot study examining micturition volumes, no difference in bladder capacity was found in women treated for uterine cancer and only insignificant changes in those treated for rectal cancer were documented. However, in men treated for prostate cancer there was a reduction in volume from week 2 and a significant change by weeks 5 to 6 (Hanfmann, Engels, & Dorr, 1998). Recently, Miyanaga et al. (2000) explored the possibility of bladder preservation for patients with locally invasive bladder cancer stage $T_{2-3}N_OM_O$ using intra-arterial chemotherapy and radiation therapy ($n = 42$). Bladder capacity was maintained in almost all cases. However, bladder function did decrease slightly. Further investigation is required to determine the precise effects of radiation therapy on bladder capacity and the resulting symptoms.

■ *Tenesmus* is the persistent sensation of the need to empty the bladder or bowel resulting from irritation of the sphincter. It is seen in women who receive radiation therapy for cervical cancer (Lamb & Moore, 1997). Tenesmus is a localized response to treatment that has a major systemic impact both physically and psychologically. Frequent trips to the bathroom and the discomfort interfere with the patient's rest/sleep pattern. Fear of not being accessible to a bathroom can be very disruptive to the patient's and family's lifestyle patterns. These responses to this distressing symptom place a great deal of stress on the patient and his or her family and should not be minimized (Cook, Brown, & Redding, 1997).

■ *Nocturia* is seen in a select group of patients undergoing lower pelvic radiation therapy. Men who are treated with prostate brachytherapy usually develop urinary irritative or obstructive symptoms. Urinary irritative symptoms may consist of dysuria, increasing nocturia, urgency, frequency, some difficulty starting a stream, and a weaker or interrupted stream to some degree (Abel et al., 2000).

■ Crooke et al. (1996) studied the patient's perspective to determine effects of pelvic radiation therapy at a dosage rate of 6,000 to 6,600 cGy delivered over 6.5 weeks for prostate cancer on the bladder (*n* = 192). The incidence of symptom occurrence was relatively low. The following urinary symptoms and incidence rates were reported: urinary stream was unchanged or improved in 83%, 2% required the use of pads for incontinence, 0.5% had frequent hematuria, and 2% experienced moderate to severe dysuria.

Urinary Incontinence

■ Urinary incontinence may be a direct effect of cystitis as seen in the acute phase of treatment or it can appear as a late side effect of radiation therapy in both men and women. A patient who has had radiation to the lower pelvic region may experience any stress, urge incontinence, or combination depending on the extent and type of damage experienced during or following the treatment.

■ *Stress incontinence* is the loss of small amounts of urine as the result of increased intra-abdominal pressure from sneezing, coughing, or laughing. Stress incontinence, often seen during the acute phase of radiation therapy, is the result of intrinsic sphincter dysfunction. It occurs in women who receive pelvic radiation therapy for cervix, uterus, and bladder cancers, and in men treated for prostate and bladder cancers.

■ *Urge incontinence* is the involuntary loss of urine following a strong sensation of urgency produced by hyperreflexic bladder (uncontrolled bladder spasms) or an unstable detrusor muscle. Urge incontinence can also be seen during the acute phase and 4 to 10 months postradiation of the female pelvic organs and is usually associated with cystitis.

■ Radiation therapy offers an alternative to surgery that may be associated with a lower incidence of incontinence. McCammon, Kolm, Main, and Schellhammer (1999) compared the quality of life of 460 men treated for localized prostate cancer at 12-month follow-up. Approximately half had Radical prostatectomy and the other half were treated with external-beam radiation. Men who received radiation therapy to the prostate had a markedly lower incidence of incontinence than men who underwent radical prostatectomy. Yarbro and Ferrans (1998) also found that the incidence of incontinence in men who received radiation therapy to the prostate was significantly less.

■ Incontinence occurs more frequently in men who have had a TURP (transurethral resection of the prostate) and are then treated with brachytherapy techniques.

Decreased Urinary Flow

■ *Decreased urinary flow* occurs most often as an acute phase problem in conjunction with prostate brachytherapy. During the immediate postoperative period following radiation implants for the treatment of prostate cancer, a patient receiving a large number of implants may experience decreased urinary flow related to clot retention or bladder outlet obstruction produced by edematous prostate tissue.

■ *Obstructive uropathy* is a potential late effect of radiation therapy to the lower pelvic area. The blockage of one or both ureters can result from retroperitoneal fibrosis secondary to pelvic irradiation, especially if the patient has had additional chemotherapy and surgery. McIntyre, Eifel, Levenback, and Oswald (1995) calculated the continuous actuarial risk of developing ureteral stricture in women with stage IB cervical cancer treated with external-beam radiation therapy to be 0.15% per year. It can result from fistula formation such as vesicocutaneous fistula (from bladder to skin) or vesicovaginal fistula (from bladder to vagina). Although rare, long-term surveillance is recommended for this serious late complication.

ASSESSMENT—ALTERED URINARY ASSESSMENT

The effect of radiation therapy on the genitourinary system impacts the flow of urine either by increasing, disrupting, or inhibiting the flow. The patient will present with urinary frequency, retention, or incontinence. A careful assessment must be performed to identify the causative factor(s) and any other contributing factors to construct an appropriate management plan.

MEDICAL HISTORY

Risk Factors
■ Preexisting urinary conditions (e.g., incontinence prior to lower pelvic radiation therapy, history of urethral stricture, history of chronic bladder infections, stones).
■ Age.
■ Previous surgery to the genitourinary system (e.g., TURP, hysterectomy).
■ Presence of comorbidities such as diabetes mellitus, alcoholism, and Parkinson's disease.

Clinical Manifestations
■ Recent changes in urinary elimination pattern (e.g., frequency, presence/absence of nocturia, urgency, hesitancy, dysuria (painful urination), sensation of incomplete emptying, change in force or caliber of flow).
■ Onset and intensity of any identified changes.
■ Presence of incontinence (under what circumstances does it occur, how often, is intervention required, if so, how many pads over a 24-hour period).
■ Aggravating or alleviating factors (types and amounts of fluids taken in, time of day, change in position).
■ Presence of other associated or coexisting signs and symptoms (dehydration, fever, rigor, constipation).
■ Review of medications to determine impact on incontinence (e.g., timing of diuretic administration).

Physical Examination
■ Baseline data
• Usual urinary elimination pattern (e.g., frequency, presence/absence of nocturia, urgency, hesitancy, painful urination,

sensation of incomplete emptying, amount of urine per void)
- Change in force or caliber of urinary flow
- Color and amount of urine excreted in 24 hours
- Fluid intake pattern (e.g., type of fluid ingested, volume, and schedule)
- Usual bowel elimination pattern (e.g., time and consistency of last bowel movement, frequency of movements)

■ Examination
- Vital signs
- Palpate abdomen and suprapubic area to assess presence of bladder distention or tenderness
- Gynecological exam in women with careful inspection of vagina and urethral opening for skin/mucosal damage and the presence of fistulas
- Prostatic examination in men for enlarged prostate. Visual inspection of perianal areas and urethral opening for skin damage
- Evaluation of hydration status (skin turgor, intake and output comparisons, urine-specific gravity and osmolality)
- Auscultate abdomen for presence of bowel sounds and palpate for presence of stool in the bowel

Laboratory and Diagnostic Evaluations

■ Urinalysis and urine cultures to rule out an infectious process.

■ Serum BUN and creatinine to determine renal function.

■ Serum electrolytes to ascertain degree of dehydration/electrolyte imbalance.

■ CBC (complete blood count) to evaluate for an elevated white blood cell count. If hematuria or hemorraghic cystitis is present, to determine extent of blood loss.

■ Cystoscopy to determine status of bladder lining.

■ Retrograde urethrogram if urethral stricture is suspected.

■ Cystometrogram to measure the intravesical pressure during passive filling and active contraction.

■ Pressure flow studies with fluoroscopy to measure voiding pressure and flow rate for assessing incontinence.

■ Postvoid residual.

■ CT of the pelvic area if obstructive outlet symptoms are present to determine the cause.

EXPECTED OUTCOMES

RESTORATION/MAINTENANCE OF NORMAL URINARY ELIMINATION PATTERN

- Most urinary complications are self-limiting. Acute cystitis is usually reversible and resolves within a few months of the completion of treatment. Anticipation of its occurrence and symptom distress management are the primary concerns.
- Dysuria is often present with cystitis. The goal of treatment is to achieve an acceptable level of comfort as reported by the patient.
- Symptoms of urinary frequency, incontinence, or retention have a major impact on an individual's quality of life. These symptoms could interfere with the patient's desire and his or her ability to socialize because of concerns of accessibility to the bathroom. They could interfere with the patient's desire or ability to be intimate and sexually active. All interventions should be directed toward maintaining the individual's quality of life.

OUTCOMES MEASURES

- The primary measurement of the effectiveness of an intervention will be based on the patient's self-report of improvement. A more accurate picture would be obtained by using a tool that quantifies the patient's report of improvement.
- The American Urological Association (AUA) Symptom Index was designed to measure symptomatic relief following prostatectomy for benign prostatic hypertrophy and may serve as a valuable tool for patients undergoing Radiation Therapy to the lower pelvic area. Abel et al. (2000) utilized this tool to evaluate men undergoing prostate brachytherapy as a pre- and postintervention assessment. The AUA index covers seven areas: frequency, nocturia, weak urinary stream, hesitancy, intermittence, incomplete emptying, and urgency. They found comfort levels could be improved by treatment changes based on frequent assessments using this tool. Although the tool was designed to be self-administered, it could also be administered over the telephone.

- The National Cancer Institute Common Toxicity Criteria (NCI, 1998) four-point grading system covers many of the following urologic symptoms:
  - *Dysuria* (range from none to unrelieved symptoms with therapy)
  - *Urinary retention* (range from normal to bladder rupture)
  - *Urinary frequency/urgency* (range from normal to urgency requiring a catheter)
  - *Ureteral obstruction* (range from none to stent or tube placement or surgery)
  - *Hematuria* (range from none to deep bladder ulceration)
  - *Incontinence* (range from none to no control, in the absence of a fistula)
- Pain assessment can be achieved by a simple tool such as the Visual Analog Scale, which is a 10 cm line on which the patient marks his or her rating of pain from 0 to 10 (McCaffery & Pasero, 1999).
- Numerical Rating Scale refers to a verbal rating of pain by the patient on a 0 (no pain) to 10 (worst possible pain) scale.
- Brief Pain Inventory (BPI) focuses on pain over the last 24 hours. This tool was designed for research but has been used in the clinical setting (Cleeland et al., 1994).
- A patient diary regarding pain and effectiveness of interventions as well as frequency, duration, and intensity of other distressful symptoms is often a useful measuring tool.
- Ferrans and Powers Quality of Life Index Cancer Version (Ferrans & Powers, 1985; Yarbro & Ferrans, 1998) assesses four domains: health and functioning, social and economic, psychological/spiritual, and family. Section I measures satisfaction and section II measures importance of the domains to the patient.
- Prostate Cancer Index from the University of California (Litwin et al., 1995) examines the functioning level of urinary, bowel, and sexual organ systems and the impact of urinary dysfunction on the patient's daily life.

OUTCOMES MANAGEMENT

Both pharmacologic and nonpharmacologic interventions play a role in relieving the symptoms associated with urinary alterations as a result of radiation therapy.

PHARMACOLOGIC INTERVENTIONS

Analgesics

- Oral analgesics offer minimal relief from bladder discomfort.
- Vasodilating agents instilled intravesically may be more effective in reducing severe pain.

Agents

- Phenazopyridine hydrochloride is the most commonly used oral agent.
- Agents used for intravesical instillation include dimethylsulfoxide, silver nitrate, steroids.

Nonsteroidal Anti-inflammatory Agents

- Effective treatment for radiation-induced dysuria.
- These agents decrease urethral and prostate edema and inflammation.
- Certain patients will not be able to take these agents because of gastrointestinal discomfort and risk for bleeding.

Agent

- Ibuprofen

Antimicrobial Therapy

- Bacterial infection can occur in the presence of radiation-induced cystitis and must be treated promptly.
- Antimicrobial therapy should be based on the culture and sensitivity results.
- Prophylaxis antimicrobial therapy may be considered in those patients who are prone to infections or at extremely high risk to contract an infection (i.e., patients receiving concurrent chemotherapy and radiation therapy).

Agents

- Trimethoprim-sulfamethoxazole
- Ciprofloxacin

Anticholinergics

- Effective treatment for urge incontinence.
- Inhibit normal bladder contractions and unstable detrusor contractions thereby increasing bladder capacity.
- Potential side effects include increased heart rate, dry mouth, constipation, confusion, blurred vision. These agents are contraindicated in patients with narrow-angle glaucoma.

Agents
- Hycosamine
- Propantheline
- Belladonna and opium suppositories

Tricyclic Antidepressants
■ Used to treat mixed, urge, or stress incontinence.
■ Exhibit anticholinergic properties decreasing unstable bladder contractions and increasing bladder outlet resistance.
■ Potential side effects include weakness, fatigue, postural hypotension, headaches, tremors, diaphoresis, and epigastric distress.

Agents
- Imipramine (most commonly used)
- Amitriptyline
- Chlorpromazine

Antispasmodics
■ Effective agents for the treatment of urge incontinence.
■ Inhibit unstable detrusor contractions thereby increasing bladder capacity.
■ Potential side effects include dry mouth, leukopenia, eosinophilia, convulsions, blurred vision, increased heart rate, and orthostatic hypotension.

Agents
■ Oxybutynin
■ Dicyclomine
■ Flavoxate

Alpha-Adrenergic Agonists
■ Effective for short-term management of stress incontinence.
■ Act by inducing muscle contractions at the base of the bladder and in the urethra.
■ Contraindicated in hypertensive patients. Because of the side effects short-term use is recommended.
■ Potential side effects include anxiety, insomnia, agitation, difficulty breathing, headache, hypertension, and cardiac arrhythmias.

Agents
- Pseudoephedrine
- Phenylpropanolamine

Alpha-Adrenergic Blocking Agents

- Used to treat overflow of urge incontinence as a result of prostatic enlargement.
- Decrease bladder outlet resistance.
- Potential side effects include postural hypertension, drowsiness, fatigue, impotence, tachycardia, constipation, and urinary frequency.

Agents

- Terazosin
- Tamsulosin
- Doxazosin

NONPHARMACOLOGIC INTERVENTIONS

A combination of nonpharmacologic interventions with or without pharmacologic interventions may achieve the desired goal more effectively than a single intervention. The Agency for Health Care Policy and Research (AHCPR) updated guideline for urinary incontinence is a useful reference in identifying the different options available for the specific types of incontinence (Newman, 1996). Further research is needed to determine which patients will benefit from which intervention or combination of interventions. Weinberger, Goodman, and Carnes (1999) explored the efficacy of nonsurgical interventions for incontinence in elderly women. The women in this study found that the combination of pelvic muscle exercises, delayed voiding, and caffeine restriction was most helpful.

Fluid Management

This management method is based on the urinary symptom, the existence of any comorbidities (i.e., cardiovascular or renal disorders) that may exist, and accessibility to a bathroom.

1. Instruct patient to drink 1 to 2 liters of fluid a day to minimize the irritative symptoms and to decrease the risk of developing constipation.
2. Decrease or eliminate liquids that are irritating to the bladder (e.g., tea, coffee, and alcohol).
3. For those patients experiencing nocturia, they should be instructed to limit fluid intake 2 to 3 hours prior to bedtime.

BEHAVIORAL INTERVENTIONS

Many behavioral interventions exist for the management of urinary incontinence. All of these interventions require patient motivation and commitment for success. Success will be based on preintervention patient education and goal setting (Foster, 1998).

Non-surgical

Pelvic Muscle Exercises (PMEs)

- PMEs are useful in managing stress, urge, and a combination of the two.
- A PME program must be individualized to the specific patient's needs and capabilities.
- The goal of PME is to increase the patient's awareness of the pelvic muscles and increase the contractility of these muscles.

Biofeedback Therapy

- Biofeedback therapy is most productive if done in conjunction with PME.
- Useful in the management of stress and urge incontinence.
- Should include visualization or auditory feedback of the contractions of the abdominal and pelvic muscles.
- Success is measured by the increase in strength of the pelvic muscles, the reduction in the number of episodes, and the degree of incontinence.
- Takes approximately from 2 months to 1 year depending on the patient's age to see improvement.
- Most of the information in the literature is about incontinence resulting from surgical interventions (i.e., prostatectomy, total abdominal hysterectomy). The effectiveness of PME and biofeedback in men who have had a prostatectomy remains unclear. Further research is needed to determine the value of PME and biofeedback in this population (Mathewson-Chapman, 1997).

Bladder Retraining

- The goal of bladder retraining is to increase the intervals between micturation. If the patient's bladder capacity is known and a schedule is established to reflect the capacity, incontinence can be avoided.
- Requires patient education, reinforcement, and an agreeable toileting schedule. Patient compliance can be related to many factors (lack of understanding of process, impatience because of delayed goal achievement). Even with a structured bladder retraining program, compliance can remain low (Visco, Weidner, Cundiff, & Bump, 1999).

- If successful, bladder retraining can lead to improved quality of life (Wyman et al., 1997).

Additional Options

- *Absorbent aids* exist in many forms (pads, diapers, and underpants). Their capability to hold urine depends on the product and the degree of incontinence. This management method can be very expensive and can have a negative impact on one's quality of life.
- *Weighted cones* can be used to improve the strength of the pelvic floor muscles.
- *Pessaries* come in many different shapes and sizes. They are devices designed to correct the angle between the bladder and the urethra increasing outflow resistance.
- An *indwelling catheter* is another method of containing the urine. Catheters can be placed intermittently or continuously. If other methods have failed and there is severe perineal skin impairment, catheter placement may be necessary. Long-term use of indwelling catheters can lead to urethra erosion and an increased risk for chronic infections. Intermittent catheterization has a reduced risk of infection and may allow for more comfort and flexibility depending on the individual.

Surgical

Most patients receiving radiation to the lower pelvic area have also received other therapies such as chemotherapy and surgery. Surgery may be considered an option to treat outflow obstruction, hemorrhagic cystitis, or incontinence if other interventions have failed.

- ■ *Fistula repair* (vesicovaginal) requires surgical intervention. Unfortunately, success of this intervention is compromised because of the prior radiation to this tissue.
- ■ *Cystoplasty* to augment the bladder capacity is another surgical option. It can be achieved in many different ways using different sections of the bowel or stomach.
- ■ *Urinary diversion* should be considered only in severe cases of uncontrolled incontinence. Consideration should be given to the impact of this intervention on the person's quality of life.

REFERENCES

Abel, L. J., Blatt, H. J., Stipetich, R. L., Fuscardo, J. A., Dafoe-Lambie, J. C., Dorsey, A. T., Butler, W. M., & Merrick, G. S. (2000). The role of urinary assessment scores in the nursing management of patients receiving prostate brachytherapy. *Clinical Journal of Oncology Nursing, 4*(3), 126–129.

Bruner, D. W., Bucholtz, J. D., Iwamoto, R., & Strohl, R. (1998). *Manual for radiation oncology nursing practice and education.* Pittsburgh, PA: Oncology Nursing Press.

Bruner, D. W., Scott, C., Byhardt, R., Coughlin, C., Friedland, J., DelRowe, J. (1994). *Changes in Urinary Function (CUF): Pilot data on the development and validation of a measure of the intrusion on quality of life caused by changes in urinary function after cancer therapy* (RTOG 9116, 9020).

Burns, P. E., & Jairath, N. (1994). Diarrhea and the patient receiving enteral feedings: A multifactorial problem. *Journal of Wound, Ostomy, and Continence Nursing, 21,* 257–263.

Bye, A., Ose, T., & Kaasa, S. (1995). Quality of life during pelvic radiotherapy. *Acta Obstetricia et Gynecologica Scandinavica, 74,* 147–152.

Cascinu, S. (1995). Drug therapy in diarrheal diseases in oncology and hematology patients. *Critical Reviews in Oncology/Hematology, 18,* 37–50.

Cella, D. F., Tulsky, D. S., Gray, G. et al. (1993). The Functional Assessment of Cancer Therapy scale: Development and validation of the general measure. *Journal of Clinical Oncology, 11* (3), 570–579.

Chang, E. (1994). *Secretory diarrhea: Overview of pathophysiology, diagnosis, and management.* Hanover, NJ: Sandoz Pharmaceuticals Corporation.

Cleeland, C. S., Gonin, R., Hatfield, A. K., Edmonson, J. H., Blum, R. H., Stewart, J. A., Pandya, K. J. (1994). Pain and its treatment in outpatients with metastatic cancer. *New England Journal of Medicine, 330,* 592–596.

Coe, F. L. (1991). Alterations in urinary function. In J. Wilson, E. Braunwald, K. J. Isselbacher, R. G. Petersdorf, J. B. Martin, A. S. Fauci, & R. K. Root, (Eds.), *Harrison's principles of internal medicine,* (pp. 271–278). New York: McGraw-Hill.

Cook, R. V., Brown, D., & Redding, L. (1997). Radiotherapy. In G. J. Moore, (Ed.), *Women and cancer: A gynecologic oncology nursing perspective,* (pp. 439–539). Sudbury, Massachusetts: Jones and Bartlett Publishers.

Craighead, P. S., & Young, S. (1998). Phase II study assessing the feasibility of using elemental supplements to reduce acute enteritis in patients receiving radical pelvic radiotherapy. *American Journal of Clinical Oncology, 21,* 573–578.

Crook, J., Esche, B., & Futter, N. (1996). Effect of pelvic radiotherapy for prostate cancer on bowel, bladder, and sexual function: The patient's perspective. *Urology, 47,* 387–394.

Dahlberg, M., Glimelius, B., Graf, W., & Pahlman, L. (1998). Preoperative irradiation affects functional results after surgery for rectal cancer:

Results from a randomized study. *Diseases of the Colon and Rectum*, 41, 543–549.

DeMaria, D., Falchi, A. M., & Venturino, P. (1992). Adjuvant radiotherapy of the pelvis with or without reduced glutathione: A randomized trial in patients operated on for endometrial cancer. *Tumori*, 78, 374–376.

Dorr, W., Eckhardt, M., Ehme, A., & Koi, S. (1998). Pathogenesis of acute radiation effects in the urinary bladder: Experimental results. *Strahlentheryapie und Onkologie*, 174 (Suppl. 3), 93–95.

Engelking, C. (1998a). Cancer-related diarrhea: A neglected cause of symptom distress. *Oncology Nursing Forum*, 25, 859–860.

Engelking, C. (1998b). Cancer treatment-related diarrhea: Challenges and barriers to clinical practice. *Oncology Nursing Updates*, 2, 1–16.

Engelking, C., Wickham, R., & Iwamoto, R. (1996). Cancer-related gastrointestinal symptoms: Dilemmas in assessment and management. *Developments in Supportive Cancer Care*, 1, 3–10.

Ferrans, C., & Powers, M. (1985). Quality of life index: Development and psychometric properties. *Advances in Nursing Science*, 8(1), 15–24.

Foster, P. (1998). Behavioral treatment of urinary incontinence: A complementary approach. *Ostomy Wound Management*, 44(6), 62–66, 68, 70.

Fruto, L. V. (1994). Current concepts: Management of diarrhea in acute care. *J Wound, Ostomy, and Continence Nursing*, 21, 199–205.

Hanfmann, B., Engels, M., & Dorr, W. (1998). Radiation-induced impairment of urinary bladder function. Assessment of micturition volumes. *Strahlentherapie und Onkologie*, 174 (Suppl. 3), 96–98.

Henriksson, R., Franzen, L., & Littbrand, B. (1992). Prevention and therapy of radiation-induced bowel discomfort. *Scandinavian Journal of Gastroenterology*, 27 (Suppl. 191), 7–11.

Jensen, L. L. (1997). Fecal incontinence: Evaluation and treatment. *Journal of Wound, Ostomy and Continence Nursing*, 24, 277–282.

Jonler, M., Ritter, M. A., Brinkmann, R., Messing, E. M., Rhodes, P. R. & Bruskewitz, R. C. (1994). Sequelae of definitive radiation therapy for prostate cancer localized to the pelvis. *Urology*, 44, 876–882.

Kollmorgen, C. F., Meagher, A. P., Wolff, B. G., Pemberton, J. H., Martenson, J. A., Illstrup, D. M. (1994). The long-term effect of adjuvant postoperative chemoradiotherapy for rectal carcinoma on bowel function. *Annals of Surgery*, 220, 676–682.

Lamb, M., & Moore, M. (1997). Invasive cancer of the cervix. In G. J. Moore, (Ed.),*Women and cancer: A gynecologic oncology nursing perspective*. (pp. 95–127). Sudbury, Massachusetts: Jones and Bartlett Publishers.

Lawton, C. A., Won, M., Pilepich, M. V., Asbell, S. O., Shipley, W. U., Hanks, G. E., Cox, J. D., Perez, C. A., Sause, W. T., Doggett, S. R. L. and Rubin, P. (1991). Long term treatment sequelae following external beam irradiation for adenocarcinoma of the prostate: an analysis of RTOG studies 7506 and 7706. *International Journal of Radiation Oncology, Biology, Physics*, 21, 935–939.

Levy, M. H. (1992). Constipation and diarrhea in cancer patients. *Cancer Bulletin*, 43, 412–422.

Litwan, M. S., Hays, R. D., Fink, A., Ganz, P. A., Leake, B., Leach, G. A., & Brook, R. H. (1995). Quality-of-life outcomes in men treated for localized prostate cancer. *JAMA, 273,* 129–135.

Martenson, J. A., Bollinger, J. W., Sloan, J. A., Novotny, P. H., Urias, R. E., Michalak, J. C., Shanahan, T. G., Mailliard, J. A., & Levitt, R. (2000). Sucralfate in the prevention of treatment-induced diarrhea in patients receiving pelvic radiation therapy: A north central cancer treatment group phase III double-blind placebo-controlled trial. *Journal of Clinical Oncology, 18,* 1239–1245.

Martz, C. H. (1996). Diarrhea. In S. H. Groenwald, M. H. Frogge, M. Goodman, & C. H. Yarbro (Eds.), *Cancer symptom management.* (pp. 498–520). Boston: Jones & Bartlett.

Mathewson-Chapman, M. (1997). Pelvic muscle exercise/biofeedback for urinary incontinence after prostatectomy: An education program. *Journal of Cancer Education, 12,* 218–223.

McCaffery, M., & Pasero, C. (1999). Assessment underlying complexities, misconceptions, and practical tools. In M. McCaffery & C. Pasero (Eds.), *Pain clinical manual.* (pp. 35–102). St. Louis: Mosby.

McCammon, K. A., Kolm, P., Main, B., & Schellhammer, P. F. (1999). Comparative quality-of-life analysis after radical prostatectomy or external beam radiation for localized prostate cancer. *Urology, 54*(3), 509–516.

McCarthy, C. P. (1992). Altered patterns of elimination. In K. H. Dow & L. J. Hilderly (Eds.), *Nursing care in radiation oncology,* (pp. 126–148). Philadelphia: W.B. Saunders.

McIntyre, J. F., Eifel, P. J., Levenback, C., & Oswald, M. J. (1995). Ureteral stricture as a late complication of radiotherapy for stage IB carcinoma of the uterine cervix. *Cancer, 75,* 836.

Mennie, A. T., Dalley, V. M., Dineen, L. C., Collier, H. O. Treatment of radiation-induced gastrointestinal distress with acetylsalicilate. Lancet 1975; 2:942–943.

Mercadante, S. (1995). Diarrhea in terminally ill patients: Pathophysiology and treatment. *Journal of Pain and Symptom Management, 10,* 298–309.

Mertz, H. R., Beck, C. K., Dixon, W., Esquivel, M. A., Hays, R. D., & Shapiro, M. F. (1995). Validation of a new measure of diarrhea. *Digestive Diseases and Sciences, 40,* 1873–1882.

Miyanaga, N., Akaza, H., Okumura, T., Sekido, N., Kawai, K., Shimazui, T., Kikuchi, K., Uchida, K., Takeshima, H., Ohara, K., Akine, Y., & Ita, Y. (2000). A bladder preservation regimen using intra-arterial chemotherapy and radiotherapy for invasive bladder cancer: A prospective study. *International Journal of Urology, 7,* 41–48.

National Cancer Institute. (1998). *Investigator's handbook: A manual for participants in clinical trials of investigational agents sponsored by the division of cancer treatment.* Rockville, MD: National Cancer Institute.

Newman, D. K. (1996). What's new: The AHCPR guidelines update on urinary incontinence. *Ostomy Wound Management, 42*(10), 46–50, 52–54.

Ogino, I., Kitamura, T., Okamoto, N. (1995). Late rectal complications following high dose rate intracavity brachytherapy in cancer of the cervix. *International Journal of Radiation Oncology, Biology, Physics, 31*(4), 725–734.

Ooi, B. S., Tjandra, J. J., & Green, M. D. (1999). Morbidities of adjuvant chemotherapy and radiotherapy for resectable rectal cancer: An overview. *Diseases of the Colon and Rectum*, 42, 403–418.

Pearson, B. D., & Kelber, S. (1996). Urinary incontinence: Treatments, interventions and outcomes. *Clinical Nurse Specialist*, 10, 177–182.

Perez, C. A., Fox, S., Lockett, M. A., Grigsby, P. W., Camel, H. M., Galakatos, A., Kao, M. S. and Williamson, J. (1991). Impact of dose in outcome of irradiation alone in carcinoma of the uterine cervix: Analysis of two different methods. *International Journal of Radiation Oncology, Biology, Physics*, 21, 885–898.

Rothenberger, D. A. (1989). Anal incontinence. In J. L. Cameron (Ed.), *Current surgical therapy* (3rd ed., pp. 185–194). Philadelphia: B. C. Cecker.

Rutledge, D., & Engelking, C. (1998). Cancer-related diarrhea: Selected findings of a national survey of oncology nurse experiences. *Oncology Nursing Forum*, 25, 861–873.

Sedgwick, D. M., Howard, G. C., & Ferguson, A. (1994). Pathogenesis of acute radiation injury to the rectum. *International Journal of Colorectal Disease*, 9, 23–30.

Toner, B. B., Stuckless, N., Ali, A., Downie, F., Emmott, S., & Akman, D. (1998). The development of a cognitive scale for functional bowel disorders. *Psychosomatic Medicine*, 60, 492–497.

Visco, A. G., Weidner, A. C., Cundiff, G. W., & Bump, R. C. (1999). Observed patient compliance with a structured outpatient bladder retraining program. *American Journal of Obstetrics and Gynecology*, 181(6), 1392–1394.

Wadler, S., Benson, A. B., Engelking, C., Catalano, R., Field, M., Kornblau, S. M., Mitchell, E., Rubin, J., Trotta, P., Yokes, E. (1998). Recommended guidelines for the treatment of chemotherapy-induced diarrhea. *Journal of Clinical Oncology*, 16, 3169–3178.

Weinberger, M. W., Goodman, B. M., & Carnes, M. (1999). Long-term efficacy of nonsurgical urinary incontinence treatment in elderly women. *Journal of Gerontology*, 54(3), M117–121.

Wyman, J. F., Fantl, J. A., McClish, D. K., Harkins, S. W., Uebersax, J. S. & Ory, M. G. (1997). Quality of life following bladder training in older women with urinary continence. *International Urogynecologic Journal of Pelvic Floor Dysfunction*, 8(4), 223–229.

Yarbro, C. H., & Ferrans, C. E. (1998). Quality of life of patients with prostate cancer treated with surgery or radiation therapy. *Oncology Nursing Forum*, 25(4), 685–693.

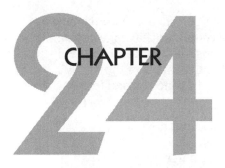

CHAPTER 24

DISTRESS/COPING

Deborah Watkins Bruner
Michael Diefenbach

PROBLEM

Current cancer treatments including radiation therapy can cure or prolong patients' lives, and in fact only half of those diagnosed with cancer will die of the disease. However, the associated physical symptoms and psychosocial problems can detrimentally affect patients' adherence with treatment. This, in due course, may negatively impact patient outcomes such as survival, functional status, and quality of life. In addition, the trend toward outpatient delivery of cancer treatment as a result of improved technology and changing reimbursement, and the longer survival time for patients with cancer, have shifted the economic and social burden of the disease to the patient and family. Not surprisingly, studies show that the prevalence of depression and anxiety among cancer patients is higher than baseline rates in the general population, particularly during the period of cancer treatment decision making and therapy (Cordova et al., 1995; Greer et al., 1992). These elevated levels of distress together with changing patterns in cancer care have left enormous need for psychosocial interventions to improve the psychological or functional status of those coping with the disease.

To improve the psychological status of those coping with the cancer, it has been suggested that a nonstigmatizing word that encompasses all levels of psychological problems—from those considered normal to diagnosable psychiatric disorders—is needed. The ensuing interest in this field has led to the common use of the word *distress* as an objective and nonjudgmental term representing the range of concerns that challenge coping (Holland, 1997).

Cancer diagnosis and cancer therapies including radiation therapy challenge the patient's and the family's coping skills in a number of ways. Patients' concerns and fears include the following:

- Fear of death
- Fear of discomfort
- Fear of disability
- Fear of disfigurement
- Fear of dismemberment

Family/relationship concerns that further tax coping include the following:

- Fear of losing role function within the family
- Fear of losing role function in the workplace
- Fear of losing role function within the social structure
- Fear of becoming a physical burden
- Fear of becoming a financial burden
- Fear of genetically passing on the cancer

The general side effects associated with radiation therapy (covered in other chapters throughout this book) that require coping efforts include:

- General side effects of therapy that assault functional status, primarily fatigue.
- Site-specific reactions that further impair functional status such as diarrhea or urinary incontinence, and assaults on body image such as alopecia.

Indeed, fatigue has been well documented as the number one most distressing radiation therapy–related symptom (Kubricht, 1989; Nail, King, & Johnson, 1986; Oberst, Change, & McCubbin, 1991). Fortunately, these concerns tend to recede over time for most patients with early-stage disease, however mild to moderate levels of distress may persist for more than a year after therapy. And although the minority, a significant number of patients may remain emotionally distressed even longer (Simonton & Sherman, 1998).

In addition to the stressors from diagnosis and treatment, additional strain may come from the psychosocial aspects of dealing with complicated referral and payment requirements of health insurance in general, and inadequate coverage in particular. Health insurance can influence the patient's decision making regarding choice of physician, treatment, and hospital. The challenge to coping for the patient and the family arises from the physical, emotional, financial, social, and employment consequences of inadequate insurance coverage (Glajchen, 1994).

EVIDENCE OF STRESS AMONG CANCER PATIENTS

One recent study documented diagnosable levels of adjustment disorders in 30% of patients treated with radiation therapy with a mean time since treatment of 4 months (range 2 weeks to 7 years) (Montgomery, Lydon, & Lloyd, 1999). This extent of distress is congruent with several other reports of distress in cancer patients regardless of treatment modality:

- One report estimated that about one-third of cancer patients experience significant distress. However, only 10% to 25% of those at high risk for psychosocial problems will eventually use psychosocial oncology services (Cwikel & Behar, 1999; Holland, 1997).
- A study seeking to document the most frequent reasons for referral for psycho-oncology services found five major diagnoses/reasons. Based on a review of 102 psychiatric nurse-generated referrals from an inpatient adult oncology unit, the following reasons for referral were given: depression (31%), anxiety (26%), adjustment disorder (24%), "difficult to care for" (13%), and delirium (6%) (Fincannon, 1995).
- A report of the frequency of psycho-oncology referrals to the Psychiatric Group at Memorial Sloan-Kettering Cancer Center broke the diagnoses into seven levels: reactive anxiety ± depression (35%), major depression (25%), delirium (15%), anxiety disorders (10%), and dementia, psychotic disorders, and substance abuse (5% each) (Holland, 1997).

BARRIERS TO UNDERSTANDING/IMPROVING COPING

Adding to the problem of understanding and improving coping skills is the lack of knowledge of the multifaceted nature of cancer distress, as well as the fact that coping strategies have been related to cancer outcomes in some studies but not others, and reports of effective interventions have been variable. Furthermore, a recent review of the inclusion of minorities and nontraditional, non-middle-class groups showed that they are not adequately represented in current intervention research in psychosocial oncology (Cwikel & Behar, 1999).

Moreover, gender differences in coping with cancer have only recently gained attention (Sormanti, Kayser, & Strainchamps, 1997).

- ■ Antiquated attitudes of patients, staff, and institutions about psychological issues, and stigmatizing labels for those who access psychological therapy have created barriers to the prompt recognition and treatment of distressed cancer patients (Holland, 1997).
- ■ It has been reported that cancer-related distress is often undetected by staff even in patients referred for counseling. A survey was conducted of a sample of oncology patients representative of the workload of the oncology department from which 51 oncology patients' referrals for clinical psychology service came. The aim of the study was to determine the prevalence of comparable psychosocial problems among patients who were not referred for help and to assess whether doctors were aware of the problems patients reported. Referred patients were significantly more anxious and depressed and showed poorer adjustment than the surveyed sample, but 30% of the latter group warranted assessment for anxiety and 23% for depression (Cull, Stewart, & Altman, 1995).
- ■ A corroborating report came from a more recent study that assessed physical symptoms, anxiety, depression, and perceived needs among 204 patients visiting an outpatient oncology department. Participating patients and their medical oncologists completed a survey in which the oncologists indicated their perception of each patient's level of symptoms and affective functioning. The oncologists' and patients' responses were most congruent (80%) for the major physical symptoms of fatigue, nausea, vomiting, and hair loss. However, for all other physical symptoms, physician awareness was less than 50%. Physician awareness was lowest for distress, with only 17% of patients classified as clinically anxious and 6% of those classified as clinically depressed, perceived as such by their oncologists (Newell, Sanson-Fisher, Girgis, & Bonaventura, 1998).

Additional barriers to understanding cancer distress and improving coping are findings that indicate that coping strategies, if broached at all, tend to remain an implicit topic in physician-patient interactions. Yet, some patients consider emotional components of physician behavior to be significant for their coping (Finset, Smedstad, & Ogar, 1997).

The following are factors associated with coping with cancer:

■ Problem and emotion-focused coping—Self-efficacy beliefs and beliefs about treatment efficacy are integrated into the individual's representational view of his or her threat. Altogether, these beliefs along with emotional reactions determine a person's coping and appraisal response to the health threat (Lau & Hartman, 1983; Leventhal & Diefenbach, 1991; Leventhal, Diefenbach, & Leventhal, 1992).

■ A fighting spirit—A study of women with breast cancer found improved psychological adjustment in women who used coping strategies characterized as a fighting spirit (Schnoll, Harlow, Stolbach, & Brandt, 1998; Watson, Pruyn, Greer, & van den Borne, 1990).

■ Optimism has been linked to improved adaptation to chronic disease in general (Scheier & Carver, 1992; Shifren, 1996), and radiation therapy in particular (Johnson, 1996). Optimism has been incorporated into at least one successful program for assisting family members cope with a loved one's chronic disease and improve caregiving (Houts, Nezu, & Bucher, 1996).

■ Spiritual and religious beliefs—Several studies have found a positive correlation between greater reliance on spiritual and religious beliefs and use of an active-cognitive coping style (Fehring, Miller, & Shaw, 1997; Holland et al., 1999). The relationship is more prevalent among African Americans and Hispanics than their White counterparts (Bourjolly, 1998; Mickley & Soeken, 1993; Stolley & Koenig, 1997).

Factors associated with maladaptive coping include the following:

■ A monitoring coping style that is characterized by cognitive vigilance to and amplification of potentially threatening information. High monitors experience greater disease-related intrusive ideation, which usually leads to ineffective defensive strategies (i.e., denial and mental and behavioral disengagement) (Miller, Rodoletz, Mangan, Schroeder, & Sedlacek, 1996).

■ Hopelessness/helplessness—Several studies have documented hopelessness/helplessness as being associated with lower levels of psychological adjustment as well as with cancer progression (Akechi et al., 1998; Garssen & Goodkin, 1999; Schnoll et al., 1998).

- Fatalism/Pessimism—In particular, a pessimistic explanatory style, has been related to hopelessness/helplessness (Burns & Seligman, 1989; Peterson, Seligman, & Vaillant, 1988). A pessimistic explanatory style refers to a patient's tendency to perceive and interpret events in such a fashion. Although no evidence has been found for a relationship between a pessimistic explanatory style and cancer progression, a pessimistic style has been associated with poorer coping and reduced immunocompetence (Kamen-Seigel, Rodin, Seligman, & Dwyer, 1991; Schnoll et al., 1998).
- Low Level of Social Support—Some evidence has been found indicating that a low level of social support may be a factor in poorer coping and cancer progression (Akechi et al., 1998; Garssen & Goodkin, 1999).
- Repression of negative emotions are factors that have also been associated with poorer coping and the promotion of cancer progression (Garssen & Goodkin, 1999).

ASSESSMENT

Multiple conceptual frameworks for the assessment of coping with cancer exist, many of which are built on Folkman and Lazarus' transactional model of stress (Lazarus & Folkman, 1984) as well as Leventhal's Common-Sense Model of Illness Representation (Figure 24–1) (Diefenbach & Leventhal, 1996; Leventhal & Diefenbach, 1991). In this parallel processing framework, a person's belief and expectations about a health threat (i.e., the illness representation) as well as the emotional reaction to the threat are centrally important. Illness representations consist of beliefs about the identity or label of the threat (e.g., "the lump that I feel in my breast must be cancerous"), beliefs about cause (e.g., "cancer is inherited and there is nothing that I can do about my risk"), beliefs about consequences (e.g., "cancer is a serious, deadly disease"), beliefs about the time-course (e.g., "I shall have to face cancer for the rest of my life"), and beliefs about control (e.g., "my doctors know about the best treatment options for me" (Leventhal & Diefenbach, 1991; Leventhal et al., 1992; Miller, 1979). In addition, self-efficacy beliefs (e.g., "I am able to comply with all treatment recommendations, even if they are aversive") and beliefs about treatment efficacy (e.g., "surgery will get rid of the cancer") are integrated into the individual's representational view of the

FIGURE 24–1   THE COMMON-SENSE MODEL OF ILLNESS REPRESENTATION

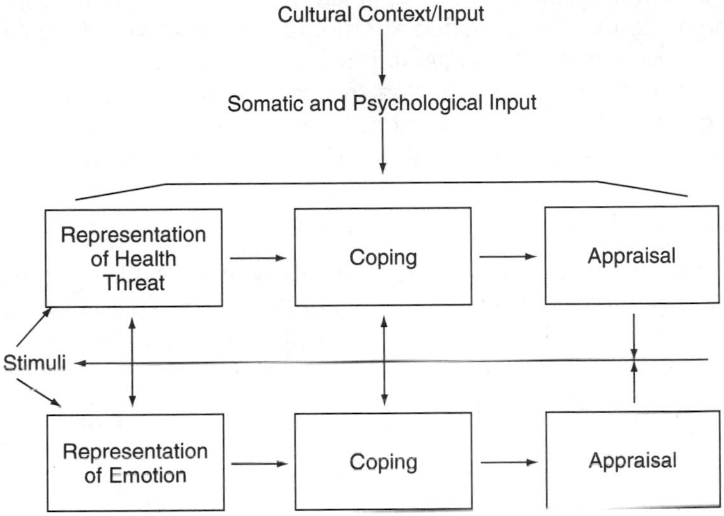

From H. Leventhal, M. A. Diefenbach, & E. A. Leventhal (1992). Illness Cognition: Using Common Sense to Understand Treatment Adherence and Affect Cognition Interactions. *Cognitive Therapy and Research*, 16, 143–163 and M. A. Diefenbach, & H. Leventhal (1996). The Common-Sense Model of Illness Representation: Theoretical and Practical Considerations. *Journal of Social Distress and the Homeless*, 5, 1–25.

threat (Lau & Hartman, 1983; Leventhal & Diefenbach, 1991; Leventhal et al., 1992). Accordingly, these beliefs together with emotional reactions determine a person's coping and appraisal response to the health threat.

Figure 24–1 demonstrates the interaction of illness representations and emotional response to a health threat. On the cognitive level external or internal stimuli evoke the illness representation, which determines a person's coping action and the appraisal of the implemented coping action. Simultaneously, emotional reactions to a threat are triggered. For example, the realization that a lump detected during breast self-examination might be cancerous will certainly evoke feelings of horror and dread. The individual then not only has to cope with the "practical" aspects of the disease but with its emotional aspects as well. This has been termed in the literature as problem-solving coping versus emotion-focused coping (Lazarus & Folkman, 1984; Leventhal, 1970) (see Leventhal, 1970 and Lazarus & Folkman, 1984, for a more detailed discussion between problem and emotion-focused coping).

Other theoretical frameworks have been developed for the assessment and study of coping, illness attribution, health behavior, and outcomes. These models attempt to take into account the complexities involved in coping and outcomes and the situation (e.g., cancer diagnosis and radiation treatments) and person variables (e.g., socioeconomic factors, social support, social norms, and coping style) on which they depend (Molassiotis, 1997; Shaw, 1999).

RISK FACTORS

To maximize the effectiveness of an individual's coping potential, a comprehensive history of sociodemographic, cognitive, and emotional variables that could put a patient with cancer at risk for significant distress includes the following factors:

- ■ Age—Younger age has been associated with higher levels of anxiety/depression at time of diagnosis (Epping-Jordan et al., 1999). However certain levels of anxiety, followed by problem-focused coping strategies, have been associated with more effective posttreatment coping in both patients treated with and without radiation therapy (Dropkin, 1997).
- ■ Gender—In the United States, depressive disorders are generally more common in women than in men. It has been estimated that in women with cancer, approximately 20% to 25% experience clinically significant depression and/or anxiety at some point during the course of medical treatment. Depression left untreated in women with cancer may be associated with a cascade of poor outcomes including significant emotional suffering, slower medical recovery, less adaptive health behaviors, and a negative effect on medical outcome and, potentially, on survival (Strouse, 1997).
  - • Several studies have suggested that men employ better coping strategies when dealing with cancer than women, although the research is scant (Akechi et al., 1998; Dropkin, 1997; Walker, Nail, Larsen, Magill, & Schwartz, 1996). A recent study found gender differences, as well as some similarities, in a sample of 149 married cancer patients (82 men, 67 women) undergoing outpatient chemotherapy for a variety of tumor sites and stages of disease. Women reported more symptoms and higher overall distress than men did. However, general satisfaction with life did not differ between genders, suggesting comparable adjustment. Further analyses indicated that physical impair-

ment, such as older age, primarily explained women's distress, whereas men's distress was closely linked to their psychological condition. Men and women also differed in their use of social support (Keller & Henrich, 1999).

■ Coping style—Two main psychological coping styles for dealing with cancer and other health threats have been identified: monitoring (attending to) or blunting (avoiding) potentially threatening information. Although "Monitors" are generally more knowledgeable about their medical situation than "Blunters," they are also more concerned and distressed about their cancer risk, experience greater treatment side effects, and are less satisfied with and more demanding about the psychosocial aspects of their care. They also prefer a more passive role in clinical decision making, are more compliant with medical recommendations, and display greater psychological morbidity in response to cancer-related threats (Miller, 1995; Ong et al., 1999).

■ Poor pretreatment coping ability has been associated with posttreatment maladaptive coping (Dropkin, 1997; Holland, 1997).

■ Concomitant psychological illness—A history of psychiatric problems is associated with an increased risk of maladaptive coping. For example, depressed patients are less successful in their coping efforts than nondepressed patients (Marx, Williams, & Claridge, 1992).

■ Social support—An association between high levels of social support and favorable coping and conversely between low levels of social support and poorer coping with cancer has been well documented (Akechi et al., 1998; Penninx et al., 1998; Sollner et al., 1999).

■ Health beliefs/locus of control—Several studies have documented strong negative correlations among attributions of responsibility for the cancer to the self, environment, another person, or chance and the adjustment to cancer (Berckman & Austin, 1993). In contrast, once the cancer is diagnosed, the belief that one could control one's cancer and the belief that others (e.g., the physician) could control the cancer have been significantly associated with good adjustment (Marks, Richardson, Graham, & Levine, 1984; Taylor, Lichtman, & Wood, 1984). Of the different types of control, cognitive control has been most strongly associated with adjustment, behavior control less strongly associated with adjustment, and information control and retrospective control (in at least one study) unassociated with adjustment (Taylor et al., 1984).

■ Experience with other life-threatening situations—Studies have shown that survivors of events or illnesses that caused post-traumatic stress disorder are likely to experience significant distress when faced with cancer and therapy (Holland, 1997). For example, a study of Holocaust survivors found that as they dealt with their cancer diagnosis and treatments they were unable to mobilize partial denial and their psychological distress was much higher yet their functioning did not significantly differ from that of the comparison group (Baider, Peretz, & Kaplan De-Nour, 1992).

EXPECTED OUTCOMES

Documentation of successful interventions that support or foster adaptive coping skills has been weak and contradictory. It has been suggested that the reason for this is the disregard of the complexity or diversity of demands that arise from the diagnosis and treatment of cancer (Parle, Jones, & Maguire, 1996).

■ Several authors have reported an improved survival benefit to psychosocial interventions that encourage the expression of emotions, provide social support, and teach coping skills. Among those reporting such a benefit is the now classic study by Spiegel and colleagues (1989) who found a survival benefit for those participating in a weekly supportive group therapy with self-hypnosis for pain, for 1 year. Eighty-six women with metastatic breast cancer (50 in the intervention group and 36 in the control group) were studied prospectively. Both groups had routine oncologic care. Survival from time of randomization and onset of intervention was a mean 36.6 (SD 37.6) months in the intervention group compared with 18.9 (SD10.8) months in the control group, a significant difference. Further analysis indicated that the divergence in survival began at 20 months after entry, or 8 months after intervention ended (Spiegel, Bloom, Kraemer, & Gottheil, 1989). However these study results have been strongly refuted and on reanalysis one author suggested that the 12 control patients surviving for more than 20 months were an extremely aberrant sample, being subject to the strong bi-asing influence of possible confounders. The author further suggests that the intervention had no effect and, in fact, that the intervention survival curve was equivalent to a control survival curve (Fox, 1998).

■ On the other hand, supporting the work by Spiegel et al. (1989), a case control study investigated the effects of a 6-week psychosocial intervention on survival among patients with breast and prostate cancer. The intervention group consisted of 21 breast and 29 prostate stage I cancer patients, and the control group consisted of 74 breast and 65 prostate stage I cancer patients from the same hospitals. The intervention consisted of six 2-hour health psychology classes conducted by a psychologist. The results indicated that the intervention group lived significantly longer than did matched controls. At 4- to 7-year follow-up (median = 4.2 years) of the breast cancer patients, none of the women in the intervention group had died, whereas 12% of those in the control group had died. At the same follow-up period, twice as many control prostate cancer patients had died compared with those in the intervention group (28% vs. 14%). Furthermore, control group survival was similar to national norms. Although the authors concluded that their results were consistent with prior clinical trials, they recognized that self-selection bias could not be ruled out as an alternative explanation for the results (Shrock, Palmer, & Taylor, 1999).

■ In addition to psychosocial interventions, the expression of negative feelings has been associated with a better survival outcome in at least one patient population. A study that examined correlations between psychosocial factors and survival in 133 consecutive patients with head and neck cancer reported that patients who expressed intense psychosocial complaints prior to treatment had a better prognosis than had those who did not express such negative feelings (De-Boer et al., 1998).

Social support including marriage, frequent daily contact with others, the presence of a confidant, and support from health care professionals can improve coping and adaptive outcomes after cancer therapy, as well as have protective value against cancer progression.

■ There is some retrospective data that suggests that major stressful life events are more prevalent in patients with cancer relapse, and that these stressful events may be associated with cancer morbidity. Furthermore, a body of evidence suggests that psychosocial factors have potentially powerful modulating effects on cancer progression. It has been suggested that a neuroimmune link may be one possible mechanism whereby psychosocial factors influence disease-resistance capabilities. Suppression of the immune system by stress has been well documented, and these effects have been modulated by social support. Therefore, several authors have hypothesized that supportive social relationships may buffer the effects of cancer-related stress on immunity, and thereby facilitate the recovery of immune mechanisms that may be important for cancer resistance (Spiegel & Kato, 1996; Spiegel, Sephton, Terr, & Stites, 1998).

■ In a recent study of an underserved population of newly diagnosed cancer patients who were treated with radiation therapy, changes in social support were documented. The impact of cancer on the psychological well-being before and during the course of radiation therapy was assessed in 70 consecutive cancer patients, most of whom were over 40 years of age, women, illiterate, and from a lower-socioeconomic group. During the course of treatment there was a decrease in the well-being scores on some dimensions such as perceived family and primary group support. Even so, outcome improvements were seen in the dimensions of positive feelings, coping, spiritual well-being, and social support other than the family. Interestingly, there were no changes in negative feelings and perceived ill health (Chandra et al., 1998). It may be that any social support is more important than from whom the support comes, or that other coping modifiers such as spirituality may compensate for a lack of social support.

■ In contrast to the previous study, a study of 53 middle-class women who were receiving treatment for breast cancer demonstrated significant negative feelings, in particular depression and anxiety, after surgery and/or radiation therapy. Depression and anxiety each were negatively associated with overall quality of life at all time points studied (Longman, Braden, & Mishel, 1999).

■ In order to make sense of these conflicting reports of psychosocial interventions and outcomes, a meta-analysis was undertaken. The meta-analysis of published randomized, controlled-outcome studies of psychosocial interventions with adult cancer patients identified 45 studies reporting 62 treatment-control comparisons. Subjects were predominantly White, female, and from the United States. The effect on survival was not statistically significant for the few reporting studies. No beneficial effect of psychosocial interventions was found for treatment-control comparisons among several categories of treatment including behavioral interventions, nonbehavioral counseling and therapy, informational and educational methods, and organized social support provided by other patients (Meyer & Mark, 1995). However, beneficial effects of psychosocial interventions were noted for emotional and functional adjustment measures, treatment- and disease-related symptoms, and for global measures of psychological functioning.

OUTCOMES MEASURES

In order to measure psychosocial concepts associated with distress and coping, multiple instruments have been developed. In the perfect world, changes from pre-illness baseline would be the desired outcomes measure, however since we rarely have pre-illness measures on cancer patients, changes from diagnosis through some predetermined follow-up time point become the critical outcome. A select list of psychosocial outcome measures include the following:

- The Hospital Anxiety and Depression Scale (HADS), developed for use with the physically ill, is an easily administered tool that demonstrates clinically meaningful results as a psychological screening tool in clinical group comparison studies with several aspects of disease and quality of life. In a study of 930 inpatients and outpatients with cancer, 47.6% of this population would warrant further psychiatric evaluation using the suggested cutoff score of 8 for the anxiety and depression subscales. Based on standard psychological criteria, 23% had scores 11 or greater and would be the most likely to have had anxiety (18%) or depressive (10%) disorders. Patients with active malignant disease and inpatient status were more likely to have higher depression scores. Furthermore, the HADS is sensitive to changes both during the course of diseases and in response to psychotherapeutic and psychopharmacological intervention. Finally, HADS scores predict psychosocial and some physical outcomes (Carroll, Kathol, & Noyes, 1993; Herrmann, 1997).

- The Hospital Anxiety and Depression Scale (HADS) has been combined with the "Distress Thermometer" as a rapid screen for cancer patients. The concern that managed care pressures health care practitioners to reduce time spent with each patient, and that a distressed patient will not receive proper assessment or be recognized, spurred researchers to develop a rapid means for oncology professionals to identify patients with significant distress. Two self-report measures were piloted in a prostate cancer clinic to detect psychologic distress. Patients who scored above 15 on the HADS scale and above 5 on the Thermometer were referred to the psychiatric liaison for evaluation. There was a 93% compliance rate in filling out the measures, with older men more reluctant to agree to evaluation and treatment. Based on elevated scores from this rapid screening method, 31% of patients evaluated were referred for psychosocial counseling, 59% of those referred agreed to evaluation, and 47% (8/17) of those evaluated met criteria for psychiatric disorders. This approach for rapid screening for distress was acceptable in men with prostate cancer and may have application in other fast-paced oncology clinics such as radiotherapy clinics (Roth et al., 1998).

- The Center for Epidemiological Studies Depression Scale (CES-D). This scale is commonly used to measure depressive symptomatology in cancer patients. Validity and reliability have been established in a number of populations including a breast cancer population and a comparison group of women with no history of cancer. (Hann, Winter, & Jacobsen, 1999; Orme, Reis, & Herz, 1986).

- The Spielberger State-Trait Anxiety Inventory (STAI) (Spielberger, Lushene, Vagg, & Jacobs, 1985). This commonly used scale comes in two versions: the original and short form. The use of a six-item short-form produced scores similar to those obtained using the full-form with acceptable reliability and validity (Marteau & Bekker, 1992).

- The Monitor-Blunter Style Scale (MBSS) has been developed to identify high monitors (who attend to and scan for threatening cues) and low monitors or "blunters" (who distract from and minimize such cues). These attentional differences have been found during decision making and cognitive-emotional coping, especially in the cancer context (Miller, 1995). High monitors have a tendency to amplify and to exaggaerate health-threat information and often experience high levels of intrusive ideation about their cancer risk (e.g., expectations and fear about painful consequences of cancer treatment and poor quality of life). The experience of dealing with cancer often is accompanied with increased psychological distress reactions that interfere with health-protective behaviors (Miller et al., 1996; Miller, Roussi, Altman, Helm, & Steinberg, 1994). Low monitors (i.e., blunters) are more likely to avoid, ignore, and distance themselves from cancer threats. Low monitors are more likely to refuse to attend to health-relevant information that runs counter to their belief that everything will be OK (Miller et al., 1996). Therefore, they are less likely to execute appropriate cancer prevention-control behaviors.
- A tool to assess religious and spiritual beliefs as potentially mediating variables in coping with life-threatening illness has been developed by Holland and colleagues (1998a). The Systems of Belief Inventory (SBI-15R) was designed to address the need for greater exploration of spiritual and religious beliefs in QOL, stress, and coping with illness. The SBI measures spiritual beliefs and practices and social support related to the respondent's religious community. The SBI has 15 items and is reliable and valid in both physically healthy and physically ill individuals (Holland et al., 1998a).

OUTCOMES MANAGEMENT

The diagnosis and treatment of cancer are known to cause distress and challenge coping. It has been shown that psychological therapies improve the quality of life of many participating cancer patients, and there is preliminary evidence that it may prolong life in some cases. Yet despite an array of available treatments, distress in the form of depression and anxiety in patients with cancer remains underdiagnosed and undertreated. This has led several authors to propose that it is time to consider psychological therapy as an adjuvant in cancer management, analogous to adjuvant chemotherapy (Cunningham & Edmonds, 1996).

Health care professionals in general, and the radiation oncology staff in particular, can do much to enhance coping and promote adjustment by establishing good rapport, providing appropriate information, involving patients in management decisions if they choose, and by early and rapid identification and treatment of distress.

- The importance of physician understanding and awareness of cancer-related distress has been highlighted by several authors who have suggested that the central event initiating a cancer-related stressful response is the interaction between the patient and physician conveying the diagnosis, prognosis, or treatment plan. These authors further suggest that addressing the initial event in a cascade of responses is an important prerequisite for progress in this area (Ruckdeschel, Blanchard, & Albrecht, 1994).
- Fears, anxieties, and depression related to diagnosis and cancer therapy need to be addressed in order to achieve the expected outcome.
- Open communication with one's partner or family should be encouraged. With the consent of the patient, including the partner in discussion of outcomes management should be a standard practice.
- Management of radiation-related side effects including the general effects of fatigue and skin discomfort, as well as the site-specific side effects, is required in order to maintain coping skills (management is addressed throughout this book).

There are five main kinds of psychological therapy that can improve coping outcomes including: providing information, emotional support, behavioral training in coping skills, psychotherapy (of various kinds), and more speculatively, spiritual/existential therapy (Cunningham & Edmonds, 1996). Guidelines for the treatment of distress related to cancer have been developed (National Comprehensive Cancer Network, 1999). These guidelines include suggestions for the process of psychological and psychiatric evaluation, treatment, and follow-up of the general cancer patient, as well as specific information for the management of cancer patients with adjustment disorders, major depressive disorder, delirium, anxiety, dementia, substance abuse disorder, or personality disorders.

■ It has been demonstrated that patients' psychological, behavioral, and physiological outcomes are improved when the information they receive about their medical condition is tailored to their own coping styles. Generally, those with a monitoring style tend to do better when given more information, and those with a blunting style do better with less information. However, patients with a monitoring style who are pessimistic about their future or who face long-term, intensely threatening, and uncontrollable medical situations may require not just more information, but also more emotional support to help them deal with their disease (Miller, 1995).

■ Two studies have documented improved psychosocial outcomes after radiation therapy related to individual nursing consultation sessions and group sessions. In a study of nursing consultation sessions on anxiety, side effects experienced, and helpfulness of self-care strategies used by patients receiving radiation therapy, mean state-anxiety scores were consistently lower for the nursing consultation group. This finding suggests that radiation oncology nurses can have a positive impact on patient anxiety at a time when anxiety is often known to interfere with patients' well-being (Grant, 1990). A second study of formal nurse-led cancer support groups for women with breast cancer found that almost three-quarters of the women expressed a positive change in attitude toward breast cancer, and all regarded participation in the groups as positive. A majority of the women reported improved outcomes in terms of adaptive physical and role function (Samarel et al., 1998).

■ Alternative methods to minimize cancer-related distress and promote coping have been tested. One study compared outcomes between a group of women who received an intervention that included imagery and support to a control group. Outcome variables included coping, life attitudes, immune function, quality of life, and emotional well-being after breast cancer. Compared with standard care, both interventions improved immune function, coping skills (seeking support), and perceived social support. Support (but not imagery) improved overall coping and death acceptance. When comparing imagery with support, imagery participants tended to have less stress, increased vigor, and improved functional and social quality of life. However, both imagery and support improved coping, attitudes, and perception of support (Richardson et al., 1997).

In addition to behavioral and psychosocial intervention, pharmacotherapy has shown promising (if underused) results in treating distress in cancer patients. Serotonin reuptake inhibitors (SSRIs) have emerged as the mainstay of drug therapy. Furthermore, numerous studies have compared the relative effectiveness of psychotherapy, pharmacotherapy, and concurrent therapeutic approaches in treatment of common comorbid psychiatric disorders, such as depression and anxiety. Generally, these studies have demonstrated that the combined approach is somewhat more effective in treating the disorder in question, as well as in preventing the relapse of distress in cancer patients (Twillman & Manetto, 1998).

■ Tricyclic antidepressants have shown effectiveness and can improve quality of life for patients with cancer. However, selective serotonin reuptake inhibitors (SSRIs) may be better suited for use in depressed patients with cancer because they lack the significant adverse anticholinergic and cardiovascular effects of tricyclic antidepressants and other classes of antidepressants (Evans et al., 1996).

■ A prospective 6-week, double-blind, placebo-controlled trial of SSRIs fluoxetine and desipramine was conducted to determine their efficacy and tolerability in treating depressive symptoms in women with cancer. Both fluoxetine and desipramine were found to be effective and well tolerated in improving depressive symptoms and quality of life in women with advanced cancer. Fluoxetine may offer greater benefit to these patients, as evidenced by greater improvements in fluoxetine-treated patients on several quality-of-life measures (Holland, Romano, Heiligenstein, Tepner, & Wilson, 1998b).

■ Antidepressants have been shown to have serendipitous benefits that minimize distress related to cancer treatment side effects. For example, venlafaxine has been found to ameliorate hot flashes in both breast cancer survivors and prostate cancer survivors who undergo androgen-deprivation therapy. In patients who received venlafaxine 12.5 mg orally twice daily, 58% of patients who completed the study had a greater than 50% reduction in hot flash scores (frequency times severity) during the fourth treatment week as compared with the baseline week. Therapy was generally well tolerated and appeared to alleviate fatigue, sweating, and trouble sleeping (Loprinzi et al., 1998; Roth & Scher, 1998).

■ In addition, the analgesic effectiveness of tricyclic antidepressants in improving pain outcomes related to neuropathic pain syndromes as a result of tumor infiltration, phantom or stump pain, and postherpetic neuropathy, has been established (Kloke, Hoffken, Olbrich, & Schmidt, 1991). A randomized, placebo-controlled study in cancer patients suffering from central pain was carried out to assess both the analgesic effect of tricyclic antidepressants and the possible relationship between their antidepressant effect and the relief of central pain. The results clearly indicated the superior analgesic effect of tricyclic antidepressants over placebo. Within the antidepressants tested, chlorimipramine, a blocker of serotonin reuptake, was statistically significantly more effective than nortriptyline, a blocker of noradrenaline reuptake. The antinociceptive effect was independent of the effects of the two drugs on the symptoms of depression (Panerai et al., 1990).

■ Furthermore, in treating a major depressive episode in an elderly patient with small cell lung cancer a case report has described possible antiemetic properties of certain antidepressant therapies. During the course of antidepressant therapy with nefazodone, the patient also experienced a remission of cancer chemotherapy-induced emesis (Khouzam, Monteiro, & Gerken, 1998).

■ Panic attacks have been successfully treated with fluoxetine at 10 to 20 mg/day. In a study comparing fluoxetine to placebo, fluoxetine, particularly the 20-mg/day dose, was associated with more improvement than was placebo in patients with panic disorder across multiple symptom measures including global improvement, total panic attack frequency, phobic symptoms, and functional impairment (Michelson et al., 1998).

■ Supporting the earlier discussion of the relationship between distress and coping and the immune system, a recent study reported improved neuroimmune outcomes with the treatment of anxiety/depression in a group of cancer patients. Cancer patients receiving treatment for at least 6 months were asked to take the antidepressant, fluvoxamine, for 28 days. Before and at the end of the study, physical and psychiatric examinations were performed. In addition, subjects' blood samples were examined for total leukocyte and lymphocyte counts, T_4, T_8, and Natural Killer cells. Ten adult cancer patients completed the study. Five of the 10 responded favorably to fluvoxamine treatment. Mean improvement at follow-up was 50% from the baseline anxiety/depression score. There was a significant correlation between the change in the anxiety/depression score of the responders and the change in Natural Killer cell counts, with a mean increment in the responders' Natural Killer cell number of 53%. In four of the five nonresponders, Natural Killer cell number dropped on average by 65%. No correlation between the change in anxiety/depression score and any other immunological parameters were detected (Ballin et al., 1997).

■ Of additional interest, management of cancer-related distress in terms of depression appears to be cost-effective. In a retrospective study of claims data from a large health insurer in New England, cancer patients treated for depression with selective serotonin reuptake inhibitors or tricyclic antidepressants for at least 6 months were more likely to experience significant reductions in the costs of medical care services (Thompson et al., 1998).

■ Antidepressants have shown remarkable success in assisting the terminally ill to adapt, even to the point of alleviating the desire for death because of major depression. In one study, six cancer patients with suicidal ideas thought to be the result of major depression, were treated with tricyclic antidepressants. Three had requested terminal sedation to relieve them from their suffering. The median survival was 4 weeks after diagnosis. One week after the start of treatment with antidepressants, five of the six patients showed a marked improvement in their mood and showed no further suicidal thoughts or requests for terminal sedation, indicating a need for the treatment of distress at all stages of cancer (Kugaya et al., 1999).

■ Regardless of stage of disease, any patient who does not respond to conventional treatment approaches should be referred to a consulting psychiatrist for confirmation of diagnosis and consideration of other treatment options (Strouse, 1997).

RESOURCES

The Internet is replete with resources for coping and can be accessed by simply searching "Coping with Cancer." Some of the standard resources include:

- The American Cancer Society
  http://www2.cancer.org/patientGuides/index.cfm
- The National Cancer Institute-sponsored Cancer Net
  http://cancernet.nci.nih.gov

Many cancer centers, institutions, pharmaceutical firms, and independent organizations offer social support on-line as well, two examples are as follows:

- OncoLink: Psychosocial Support and Personal Experiences
  http://www.oncolink.upenn.edu/psychosocial
- EduCare's Breast Health and Breast Cancer Network
  http://www.cancerhelp.com

Resources for coping with site-specific cancers can easily be found on-line also. Examples include:

- Thyroid Cancer—Patient Information
  http://www.thyroid.com/guide.htm
- Ovarian Cancer—Conversations
  http://www.ovarian-news.com

Published pamphlets and resources to assist with coping with cancer can be found by contacting your local American Cancer Society or through literature such as the following:

- The *Resource Kit for Women With Breast Cancer*, designed to facilitate adaptation to diagnosis, treatment, and recovery, was developed for women with newly diagnosed breast cancer and may be helpful, particularly for women who are too overwhelmed by their situations to retain the vast amount of new information to which they are exposed (Samarel et al., 1999).

REFERENCES

Akechi, T., Kugaya, A., Okamura, H., Nishiwaki, Y., Yamawaki, S., & Uchitomi, Y. (1998). Predictive factors for psychological distress in ambulatory lung cancer patients. *Supportive Care in Cancer, 6*(3), 281–286.

Baider, L., Peretz, T., & Kaplan De-Nour, A. (1992). Effect of the Holocaust on coping with cancer. *Social Science and Medicine, 34*(1), 11–15.

Ballin, A., Gershon, V., Tanay, A., Brener, J., Weizman, A., & Meytes, D. (1997). The antidepressant fluvoxamine increases natural killer cell counts in cancer patients. *Israel Journal of Medical Sciences*, 33(11), 720–723.

Berckman, K. L., & Austin, J. K. (1993). Casual attribution, perceived control, and adjustment in patients with lung cancer. *Oncology Nursing Forum*, 20(1), 23–30.

Bourjolly, J. N. (1998). Differences in religiousness among black and white women with breast cancer. *Social Work in Health Care*, 28(1), 21–39.

Burns, M. O., & Seligman, M. E. P. (1989). Explanatory style across the life span: Evidence for stability over 52 years. *Journal of Personality and Social Psychology*, 56, 471–477.

Carroll, B. T., Kathol, R. G., & Noyes, R. J. (1993). Screening for depression and anxiety in cancer patients using the Hospital Anxiety and Depression Scale. *General Hospital Psychiatry*, 15(2), 69–74.

Chandra, P. S., Chaturvedi, S. K., Channabasavanna, S. M., Anantha, N., Reddy, B. K., Sharma, S., & Rao, S. (1998). Psychological well-being among cancer patients receiving radiotherapy—a prospective study. *Quality Life Research*, 7(6), 495–500.

Cordova, M. J., Andryowski, M. A., Kennedy, D. E., McGrath, P. C., Sloan, D. A., & Redd, W. H. (1995). Frequency and correlates of post-tramatic-stress disorder-like symptoms after treatment for breast cancer. *Journal of Consultative Clinical Oncology*, 63, 981–986.

Cull, A., Stewart, M., & Altman, D. G. (1995). Assessment of and intervention for psychosocial problems in routine oncology practice. *British Journal of Cancer*, 72(1), 229–235.

Cunningham, A. J., & Edmonds, C. V. (1996). Group psychological therapy for cancer patients: A point of view, and discussion of the hierarchy of options. *International Journal of Psychiatry in Medicine*, 26(1), 51–82.

Cwikel, J. G., & Behar, L. C. (1999). Organizing social work services with adult cancer patients: Intergrating empirical research. *Social Work in Health Care*, 28(3), 55–76.

DeBoer, M. F., Van den Borne, B., Pruyn, J. F., Ryckman, R. M., Volovics, L., Knegt, P. P., Meeuwis, C. A., Mesters, I., & Verwoerd, C. D. (1998). Psychosocial and physical correlates of survival and recurrence in patients with head and neck carcinoma: Results of a 6-year longitudinal study. *Cancer*, 83(12), 2567–2579.

Diefenbach, M. A., & Leventhal, H. (1996). The Common-Sense Model of Illness Representation: Theoretical and practical considerations. *Journal of Social Distress and the Homeless*, 5, 1–25.

Dropkin, M. J. (1997). Coping with disfigurement/dysfunction and length of hospital stay after head and neck cancer surgery. *ORL—Head and Neck Nursing*, 15(1), 22–26.

Epping-Jordan, J. E., Compas, B. E., Osowiecki, D. M., Oppedisano, G., Gerhardt, C., Primo, K., & Krag, D. N. (1999). Psychological adjustment in breast cancer: Processes of emotional distress. *Health Psychology*, 18(4), 315–326.

Evans, D. L., Staab, J., Ward, H., Leserman, J., Perkins, D. L., Golden, R. N., & Petitto, J. M. (1996). Depression in the medically ill: Management considerations. *Depression and Anxiety*, 4(4), 199–208.

Fehring, R. J., Miller, J. F., & Shaw, C. (1997). Spiritual well-being, religiosity, hope, depression, and other mood states in elderly people with cancer. *Oncology Nursing Forum*, 24(4), 663–671.

Fincannon, J. L. (1995). Analysis of psychiatric referrals and interventions in an oncology population. *Oncology Nursing Forum*, 22(1), 87–92.

Finset, A., Smedstad, L. M., & Ogar, B. (1997). Physician-patient interaction and coping with cancer: The doctor as informer or supporter. *Journal of Cancer Education*, 12(3), 174–178.

Fox, B. H. (1998). A hypothesis about Spiegel et al.'s 1989 paper on psychosocial intervention and breast cancer survival. *Psycho-Oncology*, 7(5), 361–370.

Garssen, B., & Goodkin, K. (1999). On the role of immunological factors as mediators between psychosocial factors and cancer progression. *Psychiatry Research*, 85(1), 51–61.

Glajchen, M. (1994). Psychosocial consequences of inadequate health insurance for patients with cancer. *Cancer Practice*, 2(2), 115–120.

Grant, M. (1990). The effect of nursing consultation on anxiety, side effects, and self-care of patients receiving radiation therapy. *Oncology Nursing Forum*, 17(3 Suppl.), 31–36.

Greer, S., Moorey, S., Baruch, J., Watson, M., Robertson, B., Mason, A., Rowden, L., Law, M., & Bliss, J. M. (1992). Adjuvant psychological therapy for patients with cancer: A prospective randomized trial. *British Medical Journal*, 304, 675–680.

Hann, D., Winter, K., & Jacobsen, P. (1999). Measurement of depressive symptoms in cancer patients: Evaluation of the Center for Epidemiological Studies Depression Scale (CES-D). *Journal of Psychosomatic Research*, 46(5), 437–443.

Herrmann, C. (1997). International experiences with the Hospital Anxiety and Depression Scale—a review of validation data and clinical results. *Journal of Psychosomatic Research*, 42(1), 17–41.

Holland, J. C. (1997). Preliminary guidelines for the treatment of distress. *Oncology*, 11(11A), 109–114.

Holland, J. C., Kash, K. M., Passik, S., Gronert, M. K., Sison, A., Lederberg, M., Russak, S. M., Baider, L., & Fox, B. A. (1998a). A brief spiritual beliefs inventory for use in quality of life research in life-threatening illness. *Psycho-Oncology*, 7(6), 460–469.

Holland, J. C., Passik, S., Kash, K. M., Russak, S. M., Gronert, M. K., Sison, A., Lederberg, M., Fox , B., & Baider, L. (1999). The role of religious and spiritual beliefs in coping with malignant melanoma. *Psycho-Oncology*, 8(1), 14–26.

Holland, J. C., Romano, S. J., Heiligenstein, J. H., Tepner, R. G., & Wilson, M. G. (1998b). A controlled trial of fluoxetine and desipramine in depressed women with advanced cancer. *Psycho-Oncology*, 7(4), 291–300.

Houts, P. S., Nezu, A. M., & Bucher, J. A. (1996). The prepared family caregiver: A problem-solving approach to family caregiver education. *Patient Education and Counseling*, 27(1), 63–73.

Johnson, J. E. (1996). Coping with radiation therapy: Optimism and the effect of preparatory interventions. *Research in Nursing and Health*, 19(1), 3–12.

Kamen-Seigel, L., Rodin, J., Seligman, M., & Dwyer, J. (1991). Explanatory style and cell-mediated immunity in elderly men and women. *Health Psychology*, 10, 229–235.

Keller, M., & Henrich, G. (1999). Illness-related distress: Does it mean the same for men and women? Gender aspects in cancer patients' distress and adjustment. *Acta Oncologica*, 38(6), 747–755.

Khouzam, H. R., Monteiro, A. J., & Gerken, M. E. (1998). Remission of cancer chemotherapy-induced emesis during antidepressant therapy with nefazodone. *Psychosomatic Medicine*, 60(1), 89–91.

Kloke, M., Hoffken, K., Olbrich, H., & Schmidt, C. G. (1991). Antidepressants and anticonvulsants for the treatment of neuropathic pain syndromes in cancer patients. *Onkologie*, 14(1), 40–43.

Kubricht, D. (1989). Therapeutic self-care demands expressed by outpatients receiving external radiation therapy. *Cancer Nursing*, 12, 21–27.

Kugaya, A., Akechi, T., Nakano, T., Okamura, H., Shima, Y., & Uchitomi, Y. (1999). Successful antidepressant treatment for five terminally ill cancer patients with major depression, suicidal ideation and a desire for death. *Supportive Care in Cancer*, 7(6), 432–436.

Lau, R. R., Bernard, T. M. & Hartman, K. A. (1989). Further explorations of common sense representations of common illnesses. *Health Psychology*, 8(2) 195–219.

Lazarus, R., & Folkman, S. (1984). *Stress, appraisal, and coping*. New York: Springer-Verlag.

Leventhal, H. (1970). Findings and theory in the study of fear communications. *Advances in Experimental Social Psychology*, 5, 119–186.

Leventhal, H., & Diefenbach, M. A. (1991). The active side of illness cognition. *Mental representation in health and illness*. New York: Springer-Verlag.

Leventhal, H., Diefenbach, M. A., & Leventhal, E. A. (1992). Illness cognition: Using common sense to understand treatment adherences and affect cognition interaction. *Cognitive Therapy and Research*, 16, 143–163.

Longman, A. J., Braden, C. J., & Mishel, M. H. (1999). Side-effects burden, psychological adjustment, and life quality in women with breast cancer: Pattern of association over time. *Oncology Nursing Forum*, 26(5), 909–915.

Loprinzi, C. L., Pisansky, T. M., Fonseca, R., Sloan, J. A., Zahasky, K. M., Quella, S. K., Novotny, P. J., Rummans, T. A., Kumesic, D. A., & Perez, E. A. (1998). Pilot evaluation of venlafaxine hydrochloride for the therapy of hot flashes in cancer survivors. *Journal of Clinical Oncology*, 16(7), 2377–2381.

Marks, G., Richardson, J. L., Graham, J. W., & Levine, A. (1984). A role of health locus of control beliefs and expectations of treatment efficacy in adjustment of cancer. *Journal of Personality and Social Psychology*, 51(2), 443–450.

Marteau, T. M., & Bekker, H. (1992). The development of a six-item short-form of the state scale of the Spielberger State-Trait Anxiety Inventory (STA1). *British Journal of Clinical Psychology*, 31(Pt. 3), 301–306.

Marx, E. M., Williams, J. M., & Claridge, G. C. (1992). Depression and social problem solving. *Journal of Abnormal Psychology*, 101, 78–86.

Meyer, T. J., & Mark, M. M. (1995). Effects of psychosocial interventions with adult cancer patients: A meta-analysis of randomized experiments. *Health Psychology*, 14(2), 101–108.

Michelson, D., Lydiard, R. B., Pollack, M. H., Tamura, R. N., Hoog, S. L., Tepner, R., Demitrack, M. A., & Tollefson, G. D. (1998). Outcome assessment and clinical improvement in panic disorder: Evidence from a randomized controlled trial of fluoxetine and placebo. The Fluoxetine Panic Disorder Study Group. *American Journal of Psychiatry*, 155(11), 1570–1577.

Mickley, J., & Soeken, K. (1993). Religiousness and hope in Hispanic and Anglo-American women with breast cancer. *Oncology Nursing Forum*, 20(8), 1171–1177.

Miller, S. M. (1979). Controllability and human stress: Method, evidence and theory. *Behavior Research Therapy*, 17, 287–304.

Miller, S. M. (1995). Monitoring versus blunting styles of coping with cancer influence the information patients want and need about their disease. Implications for cancer screening and management. *Cancer*, 76(2), 167–177.

Miller, S. M., Rodoletz, M., Mangan, C. E., Schroeder, C. M., & Sedlacek, T. V. (1996). Applications of the monitoring process model to coping with severe long-term medical threats. *Health Psychology*, 15(3), 216–225.

Miller, S. M., Roussi, P., Altman, D., Helm, W., & Steinberg, A. (1994). The effects of coping style on psychological reactions to colposcopy among low-income minority women. *Journal of Reproductive Medicine*, 39, 711–718.

Molassiotis, A. (1997). A conceptual model of adaptation to illness and quality of life for cancer patients treated with bone marrow transplants. *Journal of Advanced Nursing*, 26(3), 572–579.

Montgomery, C., Lydon, A., & Lloyd, K. (1999). Psychological distress among cancer patients and informed consent. *Journal of Psychosomatic Research*, 46(3), 241–245.

Nail, L., King, K., & Johnson, J. (1986). Coping with radiation treatment for gynecologic cancer: Mood and disruption of usual function. *Journal of Psychosomatic Obstetrics and Gynecology*, 5, 271–281.

National Comprehensive Cancer Network. (1999). NCCN practice guidelines for the management of psychosocial distress. *Oncology*, 13(5A), 113–147.

Newell, S., Sanson-Fisher, R. W., Girgis, A., & Bonaventura, A. (1998). How well do medical oncologists' perceptions reflect their patients' reported physical and psychosocial problems. *Cancer*, 15(8), 1640–1651.

Oberst, M. T., Change, A. S., & McCubbin, M. A. (1991). Self-care burden, stress appraisal, and mood among persons receiving radiotherapy. *Cancer Nursing*, 14(2), 71–78.

Ong, L. M., Visser, M. R., van Zuuren, F. J., Rietbroek, R. C., Lammes, F. B., & de Haes, J. C. (1999). Cancer patients' coping styles and doctor-patient communication. *Psycho-Oncology*, 8(2), 155–166.

Orme, J. G., Reis, J., & Herz, E. J. (1986). Factorial and discriminant validity of the Center for Epidemiological Studies Depression (CES-D) Scale. *Journal of Clinical Psychology*, 42(1), 28–33.

Panerai, A. E., Monza, G., Movilia, P., Bianchi, M., Francucci, B. M., &
  Tiengo, M. (1990). A randomized, within-patient, cross-over, placebo-
  controlled trial on the efficacy and tolerability of the tricyclic antidepressant chlorimipramine and nortriptyline in central pain. Acta Neuro-
  logica Scandinavica, 82(1), 34–38.

Parle, M., Jones, B., & Maguire, P. (1996). Maladaptive coping and affective
  disorders among cancer patients. Psychological Medicine, 26(4) 735–744.

Penninx, B. W., van Tilburg, T., Boeke, A. J., Deeg, D. J., Kriegsman, D. M., &
  van Eijk, J. T. (1998). Effects of social support and personal coping resources on depressive symptoms: Different for various chronic diseases. Health Psychology, 17(6), 551–558.

Peterson, C., Seligman, M. E. P., & Vaillant, G. E. (1988). Pessimistic explanatory style is a risk factor for physical illness: A thirty-five year
  longitudinal study. Journal of Personality and Social Psychology, 55, 23–27.

Richardson, M. A., Post-White, J., Grimm, E. A., Moye, L. A., Singletary,
  S. E., & Justice, B. (1997). Coping, life attitudes, and immune re-
  sponses to imagery and group support after breast cancer treatment.
  Alternative Therapies in Health and Medicine, 3(5), 62–70.

Roth, A. J., Kornblith, A. B., Batel-Copel, L., Peabody, E., Scher, H. I., & Holland, J. C. (1998). Rapid screening for psychologic distress in men with
  prostate carcinoma: A pilot study. Cancer, 82(10), 1904–1908.

Roth, A. J., & Scher, H. I. (1998). Sertraline relieves hot flashes secondary to
  medical castration as treatment of advanced prostate cancer. Psycho-
  Oncology, 7(2), 129–132.

Ruckdeschel, J. C., Blanchard, C. G., & Albrecht, T. (1994). Where we have
  been, where we are going, and why we will not get there. Cancer, 74(4
  Suppl.), 1458–1463.

Samarel, N., Fawcett, J., Krippendorf, K., Piacentino, J. C., Eliasof, B.,
  Hughes, P., Kowitski, C., & Ziegler, E. (1998). Women's perceptions of
  group support and adaptation to breast cancer. Journal of Advanced
  Nursing, 28(6), 1259–1268.

Samarel, N., Fawcett, J., Tulman, L., Rothman, H., Spector, L., Spillane,
  P. A., Dickson, M. A., & Toole, J. H. (1999). A resource kit for women
  with breast cancer: Development and evaluation. Oncology Nursing Forum, 26(3), 611–618.

Scheier, M. F., & Carver, C. S. (1992). Effects of optimism on psychological
  and physical well-being: Theoretical overview and empirical update.
  Cognitive Therapy and Research, 16, 201–228.

Schnoll, R. A., Harlow, L. L., Stolbach, L. L., & Brandt, U. (1998). A structural model of the relationships among stage of disease, age, coping,
  and psychological adjustment in women with breast cancer. Psycho-
  Oncology, 7, 69–77.

Shaw, C. (1999). A framework for the study of coping, illness behaviour and
  outcomes. Journal of Advanced Nursing, 29(5), 1246–1255.

Shifren, K. (1996). Individual differences in the perception of optimism and
  disease severity: A study among individuals with Parkinson's disease.
  Journal of Behavioral Medicine, 19(3), 241–271.

Shrock, D., Palmer, R. F., & Taylor, B. (1999). Effects of a psychosocial intervention on survival among patients with stage I breast and prostate cancer: A matched case-control study. *Alternative Therapies in Health and Medicine*, 5(3), 49–55.

Simonton, S. S., & Sherman, A. C. (1998). Psychological aspects of mind-body medicine: Promises and pitfalls form research with cancer patients. *Alternative Therapies*, 4(4), 50–67.

Sollner, W., Zschocke, I., Zingg-Schir, M., Stein, B., Rumpold, G., Fritsch, P., & Augustin, M. (1999). Interactive patterns of social support and individual coping strategies in melanoma patients and their correlations with adjustment to illness. *Psychosomatics*, 40(3), 239–250.

Sormanti, M., Kayser, K., & Strainchamps, E. (1997). A relational perspective of women coping with cancer: A preliminary study. *Social Work in Health Care*, 25(1–2), 89–106.

Spiegel, D., Bloom, J. R., Kraemer, H. C., & Gottheil, E. (1989). Effect of psychosocial treatment on survival of patients with metastatic breast cancer. *Lancet*, 2(8668), 888–891.

Spiegel, D., & Kato, P. M. (1996). Psychosocial influences on cancer incidence and progression. *Harvard Review of Psychiatry*, 4(1), 10–26.

Spiegel, D., Sephton, S. E., Terr, A. I., & Stites, D. P. (1998). Effects of psychosocial treatment in prolonging cancer survival may be mediated by neuroimmune pathways. *Annals of the New York Academy of Sciences*, 840, 674–683.

Spielberger, C. D., Lushene, R. E., Vagg, B. A., & Jacobs, E. (1985). *State-trait anxiety inventory*. Palo Alto, CA: Consulting Psychologist Press.

Stolley, J. M., & Koenig, H. (1997). Religion/spirituality and health among elderly African-Americans and Hispanics. *Journal of Psychosocial Nursing and Mental Health Services*, 35(11), 32–38.

Strouse, T. (1997). Identifying and treating depression in women with cancer: A primary care approach. *Medscape Women's Health*, 2(9), 3–5.

Taylor, S. E., Lichtman, R. R., & Wood, J. V. (1984). Attributions, beliefs about control, and adjustment to breast cancer. *Journal of Personality and Social Psychology*, 46(3), 489–502.

Thompson, D., Hylan, T. R., McMullen, W., Romeis, M. E., Buesching, D., & Oster, G. (1998). Predictors of a medical-offset effect among patients receiving antidepressant therapy. *American Journal of Psychiatry*, 155(6), 824–827.

Twillman, R. K., & Manetto, C. (1998). Concurrent psychotherapy and pharmacotherapy in the treatment of depression and anxiety in cancer patients. *Psycho-Oncology*, 7(4), 285–290.

Walker, B. L., Nail, L. M., Larsen, L., Magill, J., & Schwartz, A. (1996). Concerns, affect, and cognitive disruption following completion of radiation treatment for localized breast or prostate cancer. *Oncology Nursing Forum*, 23(8), 1181–1187.

Watson, M., Pruyn, J., Greer, S., & van den Borne, B. (1990). Locus of control and adjustment to cancer. *Psychological Reports*, 66(1), 39–48.

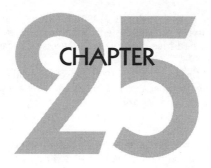

CHAPTER 25

MAINTENANCE OF EFFICIENT VENTILATION

Audrey G. Gift, PhD, RN

PROBLEM

Dyspnea is defined as "a subjective experience of breathing discomfort that consists of qualitatively distinct sensations that vary in intensity. The experience derives from interactions among multiple physiological, psychological, social, and environmental factors, and may induce secondary physiological and behavioral responses" (Meek etal., 1999, p. 322). It has been estimated that dyspnea occurs in 21% to 78.6% of patients with advanced cancer and is reported to be at the moderate to severe level in 10% to 63% of patients (Ripamonti, 1999). These symptoms, however, have been vastly underreported by patients and unnoticed by health care professionals, especially in late-stage cancer (Roberts, Thorne, & Pearson, 1993). Those with late-stage cancer report having significant, prolonged dyspnea lasting 3 months or more (Dudgeon et al., 1999). It is accompanied by feelings of fear, extreme fatigue, loss of memory, concentration, and appetite (Brown, Carrieri, Janson-Bjerklie, & Dodd, 1986). A study of terminally ill cancer patients showed them to be troubled by dyspnea and pain, with the pain being relieved soon after referral, but the dyspnea increasing until the time of death (Higginson & McCarthy, 1989). Unrelieved dyspnea is very frightening for both the patient and family and is one of the main reasons for families to hospitalize cancer patients. Unrelieved symptoms requiring emergency room treatment have been shown to be predictive of impending death (Escalante et al., 1996). Even without emergency room treatment the presence of dyspnea is of deep concern because it has been associated with loss of function and increased mortality (Reuben & Mor, 1988). The problem is complicated by the lack of an understanding of strategies to relieve symptoms on the part of physicians (Sloan, Donnely, Schwartz, & Sloan, 1997).

MECHANISMS OF DYSPNEA

Physiological Mechanisms

Neuromechanical or efferent-reafferent dissociation theory of dyspnea states that dyspnea is caused by a dissociation or mismatch between central respiratory motor activity and incoming afferent information from receptors in airways, lungs, and chest wall. Therefore, dyspnea is intensified when changes in airflow, respiratory pressure, or respiratory movement are not appropriate for the outgoing motor command (Meek et al., 1999). Dyspnea can be caused by heightened ventilatory demand, respiratory muscle abnormalities, abnormal ventilatory impedence, and abnormal breathing patterns.

Neurochemical changes in blood gases resulting in hypoxemia and hypercapnia stimulate chemoreceptors and result in respiratory motor activity. They may also have a direct dyspneogenic effect, since dyspnea can occur even without ventilatory changes.

Dyspnea after radiation therapy is related to the percent of total lung irradiated as well as the dose of radiation. The reaction is bimodal with early and late characteristics. A few weeks to months after exposure to radiation the lung reacts with congestion and intraalveolar edema. The edema then organizes into collagen fibriles, which eventually leads to thickening of the alveolar septa. This is the stage known as acute radiation pneumonitis. It is believed that damage to the type II pneumocyte, which produces surfactant, and the endothelial cell is closely linked to this process. Changes in the surfactant system, leading to alterations in alveolar surface tension and low lung compliance are most likely a direct result of the radiation. The late lung injury is characterized by progressive fibrosis of alveolar septa that become thickened by bundles of elastic fibers and collagen. The alveoli later collapse and are obliterated by connective tissue (McDonald, Rubin, Phillips, & Marks, 1995).

Psychosocial Mechanisms

There are affective influences on dyspnea perception. The correlation between dyspnea and anxiety has been demonstrated in a number of studies (Carrieri, Kohlman, Gormley, Douglas, Paul, & Stulbarg, 1996; Gift, 1991; Gift, Plaut, & Jacox, 1986). While found to be related, there are no studies demonstrating a cause and effect relationship between dyspnea and anxiety. Coping strategies have been found to effect the perception of dyspnea (Carriere, Jansen-Bjerklie, 1986).

Cognition, judgment, and attention have also been shown to influence the perception of dypsnea. The interpretation or meaning of dyspnea influences the patient's perception of severity (Teel, Meek, McNamara, Watson, 1997). There have not been any studies in cancer patients to determine if a diagnosis of cancer or advanced cancer enhances the perception of dyspnea intensity.

Mechanism Causing Insufficient Ventilation in Cancer

■ Insufficient ventilation is most commonly associated with breast, lung, and colorectal cancer (Acheson & MacCormack, 1997). It has been shown to be related to the space occupying tumor directly, indirectly because of the debilitating nature of the disease, or to the treatment modalities used in cancer.

■ Insufficient ventilation directly related to cancer tumor includes the following:

   a. Bronchial or airway obstruction
   b. Superior vena cava syndrome obstruction
   c. Tumor invasion of lung tissue
   d. Lymphatic spread
   e. Phrenic nerve paralysis
   f. Pleural effusion(s)
   g. Pericardial effusion
   h. Ascites
   i. Hepatomegaly

■ Insufficient ventilation indirectly related to cancer such as that resulting from other disease effects or debilitation includes the following (Acheson & MacCormack, 1997):

   a. Anemia
   b. Cachexia
   c. Pulmonary embolism
   d. Pulmonary aspiration
   e. Pneumonia
   f. Electrolyte imbalance
   g. Mucositis
   h. Infection

- Insufficient ventilation can also be related to radiation therapy (Acheson & Beinert et al., 1999; MacCormack, 1997). In addition to the disease of cancer, the effects of the treatment can also result directly in ventilatory impairment. Radiation therapy can result in destruction of the lung parenchyma and result in impairment in ventilation. The clinical pathologic course is biphasic and is dependent on the dose and volume of lung exposed to the radiation as well as the patient's preexisting pulmonary reserves. The process involves changes in the surfactant system, leading to alterations in alveolar surface tension and low compliance, which are the direct results of the radiation and become evident within weeks to months after exposure. These changes usually resolve within a few weeks or months, but can lead to acute radiation pneumonitis (McDonald et al., 1995).
- Classical radiation pneumonitis is characterized by a threshold dose of radiotherapy, a narrow sigmoid dose-response relation, and an inflammatory reaction confined to the lung volume irradiated. Radiation pneumonitis and pulmonary fibrosis are thought to be caused by reactive oxygen species (ROS) by causing cell component alterations and changing cellular protein expression. In complex cell-cytokine-interactions, ROS give rise to a self-amplifying cascade of tissue damage, inflammation, and finally fibroblast activation with development of pulmonary fibrosis (Beinart et al., 1999).
- Sporadic radiation pneumonitis represents an out-of-field, lymphocytic inflammation, and seems to be an immunologically medicated process because of the vast amounts of lung antigens that are released with tissue damage. Severity of this type of radiation pneumonitis does not clearly follow a dose-effect relationship and shows lesser fibrogenic tendencies (Beinart et al., 1999). The cytokine transforming growth factor beta$_1$ has been implicated in the development of normal tissue injury after irradiation in several organs including the lung (Anscher, Kong, & Jirtle, 1998).
- The late lung injury is characterized by progressive fibrosis. The mechanisms of chronic complications are believed by some to be related to the effects of radiation on the vascular tissue and may be evident months to years following treatment (McDonald et al., 1995).

ASSESSMENT

The assessment of the patient needs to be a comprehensive evaluation of the patient's pretreatment pulmonary function including comorbid conditions such as respiratory disease, cardiac disease, anemia, obesity, or other factors that may contribute to respiratory compromise. The patient's response to radiation therapy is also important.

MEDICAL HISTORY

The medical history should include an assessment of the type, location, size, and stage of the cancer as well as other comorbidities the patient may have. The specifics of the radiation therapy such as the site, dose, and extent of the area irradiated need to be determined. In radiation therapy–induced dyspnea, especially the classical radiation pneumonitis, the severity of lung injury is highly correlated with the extent of lung volume incorporated in the field of radiation (Shulimzon et al., 1996).

Dyspnea should be characterized by assessing its onset, either sudden or gradual, factors precipitating dyspnea, its frequency, duration, quality, and the distress the patient feels as a result of the dyspnea (Meek et al., 1999). Dyspnea cannot be assessed in isolation, in fact many recommend that it be assessed by inquiring about the activities that precipitate the dyspnea or the effort required to perform those activities (Mahler, Weinberg, Wells, & Feinstein, 1984).

Radiation pulmonary impairment is characterized by the symptoms of fever, cough, and shortness of breath. The signs of respiratory rate include signs on percussion of pleural effusion, signs on auscultation, and occasionally of rales or rhonchi (McDonald et al., 1995). Symptoms are often not reported by the patient until 1 to 3 months after completion of radiation and occur in only 5% to 15% of patients. Symptoms are most likely to appear in patients who have mediastinal irradiation, such as those treated for lymphoma, lung, or breast cancer. The severity of the symptoms is related to the degree of pulmonary involvement. There may be low-grade fever, dyspnea, cough, congestion, or fullness in the chest. Physical signs are usually absent in the chest except for consolidation in the area of injury. Generally, this phase with acute symptoms is relatively short in duration and is followed by an intermittent phase during which the histological changes progress but the symptoms are not as marked.

This progresses to the eventual fibrotic phase that is characterized by minimal symptoms unless more than 50% of the lung is involved (McDonald et al., 1995).

Pulmonary Function Tests

The ratio of forced expiratory volume to forced vital capacity (FEV_1/FVC) is the accepted standard measure of obstructive pulmonary disability when compared with the predicted normal values (Knudson, Slatin, Lebowitz, & Burrows, 1976; Thurlbeck, 1983). Spirometry is the best technique for obtaining the two diagnostic parameters, the FEV_1 and vital capacity (FVC). Pulmonary function laboratories should meet the criteria for accuracy established by the American Thoracic Society (1991) (Gardner & Hankinson 1987). The relationship between pulmonary function tests (PFTs) and dyspnea varies with the disease being studied. In chronic obstructive pulmonary disease (COPD) a low relationship was found, while in cancer 93% of cancer patients with dyspnea were found to have abnormal PFTs (Dudgeon, Lertzman, 1998). It has been shown that the forced vital capacity and total lung capacity have been found by some to decrease between 6% and 8% after radiation therapy (Abratt & Willcox, 1995), while others examining changes after local irradiation of the chest have not found such decreases (Hardman et al., 1994). There are, however, changes seen in lung perfusion that develop over 3 to 6 months following regional lung radiation and are dose-dependent (Marks et al., 1997). It is important for the clinician to determine the pretreatment diffusion capacity because it has been found to be predictive of clinical tolerance to irradiation (Abratt & Willcox, 1995). After radiation therapy patients should be assessed using ventilation-perfusion scintigraphy to differentiate between radiation pneumonitis and other causes of dyspnea (Chin, Welsh, Kleinberg, Ettinger, & White, 1999). Radiation pneumonitis often mimics infectious pneumonitis because they share many clinical symptoms. It is recommended that differentiation involve first chest radiograph to detect a sharp margin conforming to the port of irradiation. If the x-ray is not characteristic, it will be necessary to rule out infection by conventional measures or perhaps bronchoscopy (Salinas & Winterbauer, 1995). Asessment of respiratory muscle function is also important in determining patient potential for ventilatory impairment, since diminished maximum inspiratory pressure (MIP) can be present in those cancer patients with severe dyspnea (Dudgeon & Lertzman, 1998).

In radiation pneumonitis, abnormalities relate to the volume of irradiated lung tissue and consist of decreases in the vital capacity, residual volume, and the FEV_1. Decreases in lung compliance will also be noted. The diffusion capacity appears to be the most sensitive parameter in this situation (McDonald et al., 1995).

ARTERIAL BLOOD GASES

Arterial blood gases (ABGs) are important in the assessment of dyspnea. These can be taken at rest without supplemental oxygen if possible. The parameters used include partial pressure of oxygen and carbon dioxide as well as oxygen saturation. Since dyspnea is contextual and related to exercise, oxygen saturation during graded exercise is a particularly useful parameter. Abnormalities seen after radiation therapy include a fall in diffusion capacity, mild arterial hypoxemia, often manifested only with exercise and normal or low PCO_2 (McDonald et al., 1995).

BRONCHOALVEOLAR LAVAGE

In addition to the ABGs, patients with suspected lung injuries after radiation therapy should have a bronchoalveolar lavage to determine the level of accumulated activated T-cells (HLADR and ICAM-1 positive T-cells) in the lung since they have been found to be a marker of radiation pneumonitis (Nakayama et al., 1996). Other experimental methods such as the use of 99mTc-DTPA aerosol lung clearance, which has been found to be sensitive to early changes in radiation pneumonitis, are being explored (Susskind et al., 1997).

The only physical sign that is related to dyspnea is *accessory muscle use*. In a clinical setting, it can be determined while the subject is in a sitting position and observing for the rise of the clavicle during inspiration. If it is not detected, it can be described as absent; if it is seen to rise but it is bearly perceptible, it can be described as mild; and if it is pronounced, it can be described as severe. In a study of 20 COPD patients measured at a time of high, medium, and low dyspnea, the only clinical sign found to be significantly increased as dyspnea increased was the retraction of the sternomastoid muscle (Gift et al., 1986). Sternomastoid muscle use is also greater during high dyspnea when compared with low dyspnea in a study of 36 asthmatic patients (Gift, 1991). The use of accessory muscle use as an indicator of dyspnea has also been validated in a laboratory setting with 18 normal subjects by adding an inspiratory resistance at 60% of the subjects' maximal inspiratory pressure (Breslin, Garoutte, Carrieri, & Celli,

1990). Comparing breathing during the resistive load with breathing under controlled, normal conditions, they found that it was the increased recruitment of the sternomastoid muscle, not the diaphragm, that was associated with dyspnea. Thus, accessory muscle use appears to be the most appropriate clinical sign of dyspnea.

ASSESSMENT OF CAREGIVER NEEDS

Providing care in the home to a terminally ill loved one is very stressful (Neundorfer, 1991; Norbeck, Chaftez, Wilson, & Weiss, 1991). The caretaker becomes increasingly stressed and reports an increase in physical and emotional symptoms during this time. In an interview with caregivers of psychiatric patients, content analysis revealed the need for emotional, informational, instrument, and feedback support (Norbeck ct al., 1991). Family members who are competent to care for chronically ill individuals report the need for more information about providing care that will relieve the stress of the illness on themselves and their loved ones (Neundorfer, 1991; Norbeck et. al., 1991). Reinhard (1994) recommends that the need of the patient and family for more caregiving information be provided by the nurse.

But with the dyspneic lung cancer patient, many home care nurses lack sufficient information to teach family members. The lack of research testing interventions to relieve dyspnea has led nurses to ignore this distressing symptom. Only 10% of lung cancer patients reported having received any education by health care professionals in relation to their shortness of breath (Brown et al., 1986). Thus, they do not report the presence of dyspnea. In a recent study it was found that 76.7% of the lung cancer patients claimed to experience dyspnea, yet only 38.8% of their charts showed any evidence of nurses noting the symptom (Roberts et al., 1993). Patients reported feeling isolated and being left to cope with their dyspnea in their own manner. It is imperative that interventions be tested for their effectiveness in relieving dyspnea as well as their acceptance by the family caregivers who are to use them in the care of terminally ill lung cancer patients.

EXPECTED OUTCOMES AFTER RADIATION THERAPY

Respiratory symptoms are common in hospitalized patients. It has been found that 33% of all patients in the hospital complain of some degree of shortness of breath when asked about their subjective sensations (Farncombe, 1997). When asked about the limitation on their activities, over 75% reported significant shortness of breath interfering with their quality of life. Also, those who reported respiratory symptoms were 39% more likely to complain of other symptoms than patients with no shortness of breath, and were 55% more likely to report other symptoms as being severe (Farncombe, 1997).

While demographic variables are important in predicting respiratory distress, the age of the patient has not been shown to be predictive of the extent of pneumonitis, severity of symptoms, or time to appearance of symptoms after radiation therapy (Pignon et al., 1998).

Dyspnea after radiation therapy was found to increase over 6 to 12 weeks and then go into remission in most subjects, with a gradual progression to the stage of pulmonary fibrosis over the next 6 to 12 months in more severe cases (Beinert et al., 1999). Factors found to be predictive of patients who will have a high level of continuous respiratory distress include patients with comorbidities, recurrent cancer, those who had chemotherapy, and patients from a low-income group (Sarna, 1993). The area of lung involved in the radiation therapy and the dose of the radiation contribute to the risk for pulmonary pneumonitis and fibrosis (McDonald et al., 1995).

After irradiation for Hodgkin's disease, the 3-year actuarial probability of lung damage has been found to be 19% overall with an increased risk of damage with dose per fraction, the presence of systemic symptoms, and total mediastinal dose (Dubray et al., 1995). Age, histological type, number of nodal sites involved, and radiotherapy duration did not significantly modify the risk of lung damage (Dubray et al., 1995). The influence of gender on respiratory disease is controversial. Lund and colleagues (1996) found that 75% of women had such sequelae while only 41% of men did. Women had increased risk of heart valve regurgitation, pericardial thickening, and reduced gas transfer. Dubray and colleagues, on the other hand, did not find gender differences. The difference in these findings may be that Lund and colleagues included patients with cardiac problems while Dubray and colleagues did not. Respiratory symptoms and reduced lung function were found as late as 5 years after irradiation for Hodgkin's disease in nearly one-third of HD survivors who appeared healthy (Lund et al., 1995).

After irradiation of the chest, the cumulative rate of radiation-induced lung injury at 12 months has been shown to be 85% (Yamazaki et al., 1995). The most significant factor contributing to radiation-induced lung injury was the irradiated area of the mediastinum ($p = .03$) (Yamazaki et al., 1995). When findings in patients after radiation therapy were compared to a group of control patients, irradiated patients showed a significantly ($p < .01$) greater percentage (29.5 ± 15.7%) of bronchoalveolar lavage (BAL) lymphocytes than controls (6.2 ± 3.3%) (Martin et al., 1999). When asymptomatic patients were compared, however, with findings in a group of patients with radiation pneumonitis, the expected differences in BAL findings were not observed (Martin et al., 1999). They also found no differences between the side of the lung irradiated and the side not irradiated. Thus, chest irradiation produces changes but these changes are not indicative of the side irradiated or the presence of pneumonitis. Patient-specific factors, such as tobacco history, pre-RT diffusion capacity to carbon dioxide, cytokine transforming growth factor beta$_1$ chemotherapy exposure, disease type, and mean lung dose were not found to have a dramatic effect on radiation-induced reduction in lung perfusion (Garipagaoglu et al., 1999).

While radiation therapy has resulted in increased respiratory symptoms, it has also been shown to be effective in palliation of respiratory symptoms such as cough, hemoptysis, and dyspnea (Lutz et al., 1997), and in patients with metastatic melanoma it can decrease pain and compression (Kirova, Chen, Rabarijaona, Piedbois, & Le Bourgeos, 1999). Palliation, however, has not led to an increase in survival rate (Chang, Horwath, Peyton, & Ling, 1994).

OUTCOMES MEASURES

Dyspnea is a multidimensional subjective experience, however, the valid and reliable measures that are available focus mostly on the intensity of the sensation not its many dimensions. There is no single measure of dyspnea that takes into account the different components, such as duration, frequency, rate of onset, and quality of the sensation (van der Molen, 1995). The best measure of dyspnea depends on the purpose for the measurement. Disease-specific measures are most valuable when assessing changes in an individual patient after therapeutic interventions. More general measures, on the other hand, are particularly valuable when comparing respiratory symptoms across different patient populations (Mahler & Jones, 1997). Patient subjective report measures will be discussed first followed by more global measures such as quality of life. For a review of measures used in the assessment of dyspnea see the paper by Mancini and Body (1999) or the one by Meek and colleagues (1999), which is the position statement by the American Thoracic Society on dyspnea.

A valid measure of dyspnea intensity is a visual analogue scale, sometimes referred to as the *Visual Analogue Dyspnea Scale* (VADS). It consists of a 100 mm vertical visual analogue scale with anchors of "shortness of breath as bad as it can be" at the top and "no shortness of breath" at the bottom. Concurrent validity of this scale has been established with COPD patients using both a horizontal visual analogue scale and a measure of airway obstruction. The correlation between the two analogue scales was .97 while the correlation between the VADS and peak expiratory flow rate was $-.85$ (Gift et al., 1986). Construct validity was established using the contrasted groups approach between patients expected to have dyspnea and those not expected to have dyspnea. Differences between the two groups were significant for COPD patients ($t = 9.73, p < .01$) as they were for asthmatic subjects ($t = 12.35, p < .01$) (Gift, 1989).

The *Numeric Rating Scale* (NRS) has patients rate the intensity of their shortness of breath by choosing a number from 0 to 10 that represents the shortness of breath they are feeling right now. Zero represents no shortness of breath and 10 is shortness of breath as bad as it can be. The NRS can be administered either in the written or verbal form and is extremely easy to administer and score. This scale has been used clinically as a measure of dyspnea and was recently shown to be a valid measure of dyspnea in the COPD patient (Gift & Narsavage, 1998).

The *quality of the dyspnea* experience expressed by the descriptors is also important, but there is no validated scale to measure quality. The words used to describe dyspnea have been varied according to the disease state or cause of dyspnea (Simon et al., 1990). These descriptors have been shown to be repeatable, demonstrating their reliability as a measure of dyspnea (Mahler et al., 1996). The exact descriptors used by cancer patients, however, have not been studied in the manner as for patients with respiratory or cardiac disease. Brown and colleagues (1986) noted that cancer patients used words such as "shortness of breath," "difficulty breathing," "hard to move air," and "tired" or "fatigued" to characterize their dyspnea.

Another dimension of dyspnea in addition to its intensity and quality is the *distress* it evokes. This has been studied by a number of researchers who have found that subjects can rate dyspnea intensity separately from its distress (Carrieri-Kohlman et al., 1996; Wilson & Jones, 1991). They suggest using a visual analogue scale.

There are several scales that measure dyspnea as one of many symptoms. One example is the *Memorial Symptom Assessment Scale*, which asks for the multidimensional evaluation of 32 physical and psychological symptoms. It lists 24 symptoms that occur periodically in cancer patients and asks subjects to rate the frequency and severity of each symptom as well as how much the symptom distressed them. In addition, 8 longer-lasting symptoms are listed and the subject is requested to indicate how severe the symptom was and how much he or she was distressed by the symptom. This scale was tested on 246 patients with a variety of cancers. A factor analysis found three factors that were labeled as psychological, high-prevalence physical, and low-prevalence physical. High correlations with the clinical status and quality of life measures give further support for the validity of the scale. Reliability was established using Cronbach's alpha with coefficients of .83 to .88 (Portenoy et al., 1994).

The *Symptom Distress Scale* (SDS) is another example of a measure that includes multiple symptoms, dyspnea being one of them. In this scale patients are asked to rate each symptom on a five-point response format ranging from 1 (normal or no distress) to 5 (extensive distress). Evidence for validity and alpha reliability (.82 for the total scale) have been reported (McCorkle, 1978; McCorkle & Benoliel, 1983).

Symptoms resulting from radiation therapy are often evaluated by the grading system developed by the Radiation Oncology Group and the European Organization for Research in the Treatment of Cancer (RTOG/EORTC). This system for evaluation of acute lung injury proposes four grades. Grade 0 is no change, Grade 1 is mild symptoms of dry cough or dyspnea on exertion, Grade 2 is persistent cough requiring narcotic antitussive agents and/or dyspnea with minimal effort, Grade 3 includes severe cough unresponsive to narcotic antitussive agents, dyspena at rest, clinical or radiographic evidence of acute pneumonitis, intermittent oxygen requirements, or requirements for steroids, and Grade 4 is severe respiratory insufficiency that is unresponsive to treatment (McDonald et al., 1995). This grading system is not linear and is not related to the dose of radiation.

There are also quality-of-life measures that include shortness of breath as a dimension of quality of life. An example would be the EORTC QLQ-LC13, which includes many of the symptoms experienced by cancer patients as well as the side effects from conventional chemotherapy and radiation therapy. This is a valid measure of quality of life because of its discriminant ability among patients having different performance levels. The dyspnea subscale was shown to be reliable with a Cronbach's alpha of .70 (Bergman, Aaronson, Ahmedzai, Kaasa, & Sullivan, 1994).

A quality-of-life scale that includes a measure of dyspnea and was developed specifically to measure quality of life in cancer patients undergoing radiation is the *Lung Cancer Symptom Scale*. Symptoms are rated by patients using five descriptors with clarifying sentences. In the case of dyspnea, the clarifying sentences relate to the level of exercise needed to provoke dyspnea. The descriptors are none (scored as 100), mild (scored as 75), moderate (scored as 50), marked (scored as 25), and severe (scored as 0). This scale is sensitive to the effects of palliative radiation therapy resulting in a significant reduction in dyspnea ($p = .0003$) (Lutz et al., 1997).

OUTCOMES MANAGEMENT

At the present time there are no known therapies to protect against the development of radiation-induced lung toxicity. Experimental agents such as monoclonal anti-CD40L antibody that disrupt CD40-CD40L interactions are being studied as pulmonary radioprotectors (Adawi et al., 1998).

PHYSIOLOGIC/PHARMACOLOGIC INTERVENTIONS

There are strategies that have been recommended to maintain the ventilatory demands of the body. One of the most widely used therapies is the use of supplemental *oxygen*. In an emergency room it is the most common treatment for dyspnea, being prescribed for 34% of cancer patients. (Escalante et al., 1996). In a prospective double-blind, crossover study, Bruera and colleagues (1993) demonstrated that supplemental oxygen reduces dyspnea in cancer patients who are hypoxic and symptomatic at rest (Bruera, de Stoutz, Velasco-Leiva, Schoeller, & Hanson, 1993). Others, however, found that oxygen did not produce any lower rating of dyspnea than air administration (Booth, Kelly, Cox, Adams, & Guz, 1996). While oxygen may be vital for those who are hypoxic, its use in those who are not hypoxic may be related to the placebo effect of cool airflow through the nasal cannula (Liss & Grant, 1988).

Dyspnea resulting from radiation-induced pneumonitis is usually treated with steroids for a period of time to reduce the effects of the inflammatory process. The effectiveness of this treatment has been questioned (Kwok & Chan, 1998), but continues mostly because of the documented effectiveness of steroids in controlling inflammation and also because there is little else to offer the patient.

Opiates have been recommended in the treatment of dyspnea because of their respiratory depressant effect on the central process of neural signals within the central nervous system. Some have found them to be effective in the relief of dyspnea (Bruera, Macmillan, Pither, & MacDonald, 1990). Opiates have been shown to decrease expiratory volume (V_E) at rest and during submaximal levels of exercise. The danger with the use of these drugs is the concomitant increase in CO_2. Opioids have been described as alleviating dyspnea by blunting perceptual responses and decreasing the intensity of the respiratory sensation. They have been recommended for acute dyspnea but there is little to recommend their use in long-term, progressive dyspnea such as in cancer (Meek et al., 1999). There is some evidence to indicate that nebulized morphine is effective in the relief of dyspnea (Zeppetella, 1997), but the evidence is minimal and thus not recommended for practice (Meek et al., 1999).

Some have recommended the use of nebulized lidocaine in the treatment of dyspnea in cancer patients. This, however, has not been found to be effective (Wilcox, Corcoran, & Tattersfield, 1994).

Nonpharmacologic Interventions

The notion of oxygen blowing through a nasal cannula as a placebo effect led some to recommend the use of a fan blowing on the cheek for the relief of dyspnea. While there is no study documenting the effectiveness of this as a dyspnea-relieving strategy, it is something patients have reported using and hospital nurses have recommended for dyspnea relief (Roberts et al., 1993; Zerwekh, 1987). Schwartzstein and colleagues (1987) studied 16 normal subjects in whom dyspnea was induced by having them breathe air containing 55 torr of CO_2 through an inspiratory resistive load. Dyspnea was recorded using a Modified Borg scale comparing times when cold air was blown on the cheek with times when there was no flow and with times when cold air was blown on the leg. Dyspnea was rated as significantly lower when cold air was blown on the cheek (Schwartzstein, Lahive, Pope, Weinberger, & Weiss, 1987).

There are a variety of other nonpharmacologic interventions that have been effective in relieving dyspnea. Many take advantage of the high correlation observed between respiratory distress and anxiety. *Relaxation* techniques have been effective in reducing dyspnea and anxiety. Patients have reported using self-taught relaxation techniques for the relief of dyspnea (Carrieri & Janson-Bjerklie, 1986). Others have found that these self-management strategies are different for patients with different diseases and from different ethnic backgrounds (Nield, 2000). Renfroe (1988) was one of the first to report the effectiveness of three 45-minute sessions with an instructor teaching progressive relaxation techniques to relieve dyspnea. However, no measures were taken to document the achievement of relaxation. Gift and colleagues (1992), on the other hand, demonstrated the effectiveness of progressive muscle relaxation techniques in reducing both dyspnea and anxiety. The mean rating of dyspnea was shown to decrease from 53 to 20 (on a 0 to 100 scale) after four 20-minute relaxation sessions (Gift, Moore, & Soeken, 1992).

A *comprehensive nursing intervention* has also been effective in improving ventilation in lung cancer patients. In a multicenter randomized, controlled trial comparing a nursing clinic offering interventions for breathlessness with best supportive care, the intervention group improved significantly at 8 weeks in breathlessness, performance, depression, and physical symptom distress. The nursing interventions combined breathing control, activity pacing, relaxation techniques, and psychosocial support (Bredin et al., 1999). Others have suggested that such a comprehensive approach should include an assessment of the factors ameliorating and exacerbating dyspnea, the meaning of breathlessness for the individual, goal setting, and patient and family education alerting them to the recognition of problems that warrant pharmacological or medical intervention (Bailey, 1995). Corner and colleagues (1996) demonstrated the effectiveness of such a strategy that also included teaching patients coping and adaptation strategies. They found breathlessness to improve by a median of 53%, breathlessness at worst by 35%, and functional capacity by 21%. They suggest that the potential of this comprehensive approach needs to be explored further (Corner, Plant, A'Hern, & Bailey, 1996).

McCorkle and Benoliel (1989) compared a nursing intervention delivered in the home by oncology nurses or home health nurses with an intervention delivered in an office setting. They found no differences in the effectiveness of the intervention based on caregiver but the intervention delivered in the home was more effective in providing symptom relief than one that required the patient to come to the office setting. Thus, they recommend that care be provided in the patient's home.

Acupuncture has also been effective in the relief of dyspnea. In a trial of acupuncture involving 20 patients, it was found that 70% of them reported marked symptomatic benefit from accupuncture. Outcome measures used included breathlessness, anxiety ($p < .01$), and respiratory rate ($p < .02$) (Filshie, Penn, & Ashley, 1996).

REFERENCES

Abratt, R. P., & Willcox, P. A. (1995). The effect of irradiation on lung function and perfusion in patients with lung cancer. *International Journal of Radiation Oncology, Biology, Physics*, 31(4), 915–919.

Acheson, A., & MacCormack, D. (1997). Dyspnea and the cancer patient—an overview. *Canadian Oncology Nursing Journal*, 7(4), 209–213.

Adawi, A., Zhang, Y., Baggs, R., Rubin, P., Williams, J., Finkelstein, J., & Phipps, R. P. (1998). Blockade of CD40-CD40 ligand interactions protects against radiation-induced pulmonary inflammation and fibrosis. *Clinical Immunology and Immunopathology*, 89(3), 222–230.

American Thoracic Society. (1991). Lung function testing: Selection of reference values and interpretative strategies. *American Review of Respiratory Disease*, 144, 1202–1218.

Anscher, M. S., Kong, F. M., & Jirtle, R. L. (1998). The relevance of transforming growth factor beta$_1$ in pulmonary injury after radiation therapy. *Lung Cancer*, 19(2), 109–120.

Bailey, C. (1995). Nursing as therapy in the management of breathlessness in lung cancer. *European Journal of Cancer Care*, 4(4), 184–190.

Beinert, T., Binder, D., Stuschke, M., Jorres, R. A., Oehm, C., Fleischhacker, M., Sezer, O., Mergenthaler, H.-G., Werner, T., & Possinger, K. (1999). Oxidant-induced lung injury in anticancer therapy. *European Journal of Medical Research*, 4(2), 43–53.

Bergman, B., Aaronson, N. K., Ahmedzai, S., Kaasa, S., & Sullivan, M. (1994) The EORTC QLQ-LC13: A modular supplement to the EORTC Core Quality of Life Questionnaire (QLQ-C30) for use in lung cancer clinical trials. EORTC Study Group on Quality of Life. *European Journal of Cancer*, 30A(5), 635–642.

Booth, S., Kelly, M. J., Cox, N. P., Adams, L., & Guz, A. (1996). Does oxygen help dyspnea in patients with cancer? *American Journal of Respiratory and Critical Care Medicine*, 153(5), 1515–1518.

Bredin, M., Corner, J., Krishnasamy, M., Plant, H., Bailey, C., & A'Hern, R. (1999). Multicentre randomized controlled trial of nursing intervention for breathlessness in patients with lung cancer. *British Medical Journal*, 318(7188), 901–904.

Breslin, E. H., Garoutte, B. C., Carrieri, V., & Celli, B. R. (1990). Correlations between dyspnea, diaphragm, and sternomastoid recruitment during inspiratory resistance breathing in normal subjects. *Chest*, 98(2), 298–302.

Brown, M. L., Carrieri, V., Janson-Bjerklie, S., & Dodd, M. J. (1986). Lung cancer and dyspnea: The patient's perception. *Oncology Nursing Forum*, 13(5), 19–24.

Bruera, E., de Stoutz, N. Velasco-Leiva, A., Schoeller, T., & Hanson, J. (1993). Effects of oxygen on dyspnoea in hypoxaemic terminal-cancer patients. *Lancet*, 342(8862), 13–14.

Bruera, E., Macmillan, K., Pither, J., & MacDonald, R. N. (1990). Effects of morphine on the dyspnea of terminal cancer patients. *Journal of Pain and Symptom Management*, 5(6), 341–344.

Carrieri, V., & Janson-Bjerklie, S. (1986). Strategies patients use to manage the sensation of dyspnea. *Western Journal of Nursing Research*, 8(3), 284–305.

Carrieri-Kohlman, V., Gormley, J. M., Douglas, M. K., Paul, S. M., & Stulbarg, M. S. (1996). Differentiation between dyspnea and its affective components. *Western Journal of Nursing Research*, 18(6), 626–642.

Chang, L. F., Horvath, J., Peyton, W., & Ling, S. S. (1994). High dose rate after loading intraluminal brachytherapy in malignant airway obstruction of lung cancer. *International Journal of Radiation, Oncology, Biology, Physics*, 28(3), 589–596.

Chin, B. B., Welsh, J. S., Kleinberg, L., Ettinger, D., & White, P. (1999). Nonsegmental ventilation-perfusion scintigraphy mismatch after radiation therapy. *Clinical Nuclear Medicine*, 24(1), 54–56.

Corner, J., Plant, H., A'Hern, R., & Bailey, C. (1996). Nonpharmacological intervention for breathlessness in lung cancer. *Palliative Medicine*, 10(4), 299–305.

Dubray, B., Henry-Amar, M., Meerwaldt, J. H., Noordijk, E. M., Dixon, D. O., Cosset, J. M., & Thames, H. D. (1995). Radiation-induced lung damage after thoracic irradiation for Hodgkin's disease: The role of fractionation. *Radiotherapy and Oncology*, 36(3), 211–217.

Dudgeon, D., Kristjanson, L., Sloan, J., & Lertzman, M. (1999). Dyspnea in cancer patients: Prevalence and associated factors. *Journal of Pain and Symptom Management*, 16(4), 212–219.

Dudgeon, D. J., & Lertzman, M. (1998). Dyspnea in the advanced cancer patient. *Journal of Pain and Symptom Management*, 16(4), 212–219.

Escalante, C. P., Martin, C. G., Elting, L. S., Cantor, S. B., Harle, T. S., Price, K. J., Kish, S. K., Manzullo, E. F., & Rubenstein, E. B. (1996). Dyspnea in cancer patients. Etiology, resource utilization and survival-implications in a managed care world. *Cancer*, 78(6), 1314–1319.

Farncombe, M. (1997). Dyspnea: Assessment and treatment. *Supportive Care in Cancer*, 5(2), 94–99.

Filshie, J., Penn, K., & Ashley, S. (1996). Acupuncture for the relief of cancer-related breathlessness. *Palliative Medicine*, 10(2), 145–150.

Gardner, R, Hankinson, J. (1987). Standardization of spirometry—1987. *American Review of Respiratory Disease*, 137(2), 493–495.

Garipagaoglu, M., Munley, M. T., Hollis, D., Poulson, J. M., Bentel, G. C., Sibley, G., Anscher, M. S., Fan, M., Jaszczak, R. J., Coleman, R. E., & Marks, L. B. (1999). The effect of patient-specific factors on radiation-induced regional lung injury. *International Journal of Radiation Oncology, Biology, Physics*, 45(2), 331–338.

Gift, A. G. (1989). Validation of a vertical visual analogue scale as a measure of clinical dyspnea. *Rehabilitation Nursing*, 14(6), 323–325.

Gift, A. G. (1991). Psychologic and physiologic aspects of acute dyspnea in asthmatics. *Nursing Research*, 40(4), 196–199.

Gift, A. G., Moore, T., & Soeken, K. (1992). Relaxation to reduce dyspnea and anxiety in COPD patients. *Nursing Research*, 4(4), 242–246.

Gift, A. G. & Narsavage, G. (1998). Validation of the numeric rating scale as a measure of dyspnea. *American Journal of Critical Care*, 7(3), 200–204.

Gift, A. G., Plaut, S. M., & Jacox, A. K. (1986). Psychologic and physiologic factors related to dyspnea in subjects with chronic obstructive pulmonary disease. *Heart and Lung,* 15, 595–601.

Hardman, P. D., Tweeddale, P. M., Kerr, G. R., Anderson, E. D., & Rodger, A. (1994). The effect of pulmonary function of local and loco-regional irradiation for breast cancer. *Radiotherapy and Oncology,* 30(1), 33–42.

Higginson, I., & McCarthy, M. (1989). Measuring symptoms in terminal cancer: Are pain and dyspnea controlled? *Journal of the Royal Society of Medicine,* 82(5), 264–267.

Kirova, Y. M., Chen, J., Rabarijaona, L. I., Piedbois, Y., & Le Bourgeos, J. P. (1999). Radiotherapy as palliative treatment for metastatic melanoma. *Melanoma Research,* 9(6), 611–613.

Knudson, R. J., Slatin, R. C., Lebowitz, M. D., & Burrows, B. (1976). The Maximal Expiratory Flow-Volume Curve *American Review of Respiratory Disease* 113, 587–600.

Kwok, E., & Chan, C. K. (1998). Corticosteroids and azathioprine do not prevent radiation-induced injury. *Canadian Respiratory Journal,* 5(2), 211–214.

Liss, H. P., & Grant, B. J. B. (1988). The effect of nasal flow on breathlessness in patients with chronic obstructive pulmonary disease. *American Review of Respiratory Disease,* 137(6), 1285–1288.

Lund, M. B., Kongerud, J., Boe, J., Nome, O., Abrahamsen, A. F., Ihlen, H., & Forfang, K. (1996). Cardiopulmonary sequelae after treatment for Hodgkin's disease: Increased risk in females? *Annals of Oncology,* 7(3), 257–264.

Lund, M. B., Kongerud, J., Nome, O., Abrahamsen, A. F., Bjortuft, O., Forfang, K., Boe, J. (1995). Lung function impairment in long-term survivors of Hodgkin's disease. *Annals of Oncology,* 6(5), 495–501.

Lush, M., Janson-Bjerklie, S., Carrieri, V. K., & Lovejoy, N. (1988). Dyspnea in the ventilator-assisted patient. *Heart & Lung,* 17(5), 528–535.

Lutz, S. T., Huang, D. T., Ferguson, C. L., Kavanagh, B. D., Terceilla, O. F., & Lu, J. (1997). A retrospective quality of life analysis using the Lung Cancer Symptom Scale in patients treated with palliative radiotherapy for advanced nonsmall cell lung cancer. *International Journal of Radiation Oncology and Biological Physics,* 37(1), 117–122.

Mahler, D. A., Harver, A., Lentine, T., Scott, J. A., Beck, K., & Schwartzstein, R. M. (1996). Descriptors of breathlessness in cardiorespiratory diseases. *American Journal of Respiratory and Critical Care Medicine,* 154(5), 1357–1363.

Mahler, D. A., & Jones, P. W. (1997). Measurement of dyspnea and quality of life in advanced lung disease. *Clinical Chest Medicine,* 18(3), 457–469.

Mahler, D., Weinberg, D., Wells, C., & Feinstein, A. (1984). The measurement of dyspnea: Contents, interobserver agreement and physiologic correlates of two new clinical indexes. *Chest,* 85(6), 751–758.

Mancini, I., & Body, J. J. (1999). Assessment of dyspnea in advanced cancer patients. *Support Care Cancer* 7:229–232.

Marks, L. B., Munley, M. T., Spencer, D. P., Sherouse, G. W., Bentel, G. C., Hoppenworth, J., Chew, M., Jaszczak, R. J., Coleman, R. E., & Prosnitz, L. R. (1997). Quantification of radiation-induced regional lung injury with perfusion imaging. *International Journal of Radiation Oncology, Biology, Physics*, 38(2), 399–409.

Martin, C., Romero, S., Sanchez-Paya, J., Massuti, B., Arriero, J. M., & Hernandez, L. (1999). Bilateral lymphocytic alveolitis: A common reaction after unilateral thoracic irradiation. *European Respiratory Journal*, 13(4), 727–732.

McCorkle, R., & Benoliel, J. Q. (1989). A randomized clinical trial of home nursing care for lung cancer patients. *Cancer*, 64(6), 1375–1382.

McCorkle, R., & Benoliel, J. Q. (1983). Symptom distress, current concerns and mood disturbance after diagnosis of life-threatening disease. *Social Science and Medicine*, 17(7), 431–438.

McCorkle, R., & Young, K. (1978). Development of a symptom distress scale. *Cancer Nursing*, 1(5), 373–378.

McDonald, S., Rubin, P., Phillips, T. L., & Marks, L. B. (1995). Injury to the lung from cancer therapy: Clinical syndromes, measurable endpoints, and potential scoring systems. *International Journal of Radiation Oncology and Biological Physiology*, 31(5), 1187–1203.

Meek, P. M., Schwartzstein, R. M., Adams, L., Altose, M. D., Breslin, E. H., Carrieri-Kohlman, V., Gift, A., Hanley, M. V., Harver, A., Jones, P. W., Killian, K., Knebel, A., Lareau, S., Mahler, D., O'Donnell, D., Steele, B., Stuhlbarg, M., & Titler, M. (1999). Dyspnea: Mechanisms, assessment, and management: A consensus statement. *American Journal of Respiratory and Critical Care Medicine*, 159, 321–340.

Nakayama, Y., Makino, S., Fukuda, Y., Min, K. Y., Shimizu, A., & Ohsawa, N. (1996). Activation of lavage lymphocytes in lung injuries caused by radiotherapy for lung cancer. *International Journal of Radiation Oncology, Biology, Physics*, 34(2), 459–467.

National Cancer Institute. (1994). 1996 *Budget estimate for scientific opportunities* (pp. 359–360). National Cancer Institute. Bethesda, Maryland.

Neundorfer, M. (1991). Coping and health outcomes in spouse caregivers of persons with dementia. *Nursing Research*, 40(5), 260–265.

Nield, M. (2000). Dyspnea self-management in African Americans with chronic lung disease. *Heart & Lung*, 29(1), 50–55.

Norbeck, J., Chaftez, L., Wilson, H., & Weiss, S. (1991). Social support needs of family caregivers of psychiatric patients from three age groups. *Nursing Research*, 40(4), 208–214.

Pignon, T., Gregor, A., Schaake Koning, C., Roussel, A., Van Glabbeke, M., & Scalliet, P. (1998). Age has no impact on acute and late toxicity of curative thoracic radiotherapy. *Radiotherapy and Oncology*, 46(3), 239–248.

Portenoy, R. K., Thaler, H. T., Kornblith, A. B., Lepore, J. M., Friedlander-Klar, H., Kiyasu, E., Sobel, K., Coyle, N., Kemeny, N., Norton, L., & Scher, H. (1994). The Memorial Symptom Assessment Scale: An instrument for the evaluation of symptom prevalence, characteristics and distress. *European Journal of Cancer*, 30A (9), 1326–1336.

Reinhard, S. (1994). Perspectives on the family's caregiving experience in mental illness. *Image: Journal of Nursing Scholarship*, 26(1), 70–74.

Renfroe, K. L. (1988). Effect of progressive relaxaton on dyspnea and state anxiety in patients with chronic obstructive pulmonary disease. *Heart & Lung*, 17(4), 408–413.

Reuben, D. B., & Mor, V. (1988). Clinical symptoms and length of survival in patients with terminal cancer. *Archives of Internal Medicine*, 148(7), 1586–1591.

Ripamonti, C. (1999). Management of dyspnea in advanced cancer patients. *Supportive Care in Cancer*, 7(4), 133–143.

Roberts, D. K., Thorne, S. E., & Pearson, C. (1993). The experience of dyspnea in late-stage cancer. *Cancer Nursing*, 16(4), 310–320.

Salinas, F. V., & Winterbauer, R. H. (1995). Radiation pneumonitis: A mimic of infectious pneumonitis. *Seminars in Respiratory Infections*, 10(3), 143–153.

Sarna, L. (1993). Correlates of symptom distress in women with lung cancer. *Cancer Practice*, 1(1), 21–28.

Schwartzstein, R. M., Lahive, K., Pope, A., Weinberger, S. E., & Weiss, J. W. (1987). Cold facial stimulation reduces breathlessness induced in normal subjects. *American Review of Respiratory Disease*, 136(1), 56–61.

Shulimzon, T., Apter, S., Weitzen, R., Yellin, A., Brenner, H. J., & Wollner, A. (1996). Radiation pneumonitis complicating mediastinal radiotherapy postpneumonectomy. *European Respiratory Journal*, 9(12), 2697–2699.

Simon, P. M., Basner, R. C., Weinberger, S. E., Fencl, V., Weiss, J. W., Schwartzstein, R. M. Wilkie, D., Lovejoy, N., Dodd, M., & Tesler, M. (1990). Cancer pain intensity measurement: Concurrent validity of three tools—finger dysnamometer, pain intensity number scale, visual analogue scale. *The Hospice Journal*, 6(1), 1–13.

Sloan, P. A., Donnely, M. B., Schwartz, R. W., & Sloan, D. A. (1997). Residents' management of the symptoms associated with terminal cancer. *The Hospice Journal*, 12(3), 5–15.

Susskind, H., Weber, D. A., Lau, Y. H., Park, T. L., Atkins, H. L., Franceschi, D., Meek, A. G., Ivanovic, M., & Wielopolski, L. (1997). Impaired permeability in radiation-induced lung injury detected by technetium-99m-DTPA lung clearance. *Journal of Nuclear Medicine*, 38(6), 966–971.

Teel, C. S., Meek, P., McNamara, A. M., & Watson, L. (1997). Perspectives unifying symptom interpretation. *Image, Journal of Nursing Scholarship* 29(2), 175–81.

Thurlbeck, W. (1983). Overview of the pathology of pulmonary emphysema in the human. *Clinics in Chest Medicine*, 4 (3), 337–350.

Van der Molen, B. (1995). Dyspnea: A study of measurement instruments for the assessment of dyspnea and their application for patients with advanced cancer. *Journal of Advanced Nursing*, 22(5), 948–956.

Wilcox, A., Corcoran, R., & Tattersfield, A. E. (1994). Safety and efficacy of nebulized lignocaine in patients with cancer and breathlessness. *Palliative Medicine*, 8(1), 35–38.

Wilson, R. C., & Jones, P. W. (1991). Differentiation between the intensity of breathlessness and the distress it evokes in normal subjects during exercise. *Clinical Science*, 80(1), 65–70.

Wolkove, N., Dajczman, E., Colacone, A., & Kreisman, H. (1989). The relationship between pulmonary function and dyspnea in obstructive lung disease. *Chest*, 96(6), 1247–1251.

Yamazaki, H., Tank, J. T., Inoue, T., Teshima, T., Ohtani, M., Ikeda, H., Itou, M., Takeuchi, E., & Inoue, T. (1995). Radiographic changes following radiotherapy in the patients with lung cancer. Is the irradiated area of the mediastinum in the simulation film a significant factor? *Strahlentherapie und Onkologie*, 171(5), 272–277.

Zeppetella, G. (1997). Nebulized morphine in the palliation of dyspnea. *Palliative Medicine*, 11(4), 267–275.

Zerwekh, J. V. (1987). Comforting the dying dyspneic patient. *Nursing 87*, 17(11), 66–69.

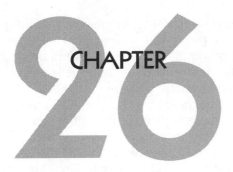

CHAPTER 26

Maintenance of Body Image and Sexual Function

Deborah Watkins Bruner

Problem

Radiation therapy assaults the patient's body image and sexual function both indirectly and directly. Indirect effects are associated with the general side effects of radiation therapy.

- General side effects of therapy that cause discomfort including skin reactions and fatigue, as well as site-specific reactions that may include alopecia, nausea, diarrhea, urinary incontinence, or dysuria, may impact how the patient perceives his or her body.
- Negative body perceptions impact intimacy and sexual function.
- Direct effects of therapy are site specific.

Breast Cancer

Women treated for breast or gynecologic malignancies face a potential fourfold assault on their sexual being: body image (i.e., weight gain/loss, disfigurement), gender role functioning (i.e., mother, wife), sexual functioning (i.e., desire, arousal, orgasm, etc.), and fertility (i.e., actual or potential desire for childbearing) (Bruner & Boyd, 1999).

- Sexual dysfunction in women treated for breast cancer has been estimated at 21% to 39%, regardless of treatment modality (Lamb, 1995). Women treated with external-beam radiation therapy in combination with lumpectomy for breast cancer may experience disruption in sexual activity, probably as a result of temporary effects of skin discomfort and fatigue (Bruner & Iwamoto, 1999).

■ Most studies have reported a more positive sexual outcome for women treated with breast-conserving therapy (lumpectomy and radiation therapy) as opposed to mastectomy in terms of body image, comfort with nudity, and frequency of intercourse (Fallowfield & Hall, 1991; Mock, 1993). Significant benefit in body image and satisfaction with treatment were observed in a recent study of women who received breast-conserving therapy. However, ratings of cosmetic results decreased with time, in line with clinical observations of long-term side effects of radiotherapy. Wide excision appeared to be the most important predictive factor for poor cosmetic result after breast-conserving therapy (Curran et al., 1998).

■ A recent study found that breast cancer survivors treated with either breast-conserving therapy or mastectomy had overall health-related quality of life and sexual functioning comparable to age-matched, healthy controls despite more frequent physical and menopausal symptoms. Ranked among the 10 most reported symptoms in this study were being unhappy with body appearance and breast sensitivity (Ganz, Rowland, Desmond, Meyerowitz, & Wyatt, 1998).

■ At least two studies have reported better body image and clothing fit outcomes in women receiving breast-conserving surgery and radiation therapy as compared with mastectomy with reconstruction or mastectomy alone (Ganz et al., 1998; Ganz, Schag, Lee, Polinsky, & Tan, 1992).

■ In a study that assessed sexuality after breast cancer based on survey responses from 863 breast cancer survivors, one-third of the women reported that breast cancer had had a negative impact on their sex life, and most reported negative changes in at least some areas. However, breast cancer survivors did not differ from age-matched, healthy controls in their report of sexual function. Breast cancer survivors who were most likely to report a negative impact on sexuality from therapy were those who had experienced changes in hormonal status, problems in their relationships, and difficulties with vaginal dryness (Meyerowitz, Desmond, Rowland, Wyatt, & Ganz, 1999).

■ A study conducted to investigate the influence of cosmetic outcome on psychosocial morbidity in patients who had undergone breast-conserving therapy for primary breast cancer found significant correlations. In 254 women aged 20 to 69 years who underwent breast-conserving therapy for operable primary breast cancer ($\leq$3 cm in diameter), satisfaction with cosmetic outcome was high (90.5% of the patients were very or moderately satisfied). There was an excellent correlation between women's perceptions of their cosmetic outcome and levels of anxiety ($r = -0.81$, $p < 0.001$) and depression ($r = -0.7$, $p < 0.001$) and between cosmesis and body image ($r = -0.4$, $p < 0.001$), sexuality ($\chi^2 = 22$, $p = 0.001$) and self-esteem ($r = -0.64$, $p < 0.001$) (Al-Ghazal, Fallowfield, & Blamey, 1999).

GYNECOLOGIC CANCERS

Pelvic radiation therapy causes premature menopause at relatively low doses. Menopause is associated with anatomical, physiological, and psychological changes that often influence sexuality. This is usually attributed to the decreased estrogen levels, which have a multitude of effects on sexual function, including decreased support of female pelvis, loss of ability to adequately lubricate the urogenital tissue, and changes in body configuration. Sexual dysfunction is further aggravated by the alterations in the skin, breasts, muscles, and skeleton caused by estrogen loss. For many women, these changes translate into a poorer self-image, diminution of self-esteem and, eventually, a loss of sexual desire (Bachmann, 1995).

■ Dyspareunia and decreases in sexual satisfaction have been reported to occur in women treated with external-beam and intracavitary radiation therapy for cervical cancer or endometrial cancer. Up to 22% of women have reported a decrease in sexual frequency and 37% reported a decrease in sexual satisfaction (Bruner et al., 1993).

■ This may be related to vaginal stenosis, which has been reported in up to 88% of women following intracavitary implants. Intracavitary radiation therapy denudes the vaginal epithelium by direct effect on the basal layer of the mucosa, the endothelium of the small vessels, and on the fibroblasts of the connective tissue in the submucosa. Indirectly, vaginal mucosa is further devitalized by narrowing and obliteration of the small vessels and circumferential fibrosis of the perivaginal tissues (Abitbol & Davenport, 1974b).

- Vaginal length after radiation implant has been reported to range from approximately 7.75 cm at 6 to < 12 months, to 7.05 cm at 12 to < 24 months, to 6.2 cm at > 24 months (Bruner et al., 1993). Masters and Johnson reported normal vaginal length as 8 to 9 centimeters (Masters & Johnson, 1966).
- Sexual dysfunction has generally been reported at higher rates in women treated with radiotherapy versus women treated with surgery for cervical carcinoma (Schrover, Fife, & Gersheson, 1989; Seibel, Graves, & Freeman, 1980), with the exception of a recent report indicating that surgery and not radiotherapy accounted for the majority of risk of vaginal stenosis as well as insufficient lubrication, and reduced vaginal elasticity (Bergmark, Avall-Lundqvist, Dickman, Henningsohn, & Steineck, 1999).
- In a study of 21 women with cervical cancer treated with radiation therapy, statistically significant changes were found in sexual function. The majority of women reported decreased frequency of masturbation and intercourse, decreased frequency of orgasm through noncoital sexual activities, less satisfaction with sex, and less enjoyment of intercourse. In addition, decreased feelings of self-esteem, sexual desirability, and attractiveness were reported. The majority believed that these changes were due to radiation therapy. The women who did not follow advice regarding use of vaginal dilators or did not resume their pre-illness level of sexual function were more likely to develop physical and sexual changes (Krumm & Lamberti, 1993).
- Sexual dysfunction in women treated for gynecologic malignancies has a documented impact on their partners. In a study of social, psychological, and sexual experiences of 47 men before their partner was treated for cervical or endometrial cancer and 1 year later, a variety of concerns were reported. In the endometrial group, men had intrapsychic problems, while interpersonal problems were more common in the cervical group. Communication with their partner, friends, and acquaintances was reported as a major problem in both groups, and the majority of men felt they had nobody to whom they could speak honestly. Most did not obtain even basic information about their partner's disease. Both groups reported that intercourse was a much more negative experience after completed treatment and a majority described impaired sexual desire (Lalos, Jacobsson, Lalos, & Stendahl, 1995).

GENITOURINARY CANCERS

■ In men, radiation therapy to the prostate carries about a 40% risk of erectile dysfunction (ED). In comparison, radical surgery and nerve-sparing surgery have about an 85% and 79% risk of ED, respectively (Green, Treible, & Wallack, 1990; Talcott et al., 1997).

  • Men treated with radiation therapy for prostate cancer have reported significantly inferior sexual arousal, function, and frequency, but not desire or enjoyment, compared with controls (Bruner, Hanlon, Nicolaou, & Hanks, 1997).

  • For men treated with the combination of radiation and androgen deprivation therapy (RT/ADT) the risk of ED is 60%. ED continues even after ADT is discontinued (Bruner et al., 1997).

  • Other sexual sequelae with combination ADT include diminished libido, phallic atrophy, and body image concerns with gynecomastia.

  • Although the specific mechanism by which radiation therapy reduces erections is still unknown, it has been suggested that radiation therapy accelerates atherosclerotic disease. This, in time, interferes with the arterial blood supply of the penis and results in erectile dysfunction (Goldstein, Feldman, Deckers, Babayan, & Kranc, 1984).

■ In a rare study of sexual function in males treated with radiation therapy for bladder cancer, 71% felt their sex life was worse following radiation therapy but only 56% were concerned about the deterioration (Little & Howard, 1998).

■ Patients treated for testicular cancer with radiation therapy have reported multiple areas of sexual dysfunction including loss of sexual desire (17%), reduced erectile potential (48%), reduced intensity of orgasm (38%), inability to ejaculate (5%), reduced semen volume (60%), and premature ejaculation (40%). In spite of these findings, only 8% of the men treated with radiation therapy reported a decrease in sexual satisfaction from prior to therapy and findings were not statistically significantly different from patients treated with chemotherapy for testicular cancer (Arai, Kawakita, Okada, & Yoshida, 1997).

OTHER SITES

■ Radiation therapy used in the treatment of head and neck cancers may cause permanent xerostomia affecting comfort, and libido, and impairing the ability for oral sexual contact (Bruner & Iwamoto, 1999).

- One study of sexual functioning in 55 head and neck cancer patients following radiation therapy with or without surgery, found 85% to still be interested in sex although a majority reported arousal problems, and 58% had orgasmic problems. Fifty-eight percent did not participate in sexual intercourse, yet 49% were satisfied with their current sexual functioning. Of note was that younger patients (< 65 years of age) had more advanced disease, lower performance status, and significantly poorer sexual functioning; those older than 65 years were more satisfied with their sexual partner and current sexual functioning (Monga, Tan, Ostermann, & Monga, 1997).

■ Radiation therapy increases the already high incidence (25–75%) of sexual dysfunction in patients treated with surgery for colorectal cancer.

■ In a classic study of quality of life after cancer therapy, radical radiation therapy in combination with chemotherapy for sarcoma was found to result in worse sexual function than in those accepting amputation (Sugarbaker et al., 1982).

■ The use of inverted Y irradiation in the treatment of Hodgkin's disease with pelvic lymph node involvement can cause early menopause in young women as a result of ovarian exposure to radiation (Classe et al., 1998). Patients with Hodgkin's disease reported decreased energy and sexual desire (Cella & Tross, 1986).

- A study that compared the long-term psychosocial adaptation of Hodgkin's disease and adult acute leukemia survivors found Hodgkin's disease survivors at a greater risk for problems in long-term adaptation than acute leukemia survivors. This included poorer sexual functioning in the Hodgkin's disease survivors ($p = 0.0001$) than acute leukemia survivors (Kornblith et al., 1998).

■ Many patients experience chronic pain associated with cancer. A recent study was conducted to assess sexual functioning and its relationship with psychological measures in 70 chronic pain patients (mean age was 49.9 years; range 29–74), with a mean pain duration of 146.7 months (range 6–624). The participants reported a wide variety of pain conditions. While 66% of patients were interested in sex, only 20% considered their current sexual life to be adequate.

Only 44% experienced normal arousal during intercourse, 33% practiced masturbation, and 47% were involved in sexual intercourse or oral sex at least once a month, and most were dissatisfied with orgasmic activities. No relationship was found between pain severity, duration, frequency, and sexual functioning, however a relationship was found between disability status, age, and sexual functioning. As would be expected, patients who reported symptoms of depression and distress had more sexual problems (Monga, Tan, Ostermann, Monga, & Grabois, 1998).

Sterility Can Occur at Relatively Low Doses of Radiation

The germinal epithelium is very sensitive to radiation-induced damage, with changes to spermatogonia occurring following as little as 0.1 Gy and permanent infertility after fractionated doses of 2 Gy and above. Total-body irradiation, and irradiation at an ovarian dose above 6 Gy usually result in permanent ovarian failure (Howell & Shalet, 1998).

- This may be of major concern for young patients treated for Hodgkin's disease. Whole mantle irradiation with inverted Y technique can cause premature menopause and infertility.
- Women may experience irregular menstrual periods or even early menopause, including the potential for hot flashes, insomnia, irritability, depression, vaginal dryness, dyspareunia, infertility, and osteoporosis (Bruner & Iwamoto, 1999).

Concomitant illnesses such as hypertension, diabetes, and some psychiatric disorders (among others) and many commonly used prescription medications may adversely affect sexual function. This further complicates determining radiation versus other causes of sexual problems posttherapy.

ASSESSMENT

In order to assess the impact of cancer therapies on sexual function, at least a rudimentary understanding of how sexuality is incorporated into a person's self-concept is required. Much of the work done in the field of sexual self-concept and cancer has been conducted by Andersen and colleagues.

- A sexual self-view or self-schema is defined as a cognitive generalization about aspects of the self and is derived from past experience, manifest in current experience. This schema influences the processing of sexually relevant social information and guides sexual behavior (Andersen & Cyranowski, 1994).

■ There are gender differences in sexual self-schema that correlate with the body of literature on gender differences in personality (e.g., men more frequently report gender-specific personality/sexual traits such as aggressive, powerful, experienced, domineering and individualistic, whereas women report more traits that exemplify extraversion, anxiety, and trust) (Andersen, Cyranowski, & Espindle, 1999).

■ Sexual self-schema may help in predicting sexual dysfunction after cancer therapy (Andersen, 1999) and may guide the individualization of interventions to improve sexual function.

A comprehensive sexual history is described in further detail elsewhere (Bruner & Iwamoto, 1999) and includes the following:

■ Age—Physiologic changes that affect sexual function occur with age (Shell & Smith, 1994). Age also is the single best predictor of ED postradiation for prostate cancer (Bruner et al., 1998a).

   • As adults pass through different developmental stages so too do they pass through different phases in sexual growth and development. For example, women in middlescence (the years between 35 and 60) undergo psychologic growth and alteration in the hormonal environment. Successful negotiation through this developmental stage includes disassembling and evaluating the self, adjusting to the changing self, adapting to alterations in sexuality caused by hormonal shifts, and finally, acknowledging the new self that has evolved (Wilmoth, 1996).

   • Men may experience andropause, a term used to describe a collection of symptoms including decreasing libido, difficulty with arousal, and fatigue, possibly related to declining androgen levels. Andropause had been compared to female climaterium, but there is a great deal of controversy over whether this is a real phenomenon. There is some evidence that these symptoms are more an identification process with the climacteric partner. Sexual function decreases with age but hormonal changes are not the major determining factor in this decline (Burns-Cox & Gingell, 1997).

■ Cultural/ethnic background—Sexual values and norms vary widely among cultures.
  - Ethnic differences in sexual socialization and attitudes, sexual history, and current practices were documented in 147 African American and White breast cancer survivors. Although there were few differences between the two ethnic groups in a predominantly well-educated, high-income, highly functional sample, African American women were however significantly less likely to be comfortable with and to practice oral sex, self-touching, and masturbation. White women were more likely to report that breast cancer had a negative impact on their sex lives (Wyatt et al., 1998).
  - There were significant differences in levels of interpersonal sexual behavior (e.g., petting, intercourse), intrapersonal sexual behavior (e.g., fantasy, masturbation), and sociosexual restrictiveness (e.g., lifetime number of partners, number of "one-night stands") between Asian and non-Asians living in North America. Asians were significantly more conservative than non-Asians on all measures of interpersonal sexual behavior and sociosexual restrictiveness (Meston, Trapnell, & Gorzalka, 1996).
  - Lavee (1991) suggests four culturally determined factors that should be assessed in order to improve outcomes of therapy: the meaning of sexuality, the definition of normal sexual relationship, the perception and meaning of sexual dysfunctions, and the role of the therapist and therapist-client relations (Lavee, 1991).

■ Sexual orientation.
  - There are scientists who believe that sexual orientation is, at least in part, biologically determined (Weinrich, 1995). This theory has been hotly refuted by others (Byne, 1995).
  - Regardless of the debate, health care professionals must be prepared to assess and respect the individual sexual orientation and needs of homosexual or bisexual patients as well as heterosexual patients treated with radiation therapy.

■ Pre-illness sexual functioning—This has been found to be the best predictor of posttreatment functioning (Andersen, 1990).

■ Pre-illness sexual relationship(s)—Poor or dysfunctional premorbid sexual relationships are not likely to improve after cancer diagnosis or therapy. Good, healthy premorbid sexual relationships are likely to endure or even improve posttherapy despite significant sexual dysfunction related to disease and treatment.

■ Body image as it contributes to the larger concept of self-esteem should be assessed using verbal and nonverbal cues.

■ Concomitant chronic illness may have an impact on sexual functioning as a result of effects on the muscular, neurologic, and/or vascular systems (e.g., diabetes, hypertension, arthritis, urologic problems).

■ Concomitant psychologic illness—A history of psychiatric problems or sexual abuse may have an impact on sexual functioning. More commonly with cancer patients, the psychological trauma of the cancer diagnosis can cause dysfunction. Anxiety, fear of pain, amputation, death, depression, financial worries, and grieving over loss of role functioning can all negatively affect sexual function.

■ Medications such as antihypertensives, antipsychotics, antidepressants, opiates, cocaine, tobacco, marijuana, sedatives, and alcohol may cause decreased libido and erectile dysfunction (Wilson, 1991). Finger and colleagues compiled a comprehensive list of medications that may adversely affect sexual function (Finger, Lund, & Slagle, 1997).

■ History of sexual abuse—A subject usually ignored by oncology specialists is nevertheless of extreme importance to many patients treated with cancer. This may be particularly relevant to patients with pelvic cancers that may be seen as yet another direct assault on their body and sexuality.

  • A United States Department of Justice, Bureau of Statistics 1996 survey estimated that the percent of persons raped during their lifetime included: attempted rape, 2.8% of females and 0.9% of men; completed rape, 14.8% of females and 2.1% of men; and total rape, 17.6% of females and 3.0% of males. This roughly translates into over 300,000 women becoming victims of rape each year (U.S. Department of Justice, 1998).

  • One study reported that 16% of women treated for gynecologic malignancies had been sexually abused (Bergmark et al., 1999).

■ An assessment of the quality of the relationship the patient is in is important because a long history of marital discord, for example, would negatively impact sexual function unrelated to radiation therapy.

Barriers to improving sexual outcomes include the following:

■ Although little research has been done to document oncology professionals' attitudes and clinical practice regarding sexuality, what is reported in the literature consistently shows a lack of knowledge and little interaction with patients regarding sexual function (Fisher, 1985; Williams, Wilson, Hongladarom, & McDonnell, 1986; Wilson & Williams, 1988).

■ This is congruent with the body of literature on how health care professionals in general deal poorly, if at all, with sexual function in their patients. Physicians have identified several barriers to addressing the sexual health of patients including lack of time, fear of intrusion, age and sex of both the general practitioner (GP) and the patient, fear of inadequacy, patients' offending behaviors, cultural differences (ethnic, gay, and youth), and the presence of a third party (Haley, Maheux, Rivard, & Gervais, 1999; Temple-Smith, Hammond, Pyett, & Presswell, 1996).

■ Methods for overcoming these barriers include better human sexuality curriculum in health education and continuing education as well as scripted role play to enhance comfort with taking a sexual history (Schweickert & Heeren, 1999).

EXPECTED OUTCOMES

The sexual and body image outcomes of cancer treatments fall into three categories: physiological, psychological, and interpersonal.

Physiological outcomes include a decrease in sexual desire and activity, orgasmic difficulty and pain, vaginal stenosis and dyspareunia, erectile dysfunction, retrograde ejaculation, premature ejaculation, decreased semen volume, neurological deficits that diminish or cause uncomfortable sensations, and menopausal symptoms.

Psychological outcomes include decreased body image, self-esteem, and self-concept, decreased sexual satisfaction, depression, performance anxiety, and fear of infertility (Lamb, 1995).

Interpersonal outcomes include disruptions in intimacy and loss of social support. For the partner without cancer, feelings of guilt and role confusion in initiating sexual contact, fear of causing pain during sexual contact, and fear of catching the cancer or effects of the therapy (i.e., radioactivity from radiation implants) may potentially result in deterioration of relationships.

MAINTENANCE OF PRE-ILLNESS LEVELS OF BODY IMAGE AND SEXUAL FUNCTION

- It is unlikely that cancer or cancer therapy would improve sexual function. It is therefore a reasonable goal for health care professionals in radiation therapy to try and maintain pre-illness levels of sexual function as opposed to improving sexual function to levels higher than pretreatment.
- Patients with a pre-illness history of sexual dysfunction, marital or relationship dysfunction, or sexual abuse need to be referred to a professional counselor or psychologist.

OUTCOMES MEASURES

Patient self-assessment questionnaires or patient interviews should be used to assess, at minimum, the following factors (*changes* from pre-illness baseline are the critical outcome measure):

- Body image
- Desire (level)
- Activity (i.e., type—oral, genital, anal, and frequency)
- Ability (e.g., erectile function, vaginal function)
- Satisfaction

Measures of sexual function exist but have mainly been used for research versus clinical assessments.

- Andersen has developed measures of sexual self-schema in male and female versions (Andersen & Cyranowski, 1994; Andersen et al., 1999).
- Watts's Sexual Function Questionnaire (WSFQ) (Watts, 1982), is a 17-item, five-point, Likert-type self-assessment instrument. WSFQ content includes the psychophysiologic component of desire as well as arousal and orgasm. In addition, items related to satisfaction were added. The scale has been tested in both patients with hypertension and women with cancer. The WSFQ was able to differentiate significantly

between healthy women and women with breast cancer (Wilmoth, 1993).

■ International Index of Erectile Dysfunction (IIEF) (Rosen et al., 1997) was developed as a measure of erectile function. Relevant cross-cultural domains of sexual function were identified via the literature, and the resulting 15-item questionnaire underwent linguistic validation in 10 languages. Five domains are assessed by the questionnaire: erectile function, orgasmic function, sexual desire, intercourse satisfaction, and overall satisfaction. The instrument demonstrated acceptable psychometric properties and was able to differentiate between patients with ED and age-matched controls.

■ Cancer-specific assessments include the following:

• The Sexual Adjustment Questionnaire (SAQ) was designed to assess the impact of cancer and/or surgery on sexual function (Waterhouse & Metcalfe, 1986). SAQ is a self-administered measure assessing desire, activity level, relationship, arousal, sexual techniques, and orgasm. The questionnaire rates most responses on a five-point Likert-type scale. The instrument comes in male and female as well as baseline and follow-up versions. The female baseline version has 37 items with 30 items in the follow-up version. Persons with cancer were found to have significantly ($p \leq .05$) lower scores on the subsections testing activity level and relationships. For the remaining subscales, over 95% of the mean scores for the healthy subjects were greater than the mean scores for cancer patients although the differences were not significant. A modified SAQ short-form has been further evaluated in over 700 prostate cancer patients treated with radiation therapy. The modified version demonstrated acceptable psychometric properties (Bruner, Scott, McGowan, Lawton, Hanks, Prestidge, Han, Gore, Asbell, 1998).

• The Sexual Behaviors Questionnaire (SBQ) (Wilmoth, 1993) is a 49-item self-assessment questionnaire measured on a six-point Likert-type scale (Wilmoth, 1993). The SBQ was developed based on Johnson's Behavioral Systems Model and further supported the model. Construct validity was determined by comparing differences in the mean score on the SBQ between 165 women diagnosed at least 6 months previously with breast cancer and 145 healthy women. The SBQ was able to differentiate significantly between the two groups. Further testing showed that based on factor analysis the SBQ is divided into seven subscales: communication, sexual response, self-touch, relationship quality, techniques, body-scar, and masturbation.

- The Sexual Function After Gynecologic Illness Scale (SFAGIS) (Bransfield, Horiot, & Nadib, 1984) is a 30-item, site-specific, self-report scale. All items are scored on a 0 to 4 Likert-type scale. Content was developed based on an extensive review of the literature about sexual functioning and gynecologic cancer. Fifteen themes were identified and incorporated into the item pool including sexual desire, unavailability of a partner, patient's fears about sexual activity, partner's fears about sexual activity, sexual satisfaction, initiation of sexual activity, affectionate behavior, frequency of sexual intercourse, frequency of orgasm, vaginal dimensions and mucosal conditions, potential for vaginal lubrication, intervention of the health provider, desire for sexual information, changes in sexual activity after therapy, and compliance with a prescription for a dilator. Face and content validity were reported as satisfactory based on the review of an undetermined number of oncologists. Psychometric data was based on 30 women with gynecologic malignancies who underwent radiotherapy.

OUTCOMES MANAGEMENT

Fears, anxieties, and depression related to diagnosis and cancer therapy need to be addressed to achieve the expected outcome. Open communication with one's partner regarding sexual function or fears of performance difficulties should be encouraged. Including the partner in discussion of sexual outcomes management should be a standard practice. Management of radiation-related side effects including psychological, behavioral, and medical interventions is required to maintain intimacy and sexual function (Bruner, Bucholtz, Iwamoto, & Strohl, 1998b).

- ■ Comfort—Fatigue may be minimized with rest prior to activity and pain medication may be taken prior to sexual activity. Achieving pain control without causing drowsiness may require dosage adjustments. Relaxation techniques, warm baths or soaks, and massage may be helpful.

- Nausea—Medication or a light meal prior to sexual activity may be helpful. Odors associated with sexual activity that increase nausea should be avoided and may include perfumes, colognes, and lotions.
- For additional comfort and symptom management measures prior to sexual activity see the chapter on comfort.
- Positions for sexual activity that minimize discomfort and enhance sexual activity can be suggested. Pictures of sexual positions may be easier for patients to understand than verbal explanations and have been published elsewhere (Bruner & Iwamoto, 1999).

Activities that maintain a positive body image should be encouraged.

- Good hygiene can be maintained with bathing, deodorants, and perfumes.
- Attractive clothing and wigs (with wig tape) assist in promoting a positive body image.

Activities that create a sensual environment with whatever appeals to the patient and his or her partner should be suggested.

- Mood-setting activities include candlelight, wine, massage, bathing together, sensual or erotic clothing, erotic pictures, and movies.
- Alternative forms of sexual expression can be explored. Suggestions could include trying new sexual positions (Bruner & Iwamoto, 1999) or sexual activities such as oral-genital sex or mutual masturbation.

For women experiencing sexual dysfunction after radiation therapy several management strategies should be considered.

- For women who have experienced dyspareunia or vaginal stenosis after intracavitary radiation therapy, anal intercourse may be an alternative. This may require education about the use of lubricants and gentle dilation.
- Women at risk for vaginal stenosis are usually instructed to have either a penis, vibrator, or dilator dilate the vagina at least three times per week, however, there is no research to date that

supports this intervention. Patient instructions for use of a vaginal dilator have been published (Bruner & Iwamoto, 1999).

■ Dyspareunia following intracavitary implant may also be minimized with the use of vaginal lubrication. Instructions for vaginal lubrication have also been published (Bruner & Iwamoto, 1999).

Hormone replacement therapy should be recommended to eligible women who have experienced premature menopause as a result of radiation therapy–related ovarian ablation. Hormone replacement therapy not only ameliorates the local anatomic and physiologic changes and prevents atrophic vaginitis and dyspareunia, but may also have positive psychological benefits such as the maintenance of libido and prevention of postmenopausal depression (Bachmann, 1995; Huppert, 1987). Progesterone may not be necessary after uterine irradiation.

■ Surgical relocation, either laterally or centrally, and shielding during abdominopelvic radiation therapy can assist in ovarian preservation. Ovarian transposition, initially performed by laparotomy, can now be done by laparoscopy. In a study of 4 young women with Hodgkin's disease who had laparoscopic ovarian transposition performed 1 week before inverted Y radiotherapy, the mean duration of hospitalization was 4 days, and there were no postoperative complications. Iatrogenic menopause did not occur in any of the women during the mean follow-up period of almost 21 months (range, 6–35 months) (Classe et al., 1998). Reports of these patients' resuming normal menstruation have been variable (Thomas et al., 1976).

■ Androgens have been documented to improve low libido in some women who have undergone menopause. In a prospective 2-year, single-blind trial of 34 healthy postmenopausal women who were randomized to either estradiol implants 50 mg alone or estradiol 50 mg plus testosterone 50 mg (with cyclical oral progestins for all women with an intact uterus), all sexual parameters assessed improved significantly in both groups. The addition of testosterone resulted in a significantly greater improvement compared with estradiol alone for sexual activity ($p < 0.03$), satisfaction ($p < 0.03$), pleasure ($p < 0.01$), and orgasm ($p < 0.035$). This suggests a therapeutic value of testosterone implants for women experiencing a postmenopausal decline in libido (Davis,

McCloud, Strauss, & Burger, 1995). Women thrust into menopause by radiation treatments should be medically evaluated
for hormone replacement therapy.

For men experiencing sexual dysfunction after radiation therapy
several management strategies are also available. Pharmacologic
and nonpharmacologic interventions that can restore voluntary
erectile function for sexual intercourse have been available for years
but have gained little attention from physicians and patients alike,
probably due to inconvenience and side effects.

The American Urologic Association (AUA) Clinical Guidelines
Panel on erectile dysfunction after reviewing published outcomes
for five treatment alternatives including vacuum constriction devices, intracavernous vasoactive injections, penile prosthesis implants, venous and arterial surgery, and oral drug therapy with
yohimbine concluded that only the first three alternatives had acceptable outcomes in terms of return to intercourse, patient satisfaction, and partner satisfaction (Montague et al., 1996). (The panel
review was prior to the FDA approval of sildenafil.)

- A vacuum device is a tube placed around the penis that creates a negative pressure that allows blood flow into the corpora cavernosa. When erection results, a constriction band
  is placed around the base of the penis. Erection may be
  maintained for up to 30 minutes, but it is not recommended
  for more than once-daily use because of potential penile
  bruising. Blocked or retrograde ejaculation occurs because
  the ejaculate is trapped in the proximal urethra because of
  the constriction band (Bruner & Iwamoto, 1999).
- Vasoactive agents such as alprostadil (prostaglandin E_1)
  cause vasodilation and vasocongestion of the penis, resulting in temporary erection. The medication has to be injected
  into the shaft of the penis, resulting in erection in 8 to 10
  minutes and lasting for 30 to 90 minutes. Orgasm and ejaculation are not affected. The drug has multiple contraindications and must be monitored. Adverse effects include local pain, bruising, and priapism (prolonged erections).
  Other effects include syncope, flushing, and hypotension.
  With long-term use, scar tissue and plaques can form along
  the shaft of the penis and result in its disfigurement. Therefore, the patient is instructed to use the medications no
  more than twice a week (Bruner & Iwamoto, 1999).

■ Sildenafil is a recently approved vasoactive oral agent for the treatment of erectile dysfunction. It works by enhancing smooth muscle relaxation and inflow of blood in the corpus cavernosum. This occurs in conjunction with sexual stimulation. Sildenafil has demonstrated significant improvement in ED patients with various histories and concomitant disease states including radical prostatectomies, but has yet to be scientifically tested in men receiving radiotherapy. A flexible dosing schedule is usually recommended starting with a 50 mg dose 1 hour prior to desired sexual intercourse and increasing in 25 mg doses to a maximum of 100 mg as needed (Goldstein et al., 1998).

■ Unlike the proven benefits of hormone replacement therapy in women, the effects of testosterone supplementation in men are equivocal and recent data cannot recommend the use of hormone replacement therapy with androgens because of potential severe side effects and lack of data on long-term effects. It may increase sexual interest, but rarely to a level thought adequate by the patient and has no proven beneficial effect on erectile dysfunction (Burns-Cox & Gingell, 1997; Tserotas & Merino, 1998).

■ Penile prostheses are available in three types: malleable, semi-inflatable, and fully inflatable.

  • The malleable prosthesis consists of two solid silicone rods placed into the corpora cavernosa. These rods are firm enough to allow sexual intercourse but leave the patient with a permanent erection. The erection is sometimes difficult to conceal but may be positioned up against the abdomen and secured with elastic briefs when not in use. There is no increase in the diameter of the penis with erection.

  • Both the semi-inflatable and fully inflatable prosthesis consist of two cylinders that are placed into the corpora cavernosa, each with its own pump and reservoir. The patient pumps behind the glans penis several times to move the fluid from the reservoirs and into the two cylinders to create an erection at the site of inflation. Deflation is accomplished by holding the penis downward for 10 seconds and then releasing the penis. The semi-inflatable prosthesis allows for full erections without a permanent erection, but never becomes totally flaccid. The fully inflatable prosthesis produces more natural erections with an increased length and diameter of the penis and also allows for total flaccidity. However, with both types of prosthesis, manual dexterity is needed for the patient or partner to operate the pump skillfully (Bruner & Iwamoto, 1999).

- A survey of 52 men, 1 to 4 years after penile prosthesis surgery, and 22 of their partners documented a mixture of positive and negative outcomes. Patients tended to be negative with regard to postoperative pain, penis size, postoperative sexual frequency, and prosthesis malfunctions. Patients emphasized the positive aspects and psychological benefits of renewed masculine self-esteem, repair of humiliation, and reduction of marital guilt. Partners corroborated patients' assessments of psychological benefits, but tended to rate the mechanical benefits of the prosthesis somewhat lower. The majority of patients said they would have the surgery again (Tiefer, Pedersen, & Melman, 1988).

- Nurse researchers have addressed the issue of teaching men Kegel exercises prior to treatment interventions with good results (Sueppel, Kreder, & See, 1998).

For men experiencing impotence after radiation therapy, or in combination with hormones, the use of a vibrator can help maintain sexual gratification for the female partner who desires vaginal penetration or the homosexual partner who desires anal penetration.

■ Cancer treatments often cause sexual dysfunctions that remain severe long after therapy is over. Nevertheless, sexual counseling is not routinely provided in most oncology treatment settings. Most patients and their partners can benefit from brief counseling that includes education on the impact of cancer treatment on sexual functioning, suggestions on resuming sex comfortably and improving sexual communication, advice on how to mitigate the effects of physical handicaps, such as having an ostomy, on sexuality, and self-help strategies to overcome specific sexual problems such as pain with intercourse or loss of sexual desire. Brief counseling can be provided by one of the allied health professionals on the oncology treatment team. A minority of patients will need specialized, intensive medical or psychological treatment for a sexual dysfunction (Bell, 1993; Schover, 1999).

- Sexual dysfunction in men treated for prostate cancer has received far more attention than sexual dysfunction in women after cancer therapy (Waxman, 1993).
- Current approaches in sex therapy may de-emphasize cultural differences by offering a set of procedures and techniques that clearly are grounded in Western sexual values. Based on existing literature concerning cultural values and clinical observations, the idea that the commonly practiced sex therapy is useful for everybody is challenged (Lavee, 1991).

Pregnancy following pelvic radiation therapy, once thought impossible, has recently been reported. Technological advances in the delivery of radiation therapy enabling enhanced dosing to tumor while better sparing surrounding normal tissue coupled with advances in the science of fertility have made pregnancy following radiotherapy possible, if still improbable.

- Three case studies have reported successful live births after pelvic radiotherapy. One case was documented in a 17-year-old patient who was submitted to left adnexectomy and radiation therapy for an ovarian dysgerminoma. Following a period of amenorrhea lasting 13 years and characterized by high serum levels of gonadotropins, the patient had a spontaneous pregnancy and at 33 weeks of gestation delivered a live and vital fetus (Garcea, Campo, Marone, & Garcea, 1998).
- A second case of a young patient with stage IB_1 carcinoma of the cervix treated by radical trachelectomy and adjuvant external beam plus implant has recently been reported. Hormonal replacement of "menopause" was prescribed and she became pregnant 1 year later. She gave birth via cesarean section at 27 weeks gestation to a healthy child (Martin, Golfier, Romestaing, & Raudrant, 1999).
- The third case report is of a 27-year-old male who underwent excision and radiotherapy for a pineal gland germinoma that caused panhypopituitarism and, thus, complete azoospermia. Four years later the patient was treated with gonadotropin replacement therapy, which resulted in the production of a small number of motile spermatozoa that were used for Intracytoplasmic Sperm Injection (ICSI) into oocytes obtained from his wife. The ICSI resulted in successful fertilization and embryo transfer and the delivery of

a healthy male live infant at term (Ramsewak, Naraynsingh, Kuruvilla, & Duffy, 1999).

■ In women with cancer concerned about future fertility as they face treatments, including pelvic radiation, that impair ovarian function, cryopreservation procedures such as in vitro fertilization and embryo storage, or ovarian tissue cryopreservation have recently been used to preserve fertility. For example, it has been shown that laproscopic ovarian biopsy is a safe and efficient method for collection of ovarian tissue in cancer patients. In Hodgkin's disease, patients' ovarian cortical tissue obtained for cryopreservation does not contain malignant cells. However, it has been recommended that the risk of cryopreserving and transferring malignant cells should be tested separately for each disease according to the risk of ovarian metastasis and the ability to detect single malignant cells (Meirow, 1999).

■ For men with cancer concerned about future fertility, sperm banking (cryopreservation) has been available for several decades. Although an abstinence period of 48 to 72 hours is the most commonly prescribed interval for diagnostic semen analysis, a study of 95 men newly diagnosed with cancer who were consulting for semen banking found no difference in postthaw semen quality after 24 to less than 48 hours of abstinence. Prefreeze and postthaw motile sperm count and motion variables (motility, velocity, linearity, amplitude of lateral head movement, and motility index), and percentage decrease in sperm variables after cryopreservation did not differ significantly among men who abstained from 24 to less than 48 hours prior to donating semen (Agarwal, Sidhuy, Shekarriz, & Thomas, 1995).

REFERENCES

Abitbol, M., & Davenport, J. (1974). The irradiated vagina. *Obstetrics and Gynecology, 44,* 249–256.

Agarwal, A., Sidhuy, R. K., Shekarriz, M., & Thomas, A. J. Jr. (1995). Optimum abstinence time for cryopreservation of semen in cancer patients. *Journal of Urology, 154*(1), 86–88.

Al-Ghazal, S. K., Fallowfield, L., & Blamey, R. W. (1999). Does cosmetic outcome from treatment of primary breast cancer influence psychosocial morbidity? *European Journal of Surgical Oncology, 25*(6), 571–573.

Andersen, B. (1990). How cancer affects sexual functioning. *Oncology*, 4(6), 81–88.

Andersen, B. L. (1999). Surviving cancer: The importance of sexual self-concept. *Medical Pediatric Oncology*, 33(1), 15–23.

Andersen, B. L., & Cyranowski, J. M. (1994). Women's sexual self-schema. *Journal of Personality and Social Psychology*, 67, 1079–1100.

Andersen, B. L., Cyranowski, J. M., & Espindle, D. (1999). Men's sexual self-schema. *Journal of Personality and Social Psychology*, 74(4), 645–666.

Arai, Y., Kawakita, M., Okada, Y., & Yoshida, O. (1997). Sexuality and fertility in long-term survivors of testicular cancer. *Journal of Clinical Oncology*, 15(4), 1444–1448.

Bachmann, G. A. (1995). Influence of menopause on sexuality. *International Journal of Fertility and Menopausal Studies*, 40(Suppl. 1), 16–22.

Bell, N. (1993). Nurses address the sexual concerns of cancer patients. *Oncology*, 7(10), 19, 48.

Bergmark, K., Avall-Lundqvist, E., Dickman, P. W., Henningsohn, L., & Steineck, G. (1999). Vaginal changes and sexuality in women with a history of cervical cancer. *New England Journal of Medicine*, 340(18), 1383–1389.

Bransfield, D., Horiot, J., & Nadib, A. (1984). Development of a scale for assessing sexual function after treatment for gynecologic cancer. *Journal of Psychosocial Oncology*, 2, 3–19.

Bruner, D. W., & Boyd, C. (1999). Assessing women's sexuality after cancer therapy: Checking assumptions with the focus group technique. *Cancer Nursing*, 21(6), 438–447.

Bruner, D. W., Bucholtz, J., Iwamoto, R., & Strohl, R. (1998b). *Manual for radiation oncology nursing practice and education* (2nd ed.). Pittsburgh, PA: Oncology Nursing Press.

Bruner, D. W., Hanlon, A., Nicolaou, N., & Hanks, G. (1997). Sexual function after radiotherapy ± androgen deprivation for clinically localized prostate cancer in younger men (age 50–65). *Oncology Nursing Forum*, 24(2), 327.

Bruner, D. W., & Iwamoto, R. (1999). Altered sexuality. In S. Groenwald, M. Frogge, M. Goodman, & C. Yarbro (Eds.), *Cancer symptom management* (2nd ed.). Boston: Jones & Bartlett.

Bruner, D. W., Lanciano, R., Keegan, M., Corn, B., Martin, E., & Hanks, G. E. (1993). Vaginal stenosis and sexual function following intracavitary radiation for the treatment of cervical and endometrial carcinoma. *International Journal of Radiation Oncology, Biology, Physics*, 27, 825–830.

Bruner, D. W., Scott, C., McGowan, D., Lawton, C., Hanks, G., Prestidge, B., Han, S., Gore, E., Asbell, S., & Rotman, M. (1998a). *Factors influencing sexual outcomes in prostate cancer patients enrolled on Radiation Therapy Oncology Group (RTOG) Studies 90-20 and 94-08.* Presented at the 5th Annual Conference of the International Society for Quality of Life Research. Baltimore, MD.

Bruner, D. W., Scott, C., McGowen, D., Lawton, C., Hanks, G., Prestidge, B., Han, S., Gore, E., Asbell, S. (1998c). The RTOG modified sexual adjustment questionnaire: Psychometric testing in the prostate cancer population. *International Journal of Radiation Oncology, Biology, Physics*, 42(1) Supplement: 202.

Burns-Cox, N., & Gingell, C. (1997). The andropause: Fact or fiction? *Postgraduate Medical Journal*, 73(863), 553–556.

Byne, W. (1995). Science and belief: Psychobiological research on sexual orientation. *Journal of Homosexuality*, 28(3–4), 303–344.

Cella, D., & Tross, S. (1986). Psychological adjustment to survival from Hodgkin's disease. *Journal of Consulting and Clinical Psychology*, 54, 616–620.

Classe, J. M., Mahe, M., Moreau, P., Rapp, M. J., Maisonneuve, H., Lemevel, A., Bourdin, S., Harousseau, J. L., & Cuilliere, J. C. (1998). Ovarian transposition by laparoscopy before radiotherapy in the treatment of Hodgkin's disease. *Cancer*, 83(7), 1420–1424.

Curran, D., van Dongen, J. P., Aaronson, N. K., Kiebert, G., Fentiman, I. S., Mignolet, F., & Bartelink, H. (1998). Quality of life of early-stage breast cancer patients treated with radical mastectomy or breast-conserving procedures: Results of EORTC trial 10801. The European Organization for Research and Treatment of Cancer (EORTC), Breast cancer Co-operative Group (BCCG). *European Journal of Cancer*, 34(3), 307–314.

Davis, S. R., McCloud, P., Strauss, B. J., & Burger, H. (1995). Testosterone enhances estradiol's effects on postmenopausal bone density and sexuality. *Maturitas*, 21(3), 227–236.

Fallowfield, L., & Hall, A. (1991). Psychosocial and sexual impact of diagnosis and treatment of breast cancer. *British Medical Bulletin*, 47, 388–399.

Finger, W. W., Lund, M., & Slagle, M. A. (1997). Medications that may contribute to sexual disorders: A guide to assessment and treatment in family practice. *Journal of Family Practice*, 44, 33–43.

Fisher, S. G. (1985). The sexual knowledge and attitudes of oncology nurses: Implications for nursing education. *Seminars in Oncology Nursing*, 1(1), 63–68.

Ganz, P. A., Rowland, J. H., Desmond, K., Meyerowitz, B. E., & Wyatt, G. E. (1998). Life after breast cancer: Understanding women's health-related quality of life and sexual functioning. *Journal of Clinical Oncology*, 16(2), 501–514.

Ganz, P. A., Schag, C. A., Lee, J. J., Polinsky, M. L., & Tan, S. J. (1992). Breast conservation versus mastectomy: Is there a difference in psychological adjustment or quality of life in the year after surgery? *Cancer*, 69, 1729–1738.

Garcea, N., Campo, S., Marone, M., & Garcea, R. (1998). Spontaneous pregnancy after 13 years of amenorrhea in a patient with a voluminous ovarian dysgerminoma and submitted to left adnexectomy and radiotherapy. *Gynecologic and Obstetric Investigation*, 46(3), 214–216.

Goldstein, I., Feldman, M., Deckers, P., Babayan, R., & Krane, R. (1984). Radiation associated impotence: A clinical study of its mechanism. *Journal of the American Medical Association*, 251, 903–910.

Goldstein, I., Lue, T. F., Padma-Nathan, H., Rosen, R. C., Steers, W. D., & Wicker, P. A. (1998). Oral sildenafil in the treatment of erectile dysfunction. *New England Journal of Medicine*, 338(20), 1397–1404.

Green, N., Treible, D., & Wallack, H. (1990). Prostate cancer: Post-irradiation incontinence. *Journal of Urology*, 144, 307–309.

Haley, N., Maheux, B., Rivard, M., & Gervais, A. (1999). Sexual health risk assessment and counseling in primary care: How involved are general practitioners and obstetrician-gynecologists? *Journal of Public Health*, 89(6), 899–902.

Howell, S., & Shalet, S. (1998). Gonadal damage from chemotherapy and radiotherapy. *Endocrinology and Metabolism Clinics of North America*, 27(4), 927–943.

Huppert, L. (1987). Hormonal replacement therapy: Benefits, risks, doses. *Medical Clinics of North America*, 71(1), 23–38.

Kornblith, A. B., Herndon, N., J. E., Zuckerman, E., Cella, D. F., Cherin, E., Wolchok, S., Weiss, R. B., Diehl, L. F., Henderson, E., Cooper, M. R., Schiffer, C., Canellos, G. P., Mayer, R. J., Silver, R. T., Schilling, A., Peterson, B. A., Greenberg, D., & Holland, J. C. (1998). Comparison of psychosocial adaptation of advanced stage Hodgkin's disease and acute leukemia survivors. *Annals of Oncology*, 9(3), 297–306.

Krumm, S., & Lamberti, J. (1993). Changes in sexual behavior following radiation therapy for cervical cancer. *Journal of Psychosomatic Obstetrics and Gynecology*, 14(1), 51–63.

Lalos, A., Jacobsson, L., Lalos, O., & Stendahl, U. (1995). Experiences of the male partner in cervical and endometrial cancer—a prospective interview study. *Journal of Psychosomatic Obstetrics and Gynecology*, 16(3), 153–165.

Lamb, M. A. (1995). Effects of cancer on the sexuality and fertility of women. *Seminars in Oncology Nursing*, 11(2), 120–127.

Lavee, Y. (1991). Western and non-western human sexuality: Implications for clinical practice. *Journal of Sex and Marital Therapy*, 17(3), 203–213.

Little, F. A., & Howard, G. C. (1998). Sexual function following radical radiotherapy for bladder cancer. *Radiotherapy and Oncology*, 49(2), 157–161.

Martin, X. J., Golfier, F., Romestaing, P., & Raudrant, D. (1999). First case of pregnancy after radical trachelectomy and pelvic irradiation. *Gynecologic Oncology*, 74(2), 286–287.

Masters, W. H., & Johnson, V. E. (1966). *Human sexual response*. Boston: Little, Brown & Company.

Meirow, D. (1999). Ovarian injury and modern options to preserve fertility in female cancer patients treated with high dose radio-chemotherapy for hemato-oncological neoplasias and other cancers. *Leukemia Lymphoma*, 33(1–2), 65–76.

Meston, C. M., Trapnell, P. D., & Gorzalka, B. B. (1996). Ethnic and gender differences in sexuality: Variations in sexual behavior between Asian and non-Asian university students. *Archives of Sexual Behavior*, 25(1), 33–72.

Meyerowitz, B. E., Desmond, K. A., Rowland, J. H., Wyatt, G. E., & Ganz, P. A. (1999). Sexuality following breast cancer. *Journal of Sex and Marital Therapy*, 25(3), 237–250.

Mock, V. (1993). Body image in women treated for breast cancer. *Nursing Research*, 42(3), 153–157.

Monga, T. N., Tan, G., Ostermann, H. J., Monga, U., & Grabois, M. (1998). Sexuality and sexual adjustment of patients with chronic pain. *Disability and Rehabilitation*, 20(9), 317–329.

Monga, U., Tan, G., Ostermann, H., & Monga, T. (1997). Sexuality in the head and neck cancer patient. *Archives of Physical Medicine and Rehabilitation*, 78, 298–304.

Montague, D. K., Barada, J. H., Belker, A. M., Levine, L. A., Nadig, P. W., Roehrborn, C. G., Sharlip, I. D., & Bennett, A. H. (1996). Clinical guidelines panel on erectile dysfunction: Summary report on the treatment of organic erectile dysfunction. *Journal of Urology*, 156, 2007–2011.

Ramsewak, S., Naraynsingh, A., Kuruvilla, A., & Duffy, S. (1999). Successful pregnancy by intracytoplasmic sperm injection after radiotherapy-induced azoospermia. *West Indian Medical Journal*, 48(4), 240–241.

Rosen, R. C., Riley, A., Wagner, G., Osterloh, I. H., Kirkpatrick, J., & Mishra, A. (1997). The International Index of Erectile Function (IEFF): A multidimensional scale for assessment of erectile dysfunction. *Urology*, 49(6), 822–830.

Schover, L. R. (1999). Counseling cancer patients about changes in sexual function. *Oncology*, 13(11), 1585–1591.

Schoven, L., Fife, M., & Gersheson, D. (1989). Sexual dysfunction and treatment for early stage cervical cancer. *Cancer*, 63, 204–212.

Schweickert, E. A., & Heeren, A. B. (1999). Scripted role play: A technique for teaching sexual history taking. *Journal of the American Osteopathic Association*, 99(5), 275–276.

Seibel, M. M., Graves, W. L., & Freeman, M. G. (1980). Carcinoma of the cervix and sexual function. *Obstetrics and Gynecology*, 55, 484–487.

Shell, J., & Smith, C. (1994). Sexuality and the older person with cancer. *Oncology Nursing Forum*, 21, 553–558.

Sueppel, C., Kreder, D., & See, W. (1998). *Timing of pelvic floor muscle strengthening and return of continence in post-prostatectomy patients* [Abstract]. Disney Coronado Springs Resort, Orlando, Florida: Fourth National Multispecialty Nursing Conference on Urinary Continence.

Sugarbaker, P., Barofsky, I., Rosenberg, S., & Gianola, F. J. (1982). Quality of life assessment of patients in extremity sarcoma clinical trials. *Surgery*, 91(1), 17–23.

Talcott, J. A., Rieker, P., Propert, K. J., Clark, J. A., Wishnow, K. I., Loughlin, K. R., Richie, J. P., & Kantoff, P. W. (1997). Patient-reported impotence and incontinence after nerve-sparing radical prostatectomy. *Journal of the National Cancer Institute*, 89(15), 1117–1123.

Temple-Smith, M., Hammond, J., Pyett, P., & Presswell, N. (1996). Barriers to sexual history taking in general practice. *Australian Family Physician*, 25(9 Suppl. 2), S71–74.

Thomas, P., Winstanly, D., Peckham, M., Austin, D. E., Murray, M. A., & Jacobs, H. S. (1976). Reproductive and endocrine function in patients with Hodgkin's disease: Effects of oophoropexy and irradiation. *British Journal of Cancer, 33*, 226–231.

Tiefer, L., Pedersen, B., & Melman, A. (1988). A psychosocial follow-up of penile prosthesis implant patients and partners. *Sexual Marital Therapy, 14*(3), 184–201.

Tserotas, K., & Merino, G. (1998). Andropause and the aging male. *Archives of Andrology, 40*(2), 87–93.

U.S. Department of Justice. (1998). *Sourcebook of criminal justice statistics online.* Washington, DC. Available: http://www.albany.edu/cgi-bin/toc_search.

Waterhouse, J., & Metcalfe, M. (1986). Development of the sexual adjustment questionnaire. *Oncology Nursing Forum, 23*(3), 451–455.

Watts, R. J. (1982). Sexual functioning, health beliefs, and compliance with high blood pressure medications. *Nursing Research, 31*(5), 278–283.

Waxman, E. S. (1993). Sexual dysfunction following treatment for prostate cancer: Nursing assessment and interventions. *Oncology Nursing Forum, 20*(10), 1567–1571.

Weinrich, J. D. (1995). Biological research on sexual orientation: A critique of the critics. *Journal of Homosexuality, 28*(1–2), 197–213.

Williams, H. A., Wilson, M. E., Hongladarom, G., & McDonnell, M. (1986). Nurses' attitudes toward sexuality in cancer patients. *Oncology Nursing Forum, 13*(2), 39–43.

Wilmoth, M. C. (1993). Development and psychometric testing of the sexual behaviors questionnaire. *Dissertation Abstracts International, 54* 6137B-6138B.

Wilmoth, M. C. (1996). The middle years: Women, sexuality, and the self. *Journal of Obstetric, Gynecologic, and Neonatal Nursing, 25*(7), 615–621.

Wilson, B. (1991). The effect of drugs on male sexual function and fertility. *Nurse Practitioner, 16*(9), 12–24.

Wilson, M., & Williams, H. (1988). Oncology nurses' attitudes and behaviors related to sexuality of patients with cancer. *Oncology Nursing Forum, 15*(1), 49–53.

Wyatt, G. E., Desmond, K. A., Ganz, P. A., Rowland, J. H., Ashing-Giwa, K., & Meyerowitz, B. E. (1998). Sexual functioning and intimacy in African American and white breast cancer survivors: A descriptive study. *Women's Health, 4*(4), 385–405.

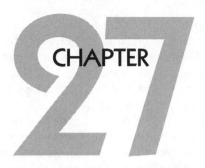

CHAPTER

MAINTENANCE OF FUNCTIONAL STATUS

Giselle J. Moore-Higgs, ARNP, MSN

PROBLEM

- Both cancer and its treatment frequently follow an unpredictable course with the potential to impact functional status and thus interfere with activities of daily living. Functional status is the performance of activities related to possible roles of spouse, parent, homemaker, community member, and worker. Roles may be altered and the ability to work and to engage in leisure activities affected. Advances in treatment technology and symptom management have improved dramatically and should alleviate the impact of many negative outcomes that prevent maintenance of a usual lifestyle. In addition to site-specific symptoms, global issues including fatigue, depression, anxiety, anorexia, cachexia, and pain may impact functional status. The following is a summary of research findings specifically related to the impact of cancer and its treatment on the activities of daily living. These factors are important considerations in the evaluation and management of all patients treated for cancer.

PHYSICAL AND PSYCHOLOGICAL ISSUES

- Quality of life as measured by the impact of illness on an individual can be predicted best by the individual's interpretation of the effect on his or her physical and functional well-being. Satisfaction with one's life can be predicted best by the individual's functional ability (Tate, Riley, Perna, & Roller, 1997).

■ Patients who receive combined-modality therapy may have a protracted course of functional loss that may be more acute and difficult to manage.

■ Disability is defined as "the expression of a physical or mental limitation in a social context—the gap between a person's capabilities and the demands of the environment" (Pope & Tarlov, 1991). One of every seven Americans has some type of disabling condition including cancer-related disabilities. The economic costs associated with disabilities are enormous. Expenditures for medical care and the indirect costs from lost productivity exceed $300 billion per year (Brandt, 1997). Persons with disabilities are often excluded from the economic and social mainstream as a result of attitude, architecture, communications, and policy barriers (O'Keefe, 1994).

■ Functional status changes with time in relation to age, stage of disease, treatment modality, and presence of comorbid disease. Several studies have identified a process of adjustment along a continuum of time. Jakobsson and colleagues (1997) interviewed 11 men with prostate cancer, focusing on functional health status in relation to daily life and life quality. The data was interpreted within the concept of transition. They found that the entry to transition was marked by an altered life continuum in terms of physical and existential fatigue, pain, micturition problems, and an altered sex life. The passage phase was marked by descriptions of a new lifestyle with hope as a central internal resource, creating a positive illusion of life in order to endure. Their external resources were wives and family who supported them physically and psychologically. The exit phase meant continuously adapting to a new lifestyle, living with a slowly deteriorating functional health status, a new sense of dependency on others, daily life routines broken by hospitalizations, treatments, and contacts with primary health care providers (Jakobson, Hallberg, & Loven, 1997).

■ Although many patients adjust to their functional deficits, many are unable to do so and their functional status progressively declines. Poor functional status has been associated with survival. Allard, Dionne, and Potvin (1995) in a study of the survival of terminally ill cancer patients found that the factor most strongly associated with shorter survival was poor performance status. There was no difference in this relationship when sex and primary cancer site were taken into account. For patients who were bedridden at the time of hospice admission, the death rate was 5.5% higher than for ambulatory patients during the first 4 days of stay, and it was 2.8 times higher subsequently (up to 19 days).

■ Fatigue is a global problem in cancer patients and is considered to be one of the major causes of distress and disability. Akechi and colleagues (1999) found that multiple factors including demographic, physical, and psychological issues impact the experience of fatigue in this population. Some of these factors include gender, education, employment status, the size of the household, the performance status, and depressive mood.

■ There is a small but growing body of work on post-traumatic stress disorder symptomatology and the experience of cancer that has been published within the past 5 years (McGrath, 1999). This work has demonstrated the unrecognized and still potentially underreported incidence of individuals coping with disabling psychological sequelae associated with their cancer experiences. Cancer patients share a common response to the diagnosis that includes painful aspects of intrusion, avoidance, numbness, and hyperarousal that may significantly impact their ability to function within their home and work environments.

FAMILY ISSUES

■ The shift of care to the outpatient setting has placed more emphasis on family-directed and self-care activities. Greimel and colleagues found that variables related to health status, disease, and treatment were highly correlated with self-care behavior, and to a lower extent to self-care preference. Age, gender, education, live-in resources, and perceived mental health were dominant predictors of self-care preferences (Greimel, Padilla, & Grant, 1997).

■ The burden of caring for a patient with cancer can place tremendous emotional and physical strain on a family and its support mechanisms. Dwyer (1995) found that a patient's functional status and length of time he or she is ill are two variables that have a significant impact on the caregiving spouse's schedule, health, and finances. The longer a patient is ill, the more negative the impact, resulting in significant burden and caregiver depression.

■ Elderly people constitute a heterogeneous group who are at an increased risk for the development of cancer (Repetto et al., 1998). Comorbidity is a frequent and often therapeutically limiting problem in older cancer patients. However, with improvements in technology and symptom management more elderly patients are being treated with curative intent.

• Goodwin, Hunt, and Samet (1991) found that functional limitations in patients aged 65 years or older and newly diagnosed with cancer included depending on others for transportation (33%), and mental incompetence or poor recent memory (42%). The percentage of patients with functional limitations increased sharply with increasing age. Also, there was evidence of poor social support networks in a substantial number of patients—26.5% lived alone and 38.9% had no children living in the vicinity. Predictors of having a poor social support network included non-Hispanic White ethnicity, advanced age, low income, and being a recent migrant to the area. Subjects with functional limitations were more likely to have poor social support networks than subjects without limitations.

• Greimel et al. (1997a) reported that age-related differences in patients with cancer were primarily in comorbidity and cancer-related impairments, with older patients having more of these problems. Despite these problems, they showed Karnofsky Performance Status (KPS) scores similar to those of their younger counterparts. Social resources, self-reported health and performance status, and complexity of care were significant predictors of the patient's ability to perform activities of daily living, but not age, comorbidity, or severity of treatment.

■ Lindsey, and colleagues (1994) evaluated 45 elderly patients receiving radiotherapy for either breast or lung cancer. Patients were found to tolerate the course of radiation with less than adequate nutritional intake for usual activity and a slight decease in mean weight, but without major disruptions in functional status despite having at least one comorbid condition.

EMPLOYMENT ISSUES

■ Approximately 25% of cancer survivors in the United States experience disparate treatment in employment solely because of their medical histories (Hoffman, 1989). Weis and colleagues found that in general most patients either take recourse to early retirement or are able to resume their occupational activity without special occupational training. Blue-collar workers returned less frequently to their former places of work, being more likely to take early retirement. From the point of view of the patients, medical rehabilitation had a negligible influence on vocational integration (Weis, Koch, Kruck, & Beck, 1994).

■ Misconceptions about cancer (contagious disease, risk of recurrence, decreased productivity, multiple absences) result in denial of employment opportunities and consequently violate the survivor's legal rights. In a survey sponsored in 1996 by *Working Woman* magazine and Amgen Inc., employees with cancer were fired or laid off at more than five times the rate of other workers (7% vs. 1.3%). Also, 14% of employees said their job responsibilities were cut as a result of their illness. Approximately one-third of the supervisors and coworkers felt that an employee with cancer could not handle job duties and illness, but only 19% of the cancer survivors expected their supervisors to feel this way. In addition, 31% of the supervisors thought an employee with cancer should be replaced compared with only 14% of survivors. Berry (1993) found that one of the most important factors in the facilitation of a person's reintegration of normal activities in the work environment is mobilization of social support by coworkers and employers.

■ Greenwald and colleagues (1989) found that the strongest predictor of work disability among cancer patients, defined as either leaving the labor force or functioning less fully at work than before becoming ill, was physical dysfunction related to the disease and stage of disease. Two job characteristics predicted work disability: physical demands of work and discretion over hours worked and how much work would be done.

■ Several characteristics of fatigue may present significant challenges for cancer patients returning to work. The fatigue experience includes a physical component of decreased functional status, an affective component of emotional distress, and a cognitive component of difficulty concentrating (Mock, 1998).

■ Several employment issues may significantly impact an employee's ability to perform including work site access, performance of essential job functions, job mastery, and job satisfaction. Satariano and DeLorenze (1996) found that "being on medical leave" was associated with the need for assistance with transportation, limitations in upper-body strength, and employment in jobs requiring physical activity.

■ Long-term survival may also impact employment. Dolgin, Somer, Buchvald, and Zaizov (1999) reported that adult survivors of childhood cancer experienced certain areas of disadvantage, such as military recruitment difficulties, lower income levels, and higher rates of workplace rejection. Significantly, almost one-half of the survivor sample reported subjective feelings that their illness experience had impaired their achievement in several domains.

FINANCIAL ISSUES

■ The enormous financial burden that accompanies the onset and subsequent treatment of cancer can become overwhelming (Berkman & Sampson, 1993). Dehospitalization of cancer treatment and the longer survival time for patients with cancer have shifted the economic and social burden of cancer to the patient and family.

■ Poverty contributes to an increase in cancer incidence and mortality. A number of factors are responsible and include a lack of employment, lack of education, inadequate housing, lack of access to medical care, chronic malnutrition, and a fatalistic attitude (Wilkes, Freeman, & Prout, 1994).

■ Absences from work can result in lost wages as well as potential loss of insurance coverage.

■ Inadequate insurance coverage can have physical, emotional, financial, social, and employment consequences.

 • Substantial gaps in insurance coverage including insurance deductibles, copayments, and medication costs can result in excessive out-of-pocket expenditures. Estimated out-of-pocket expenditures incurred during a 1-month period of chemotherapy, excluding lost income, have been reported and range widely from $12 to $3,130 (Moore, 1998). Unmet personal and family needs that arise from deficient insurance coverage can cause emotional distress for the patient and family (Glajchen, 1994).

- Health insurance can influence a patient's decision making regarding treatment, choice of physician, and hospital.
- The extent of out-of-pocket expenditures may depend on treatment protocol, ease of symptom management, functional status, and nonclinical elements such as socioeconomic factors.
- Patient and/or family may be reluctant to change or leave unsatisfactory employment or seek new employment opportunities because of potential risk of increased insurance premiums or ineligibility for a new insurance program secondary to a previous diagnosis of cancer.

GENETIC ISSUES

■ Genetic discrimination occurs when genetic information is used to differentially treat individuals, deny them normal privileges, or to treat them unfairly. Federal law (Americans with Disabilities Act 1990) prohibits discrimination in employment on the basis of disability including those with a genetic predisposition and those who are asymptomatic carriers of a late-onset disorder. Currently, the issue of discrimination occurs in the areas of employment and insurance coverage when a person's privacy rights are in conflict with the rights of the employer or insurance company to have the information needed for determining the extent of coverage.

ASSESSMENT

■ Assessment of functional status requires careful evaluation of physical, psychosocial, family, and employment issues. A multidisciplinary approach is very important in order to capture all of the information necessary to develop a comprehensive plan of care. The team should include physician, nurse, social services representative, financial counselor, and dietician.

MEDICAL HISTORY

■ The medical history should include questions regarding global symptoms such as fatigue as well as specific symptoms related to disease and/or treatment site.

PHYSICAL EXAMINATION

■ The physical examination should be thorough. Careful documentation of all physical disabilities using a qualitative approach will provide opportunity to assess response to intervention or progression of symptoms. The following is a list of assessment criteria for each treatment site:

1. Brain
   a. Cerebral function (cognitive system and mental status) including behavior, affect, thought content, intellectual functioning, memory, and judgment.
   b. Cortical function including visual, auditory, and tactile sensation; cortical motor integration; language
   c. Cranial nerve function
   d. Motor function including muscle tone, spasticity, rigidity, and abnormal movements
   e. Reflexes
   f. Cerebellar function including stance, gait, and coordination of movement
2. Head and Neck
   a. Ability to eat, drink, and swallow; xerostomia
   b. Speech
   c. Range of motion of neck
   d. Dental status
3. Breast
   a. Chest wall and/or axillary fibrosis resulting in decreased range of motion and persistent pain
   b. Lymphedema of the extremity
4. Chest
   a. Chest wall fibrosis
   b. Shortness of breath, persistent cough, oxygen supplementation requirements
5. Abdomen
   a. Chronic nausea, vomiting, enteritis
   b. Colostomy management
   c. Feeding tube management

6. GU/GYN
   a. Persistent urinary symptoms including dysuria, frequency, and incontinence
   b. Ileostomy management
   c. Urinary catheter or urostomy management
   d. Sexual dysfunction
7. Extremity
   a. Range of motion and mobility
   b. Lymphedema
   c. Fibrosis and pain

PSYCHOLOGICAL EVALUATION

■ Psychological evaluation for evidence of depression, anxiety, or other psychological sequelae should be performed. Referral to a clinical psychologist or psychiatrist may be necessary for comprehensive evaluation.

LABORATORY AND RADIOLOGY STUDIES

■ Laboratory and radiology studies may be performed depending on clinical manifestations and physical finding.

SOCIAL SERVICES EVALUATION

■ The social services evaluation should include the following:
1. Individual's Status
   a. Expectations of cancer diagnosis, treatment, and health care system
   b. Current coping mechanisms
   c. Interest in compliance with treatment plan
   d. Self-care adjustment and ability to conduct activities of daily living
2. Family Resources
   a. Housing
   b. Transportation
   c. Financial capacity for unexpected expenses
   d. Spiritual support mechanism
   e. Family relationships
      • Evidence of impaired or altered family relationships
      • Evidence of altered family or spousal roles

- Evidence of ineffective or compromised family coping skills
  f. Primary caregiver
    - Expectations related to cancer diagnosis
    - Caregiver's health and skills to conduct activities of daily living as well as care of the patient
    - Alteration of caregiver's pattern of living
    - Expectations of family members, health care system, and community
  3. Employment Status
     a. Current employment status
     b. Disability evaluation
  4. Insurance
     a. Current insurance status
     b. Potential insurance gaps that may require community resources
- Treatment factors that may influence social services include hyperfractionation regimen, multimodality therapy, and/or a protracted course of treatment.

EXPECTED OUTCOMES

MAINTENANCE OF PRE-ILLNESS LEVELS OF FUNCTIONAL STATUS

- Utilize appropriate therapeutic resources to reduce acute and chronic functional deficits.
- Utilize medical and community resources for rehabilitation of patient with functional deficits to encourage independence and improve overall quality of life.

OUTCOMES MEASURES

- A number of instruments have been developed to evaluate functional status of cancer patients. Some of the instruments are designed to be completed by proxy raters (physician, family, or friend) and others by the patient. Although it has been the belief that only a patient can provide accurate information about his or her quality of life, recent data show that proxy raters may be useful sources of information. Sneeuw et al. (1999) examined the usefulness of caregiver ratings of cancer patients' quality of life. With few exceptions, mean scores of the proxy raters were equivalent or similar to those of the patients'. Disagreement was not dependent on the type of proxy rater or on the rater's background characteristics, but was influenced by the QOL dimension under consideration and the clinical status of the patient. Better patient-proxy agreement was observed for more concrete questions and for patients with either a very good or poor performance status.

■ The following is a list of instruments available to evaluate general functional status and quality of life. There are also many instruments available for assessing specific clinical problems, health, and function that may impact quality of life and functional status (Frank-Stromborg & Olsen, 1997):

1. **Psychosocial Adjustment to Illness Scale (PAIS)** (Derogatis & Fleming, 1996)—A semistructured interview designed to assess the quality of a patient's psychosocial adjustment to a current medical illness or its residual effects.

2. **Sickness Impact Profile (SIP)** (Damiano, 1996)—A 136-item, 12 category instrument that may be used to assess the burden of illness associated with different diseases or conditions.

3. **Cancer Rehabilitation Evaluation System (CARES)** (Schag, Ganz, & Heinrick, 1991)—Evaluates physical, psychosocial, medical interaction, marital, sexual, and other common issues related to rehabilitation from cancer.

4. **Functional Living Index-Cancer (FLIC)** (Schipper, Clinch, McMurray, & Levitt, 1984)—An instrument that measures quality of life with emphasis on the extent to which the patient's normal function is affected by cancer and its treatment.

5. **Katz Index of Activities of Daily Living** (Katz, Ford, & Moskowitz, 1963)—An instrument that measures independence in six functions of daily living (bathing, dressing, going to the toilet, transferring, continence, and feeding). Developed to study the results of treatment and prognosis in the elderly and chronically ill.

6. **Karnofsky Performance Status Scale (KPS)** (Karnofsky & Burchenal, 1947)—Widely used to quantify the functional

status of cancer patients. Yates, Chalmer, and McKegney (1980) investigated the KPS and found that it has considerable validity as a global indicator of the functional status of patients with cancer. Mor, Laliberte, Morris, and Wiemann (1984) used the KPS in the National Hospice Study as both a study eligibility criterion and an outcome measure. The findings suggested that the KPS is a valuable research tool when employed by trained observers.

7. **Eastern Cooperative Oncology Group Scale of Performance Status (ECOG—PS)**—Describes the status of symptoms and functions with respect to ambulatory status and need for care. Taylor, Oliver, Sivanthan, & Purnell (1999) compared the ECOG scale and KPS and found no significant difference between the two scales in terms of individual raters. Interobserver variability was less using the ECOG scale.

8. **Inventory of Functional Status—Cancer** (Tulman, Fawcett, & McEvoy, 1991)—Developed to measure functional status in women with cancer.

9. **Edmonton Functional Assessment Tool** (Kaasa, Loomis, Gillis, Bruera, & Hanson, 1997)—Developed as a functional outcome measure for use with a palliative care population.

10. **MACE** (Monfardini, Ferruci, Fratino, del Lungo, Serraino, & Zagonel, 1996)—Multidimensional geriatric assessment tool for elderly patients with cancer. Collects information on demographics, socioeconomic status, cognitive status, depression, physical performance, disability, and tumor characteristics.

11. **Barthel Index (BI)**—A 16-item performance score of activities of daily living. In recent study of patients with high-grade gliomas (Brazil et al., 1997), the BI was found to be easy to use, reliable, and sensitive to change.

OUTCOMES MANAGEMENT

MEDICAL MANAGEMENT

Address Reversible Causes

■ Treatment side effects should be appropriately managed with early detection and intervention (see specific chapters).

■ Differentiate fatigue from depression (see Chapter 20). Refer patient for evaluation and management of depressive symptoms.

Treat Symptoms of Comorbid Disease
■ Collaboration with primary care provider to maximize overall health status.

Rehabilitation
■ Rehabilitation should be considered for all patients who have a reasonable life expectancy and may benefit from immediate rather than delayed services. Unfortunately, there is significant underuse of such services often because of the lack of services close to the patient's home or financial concerns. Such services should be offered as soon as the risk for injury has been resolved (i.e., surgical wounds have healed). For many patients, active participation in rehabilitation signifies a return to a normal life, which has been found to be an important variable in coping (Hilton, 1996). Sabers and colleagues (1999) evaluated patients who received interdisciplinary rehabilitation services (Cancer Adaptation Team) on a consultation basis during hospitalization. They found that these patients made significant functional improvement between enrollment and dismissal as compared with patients not offered services.
  • Physical Therapy—Provides an opportunity for improving range of motion, muscle strength and tone, and improving stamina. Treatment should be initiated as soon as possible to reduce the risk of contractures and other scar tissue formation.
  • Occupational Therapy—Provides opportunity to learn new skills related to activities of daily living. In particular, this may be helpful to patients who have required amputation or who have lost the function of a hand, arm, or leg. Improves skills to maintain self-care and independence. Soderback and Paulson (1997) found that many patients are not referred for occupational therapy despite the primary nursing evaluation of this therapy as potentially beneficial (26% vs. 47%).
  • Speech Therapy—Important in the rehabilitation of individuals who have suffered loss of speech because of a stroke, damage to cranial nerves, or treatment for head and neck cancer.

- Dental Evaluation—Reconstruction with dentures or dental implants may improve speech, ability to eat, and improve self-image.
- Cochlear Implants—May be considered in patients who have suffered hearing loss.
- Swallowing Clinic—Evaluation for swallowing efficiency.
- Complementary Medicine—Some patients may benefit from therapies such as massage, acupuncture, relaxation methods, and psychosocial support to enhance rehabilitation.

Patient and Family Education

- Patient education significantly improves the patient's and family's ability to cope with side effects of treatment. Johnson, Nail, Lavver, King, & Keys (1988) found that patients who received four informational messages during the course of radiotherapy reported significantly less disruption in usual activities during and following radiation therapy as compared with patients who received only limited information.
- Design a schedule during treatment that takes into account family schedule, work schedule, and fatigue patterns. Encourage energy conservation and nutritional support.

Development and Evaluation

- Participation in the development and evaluation through clinical trials to find new approaches to the treatment of cancer and decrease the impact of acute and chronic side effects.

PSYCHOSOCIAL MANAGEMENT

Psychosocial Support

1. Clinical psychology or psychiatry referral
2. Community support groups

Social Services Referral

- Social services can provide home health and community resources to assist patients in adapting to changes in functional status and encourage independence. Early recognition of problems and referral decreases the risk of chronic irreversible problems.
- Braden, Mischel, and Longman (1998) initiated a program to enhance patients' self-care abilities through intervention

that included a self-help course, uncertainty management course, or both. They found that at baseline, women having a high resourcefulness compared with women with a low resourcefulness evidenced greater self-care, self-help, psychological adjustment, and confidence in cancer knowledge. Participation in the intervention programs resulted in higher levels of function in all four variables regardless of baseline resourcefulness. Those women with a baseline low resourcefulness demonstrated the greatest change over time in the variables.

Employment

■ Early recognition of potential employment issues may influence patient behavior. Health professional's attitude and behavior toward continued employment may influence the patient's decision to work. Each patient and their employment environment should be evaluated to determine unique variables (i.e., impact on family finances, impact on physical well-being, impact on emotional well-being). Letters of support may be required including suggestions for adaptation to treatment regimens (i.e., required breaks, environmental risks to patient, flexibility of work hours).

Financial Support

■ Careful attention to the necessity of procedures and studies should be a primary responsibility of all health care providers. Patients may be too embarrassed or intimidated to verbalize concerns about financial costs of studies until they are in debt. This may be particularly true if they are led to believe that having the studies will significantly influence the outcome of their treatment.

■ Assist the patient with negotiations between insurance company and facility. Do not make patients responsible for obtaining authorization for procedures. Provide adequate documentation for requested procedures in a timely fashion. Many patients do not have a choice in their insurance carriers, and guilt regarding inadequacies of coverage increases patient stress.

■ Refer patient to social services whenever possible to determine possible financial assistance (i.e., American Cancer Society—transportation reimbursement).

REFERENCES

Akechi, T., Kugaya, A., Akamura, H., Yamawaki, S., & Uchitomi, Y. (1999). Fatigue and its associated factors in ambulatory cancer patients: A preliminary study. *Journal of Pain and Symptom Management*, 17(1), 42–48.

Allard, P., Dionne, A., & Potvin, D. (1995). Factors associated with length of survival among 1081 terminally ill cancer patients. *Journal of Palliative Care*, 11(3), 20–24.

Amgen, Inc. (1996). *Cancer discrimination in the workplace: A national assessment of survivor experiences*. Thousand Oaks, CA: Amgen.

Berkman, B. J., & Sampson, S. E. (1993). Psychosocial effects of cancer economics on patients and their families. *Cancer*, 72(Suppl. 9), 2846–2849.

Berry, D. L. (1993). Return-to-work experiences of people with cancer. *Oncology Nursing Forum*, 20(6), 905–911.

Braden, C. J., Mischel, M. H., & Longman, A. J. (1998). Self-Help Intervention Project. Women receiving breast cancer treatment. *Cancer Practice*, 6(2), 87–98.

Brandt, E. N. (1997). *Quality of life is as important as quantity*. Washington, DC: National Academy of Sciences. (Accessed from www4.nationalacademics.org on 2/8/00)

Brazil, L., Thomas, R., Laing, R., Hines, F., Guerrero, D., Ashley, S., & Brada, M. (1997). Verbally administered Barthel Index as functional assessment in brain tumour patients. *Journal of Neuro-oncology*, 34(2), 187–192.

Damiano, A. M. (1996). The Sickness Impact Profile. In B. Spilker (Ed.). *Quality of life and pharmacoeconomics in clinical trials* (2nd ed. pp. 347–354). Philadelphia: Lippincott-Raven.

Derogatis, L. R., & Fleming, M. P. (1996). Psychological Adjustment to Illness Scale: PAIS and PAIS-SR. In B. Spilker (Ed.). *Quality of life and pharmacoeconomics in clinical trials* (2nd ed. pp. 287–299). Philadelphia: Lippincott-Raven.

Dolgin, M. J., Somer, E., Buchvald, E., & Zaizov, R. (1999). Quality of life in adult survivors of childhood cancer. *Social Work in Health Care*, 28(4), 31–43.

Dwyer, T. F. (1995). *Assessing distress in couples with cancer: A life cycle review*. Purdue University PhD.

Frank-Stromborg, M., & Olsen, S. J. (1997). *Instruments for clinical health-care research* (2nd ed.). Boston: Jones & Bartlett.

Glajchen, M. (1994). Psychosocial consequences of inadequate health insurance for patients with cancer. *Cancer-Practice*, 2(2), 115–120.

Goodwin, J. S., Hunt, W. C., & Samet, J. M. (1991). A population-based study of functional status and social support networks of elderly patients newly diagnosed with cancer. *Archives of Internal Medicine*, 151(2), 366–370.

Greenwald, H. P., Dirks, S. J., Borgatta, E. F., McCorkle, R., Nevitt, M. C., & Yelin, E. H. (1989). Work disability among cancer patients. *Social Science Medical*, 29(11), 1253–1259.

Greimel, E. R., Padilla, G. V., & Grant, M. M. (1997). Physical and psychosocial outcomes in cancer patients. A comparison of different age groups. British Journal of Cancer, 76(2), 251–255.

Greimel, E. R., Padilla, G. V., & Grant, M. M. (1997). Self-care responses to illness of patients with various cancer diagnoses. Acta Oncologica, 36(2), 141–150.

Hilton, B. A. (1996). Getting back to normal: The family experience during early stage breast cancer. Oncology Nursing Forum, 23(4), 605–614.

Hoffman, B. (1989). Cancer survivors at work: Job problems and illegal discrimination. Oncology Nursing Forum, 16(1), 39–43.

Jakobsson, L., Hallberg, I. R., & Loven, L. (1997). Experience of daily life and life quality in men with prostate cancer. An explorative study. Part. I. European Journal of Cancer Care, 6(2), 108–116.

Johnson, J. E., Nail, L. M., Lauver, D., King, K. B., & Keys, H. (1988). Reducing the negative impact of radiation therapy on functional status. Cancer, 61(1), 46–51.

Kaasa, T., Loomis, J., Gillis, K., Bruera, E., & Hanson, J. (1997). The Edmonton Functional Assessment Tool: Preliminary development and evaluation for use in palliative care. Journal of Pain and Symptom Management, 13(1), 10–19.

Karnofsky, D. A. & Burchenal, J. H. (1947). The clinical evaluation of chemotherapeutic agents in cancer. In C. M. Maclead (Ed.). Evaluation of chemotherapeutic agents. New York: Columbia Press.

Katz, S., Ford, A. S., & Moskowitz, R. W. (1963). The index of ADL: A standardized measure of biological and psychosocial function. JAMA, 185(12), 914.

Lindsey, A. M., Larson, P. J., Dodd, M. J., Brecht, M. L., & Packer, A. (1994). Comorbidity, nutritional intake, social support, weight, and functional status over time in older cancer patients receiving radiotherapy. Cancer Nursing, 17(2), 113–124.

McGrath, P. (1999). Posttraumatic stress and the experience of cancer: A literature review. Journal of Rehabilitation, 3, 17–23.

Mock, V. (1998). Breast cancer and fatigue: Issues for the workplace. American Association of Occupational Health Nurses, 46(9), 425–431.

Monfardini, S., Ferruci, L., Fratino, L., del-Lungo, I., Serraino, D., & Zagonel, V. (1996). Validation of a multidimensional evaluation scale for use in elderly cancer patients. Cancer, 77(2), 395–401.

Moore, K. (1998). Out-of-pocket expenditures of outpatients receiving chemotherapy. Oncology Nursing Forum, 25(9), 1615–1622.

Mor, V., Laliberte, L., Morris, J. N., & Wiemann, M. (1984). The Karnofsky Performance Status Scale. An examination of its reliability and validity in a research setting. Cancer, 53(9), 2002–2007.

O'Keefe, J. (1994). Disability, discrimination, and the Americans with Disabilities Act. In S. M. Bruyère & J. O'Keefe (Eds.), Implications of the Americans with Disabilities Act for psychology. New York: Springer-Verlag.

Pope, A. M., & Tarlove, A. R. (Eds.). (1991). Disability in America: Toward a national agenda for presentation. Washington, DC: National Academy Press.

Repetto, L., Venturino, A., Vercelli, M., Gianni, W., Biancardi, V., Casella, C., Granetto, C., Parodi, S., Rosso, R., & Marigliano, V. (1998). Performance status and comorbidity in elderly cancer patients compared with young patients with neoplasia and elderly patients without neoplastic conditions. *Cancer*, 82(4), 760–765.

Sabers, S. R., Kodal, J. E., Girardi, J. C., Philpott, C. L., Basford, J. R., Therneau, T. M., Schmidt, K. D., & Gamble, G. L. (1999). Evaluation of consultation-based-rehabilitation for hospitalized cancer patients with functional impairment. *Mayo Clinic Proceedings*, 74(9), 855–861.

Satariano, W. A., & DeLorenze, G. N. (1996). The likelihood of returning to work after breast cancer. *Public Health Reports*, 111(3), 236–243.

Schag, C. A., Ganz, P. A., & Heinrick, R. L. (1991). Cancer Rehabilitation Evaluation System-Short Form (CARES-SF): A cancer specific rehabilitation and quality of life instrument. *Cancer*, 68(6), 1406–1413.

Schipper, H., Clinch, J., McMurray, A., & Levitt, M. (1984). Measuring the quality of life of cancer patients: The Functional Living Index-Cancer: Development and validation. *Journal of Clinical Oncology*, 2(5), 472–483.

Seegers, C., Walker, B. L., Nail, L. M., Schwartz, A., Mudgett, L. L., & Stephen, S. (1998). Self-care and breast cancer recovery. *Cancer-Practice*, 6(6), 339–345.

Sneeuw, K. C., Aaronson, N. K., Sprangers, M. A., Detmar, S. B., Wever, L. D., & Schornagel, J. H. (1999). Evaluating the quality of life of cancer patients: Assessments by patients, significant others, physicians and nurses. *British Journal of Cancer*, 81(1), 87–94.

Soderback, I., & Paulsson, E. H. (1997). A needs assessment for referral to occupational therapy. Nurses' judgement in acute cancer care. *Cancer Nursing*, 20(4), 267–273.

Tate, D. G., Riley, B. B., Perna, R., & Roller, S. (1997). Quality of life issues among women with physical disabilities or breast cancer. *Archives of Physical Medicine and Rehabilitation*, 78(12 Suppl. 5), S18–S25.

Taylor, A. E., Oliver, I. N., Sivanthan, T., Chi, M., & Purnell, C. (1999). Observer error in grading performance status in cancer patients. *Support Care Cancer*, 7(5), 332–335.

Tulman, L., Fawcett, J., & McEvoy, M. D. (1991). Development of the Inventory of Functional Status—Cancer. *Cancer Nursing*, 14(5), 254–260.

Weis, J., Koch, U., Kruck, P., & Beck, A. (1994). Problems of vocation integration after cancer. *Clinical Rehabilitation*, 8(3), 219–225.

Wilkes, G., Freeman, H., & Prout, M. (1994). Cancer and poverty: Breaking the cycle. *Seminars Oncology Nursing*, 10(2), 79–88.

Yates, J. W., Chalmer, B., & McKegney, F. P. (1980). Evaluation of patients with advanced cancer using the Karnofsky performance status. *Cancer*, 45(8), 2220–2224.

INDEX